T0210202

Diagnosis and Treatment of Movement Impairment Syndromes

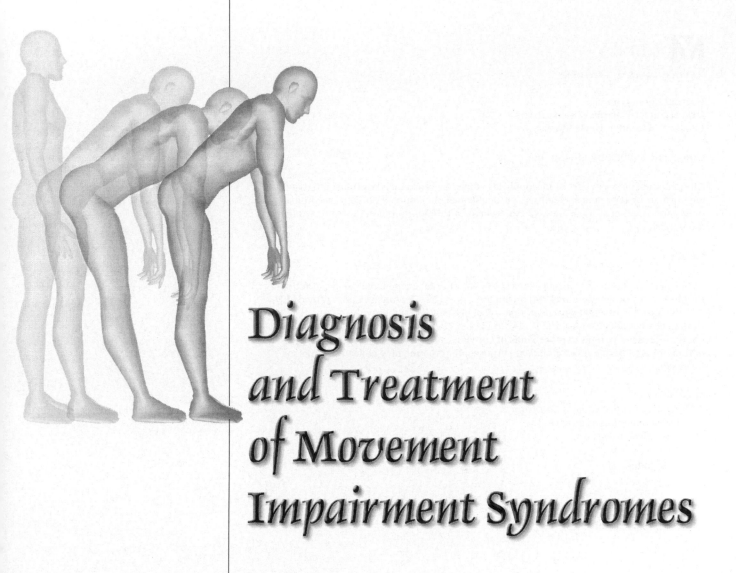

Diagnosis and Treatment of Movement Impairment Syndromes

Shirley Sahrmann, PhD, PT, FAPTA

PROFESSOR, PHYSICAL THERAPY, CELL BIOLOGY & PHYSIOLOGY
ASSOCIATE PROFESSOR, NEUROLOGY
DIRECTOR, PROGRAM IN MOVEMENT SCIENCE
WASHINGTON UNIVERSITY, SCHOOL OF MEDICINE

360 *illustrations*

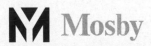 Mosby

A Harcourt Health Sciences Company

St. Louis   London   Philadelphia   Sydney   Toronto

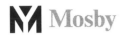

A Harcourt Health Sciences Company

EDITOR: Kellie White
DEVELOPMENT EDITOR: Christie Hart
PROJECT MANAGER: Gayle Morris

Copyright © 2002 by Mosby, Inc.

All rights reserved. No part of this publication may be reproduced or transmitted in any form or by any means, electronic or mechanical, including photocopy, recording, or any information storage and retrieval system, without permission in writing from the publisher.

NOTICE

Permission to photocopy or reproduce solely for internal or personal use is permitted for libraries or other users registered with the Copyright Clearance Center, provided that the base fee of $4.00 per chapter plus $.10 per page is paid directly to the Copyright Clearance Center, 222 Rosewood Drive, Danvers, Massachusetts 01923. This consent does not extend to other kinds of copying, such as copying for general distribution, for advertising or promotional purposes, for creating new collected works, or for resale.

Mosby, Inc.
A Harcourt Health Sciences Company
11830 Westline Industrial Drive
St. Louis, Missouri 63146

Printed in India

ISBN 0-8016-7205-8

Last digit is the print number 203 202 201

Foreword

On rare occasions, someone comes along who challenges the way we view our world. Professor Shirley Sahrmann is one of these individuals. *Diagnosis and Treatment of Movement Impairment Syndromes* is the result of many years spent simply observing and analyzing how the human body moves. Everyone who reads this text will understand the world of musculoskeletal medicine differently, and his or her world will be forever changed. I have frequently said to Dr. Sahrmann that she has given me "new eyes." After many years of observing a wide variety of musculoskeletal problems, I am now understanding them differently. I once said this to a patient and was told that "the eye can only see what the brain knows." This text will challenge its readers to observe their patients with movement system disorders with brains jammed full of new information that can be quickly incorporated into their practices. I have no doubt that perfecting the examination techniques and becoming adept at selecting and teaching the exercises outlined in this book will result in tremendous satisfaction both for the patient and the health care practitioner.

Like most of my contemporaries, I was taught assessment skills using the pathokinesiologic model. My skills were limited to telling patients what pathologic conditions they were experiencing and to hoping that they would go home happy once they knew their diagnoses. In actual fact, my patients wanted to know what caused their symptoms and pain problems. I often dismissed such requests with a perfunctory, "It is a result of overuse," hoping no more questions would follow. My tremendous frustration resulted in the beginning of my quest to find the solutions to the limitations of this education model. I remember mentioning my dilemma at the Lillehammer Olympic Games. The chief therapist for the Canadian team suggested I attend one of Dr. Sahrmann's muscle balance courses. I followed his advice and found that the assessment and treatment skills I learned and with the subsequent attendance at a number of courses perfectly met my needs. I continue to apply this knowledge with virtually every patient assessment in my practice.

Dr. Sahrmann is the first to categorize pain disorders logically into movement impairment categories. I quickly discovered that after using her assessment skills, the identical pathologic diagnosis is frequently not associated with the same movement impairment. Treating the specific impairment rather than the diagnostic label has been very rewarding in terms of outcomes. *Diagnosis and Treatment of Movement Impairment Syndromes* gives the clinician the necessary information to diagnose the various impairment syndromes with confidence. It also provides the researcher the grounding with which to perform the necessary investigations to expand the diagnostic categories and treatment protocols for the body regions not discussed in this book.

I hope this text will be followed by others from Dr. Sahrmann and her colleagues from the Washington University program in physical therapy. This information will serve as a stimulus for other researchers to test the theoretical concepts and further define the treatment protocols. The concepts have been tested by physical therapists around the world, but Dr. Sahrmann is to be commended for presenting her material in written form for all to see and evaluate, even though it remains largely a work in progress. *Diagnosis and Treatment of Movement Impairment Syndromes* has been a labor of love for Dr. Sahrmann. I, among many others, are very thankful for the years of effort it has taken to conceptualize, test, and document this information. It is an important body of work and one that will have significant effect on how we treat our patients with movement disorders. I hope all that read *Diagnosis and Treatment of Movement Impairment Syndromes* will find themselves saying, "I have seen this clinical scenario many times. With this knowledge, I now see it so differently." Thank you, Dr. Sahrmann, for sharing your knowledge with me and for helping make working with patients such a joy!

Robert Stalker, MD
Dalhousie University Health Service
Halifax, Nova Scotia
Canada

Preface

Frequently, the obvious answer to a problem is overlooked, and complex answers or explanations are pursued instead. This approach to problem solving is exemplified by the adage, "When you hear hoof beats, think horses before zebras." With this approach in mind, the simple method for controlling the spread of disease is hand washing, yet this obvious answer was overlooked for too many years. Amazingly, even today, numerous reminders are given to help people follow this important practice. I believe a parallel exists in the mechanical cause of musculoskeletal pain problems and the medical treatment of the symptoms of these conditions. Rather than addressing the obvious mechanical problems, medications are used to treat the symptomatic tissues without pursuing the precipitating factors.

Exercise is advocated because of the changes induced in the musculoskeletal system, yet everyday activities also include a key component of exercise—repeated movements. Alignment and movements patterns are carefully addressed in the training of athletes, yet little attention is given to these factors in everyday activities. Postural alignment is the basis of movement patterns, thus optimal movement is difficult if alignment is faulty. Long gone are the days when children were strongly reminded to sit and stand up straight. In years past, most men had to serve in the military, and an intrinsic part of that experience was training that required standing with good alignment. Today, the slouched or slumped position is acceptable. Furniture is shaped to accommodate and encourage the slumped posture, particularly when at home "relaxing." Acceptance of poor posture is particularly notable when, as a society, we sit more than we have in the past. Ironically, as women approach the senior status, a major concern is the development of the kyphotic posture, characteristic of "old" women. Yet, as young women, little effort is spent to prevent the development of an increased thoracic curve. Wolff's Law, which states that bones adopt the shape of the forces that are imposed on them, is a well-accepted principle of the skeletal system. The tissues controlling the alignment and stability of the joints are also influenced by the forces placed on them. In an era in which lifestyles are relatively sedentary, musculoskeletal tissue is not as well developed as it should be because of a lack of physical demands, thus predisposing the body to injury more readily than if tissues were "stronger" from responding to stress. The consequence is a greater predisposition to mechanical injuries from the repeated movements of everyday activities. Once a pattern of behavior is established, it becomes the prevailing pattern, repeated over and over. At work, repeatedly turning to one side to work on the computer, to answer the telephone, to work on an adjoining counter are typical. A mother frequently turns toward the back seat of her car to check the children in their car seats. Mothers get in and out of their cars repeatedly during the day, also turning consistently in the same direction. A dentist always works from the same side of his or her patients. Cardiologists repeatedly bend over to use their stethoscopes. Golfers and racquetball players repeatedly swing their clubs or racquets using the same patterns of movement. Even sleeping on the same side can induce alignment changes.

A major purpose of this book is to describe the changes induced in movement patterns and tissues by everyday activities. The proposed thesis is that correcting these movement patterns and tissue adaptations will not only alleviate mechanical musculoskeletal pain problems, but correction can prevent them. Correcting body mechanics should help reduce the use of medications that are designed to decrease inflammation, because the mechanical cause will, at the least, be diminished or, at the most, be alleviated. Patients can be taught to assume responsibility for their pain problems rather than depend on drugs to alleviate the symptoms, thus failing to address the actual causes. Because motions of joints are limited, common problems can develop from a wide variety of activities. Thus it has been possible to describe specific movement syndromes that can be identified by the clinician based on the patient's signs, symptoms, and results of examination. This text describes these movement impairment syndromes of the shoulder, low back, and hip.

A second purpose of this book is to describe how the basic tests and measurements of physical therapy combined with the observations of alterations in normal anatomy and kinesiology can be used to organize a classification system consisting of movement impairment syndromes. I believe the development of classification systems, which constitutes diagnoses that direct physical therapy, is essential to the continued development of the profession. The focal premise of the theory underlying the system is that a joint develops a directional susceptibility to movement, which then becomes the "weak link" and most often the site of pain.

Chapter 1 describes the historical and professional events that led to the development of the concepts of the movement system and movement impairment syndromes and the reasons the pursuit of a classification system are important.

Chapter 2 contains the concepts and principles upon which the system is based. When the field of psychiatry recognized the need to establish a common system of diagnoses for mental illnesses, behavior patterns were used as the basis. Emotional dysfunctions could not be related to specific lesions or interactions in the brain, and interactive factors in behaviors were difficult to identify. Classifications of human movement dysfunction have a distinct advantage when organizing behaviors. Because the system is biomechanical with defined anatomic and kinesiologic principles, interactions are predictable. Thus it is even possible to hypothesize a key factor that can explain the dysfunctions and the altered interactions that can contribute to the problem. In this chapter the adaptations of tissues caused by the repeated movements and sustained postures associated with everyday activities are described. The resultant effect of a joint developing a directional susceptibility to movement is explained. Three models of the movement system and their varying relationships to impairments are proposed. The kinesiologic, pathokinesiologic, and kinesiopathologic models and their elements and components are used to explain the development of impairments and the consequences of these impairments. The types and characteristics of the alterations in the components and their interactions, as well as the application to clinical patients, are described. Case examples are used to illustrate the impairments arising from tissue changes and explain how they contribute to altered movement patterns.

Chapters 3, 4, and 5 describe the movement impairment syndromes of the low back, hip, and shoulder, respectively. Each chapter provides the basic anatomy and kinesiology considered necessary to understand the normal performance of the relevant body area. Each chapter follows a format of describing the relevant symptoms and pain, as well as the impairments in movement, alignment, recruitment patterns, relative flexibility and stiffness, and muscle length and strength. Confirming tests, summary, and treatment program are described for each syndrome. Each movement impairment syndrome is illustrated by a case presentation. To assist in understanding the syndromes, each chapter has an appendix that presents a grid to explain the symptoms and history, the key tests and signs, the associated signs, the differential movement and associated diagnoses, and the potential medical diagnoses that require referral.

Chapter 6 presents the examinations for lower and upper quarter impairments, the results of which should result in the diagnosis and identification of the contributing factors that need to be addressed by the treatment program. The examinations are organized according to position and tests in the specific positions. Two forms are provided. One contains the normal or ideal standard for the test, the criteria for an impairment, and what the specific impairments could be. The other form is one that can be used as the basis of a clinical examination form. It is a checklist that enables the therapist to record the specific impairments identified during the examination and the possible joint movement directions that underlie the pain problem and thus potentially form the diagnosis. The other impairments identified by the examination are the repeated movements believed to be contributing factors that are causing pain.

Chapter 7 is a detailed explanation of the exercise program that supports the corrections in body mechanics and the performance of life activities that are important to minimizing or preventing mechanical pain problems. I believe that a simple but well-selected and precisely taught therapeutic exercise program is essential to aid in the resolution of the patient's pain problem. Therefore great detail is provided on each exercise, as well as special considerations for specific conditions. Chapter 8 consists of the illustrated exercises written in a format that can be copied and distributed to patients. As the therapist will note, the exercise program closely follows the examination. As a result, when the therapist is performing the examination, he or she is also determining the specific exercises the patient will be given for his or her treatment program. The therapist will also be acquiring the information that is necessary for patient education and, most importantly, contributing to practice based on diagnosis to direct physical therapy.

Shirley Sahrmann, PhD, PT, FAPTA

Acknowledgments

This manuscript seems to have begun with a few chisel marks on the walls of caves in the late Stone Age, to have been sustained through many ages by verbal tradition known as rumor, and to have finally become a reality in the electronic age of the twenty-first century, thus preventing its anticipated completion on a starship in another galaxy. Because she was there, I am particularly grateful to my friend and colleague, Kathleen K. Dixon, PT, for the many hours she spent reading, translating from "Shirleese," and refining the content of this book, as well as for enabling me to remain immersed in my profession. Robert Stalker, MD, also spent many hours editing and critiquing the manuscript. My appreciation is extended to Christie Hart, developmental editor, for her able assistance, to Dana Peick for editing and layout, and to others at Harcourt who assisted with this project.

Throughout my professional and academic career, I have been fortunate to be guided by individuals who have imparted their commitment to excellence in scientific thought and to the best in patient care. During my professional education, Lorraine F. Lake, PT, PhD, first imparted the need for science in physical therapy. During my graduate studies, Margaret Clare Griffin and William M. Landau, MD, set a standard to which I am still working to reach. Steven J. Rose, PT, PhD, conveyed his excitement and commitment to research in physical therapy and to the importance of classification of clinical conditions. Barbara J. Norton, PT, PhD, has been a loyal friend, colleague, supporter, and most valued critic who has pulled me back from many an intellectual limb. Nancy J. Bloom, MSOT, PT, began to put these ideas into a useful format as a student and has continued in her efforts to do so for many years. I am indebted to all my colleagues who have helped develop, refine, and teach these concepts: Cheryl Caldwell, PT, CHT; Mary Kate McDonnell, PT, OCS; Debbie Fleming, PT; Susie Cornbleet, PT; Kate Crandell, PT; Tracy Spitznagle, PT; Renee Ivens, PT; and Carrie Hall, PT. I am particularly appreciative of Linda Van Dillen, PT, PhD, and her efforts to examine the low back movement impairment classifications and to publish her findings. In addition, this work would not have been possible without the foundational knowledge and inspiration provided by the careful observations and empirical analyses of the Kendalls in their classic text, *Muscles, Testing, and Function*, and the many spirited debates that I have enjoyed with Florence Kendall throughout my career.

I am very fortunate to have been a faculty member at Washington University School of Medicine for most of my career. For more than 40 years I have worked with colleagues who are among the most outstanding and dedicated physical therapists in the profession. Because of their efforts and the able direction of Susie Deusinger, PT, PhD, the program in physical therapy has truly earned its outstanding reputation. I have been a faculty member of an institution that is without parallel in its support of its faculty and educational components, providing the environment within which we can truly strive for and achieve excellence. My hope is that this text represents another step in physical therapy's pursuit of excellence in patient care.

—SS

Contents

1 *Introduction*   1

Development of the Movement System   1
    Balance Concept
    First Era: Focus on Dysfunction   1
      of the Peripheral Neuromuscular
      and Musculoskeletal Systems
    Second Era: Focus on Central Nervous   2
      System Dysfunction
    Third Era: Focus on Joint Dysfunction   2
    Current Era: Focus on the Movement System   2
Underlying Premise of Movement   3
  as a Cause of Pain Syndromes
Overview   4
    Concepts and Principles   4
Movement Impairment Syndromes   5
    Definition   5
    Prevalence   5
    Diagnosis and Management   5
    Structures Affected   6
    Treatment Approaches Based on Intervention   6
    Cause Identification Versus Symptom Reduction   7
Need for Classification   7

2 *Concepts and Principles of Movement*   9
Kinesiologic Model   9
    Composition of the Model   9
    Clinical Relevance of the Model   10
Pathokinesiologic Model   10
    Composition of the Model   10
    Clinical Relevance of the Model   11
Kinesiopathologic Model   12
    Rationale for the Model   12
    Clinical Relevance of the Model   14
Base Element Impairments of the   16
  Muscular System
    Muscle Strength   16
    Muscle Length   17
    Case Presentation 1   18
    Case Presentation 2   19
    Case Presentation 3   24
    Case Presentation 4   27
Base Element Impairments of the Skeletal   34
  System: Structural Variations in Joint
  Alignment
    Case Presentation   34
    Hip Retrotorsion   34
Modular Element Impairments of the   35
  Nervous System
    Altered Recruitment Patterns   35
    Altered Dominance in Recruitment Patterns   35
      of Synergistic Muscles
    Recruitment and Relative Flexibility   39

    Patterns of Eccentric Contraction   40
Biomechanical Element Impairments   41
    Statics: Effects of Gravitational Forces   42
    Dynamics: The Relationship Between Motion   44
      and the Forces Producing Motion
    Kinematics and Impairments of Joint   45
      Function
    Kinesiopathologic Model Applied to   46
      Patellofemoral Joint Dysfunction
Multiple Impairments of the Components   47
  of Movement
    Case Presentation   47
Support Element Impairments   47
Summary   49

3 *Movement Impairment Syndromes*   51
  of the Lumbar Spine
Introduction   51
Normal Alignment of the Lumbar Spine   52
    Standing   52
    Sitting   54
Motions of the Lumbar Spine   57
    Path of the Instant Center of Rotation   57
    Flexion: Forward Bending   58
    Return from Flexion   60
    Extension   60
    Rotation   61
    Lateral Flexion or Side Bending   63
    Translation Motion   63
    Compression   63
    Summary   64
Muscular Actions of the Lumbar Spine   65
    Back Muscles   65
    Abdominal Muscles   69
    Summary   73
Movement Impairment Syndromes of the   74
  Low Back
    Lumbar Rotation-Extension Syndrome With   74
      or Without Radiating Symptoms
    Case Presentation 1   84
    Case Presentation 2   87
Lumbar Extension Syndrome   88
    Case Presentation   91
Lumbar Rotation Syndrome   93
    Case Presentation   96
Lumbar Rotation-Flexion Syndrome   98
    Case Presentation   100
Lumbar Flexion Syndrome   103
    Case Presentation   105
Sacroiliac Dysfunction   107
Compression   108
Additional Considerations   108

Chapter 3 Appendix   110
  Lumbar Flexion Syndrome   110
  Lumbar Extension Syndrome   112
  Lumbar Rotation Syndrome   114
  Lumbar Rotation With Flexion Syndrome   116
  Lumbar Rotation With Extension Syndrome   118

4 *Movement Impairment Syndromes of the Hip*   121
  Introduction   121
  Normal Alignment of the Hip   122
    Pelvis   122
    Hip Joint   124
    Knee Joint   129
    Foot   134
  Motions of the Hip   134
    Pelvic Girdle Motions   134
    Hip Joint Motions   134
    Hip Joint Accessory Motions   135
  Muscular Actions of the Hip   135
    Anterior Trunk Muscles Affecting the Pelvis   135
    Posterior Muscles Affecting the Pelvis   136
    Anterior Muscles Affecting the Hip Joint   136
    Posterior Muscles Affecting the Hip   137
    Medial Muscles Affecting the Hip   138
    Anterior Muscles Affecting the Hip and Knee   138
    Posterior Muscles Affecting the Hip and Knee 139
    Posterior Leg Muscles Affecting the Knee   140
      and Ankle
    Anterior Leg Muscles Affecting the Ankle   140
    Lateral Leg Muscles Affecting the Foot   142
    Posterior Leg Muscles Affecting the Foot   142
    Muscles Attached to the Foot   143
    Muscle and Movement Impairments   143
  Movement Impairment Syndromes of the Hip   144
    Femoral Anterior Glide Syndrome   144
    Case Presentation 1   148
    Case Presentation 2   150
    Femoral Anterior Glide Syndrome With Lateral 151
      Rotation
    Case Presentation   153
    Hip Adduction Syndrome   154
    Case Presentation 1   156
    Case Presentation 2   157
    Case Presentation 3   159
    Hip Extension With Knee Extension Syndrome   161
    Case Presentation   162
    Hip Lateral Rotation Syndrome   164
    Case Presentation   165
    Femoral Accessory Motion Hypermobility   166
    Case Presentation   167
    Femoral Hypomobility with Superior Glide   168
    Case Presentation   170
    Femoral Lateral Glide Syndrome With   171
      Short-Axis Distraction
    Case Presentation   172
    Conclusion   174

Chapter 4 Appendix   176
  Femoral Anterior Glide Syndrome   176
  Femoral Anterior Glide With Medial   178
    Rotation Syndrome
  Femoral Anterior Glide With Lateral   180
    Rotation Syndrome
  Hip Adduction Syndrome With Medial   182
    Rotation
  Femoral Lateral Glide Syndrome   184
  Hip Extension With Knee Extension   184
  Hip Extension With Medial Rotation   186
  Femoral Hypomobility Syndrome With   186
    Superior Glide
  Femoral Accessory Hypermobility   188
    Syndrome
  Hip Lateral Rotation Syndrome   190

5 *Movement Impairment Syndromes of the*   193
  Shoulder Girdle
  Introduction   193
  Normal Alignment of the Shoulder Girdle   194
    Shoulders   194
    Scapula   195
    Humerus   198
    Thoracic Spine   199
  Motions of the Shoulder Girdle   199
    Glossary of Scapular Motions   199
    Shoulder Girdle Movement Patterns 201
  Muscular Actions of the Shoulder Girdle   206
    Thoracoscapular Muscles   206
    Thoracohumeral Muscles   211
    Scapulohumeral Muscles   212
  Movement Impairment Syndromes of the   216
    Scapula
    Relationship Between Alignment   216
      and Movement
    Criteria for the Diagnosis of a Scapular   217
      Syndrome
    Scapular Syndromes in Observed Frequency   217
      of Occurrence
  Movement Impairment Syndromes   231
    of the Humerus
    Relationships Between Alignment   231
      and Movement
    Criteria for a Diagnosis of a Humeral Syndrome   231
    Order of Observed Frequency of Humeral   231
      Syndromes

Chapter 5 Appendix   246
  Scapular Downward Rotation Syndrome   246
  Scapular Depression Syndrome   248
  Scapular Abduction Syndrome   250
  Scapular Winging and Tilting Syndrome   252
  Humeral Anterior Glide Syndrome   254
  Humeral Superior Glide Syndrome   256

Shoulder Medial Rotation Syndrome   **258**
Glenohumeral Hypomobility Syndrome   **260**

6 Lower and Upper Quarter Movement   263
   Impairment Examinations
Introduction   **263**
Movement Impairments: Lower Quarter   **264**
   Examination
Movement Impairments: Upper Quarter   **328**
   Examination

7 Corrective Exercises: Purposes and Special   367
   Considerations
Introduction   **367**
Standing Exercises   **368**
   Forward Bending (Hip Flexion With Flat   368
      Lumbar Spine)
   Curled Forward Bending (Spinal and Hip   369
      Flexion)
   Side Bending (Lateral Spinal Flexion)   369
   Single-Leg Standing (Unilateral Hip and   369
      Knee Flexion)
   Limited Range of Hip and Knee Flexion   370
      With Trunk Erect (Small Squat)
Supine Exercises   **371**
   Hip Flexor Stretch (Hip and Knee Extension   371
      With Maximal Flexion of Contralateral
      Hip and Knee)
   Control of Pelvis With Lower-Extremity   371
      Motion (Hip and Knee Extension From
      Hip and Knee Flexion)
   Gluteus Maximus Stretch (Hip and Knee   371
      Flexion From Hip and Knee Extension)
   Gluteus Maximus Stretch (Hip and Knee   372
      Flexion From Hip and Knee Extension)
   Hip and Knee Flexion, Sliding Heel From Hip   372
      and Knee Extension (Heel Slides)
   Lower Abdominal Muscle Exercise Progression   373
   Trunk-Curl Sit-Up (Upper Abdominal   376
      Progression)
   Hip Abduction/Lateral Rotation From Hip   377
      Flexed Flexed Position
   Straight-Leg Raises (Hip Flexion With Knee   378
      Extended)
   Hip Flexor Stretch (Two-Joint)   378
   Latissimus Dorsi and Scapulohumeral Muscle   379
      Stretch (Shoulder Flexion/Elevation With
      Elbow Extended)
   Shoulder Abduction   380
   Shoulder Abduction in Lateral Rotation With   380
      Elbows Flexed
   Shoulder Rotation   381
   Pectoralis Minor Stretching   382
Side-Lying Exercises (Lower Extremity)   **382**
   Hip Lateral Rotation   382

   Hip Abduction With and Without Lateral   383
      Rotation
Side-Lying Exercises (Upper Extremity)   **384**
   Shoulder Flexion, Lateral Rotation, and   384
      Scapular Adduction
   Scapular Abduction and Upward Rotation   385
Prone Exercises (Lower Extremity)   **385**
   Knee Flexion   385
   Hip Rotation   386
   Hip Extension With Knee Extended   386
   Hip Extension With Knee Flexed   387
   Hip Abduction   387
   Isometric Hip Lateral Rotation With Hips   387
      Abducted and Knees Flexed
   Isometric Gluteus Maximus Contraction   388
Prone Exercises (Upper Extremity)   **388**
   Back Extensor Activation (Shoulder Flexion   388
      to Elicit Back Extensor Muscle Activity)
   Shoulder Flexion   388
   Trapezius Muscle Exercise Progression   388
   Shoulder Rotation   389
Quadruped Exercises   **390**
   Quadruped Rocking   390
   Limb Movement in the Quadruped Position   391
   Cervical Flexion and Extension   392
   Cervical Rotation   393
Sitting Exercises   **393**
   Knee Extension and Ankle Dorsiflexion   393
   Hip Flexion   394
Standing Exercises   **395**
   Shoulder Flexion (Back Against Wall)   395
   Shoulder Abduction (Back Against Wall)   396
   Shoulder Flexion (Other Than Back Against   396
      Wall)
   Shoulder Abduction (Facing Wall and Trapezius   397
      Exercises)
Walking Exercises   **398**
   Control of Hip and Knee Medial Rotation   398
   Limiting Hip Adduction   399
   Preventing Knee Hyperextension   399
   Limiting Knee Rotation   399
   Ankle Plantar Flexion   399

8 Exercises to Correct Movement Impairment   401
   Syndromes

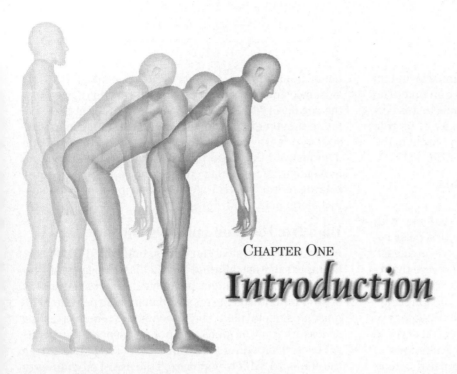

CHAPTER ONE

Introduction

Chapter Highlights

Development of the Movement System Balance Concept
Underlying Premise of Movement as the Cause of Pain
   Syndromes
Overview
Movement Impairment Syndromes
Need for Classification

Chapter Objectives

After reviewing this chapter, the reader will be able to:
1. Describe what should be valued from each of the three historical eras of physical therapy. Explain how aspects of practice of each era can be incorporated into today's practice.
2. Explain how the movement system plays the major role in the development of musculoskeletal pain syndromes.
3. Describe how physical therapists use classifications and diagnoses to direct their interventions.

Development of the Movement System Balance Concept

As a physical therapist for more than 40 years, I have witnessed the evolution of physical therapy (PT) from a technical field to a professional discipline, the advancement of which continues to demand major changes in the practice of the profession. In the twentieth century, the focus of PT can be divided into three eras. In each, the treatment of one anatomic system has been predominant, usually stemming from the prevalence of a physical disability caused by a specific medical problem. In each era, different key concepts have been developed,

which have influenced the characteristics of practice and the techniques used. These concepts have also provided an important philosophic basis for practice.

First Era: Focus on Dysfunction of the Peripheral Neuromuscular and Musculoskeletal Systems

The first era involved the treatment of patients with peripheral neuromuscular or musculoskeletal system dysfunction as a result of war injuries or poliomyelitis. Manual testing of muscle for quantitative assessment of neurologic and muscular dysfunction was key in establishing the role of PT in diagnosis. Specific tests were performed, providing evaluation information to the physician, who would then formulate the diagnosis and define the extent of the dysfunction.

The relatively clear relationship between the loss of muscle function and the impairment of movement provided the direction for treatment. Although the relationship between motor unit loss and the consequences of weakness and loss of range of motion were defined, there was controversy surrounding the best management practices for patients with poliomyelitis, particularly during the acute phase of the illness. During this phase, the primary focus of treatment was to maintain range of motion through the use of stretching exercises and braces. During the recovery phase, exercises designed to strengthen the recovering and unaffected muscles were also important parts of the management of the patient's condition. The most effective treatment included specific exercises that were based on the results of the manual muscle test. This information was also used to prescribe braces or other supports and to set expectations for functional performance. Precise exercises with careful consideration of each muscle and its directions of pull were keys to an optimal outcome. The role of the nervous system in activating muscle was certainly appreciated; however, the complexity of its role in regulating movement was not readily apparent in the patient with lower motor neuron dysfunction.

Second Era: Focus on Central Nervous System Dysfunction

With the eradication of poliomyelitis, patients with stroke, head or spinal cord injury, and cerebral palsy became the predominant patient populations receiving PT. Because the impairments in these patients were the result of central nervous system dysfunction, the previous methods used by physical therapists were no longer applicable. During this era the specific pathophysiology of movement problems that resulted from central nervous system dysfunction was not known. The methods of stretching and strengthening that were used in the treatment of the patient with poliomyelitis were considered unacceptable, because these methods were believed to augment the patient's spasticity. Similarly, manual muscle testing was not considered an accurate indicator of muscle performance because spasticity was believed to augment the muscle response. The mechanisms contributing to impairments in the patient with neurologic dysfunction were not known. Therefore traditional methods of examination and treatment that were used in the management of the patient with musculoskeletal dysfunction were not considered acceptable. The lack of agreement surrounding the underlying mechanisms of the paresis and the suitable treatment meant that specific guidelines for the management of the patient with central nervous system dysfunction were not established. As a result, treatment regimens based on the clinician's experiences and beliefs were developed. The lack of guidelines resulted in highly individual and eclectic treatment; unfortunately, this established a precedent of treatment based on loosely constructed hypotheses. This era also changed the relationship between diagnosis and treatment. The medical diagnoses of diseases of the central nervous system did not provide guidelines for PT treatment in contrast to the diagnosis of poliomyelitis in which the underlying physiologic problem was relatively well understood.

Physical therapists sought explanations for the mechanisms that contributed to the impairment of movement, as evident in the NUSTEP conference in 1967,[2] but as a result of the limited knowledge at the time, explanations that support clinical hypotheses concerning treatment mechanisms were necessarily vague and easily misconstrued. Unfortunately, the mechanisms of motor control still elude clear understanding, as do the mechanisms of the pathophysiology of move-

ment impairments associated with central nervous system lesions. It became obvious during this period that the regulatory function of the nervous system is essential to movement. Although movement impairments associated with central nervous system dysfunction demonstrate the importance of the nervous system in movement, there remained a limited appreciation of the role of motor control and its contribution to musculoskeletal pain syndromes (MPS).

Third Era: Focus on Joint Dysfunction

In the 1980s, physical therapists, influenced by physiotherapists in Australia and New Zealand, began using assessment and treatment techniques directed primarily at joint function as the means of managing patients with musculoskeletal pain. These techniques required testing accessory joint motions and noting associated pain responses. This type of treatment was a departure from the standard, which emphasized the use of modalities to alleviate inflammation and the use of general exercises to strengthen muscles related to the affected segment. Some therapists also began using clinical methods advocated by Dr. James Cyriax[3] to identify specific tissues that were the sources of the pain. Inherent in the use of these methods was a change in the role for the physical therapist. Previously, the physician prescribed treatment on the basis of the diagnosis. Although the majority of referrals merely directed the therapist to "evaluate and treat," particularly when the problem involved the central nervous system, more specific direction was frequently provided for the treatment of the patient with musculoskeletal pain. Thus when the therapist examined joints to determine the source of the pain rather than applying modalities and prescribing a generalized exercise program to improve function, it was a significant change in practice.

Evaluating assessory joint motion represented a philosophical change for the profession; the focus became the identification of soft-tissue or joint restriction as the source of dysfunction, rather than the relief of pain with palliative modalities. However, because periarticular tissues and restricted joint motions were considered the primary problem, minimal consideration was given to the role that muscle and motor control plays in causing dysfunction. Another major development during this period was the classification of patients by directing him or her to perform movements of the spine to determine those movements associated with pain.[11]

Current Era: Focus on the Movement System

During the 1990s, those with musculoskeletal pain have become the largest group of patients receiving PT.[8] Thus the management of these patients is important to the profession. Providing treatment that addresses muscular, neurologic, or skeletal problems in isolation can only be considered incomplete and inadequate. The continued evolution of PT requires that movement remain the central focus. The American Physical Therapy Association adopted a philosophical statement clearly stating that movement dysfunction is the basic problem addressed by our intervention.[1]

Movement is the action of a physiologic system that produces motion of the whole body or of its component parts.[15] These components are the musculoskeletal, neurologic, cardiopulmonary, and metabolic systems. Thus this text is about the movement system and its contribution to movement impairment syndromes.

Because of my initial clinical interest in neurologic dysfunction, observing movement patterns almost became an obsession. Eventually I realized that everyone has a characteristic movement pattern, but these patterns are exaggerated in the patient with musculoskeletal pain. For the past 20 years, I have attempted to identify the organizing principles that best explain the characteristics of these movement patterns, their contributing factors, and why they are associated with or cause pain. Most of the explanations are based on clinical observations that have been used to guide treatment.

The observed clinical outcomes of treatment interventions have been used to refine the basic principles. Currently these principles are the subject of research studies that will further refine, modify, or refute the basic assumptions or syndrome descriptions. Although research is needed to validate these principles, they are based on well-accepted anatomic and kinesiologic relationships. The concepts of anatomy, kinesiology, and physiology that form the basis of PT education are the basis for assessing the patient's muscle and movement performance.

The examination consists of (1) observing movement based on kinesiologic principles, and (2) testing muscle length and strength. Since the earliest days of the profession, physical therapists have used this type of examination to assess physical performance and to design exercise programs.[9] This approach is named movement system balance (MSB) because of the importance of precise or balanced movement to the health of the movement system and its components. The MSB diagnostic and treatment scheme used by the physical therapist organizes basic information into syndromes or diagnostic categories and identifies the factors that contribute to the syndromes. The name of the syndrome identifies the primary dysfunction, or the movement impairment, and directs treatment.[13] Neither outcome effectiveness nor cost containment will permit the physical therapist to continue to use a trial-and-error approach to patient care. This theory and the syndromes are presented with the expectation that others will join me in its validation and refinement.

Three main factors are key to the future growth of the PT profession. The first factor is developing diagnostic categories to direct treatment. The second factor is understanding and managing movement and movement-related dysfunctions and articulating the associated pathophysiology. The third factor is meeting the demands for evidence-based practice by conducting clinical trials based on diagnostic categories that direct PT treatment and knowledge of the underlying clinical science.

Underlying Premise of Movement as a Cause of Pain Syndromes

Maintaining or restoring precise movement of specific segments is the key to preventing or correcting musculoskeletal pain. This is the major premise presented in this text. The biomechanics of the movement system are similar to the mechanics of other systems. In mechanical systems, the longevity of the components and the efficiency of performance require the maintenance of precise movements of the rotating segments. In contrast to machinery, stress on the components is necessary for optimal health and graded stress can actually improve the strength of the involved tissues—two advantageous characteristics of the human body.[10] The stress requirement has upper and lower constraints that determine whether it will help or harm the health of tissues. The loss of precise movement can begin a cycle of events that induces changes in tissues that progress from microtrauma to macrotrauma.

As with any other mechanical system, alignment is important. Ideal alignment facilitates optimal movement. If alignment is faulty before motion is initiated, correction is necessary to achieve the ideal configuration that must be retained throughout the motion. Obviously the dynamic and regenerative properties of biological tissues provide more latitude than the moving segments of most mechanical systems. However, a logical assumption is that the more ideal the alignment of the skeletal segments, the more optimal the performance of the controlling elements such as the muscle and nervous systems. Similarly, if alignment is ideal, there is less chance of causing microtrauma to joints and supporting structures. Studies have shown that the spinal segments subjected to the most movement are the segments that show the greatest signs of degenerative changes.[14] When movement deviates from the ideal, it is reasonable to assume that degenerative changes will likely occur. An analogy is found in the wheel movement of an automobile. For optimal rotation, the wheels must be aligned and in balance. When aligned and balanced, the tires, as the interface between the automobile and the supporting surface, wear evenly, thus increasing the years of use. As discussed in this text, optimal muscular performance through subtle adjustments of muscular length and strength, as well as through the pattern of recruitment, produces and maintains the alignment and balance of human joint motion.

Overview

Concepts and Principles

The concepts and principles explain how repeated movements and sustained postures alter tissue characteristics, which eventually change the pattern of movement and, if less than ideal, can cause impairments. The practice of PT is based on exercises that include repeated movements and sustained postures designed to affect tissues positively. These expected positive results are to improve flexibility, strength, and movement patterns. The physical therapist expects a positive result if the exercises are practiced for 30 minutes to 1 hour each day. However, not all repeated movements and sustained postures are structured for a positive outcome; even sedentary individuals perform repeated movements or sustain postures for many hours per day as part of their daily activities.

When movements are faulty or strength and flexibility are compromised, negative changes occur in soft tissues and in bony structures. The eventual result of injury to these tissues is musculoskeletal pain or a movement impairment syndrome. A model was developed to provide a guide to the impairments produced by movement.

The kinesiologic model described in Chapter 2 incorporates the elements and components of movement and is used to describe relationships among components and the development of impairments in the components. The impairments of soft tissues induced by repeated movements and sustained postures eventually cause a joint to develop a susceptibility to movement in a specific anatomic direction. The susceptibility of a joint to motion increases the frequency of accessory and physiologic movements and is believed to cause tissue damage. Identification of the joint's *directional susceptibility to movement* (DSM) is the focus of the organization and naming of diagnostic categories. Categories named for the offending direction or directions of movement are described in detail. Future refinements are anticipated, but today's information and ideas provide a useful classification system. The classification into syndromes is an important step in outcome research. For example, as every clinician knows, determining the effectiveness of treatment of the patient with low back pain is almost impossible if the only category is the complaint of low back pain. Clearly, treatment of heart disease and other medical conditions could not have progressed to their current level of effectiveness if cardiac and other medical conditions had not been classified. The diagnoses described in this text will cover the shoulder, spine, and hip.

Examination Format

A standardized examination is used to identify the DSM and the factors that contribute to the presence of a dysfunction. Because the trunk provides the support for the limbs and their muscular attachments, its alignment affects all other body segments. Faulty alignment of the head, cervical spine, and shoulders cannot be corrected without correcting the alignment of the trunk and pelvic girdle. The alignment of the hip, knees, and joints of the ankles and feet, as well as the distribution of forces exerted on these joints, are also greatly affected by the alignment of the trunk and pelvis. Therefore a biomechanical examination of any specific anatomic region must incorporate movements of the trunk and extremities to assess their effects on the site of interest. A standard examination is used with slightly different emphases or special tests, depending on the location of the painful segment. (This standard examination is described in detail and then specifically applied to the examination of the shoulders, spine, and hip regions in the appropriate chapters.)

Corrective Exercises

Examination provides the basis for determining corrective exercise. When the patient fails a part of the examination, the test item or a modification of the item is used as part of his or her therapeutic exercise program. Therefore the basic exercises, their modifications, and their progressions are described. The treatment program also includes instructing the patient in maintaining optimal postures and using correct movement patterns for daily activities.

Routine daily movements that are repeatedly performed incorrectly result in the pain syndrome. These impairments in basic movement patterns must be identified, and correct performance patterns must be practiced. Corrective exercises are designed to help patients improve neuromuscular control of a specific muscle and movement, but they do not ensure that under more dynamic conditions, the correct patterns will be used. Patients will return to their former patterns unless they understand the importance of preventing motion in their joint's DSM. Patients must be specifically trained to move correctly during all activities and to maintain correct alignment in static positions, such as sitting and standing. Because the program must be performed daily and requires continual attention to body mechanics, performance is the responsibility of the patient. Therefore home programs are the primary method of treatment with weekly reassessments performed by the therapist of both the effectiveness of the program and the quality of patient performance.

The examination can also identify signs of muscle and movement impairments before the development of symptoms and thus can be used to design preventive programs. Educating a person about his or her specific musculoskeletal impairments and how to correct these before pain develops is part of a preventive program.

Movement Impairment Syndromes

Definition

A variety of terms have been used to describe painful musculoskeletal conditions of unknown origin. Hadler refers to these conditions as regional musculoskeletal disorders.[6] The term regional emphasizes the lack of an underlying systemic disease, supporting the belief that local mechanical trauma is the causative agent. Other common terms used to describe localized pain are musculoskeletal disorders, musculoskeletal dysfunction, myofascial syndromes, overuse syndromes, cumulative trauma, and repetitive strain injuries. Pain from major trauma to bones or from bone tumors or systemic diseases, such as rheumatoid arthritis, does not fall into this category.

In this text the term movement impairment syndrome is used synonymously with musculoskeletal pain (MSP). These syndromes are defined as localized painful conditions arising from irritation of myofascial, periarticular, or articular tissues. Their origin and perpetuation are the result of mechanical trauma, most often microtrauma. Microtrauma is often ascribed to overuse, which is the repeated use or an excessive load that causes stress that exceeds the tissue's tolerance to withstand injury. Excessive load can occur during a single episode of performing an activity or during repeated movements. Repeated use can occur in relatively short duration, such as a single episode of throwing a ball for 1 hour, many years after the cessation of a similar activity. Repeated use can also occur in long duration, such as the baseball player who performs the same activity everyday for many days. Another cause of microtrauma is the development of tissue-damaging stress as a result of a deviation in the ideal arthrokinematics and the resulting movement impairment.

Although the management described in this book is primarily applied to overuse syndromes, the treatment concepts described can be applied to any disease that causes changes in joints and muscles, such as rheumatoid arthritis. Because the concepts are applicable whenever disease affects the biomechanics of the musculoskeletal system, the standard examination and similar treatment are recommended for all patients, even those with neurologic dysfunction. However, additional factors must be considered in applying these principles when there is known dysfunction of the skeletal or nervous system.

Prevalence

Patients with pain originating from the musculoskeletal system constitute the largest group of individuals receiving PT. In a report by Jette, more than 60% of the patients discharged from a sample of PT clinics were treated for MSP, 25% were treated for low back pain, approximately 12% for cervical pain, 12% for shoulder pain, and 12% for knee or hip pain.[8] The prevalence of patients with low back pain in PT is consistent with the finding that the lower back is the most common site of musculoskeletal pain.[5] Two factors explain why the majority of PT patients have MPS. One factor is the high incidence of these syndromes in the general public; the second factor is that exercise and the correction of body mechanics are logical forms of treatment for conditions in which movement most often increases symptoms. This text discusses how movement associated with pain is impaired or causes additional stress to tissues that are already injured, thus contributing further to the trauma.

Numerous reports have cited the high cost of low back pain paid by society.[4] These expenses include direct costs for treatment, as well as indirect costs associated with lost work time. The economic effect on society is significant when the costs associated with MPS are combined with those of low back syndromes.

Diagnosis and Management

Although costly to society and compromising to the individual, the cause of mechanical MPS is poorly understood. Even after the condition has progressed sufficiently to allow identification of specific tissue damage by radiologic or neurologic examinations, diagnosis can remain inconclusive or misleading. Studies, particularly of low back syndromes, have shown positive radiologic findings without clinical symptoms and negative radiologic findings with clinical symptoms. Although specific pathologic abnormalities may be present, they may not be the cause of the pain.[7] Therefore diagnostic labels in the early stages of a painful condition may be relatively nonspecific, (e.g., low back pain or shoulder impingement). Management is most often based on symptomatic treatment of the presumed tissue inflammation, rather than on the correction of the mechanical cause of the tissue irritation. Because these conditions usually affect the quality of life rather than the quantity of life, little investigative attention has been directed to movement impairment syndromes when compared with other disease processes, such as cardiovascular, metastatic, and neurologic diseases. Management of many mechanically induced movement impairment syndromes has proven difficult, because diagnosis is often based on patient self-reporting symptoms rather than on objective tests. The subjective nature of these reports and the difficulty in relating specific tissue abnormalities to symptoms make diagnosis and treatment a difficult challenge to the practitioner. Relating the consistency of pain behavior to specific movements is a useful guide to deciphering the mechanical and subjective factors contributing to the MPS.

To provide effective treatment, the therapist must (1) develop a reasonable hypothesis of causal and contributing factors, (2) perform a specific and systematic examination to identify those factors, (3) formulate a diagnosis to direct PT treatment, (4) provide a well-designed treatment strategy based on the diagnosis and contributing factors, and (5) evaluate the outcome of treatment.

Structures Affected

Structures that are the source of symptoms are myofascial, periarticular, articular, and neurologic. Pain indicates that either mechanical deformation or an inflammatory process is affecting the nociceptors in the symptomatic structures. Although various soft tissues can be identified as the sources of pain, a more important and often ignored consideration should be to answer the question, "What caused them to become painful?" The variety of affected tissues suggests different sources, but a parsimonious explanation suggests a common cause. The likely cause is mechanical irritation or stress. Entrapment, impingement, or adhesions that are also mechanical causes of irritation can affect myofascial tissue, as well as nerves and nerve roots.

Identifying the symptomatic tissue, if possible, is only one step and not always a necessary step to correct a painful condition. For example, although the supraspinatus tendon can be identified as the source of a specific shoulder pain, the reason it became painful needs to be identified to alleviate and prevent the recurrence of the pain. One commonly used explanation is that physical stress from repetitive motion is the cause of mechanical irritation of the tendon. A more useful explanation is that motion at the glenohumeral joint is impaired—an acquired alteration in arthrokinematics —thus creating mechanical irritation of the tendon that

would not have occurred if the joint motion had been optimal. Identifying the specific characteristics of the impairment in glenohumeral motion is more informative than identifying the supraspinatus tendon as the painful structure. Knowledge of the impairment provides information that can be used to limit its progression, achieve correction of the impairment, eliminate the present pain, and prevent future recurrence of the problem.

Treatment Approaches Based on Intervention

Variations in belief about underlying causative factors have led to three basic approaches to PT treatment of MSPs. One approach focuses on the symptoms, another focuses on both the source of symptoms and restrictive tissues, and the third focuses on the cause of the symptoms and contributing factors.

The symptom-focused approach presumes that the painful tissue is the source of the problem.[3] Tissue is inflamed and relief of the inflammation will resolve the problem. In this situation the nonspecific stress that causes tissue irritation arises primarily from fatigue that occurs when abnormal stresses are imposed on a structure over a prolonged period, resulting in tissue breakdown. Overuse, defined as activity that exceeds tissue tolerance, can also be a factor that results in the breakdown of tissue or produces an inflammatory response. Management in this approach is directed at eliminating the destructive stress by rest and providing antiinflammatory treatment to allow the affected tissue to heal. An exercise program to strengthen the affected tissues is the next step in treatment after a resolution of symptoms.

The symptom source and restricted tissue approach focuses on treating the source of the symptoms, such as the painful supraspinatus tendon in a reduced subacromial space, and correcting restrictive tissues, especially those contributing to accessory joint motion impairments. Any deficits in joint movements, particularly those that are painful, are treated by mobilization or manipulation. When accessory joint mobility is within normal limits and painless after treatment, then subsequent movement will continue to be normal and the condition will be alleviated.

The third approach, and the one advocated in this text, places less emphasis on identifying the source of the symptoms and more on identifying the cause. This approach presumes that the problem occurred because patterns of movement were impaired before joint movement became painful or restricted. Restricted joint motion is considered the consequence rather than the cause of movement faults. In the case of supraspinatus tendonitis, the movements of the scapula during shoulder flexion and abduction are usually restricted. If the scapula does not sufficiently abduct or upwardly rotate to achieve 60 degrees of upward rotation, the subacromial space will be reduced and the tendon will become irritated. Although the pain is at the glenohumeral joint in this example, the movements of the entire shoulder girdle complex must be examined. Pain around the glenohumeral joint is often a result of scapular motion impairment; therefore treatment should be directed at scapular muscular control rather than just at the musculature of the glenohumeral joint.

The MSB examination attempts to identify all the factors contributing to movement pattern impairments of the shoulder girdle. These factors are alignment and neuromuscular performance. The supraspinatus tendon would not be the focus of treatment by direct application of modalities unless clear signs of inflammation are present; rather, the primary treatment would be alleviating the mechanical source of the problem. The purpose of treatment in this approach is to correct factors predisposing or contributing to movement pattern impairments, thus alleviating the stress on the painful tissues and allowing inflammation to subside. By avoiding direct treatment of symptomatic tissues, the change in symptoms can be used to assess and monitor the effectiveness of movement correction achieved with the exercise program.

Cause Identification Versus Symptom Reduction

Movement is essential for physical, economic, social, and emotional reasons. When specific movements cause pain that compromises overall function, reducing pain by correcting the movement impairment is beneficial to the patient's mental and physical health and alleviates the microtrauma affecting the painful tissues. When the patient has an understanding of how to control the factors producing his symptoms, he or she can assume an active role in treatment and prevention and not become dependent on passive treatment from the health care system. Addressing the movement source of pain contributes to a more complete and enduring correction than using an approach in which the pain is relieved by temporary measures (e.g., physical or chemical agents) and the patient remains uninformed about the cause and ways to prevent recurrence.

Need for Classification

The practice of medicine is based on classification. The goal of the physician's examination is to establish a diagnosis to prescribe treatment. Often implicit in the diagnosis is knowledge of the underlying pathophysiology. Without diagnosis-based practice, medicine would not have made the advancements in care that are evident today. The diagnosis provided by the physician is adequate to direct treatment, because it is associated with an underlying pathophysiologic condition. When the diagnosis is associated with a clear explanation of the mechanism of movement impairment, it is adequate to direct the treatment provided by a physical therapist. The physician's diagnosis of an MSP syndrome directs only the medical resolution of pain through pharmacologic or surgical intervention, but this diagnosis is not adequate to describe or direct the treatment of the biomechanical origins of the pain syndromes. Physical therapists have devised effective treatment programs for patients; unfortunately, such programs are often based on a therapist's individual judgment and not from a widely accepted or recognized diagnostic scheme with associated treatment recommendations. Impairments, as described by Nagi in his model of disablement,[12] are appropriate for diagnosis by physical therapists. Diagnostic categories consisting of impairment syndromes are consistent with the physical therapist's education and treatment focus. Nagi defines impairment as "an alteration in anatomical, physiological, or psychological structures or functions that is the result of some underlying abnormality."[12] This is distinct from pathologic conditions that arise from disease that, according to the Nagi model, are the basis of the physician's diagnosis.[12] Just as diagnostic schemes have advanced the treatment and research of a variety of conditions arising from disease, so do diagnostic schemes advance the treatment and research of conditions associated with impairments. This text presents impairments that are classified and organized into syndromes similar to the medical diagnosis used to classify disease-induced conditions. Movement impairments have been used as the focus for classification of MPS.

The approach advocated in this text is diagnosis of MPS by classification according to the directions of motion or stress that are accompanied by pain. The names of the diagnostic categories of the classification system are the names of joint motions, physiologic or accessory. In naming the syndrome, the diagnosis is given the name of the movement(s) or postural alignment during which the patient complains of pain or during which the motion is performed in a faulty (less than ideal) manner. For example, in the diagnostic category for low back pain, the pain is elicited not only with direct movements of the spine, but it is also caused by movements of the extremities that impose the same direction of stress on or movement of the spine. The lumbar flexion syndrome is characterized by pain whenever the lumbar spine is flexed, such as during forward bending or sitting in a slumped position. When the patient is instructed to maintain the lumbar spine in a neutral position and bend forward with hip flexion only, the lumbar flexion is eliminated. In the sitting position when the patient extends the knee, there is associated lumbar flexion and an increase in symptoms. Limiting the range of knee extension and preventing the lumbar motion, which decrease the syndrome, support this diagnosis.

The examination is combinatorial, because multiple test items are used to verify the presence of the DSM (e.g., lumbar flexion). Careful assessment of precise movement at specific joints is an important part of the examination. Specific tests of contributing factors, such as muscle stiffness, length, and strength, and patterns of recruitment and compensatory secondary joint movement, are also parts of the examination. Because pain is a major factor, psychological attitudes and illness behavioral information are important components in the diagnosis and management of the cases of MSP.[16] Although recognized as important, this aspect of diagnosis is not discussed in this text, and the reader is referred to other sources.

References

1. American Physical Therapy Association: Philosophical statement on diagnosis in physical therapy. In *Proceedings of the House of Delegates*, 1983, Washington, DC, APTA.
2. Bouman HD: *An exploratory and analytical survey of therapeutic exercise*, Baltimore, 1967, Waverly Press.
3. Cyriax J, Cyriax P: *Illustrated manual of orthopedic*, Boston, 1983, Butterworths.
4. Deyo RA, Cherkin DC, Douglas C, Volinn E: Cost, controversy, crisis: low back pain and the health of the public, *Ann Rev Public Health* 12:11, 1991.
5. Deyo RA, Phillips WR: Low back pain: a primary care challenge, *Spine* 21:2826, 1996.
6. Hadler N: *Medical management of regional musculoskeletal diseases*, Orlando, 1984, Grune & Stratton.
7. Haldeman S: North American Spine Society: failure of the pathology model to predict back pain [presidential address], *Spine* 15:718, 1990.
8. Jette AM, Davis KD: A comparison of hospital-based and private outpatient physical therapy practices, *Phys Ther* 74:366, 1991.
9. Kendall HO, Kendall FP: *Muscles: testing and function*, ed 1, Baltimore, 1949, Williams & Wilkins.
10. Lieber RL: *Skeletal muscle, structure and function*, Baltimore, 1992, Williams & Wilkins.
11. McKenzie RZ: *The lumbar spine: mechanical diagnosis and therapy*, Waikanae, New Zealand, 1989, Spinal Publications.
12. Nagi SZ: *Disability and rehabilitation*, Columbus, Ohio, 1969, Ohio State University Press.
13. Sahrmann SA: Diagnosis by the physical therapist—a prerequisite for treatment: a special communication, *Phys Ther* 68:1703, 1988.
14. Singer KP, Fitzgerald D, Milne N: Neck retraction exercises and cervical disk disease. In Singer KP, editor: *Biennial manipulative physiotherapist conference*. Perth, Australia; 1995.
15. Dirckx JH, editor: *Stedman's concise medical dictionary*, ed 3, Baltimore, 1997, Williams & Wilkins.
16. Waddell G et al: A new clinical model for the treatment of low-back pain, *Spine* 9:209, 1984.

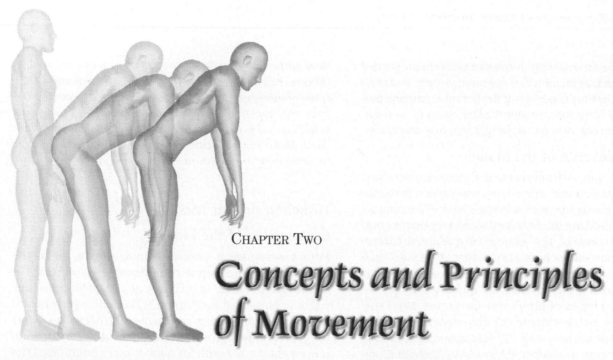

CHAPTER TWO

Concepts and Principles of Movement

Chapter Highlights

Kinesiologic Model

Pathokinesiologic Model

Kinesiopathologic Model

Base Element Impairments of the Muscular System

Base Element Impairments of the Skeletal System: Structural Variations in Joint Alignment

Modulator Element Impairment: Nervous System

Biomechanical Element Impairments

Multiple Impairments of the Components of Movement

Support Element Impairments

Chapter Objectives

After reviewing this chapter, the reader will be able to discuss:

1. The components of and differences among the three models of the movement system.
2. How the muscular, nervous, and skeletal systems are affected by repeated movements and sustained postures.
3. How repeated movements and sustained postures contribute to the development of musculoskeletal pain syndromes.
4. The concept of relative flexibility, its relationship to muscle stiffness, and its implications in the role of exercise to stretch muscles.
5. The role of a joint's directional susceptibility to movement in the development of a musculoskeletal pain syndrome.

Kinesiologic Model

Composition of the Model

This text discusses musculoskeletal pain syndromes arising from tissue alterations that are caused by move-

ment. Movement is considered a system that is made up of several elements, each of which has a relatively unique basic function necessary for the production and regulation of movement. Various anatomic and physiologic systems are components of these basic elements (Figure 2-1). To understand how movement induces pain syndromes, the optimal actions and interactions of the multiple anatomic and physiologic systems involved in motion must be considered. The optimal function and interaction of the elements and their components are depicted in the following kinesiologic model.

The elements of the model are (1) base, (2) modulator, (3) biomechanical, and (4) support. The components that form the *base* element, the foundation on which movement is based, are the muscular and skeletal systems. The components of the *modulator* element regulate movement by controlling the patterns and characteristics of muscle activation. The modulator element of motion is the nervous system, because of its regulatory functions (described in the sciences of neurophysiology, neuropsychology, and physiologic psychology). Components of the biomechanical element are statics and dynamics. Components of the *support* element include the cardiac, pulmonary, and metabolic systems. These systems play an indirect role because they do not produce motion of the segments but provide the substrates and metabolic support required to maintain the viability of the other systems.

Every component of the elements is essential to movement because of the unique contributions of each; however, equally essential is the interaction among the components. Each has a critical role in producing movement and is also affected by movement. For example, muscular contraction produces movement, and movement helps maintain the anatomic and physiologic function of muscle. Specifically, movement affects properties of muscle, such as tension development, length, and stiffness, as well as the properties of the nervous, cardiac, pulmonary, and metabolic systems. (The changes in these properties are discussed in detail later in this chapter.)

Clinical Relevance of the Model

Optimal function of the movement system is maintained when there is periodic movement and variety in the direction of the movement of specific joints. For example, a posture should not be sustained for longer than 1 hour, based on studies of the effects of sustained forces. McGill and associates have shown that 20 minutes in a position of sustained flexion can induce creep in the soft tissues, requiring longer than 40 minutes for full recovery.[41] Two types of effect on soft tissues from sustained forces are described: (1) time-dependent deformation of soft tissues, and (2) soft tissue adaptations involving protein synthesis.[23] A study by Light and colleagues demonstrates that 1 hour per day of sustained low-load stretching produces significant improvement in range-of-knee extension in patients with knee flexion contractures when compared with high-load stretching produced during short duration.[37] The implication is that short duration stretching produces temporary deformation of soft tissues, but 1 hour of stretching may

be a sufficient stimulus for long-term soft-tissue adaptations. *When there is variety in the stresses and directions of movement of a specific joint, the supporting tissues are more likely to retain optimal kinesiologic behavior (defined as precision in movement) than when there is constant repetition of the same specific movement or maintenance of the same specific position.*

Pathokinesiologic Model

Composition of the Model

Pathokinesiology is described by Hislop as the distinguishing clinical science of physical therapy, and it is defined as the study of anatomy and physiology as they relate to abnormal movement.[25] Based in part on word construction and in part on clarification of causative factors, pathokinesiology emphasizes abnormalities of movement as a result of pathologic conditions. The pathokinesiologic model (Figure 2-2) depicts the role of disease or injury as producing changes in the components of movement, which result in abnormalities of movement. In the Nagi model of disablement,[45] disease leads to impairments that cause functional limitations with the possible end result of disability. *Impairments* are defined as any abnormality of the anatomic, physio-

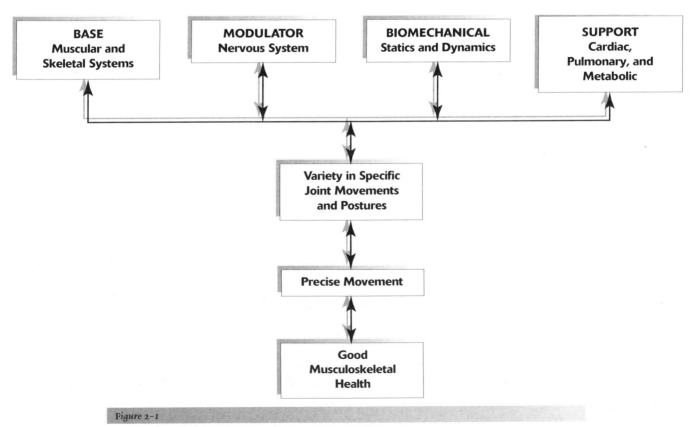

Figure 2-1

The kinesiologic model.

logic, or psychologic system. Therefore abnormalities of any component system or of any movement are considered impairments.

In the pathokinesiologic model, a pathologic disease such as rheumatoid arthritis, produces lesions in the skeletal components because of the degenerative changes in joints. The degenerative joint changes cause alterations in movement of the joint and possibly in movements involved in functions such as ambulating or self-care activities. This model suggests that in addition to the changes in skeletal components, such as joint structures and movement characteristics, there are also changes in the neurologic, biomechanical, cardiopulmonary, and metabolic components. Depending on the severity of the movement impairments, the consequence can be disability.

Similarly, a cerebral vascular accident produces pathologic abnormalities in the central nervous system with the consequence often a form of paresis and movement impairment. Although the primary lesion is in the nervous system, all secondary changes in other components of the movement system must be considered to ensure optimal management of the patient's movement impairment.

Clinical Relevance of the Model

In the pathokinesiologic model, the pathologic abnormality is the source of component impairments, which then causes movement impairments, functional limitations, and often disability. Because of the interaction of the component systems as depicted in the model, identifying the secondary changes in each system is as important as understanding the primary pathologic effect on a system component. For example, in the case of hemiparesis, the movement dysfunction is the result of an abnormality involving the nervous system. Factors

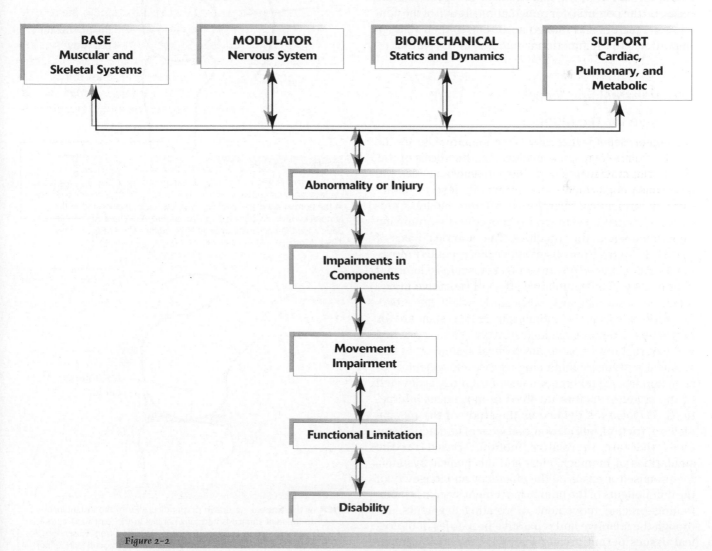

Figure 2-2

The pathokinesiologic model.

contributing to movement dysfunction include but are not limited to (1) an inability of the central nervous system to recruit and drive motor units at a high frequency,[56] (2) the co-activation of antagonistic muscles,[13] (3) a secondary atrophy of muscles that compromise contractile capacity,[7] (4) the stiffness of the muscle,[57] (5) a loss of range of motion from contracture,[21] (6) the biomechanical alterations that are the result of insufficient and inappropriate timing of muscular activity,[12,51] and (7) an internal sensory disorganization.[12] In addition, the alterations of metabolic demands during activity and the aerobic conditioning of the patient must all be considered as contributing factors in the movement impairment. The degree of involvement of each of these factors and their influence on function varies from patient to patient. Physical examination formats should address all these factors and their relative importance to the patient's functional problem. Decisions that lead to the formation of the management program must be based on the potential for remediation of each of the contributing factors and ranked according to their relative importance to the functional outcome of the patient.

Kinesiopathologic Model

Rationale for the Model

A common belief is that movement impairments are the result of pathologic abnormalities, but the thesis of this text is that movements performed in daily activities can also cause impairments that eventually lead to pathologic abnormalities. Therefore a different model is proposed to characterize the role of movement in producing impairments and abnormalities. The empirical basis of this model stems from observations that repetitive movements and sustained postures affect musculoskeletal and neural tissue. The cumulative effect of repetitive movements is tissue damage, particularly when the movements deviate from the optimal kinesiologic standard for movement. Human movements involve similar internal and external forces as do mechanical systems.[49] In mechanical systems, maintaining precise movement is of such importance that the science of tribology is devoted to the study of factors involved in movement interactions. *Tribology* is defined as the study of the mechanisms of friction, lubrication, and wear of interacting surfaces that are in relative motion.[1] Based on the similarities of biomechanical and mechanical systems, the premise for ensuring the efficiency and longevity of the components of the human movement system is maintaining precise movement of rotating segments. Although the adaptive and reparative properties of biological tissues permit greater leeway in maintaining their integrity than do nonbiologic materials, it is reasonable

to assume that maintaining precise movement patterns to minimize abnormal stresses is highly desirable.

A useful criterion for assessing precise or balanced movement is observing the path of instantaneous center of rotation (PICR) during active motion (Figure 2-3). The instantaneous center of rotation (ICR) is the point around which a rigid body rotates at a given instant of time.[48] The PICR is the path of the ICR during movement. In many joints the PICR is not easily analyzed and radiologic methods are necessary to depict the precision of the motion (Figure 2-4). These radiologic methods use

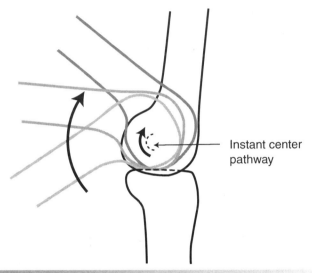

Instant center pathway

Figure 2-3

As the knee moves from flexion to extension, successive instantaneous centers can be mapped, which is known as the instant center pathway. In the normal knee, the pathway is semicircular and located in the femoral condyle. (Modified from Rosenberg A, Mikosz RP, Mohler CG: Basic knee biomechanics. In Scott WN, editor: *The knee*, St Louis, 1994, Mosby.)

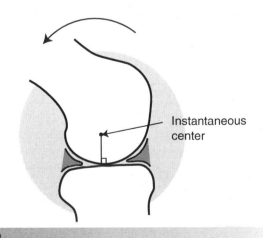

Instantaneous center

Figure 2-4

PICR of the knee. Line drawn perpendicular from the instantaneous center to the joint surface is normally parallel to the joint surface, indicative of a sliding motion between surfaces. (Modified from Rosenberg A, Mikosz RP, Mohler CG: Basic knee biomechanics. In Scott WN, editor: *The knee*, St Louis, 1994, Mosby.)

movements that are performed passively and under artificial conditions. The joints in which the PICR is difficult to observe clinically include those of the knee and spine. The PICR of the scapulothoracic (Figure 2-5) and glenohumeral (Figure 2-6) joints can be observed visually, but it cannot be easily quantified.

Knowledge of the PICR and range of motion of the joint both guide observations and judgments about movement. Although it is rarely referred to specifically, the observation of the PICR is the guideline that physical therapists use to judge whether the joint motion is normal or abnormal. Anatomic and kinesiologic factors that determine the PICR and the pattern of joint movement are (1) the shape of joint surfaces, (2) the control by ligaments, and (3) the force-couple action of muscular synergists.[73]

With normal or ideal movement of joints, the question arises, "What is the cause of deviations in joint movement when a pathologic condition or specific injury is not the problem?" Suggested causes of deviations in joint movement patterns are *repeated movements* and *sustained postures* associated with daily activities of work and recreation. For example, baseball pitchers and swimmers perform repeated motions and commonly experience shoulder pain.[16,31] Prolonged sitting has been cited as a factor in the development of back pain.[52] Cyclists who spend 3 hours riding their bicycles in a position of lumbar flexion have a reduced lumbar curve when compared with control subjects who do not ride bicycles.[10]

Therapists and other clinicians involved in exercise prescription believe that *repeated movements can be used therapeutically to produce desired increases in joint flexibility, muscle length, and muscle strength, as well as to train specific patterns of movement.* All individuals who participate in exercise accept the fact that repeated movements affect muscle and movement performance. Thus these individuals should also accept the idea that *repeated motions of daily activities, as well as those activities of fitness and sports, may also induce undesirable changes in the movement components.* Stretching and strengthening exercises performed for shorter than 1 hour are believed to produce changes in muscular and connective tissues. However, repeated movements and sustained postures associated with everyday activities that are performed for many hours each day may eventually induce changes in the components of the movement system. The inevitable result is the development of movement impairments, tissue stress, microtrauma, and eventually macrotrauma. In accordance with this proposed theory, the effects of repeated movements and sustained postures modify the kinesiologic model so that it becomes a kinesiopathologic model (Figure 2-7), that is, a study of disorders of the movement system.

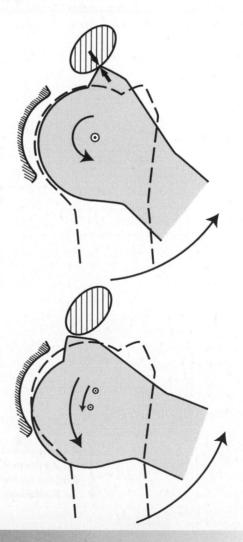

Figure 2-6

PICR of the glenohumeral joint.

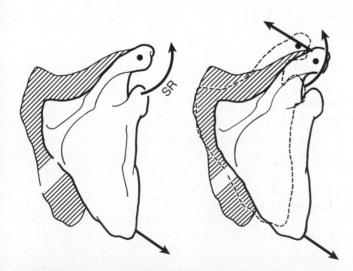

Figure 2-5

PICR of the scapulothoracic joint.

Clinical Relevance of the Model

The kinesiopathologic model serves as a general guide for identifying the components that have been altered by movement. Identifying the alterations or suboptimal functions of components provides a guide to prevention, diagnosis, and intervention. If there is suboptimal function of any component of an element, operationally defined as an impairment, it may be considered a problem and corrected before the client develops musculoskeletal pain. Identifying impairments and correcting them before they become associated with symptoms is using the information incorporated in the model as a guide to prevention. If the impairment is not corrected and the repeated movements continue, the sequence of movement impairment leading to microtrauma and macrotrauma progresses with the consequence of pain and, eventually, identifiable tissue abnormalities.

If pain is present, the kinesiopathologic model can be used to identify all the contributing factors that must be addressed in a therapeutic exercise program. Reversal of the deleterious sequence requires the identification and correction of the movement and component impairments. More important than developing a therapeutic exercise program, the performance of

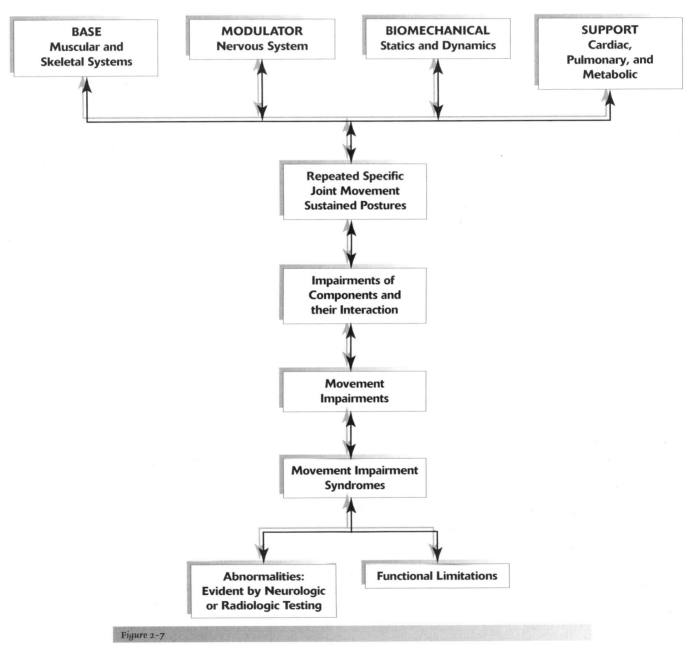

Figure 2-7

The kinesiopathologic model.

functional activities that cause pain must be identified and corrected.

Based on clinical examinations, muscular, skeletal, and neurologic component impairments have contributed to musculoskeletal pain syndromes. (Each of these impairments is individually discussed in this chapter.) The key to diagnosis and effective intervention is the identification of all impairments contributing to a specific movement impairment syndrome. (Syndromes and their multiple associated impairments are discussed in the relevant chapter on diagnostic categories.)

How do repeated movements and sustained postures cause changes in the component systems? The prevailing characteristic of the muscular system is its dramatic and rapid adaptation to the demands placed on it. Most often, adaptations such as changes in strength are considered advantageous; however, changes in strength can also be detrimental and may contribute to movement impairments. Muscles become longer or shorter as the number of sarcomeres in series increases or decreases. Everyday activities can change the strength and length of muscles that alter the relative participation of synergists and antagonists and, eventually, the movement pattern.

Identifying the types of changes that occur in muscle and the causative factors for these changes is the key to maintaining or restoring optimal musculoskeletal health. Changes in muscle occur even when an individual lives a sedentary lifestyle; muscular changes are not limited to those who perform physically demanding work. The most sedentary occupation or lifestyle is associated with some form of repeated movement or sustained posture. For example, individuals who sit at a desk during most of the day perform many rotational or side-bending movements of their spine when they move from a writing surface to the computer or when they reach for the telephone or into a file drawer.

Movements repeated at the extremes of frequency (either high or low) and movements that require the extremes of tension development (either high or low) can cause changes in muscle strength, length, and stiffness. Similarly, sustained postures and particularly those postures that are maintained in faulty alignments can induce changes in the muscles and supporting tissues that can be injurious, especially when the joint is at the end of its range.[70]

One of the most surprising characteristics of muscle performance evident to those who perform specific manual muscle testing is the presence of weakness, even in those individuals who regularly participate in physical activities. A frequently held assumption is that participation in daily activities or participation in sports places adequate demands on all muscles, ensuring normal performance. However, careful and specific muscle testing demonstrates that several muscles commonly test weak. For example, muscles frequently found to be weak are the lower trapezius, external oblique abdominal, gluteus maximus, and posterior gluteus medius. Even individuals who are active in sports demonstrate differences in the strength of synergistic muscles; one muscle can be notably weaker than its synergist.

The following example illustrates how repeated movements can alter muscle performance and lead to movement impairments. When the gluteus maximus and piriformis muscles are the dominant muscles producing hip extension, their proximal attachments provide more optimal control of the femur in the acetabulum than do the hamstring muscles. The attachments of the piriformis and gluteus maximus muscles onto the greater trochanter and intertrochanteric line of the femur provide control of the proximal femur during hip extension. The gluteus maximus through the iliotibial band also attaches on the tibia distally. Therefore this muscle is producing movement of both the proximal and distal aspects of the thigh, which reinforces the maintenance of a relatively constant position of the femoral head in the acetabulum during hip extension (Figure 2-8).

The normal pattern can become altered, particularly in distance runners who develop weakness of the iliopsoas and gluteus maximus muscles. In contrast, the tensor fascia lata (TFL), rectus femoris, and hamstring muscles often become stronger and more dominant in distance runners than in nonrunners. The lack of balance in the strength and pattern of activity among all the hip flexor and extensor muscles can contribute to movement impairments, because each muscle has a slightly different action on the joint to which it attaches. When one in the group becomes dominant, it alters the precision of the joint motion. In the scenario where the activity of the hamstring muscles is dominant and the gluteus maximus muscle is weak, the result can be hamstring strain and a variety of hip problems that are painful. One plausible reason hip joint motion becomes altered is that the hamstring muscles, with one exception, originate from the ischial tuberosity and insert into the tibia. (The exception is the short head of the biceps femoris muscle, which attaches distally on the femur.) Because the hamstring muscles, with the exception of the short head, do not attach into the femur, they cannot provide precise control of the movement of the proximal end of the femur during hip extension. When the hamstring muscular activity is dominant during hip extension, the proximal femur creates stress on the anterior joint capsule by anteriorly gliding during hip extension rather than maintaining a constant position in the acetabulum (see Figure 2-8). This situation can be ex-

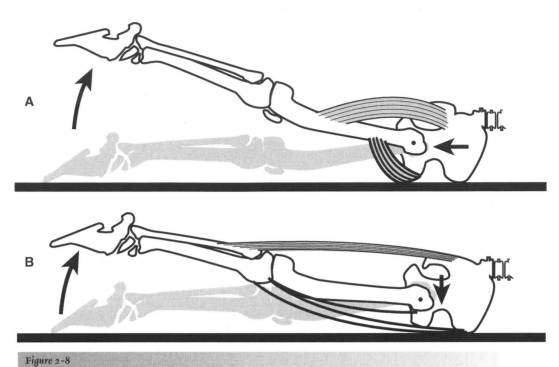

Figure 2-8

Hip extension in prone. *A*, Normal hip extension with constant position of femur in acetabulum; *B*, Abnormal hip extension because of anterior glide of femoral head.

aggerated if the iliopsoas is stretched or weak and is not providing the normal restraint on the femoral head.

These changes in dominance are not presumed; they are confirmed through manual muscle testing and careful monitoring of joint movement. Manual muscle testing[32] is used to assess the relative strength of synergists and the identification of muscle imbalances. Carefully monitoring the precision of joint motion as indicated by the PICR is also necessary when the muscle imbalance has produced a movement impairment. For example, monitoring the greater trochanter during hip extension will identify which muscles are exerting the dominant effect. The greater trochanter will move anteriorly when the hamstrings are the dominant muscles. In contrast, the greater trochanter will either maintain a constant position or move slightly posteriorly when the gluteus maximus and piriformis muscles are the prime movers for hip extension.

Muscle testing identifies the muscles that demonstrate performance deficits as a result of weakness, length changes, or altered recruitment patterns. In addition to reduced contractile capacity of muscle, other factors such as length and strain can be responsible for altered muscle performance, and the muscle can score a less than normal grade in a manual muscle test. The different mechanisms that contribute to these factors can be identified by performance variations during manual muscle testing and are discussed in this chapter.

Base Element Impairments of the Muscular System

Muscle Strength

To design an appropriate intervention program, it is necessary to identify the specific factors that are causing the impairments of the muscular system and contributing to movement impairment. Factors affecting the contractile capacity of the muscle are the number of muscle fibers, the number of contractile elements in each fiber (atrophy or hypertrophy), the arrangement (series or parallel), the fundamental length of the fibers, and the configuration (disruption, over-lengthened, or over-lapped) of the contractile elements.

Muscular force is in proportion to the physiologic cross-sectional area.[36] The physiologic cross-sectional area is a function of the number of contractile elements in the muscle (Figure 2-9). Muscle will atrophy, or lose contractile elements, when it is not routinely required to develop other than minimal tension. Conversely, the muscle cells hypertrophy when routinely required to develop large amounts of tension, as long as the tension demands are within the physiologic limit of its adaptive response. The change in size (circumference) of a muscle occurs either by a decrease in sarcomeres (atrophy) (Figure 2-10) or an increase in sarcomeres (hypertrophy) (Figure 2-11). In hypertrophy the addition of sarcomeres in parallel is accompanied by the

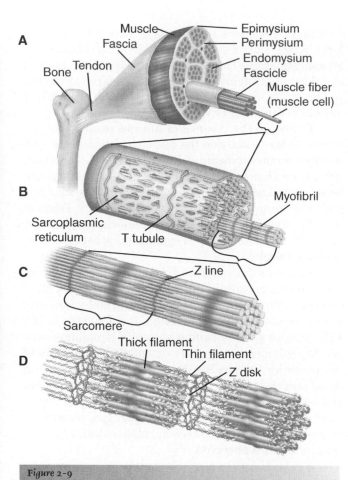

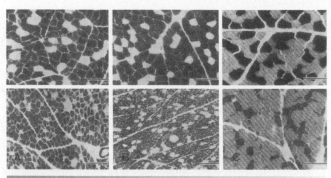

Figure 2-10

Atrophy of muscle. Micrographs from normal muscles *(top panel)*. Micrographs from immobilized muscles illustrating atrophied muscles where the sarcomeres have decreased in diameter *(bottom panel)*. (From Leiber RL et al: Differential response of the dog quadriceps muscle to external skeletal fixation of the knee, *Muscle Nerve* 11:193, 1988.)

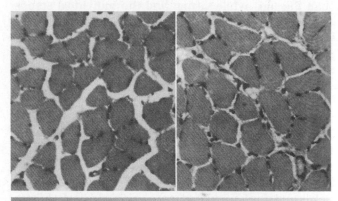

Figure 2-11

Hypertrophy of muscle. Cross-section of control rat soleus muscle *(left)*. Cross-section of hypertrophied rat soleus muscle *(right)*. (From Goldberg AL et al: Mechanism of work-induced hypertrophy of skeletal muscle, *Med Sci Sports* 3:185, 1975.)

Figure 2-9

Structure of skeletal muscle. *A,* Skeletal muscle organ, composed of bundles of contractile muscle fibers held together by connective tissue. *B,* Greater magnification of single fiber showing small fibers, myofibrils in the sarcoplasm. *C,* Myofibril magnified further to show sarcomere between successive Z lines. Cross striae are visible. *D,* Molecular structure of myofibril showing thick myofilaments and thin myofilaments. (From Thibodeau GA, Patton KT: *Anatomy & physiology,* 3e, St Louis, 1996, Mosby.)

addition of sarcomeres in series, though to a lesser extent than those added in parallel.

Decreased Muscle Strength Caused by Atrophy

One cause of muscle weakness is a deficiency in the number of contractile elements (actin and myosin filaments) that make up the sarcomere structure of the muscle. Atrophy of a muscle is not typically associated with pain during either contraction or palpation. A lack of resistive load on muscle can cause atrophy, not only by reducing the numbers of sarcomeres in parallel and, to a lesser extent, in series, but also by decreasing the amount of connective tissue.

The decreased number of sarcomeres and the decreased amount of connective tissue can affect both the active[36] and passive[9] tension of a muscle, which affects the dynamic and static support exerted on each joint it

crosses. The effect is diminished capacity for the development of active torque and less stability of the joint controlled by the muscle. For example, if the peroneal muscles of the leg are weak, the motion of eversion will be weak and the passive stability that helps restrain inversion will be diminished.

The passive tension of muscles also affects joint alignment. When the elbow flexor muscles are weak or have minimal passive tension, the elbow remains extended when the shoulder is in neutral. When the elbow flexors are hypertrophied from weight training, the resting position of the elbow joint is often one of flexion. Because atrophy means a deficiency of contractile elements, the size of a muscle (cross-sectional area) and its firmness can be used as guides to assess strength. For example, poor definition of the gluteal muscles is usually a good indication that these muscles are weak, particularly when the definition of the hamstring muscles suggests hypertrophy. Examiners should not rely solely on observation, but they should perform a manual muscle test to confirm or refute the hypothesis.

As mentioned, when muscle in the normal individual is tested, it is not uncommon to find deficient performances, even in those who exercise regularly. These deficiencies develop because subtle differences in an individual's physical structure and manner of performing activities can have a major effect on the participation of different muscles. When an individual shorter than 5 feet, 2 inches in height stands from sitting in a standard chair, the demands placed on his or her hip and knee extensor muscles are not the same as those in the individual who is 6 feet, 2 inches in height or who has long tibias that cause the knees to be higher than the hips when sitting. A greater demand is placed on the extensor musculature when the knees are higher than the hips while sitting and the individual stands from a sitting position. These differences become apparent when standing from a low chair or sofa. When individuals use their hands to push up from a chair, they also contribute to the weakness of the hip and knee extensor muscles by decreasing their participation.

Another example of altering the use of specific muscles is seen in the individual who returns to an upright position from a forward flexed position by swaying the hips forward rather than maintaining a relatively fixed position of the hips. The individual with the relatively fixed position of the hips lifts the length of the pelvis and trunk by extending the hips and back (Figure 2-12). Typically, individuals who sway their pelvis forward have weak gluteus maximus muscles. There are numerous ways in which slight subtleties in movement patterns contribute to specific muscle weaknesses. The relationship between altered movement patterns and specific muscle weaknesses requires that remediation addresses the changes to the movement pattern; the performance of strengthening exercises alone will not likely affect the timing and manner of recruitment during functional performance.

Clinical Relevance of Muscle Atrophy

Identifying specific muscle weakness requires manual testing. When a muscle is atrophied, it is unable to hold the limb in the manual test position or at any point in the range when resistance is applied. The muscle is not painful when palpated or when contracting against resistance. When a muscle tests weak, the therapist carefully examines movement patterns for subtleties of substitution. Correction of these movement patterns in addition to a specific muscle-strengthening program is required for an optimal outcome. Another factor that must be corrected is the habitual use of any position or

posture that subjects the muscle to stretching, particularly when the patient is inactive (e.g., sleeping). Sleeping postures can place the muscles of the hip and shoulder in stretched positions. (This type of stretch weakness is discussed in the section on lengthened muscle in this chapter.)

To initiate the reversal of muscle atrophy, the patient's ability to activate the muscle volitionally is augmented. Studies indicate that after 2 weeks of training, 20% of the change in muscle tension development can be attributed to muscular factors (contractile capacity) and 80% from enhanced neural activation.[43] Training specific muscles is particularly important when the problem is an imbalance of synergists rather than generalized atrophy.

Exercises that emphasize major muscle group contraction can contribute to the imbalance, rather than correct it. When the patient performs hip abduction with the hip flexed or medially rotated, the activities of the TFL, anterior gluteus medius, and gluteus minimus muscles are enhanced to a greater extent than the activity of the posterior gluteus medius muscle, even though all these muscles are hip abductors. The end result is hip abduction with hip flexion and medial rotation rather than pure abduction. Resistance exercises performed on machines can contribute to imbalances unless proper precautions are observed.

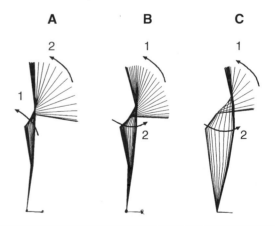

Figure 2-12

Return from forward bending using three different strategies. Optotrak depiction of movement of markers placed at the head of the fifth metatarsal, ankle joint, lateral epicondyle of the knee, greater trochanter, iliac crest, and tip of shoulder. *A*, The motion is initiated by hip extension, followed by immediate and continuous lumbar extension, and is accompanying the rest of the hip motion. *B*, The motion is initiated by lumbar extension and followed by hip extension. *C*, In the forward-bending position, the subject is swayed backward with the ankles in plantar flexion. The return motion is a combination of ankle dorsiflexion and hip extension by forward sway of the pelvis. (Courtesy of Amy Bastian, PhD, PT.)

Approximately 4 weeks of strengthening exercises are required to verify the morphologic increase in muscle cross-sectional area.[43] Studies at the cellular level suggest that change may be occurring earlier than 4 weeks, which is consistent with the metabolic properties of other proteins. Because 4 weeks is required for changes in the number of contractile elements, early improvements in muscle performance are attributed to neuromotor recruitment. The rate of recruitment and the absolute frequency of activation of muscles are important factors in the performance of producing, improving, and maintaining the tension-generating properties of muscles.

Decreased Muscle Strength Secondary to Strain

Strain can result from excessive stretching for short duration or excessive physiologic loading usually associated with eccentric contraction.[35] (Additional discussion of the cellular manifestation of strain is found in the section on increased muscle length in this chapter.) Unless there is an actual tear of muscle fibers and obvious signs of hemorrhage, strain is not readily recognized as a source of muscle weakness. The intervention is different than when the muscle is strained and not merely atrophied.

Muscles that are strained are usually painful when palpated or when contracting. As with atrophy, a strained muscle is weak and unable to hold the limb in any position when resistance is applied throughout the range of motion. The presence of pain is usually an indicator of weakness from strain rather than from atrophy. When the length of the strained muscle is not constrained by its joint attachments, it is elongated in the resting position, such as a dropped or forward shoulder with a strain of the trapezius muscle. Strained muscles need to be rested at the ideal resting length to decrease the elongation of the muscle cells. The strained muscle can be supported by external support such as tape, preferably a type that has a strong adhesive and lacks elasticity. Exercises and active motions should be pain free or cause only mild discomfort.

The same principles used to manage atrophied muscles are applied to strained muscles, once the muscle is no longer painful.

Increased Muscle Strength Caused by Hypertrophy

Studies have shown that when a muscle is subjected to overload conditions, the response is the addition of contractile and connective tissue proteins. The value of hypertrophy in increasing the tension-generating capability of muscle is well known and frequently used by those involved in rehabilitation and athletics. Less appreciated is the effect of hypertrophy on the passive-tension properties of muscle and other connective tissue. Many tissues respond to stress by adapting (see Figure 2-11), which for muscle is hypertrophy. The quantity of connective tissue proteins of ligaments, tendons, and muscle also increases with hypertrophy. Tendons and ligaments become stronger and stiffer when subjected to stress, but they grow weaker when they are not subjected to stress.[64,67,72] The result is an increase in the passive tension of these tissues, not just the active tension that is generated by muscle during contraction. (The cellular factors are described in the section on muscle stiffness in this chapter.)

The use of strengthening exercises that are based on requiring muscle to lift maximal loads is well known to physical therapists. Strengthening exercises not only increase the tension-generating capacity of the muscle, but they also increase the stiffness of the muscle and the stability of the joints. Hypertrophy is important in improving muscle control under both active and passive conditions.

Muscle Length

A muscle can become lengthened by one of the following three mechanisms:

1. ***Prolonged elongated position.*** Muscle may remain in an elongated position during a prolonged period (hours or days) of rest or inactivity (e.g., elongation of the ankle dorsiflexors by the tension of bed covers during bed rest). This condition is similar to over-stretch weakness and a mild form of strain that does not involve eccentric contraction under load as described by Kendall.[32]
2. ***Injurious strain.*** Muscle may be subjected to injurious strain, which is the disruption of the cross bridges, usually in response to a forceful eccentric contraction. The muscle may then be subjected to continuous tension.
3. ***Sustained stretching.*** Muscle may respond to sustained (many days to weeks) stretching during immobilization in a lengthened position with the addition of sarcomeres in series.[71]

Over-Stretch Weakness

Muscles become weak when they maintain a lengthened position, particularly when the stretch occurs during periods of prolonged rest. A common example is the development of elongated dorsiflexor and shortened plantar flexor muscles in the patient for whom bed rest is prescribed or in the individual who remains supine for a prolonged period without the use of a footboard. This problem is exaggerated when the sheet exerts a downward pull on the feet, causing an additional force into plantar flexion and a consequent lengthening of the dorsiflexor muscles.

Another example is the prolonged stretch of the posterior gluteus medius that occurs while sleeping. This condition is seen particularly in the woman with a broad pelvis who regularly sleeps on her side with her uppermost leg positioned in adduction, flexion, and medial rotation. During manual muscle testing, this patient is unable to maintain the hip in abduction, extension, and lateral rotation—the testing position—or at any point in the range, as the resistance is continually applied by the examiner. The resultant lengthening of the muscle can produce postural hip adduction or an apparent leg length discrepancy when the patient stands.

Another example of prolonged stretch occurs when an individual sleeps in a side-lying position with the lower shoulder pushing forward, causing the scapula to abduct and tilt forward. This prolonged position stretches the lower trapezius muscle and possibly the rhomboid muscles. In the side-lying position, the top shoulder is susceptible to problematic stretching when the arm is heavy and the thorax is large, causing the arm to pull the scapula into the abducted, forward position. This sleeping position can also cause the humeral head in the glenoid to move into a forward position.

There are several characteristics of muscles with over-stretch weakness:

1. Postural alignment that is controlled by the muscle indicates that the muscle is longer than ideal, as in depressed shoulders or in a postural alignment of the hip of adduction and medial rotation.
2. Muscle tests weak throughout its range of motion and not only in the shortened muscle test position.

Case Presentation 1

History. 20-year-old female college student has developed back pain that is partially attributable to working as a waitress. Radiologic studies indicate she has a C-curve of her lumbar spine with a right convexity. Her left iliac crest is 1 inch higher than her right, and she stands with a marked anterior pelvic tilt.

Symptoms. The patient complains that her slacks are not fitting correctly. Although she is slender, the patient has a very broad pelvis. She sleeps on her right side with her left leg positioned in hip flexion, adduction, and medial rotation.

Muscle Length and Strength. Muscle length testing indicates a shortened left TFL. Manual muscle testing indicates that the posterior portion of her left gluteus medius muscle is weak, grading 3+/5. Her external oblique abdominal muscles also test weak, grading 3+/5. In the side-lying position, her left hip adducts 25 degrees and rotates medially to the extent that the patella faces the plinth. A home exercise program that emphasizes strengthening her posterior gluteus medius muscle in the shortened position is prescribed.

In the supine position with her hips and knees flexed, she performs isometric contraction of her external oblique abdominal muscles while maintaining a neutral tilt of her pelvis. She then extends one lower extremity at a time. The position for hip flexor length testing is used to stretch the TFL. She also performs knee flexion and hip lateral rotation in the prone position. She is instructed to stand with her hips level and to contract her external oblique abdominal and gluteal muscles. She is also asked to use a body pillow to support her left leg while sleeping to prevent the adduction and medial rotation of her left hip when lying on her right side.

Outcome. On her second visit 3 weeks later, the patient's symptoms have greatly improved to only an occasional incident of discomfort. Her iliac crests are level, and her spinal lateral curvature is no longer clinically evident. The anterior pelvic tilt has resolved. She states she no longer has back pain.

Clinical relevance

This case demonstrates that when the diagnosis is over-stretch weakness, an exercise program that strengthens the muscle and alleviates the stretch can correct alignment and eliminate symptoms. The sleeping positions combined with a patient's structural characteristics can cause over-stretch weakness. A similar mechanism can also contribute to over-stretch weakness of the upper trapezius muscle. This condition can progress to painful muscle strain if not corrected immediately after the onset of the length change. A prolonged passive stretch exerted on a muscle, particularly under rest conditions, can be the precipitating factor in the development of this condition. The key factors that identify over-stretch weakness are: (1) weakness of the muscle that is evident throughout the range of motion, and (2) increased resting muscle length that is greater than its ideal anatomic length and is usually evident in the postural alignment examination.

Increased Muscle Length Secondary to Strain

Strain is discussed because of the importance of differentiating whether the cause of muscle pain is muscle shortness or excessive muscle length. A common approach to the treatment of painful muscles, particularly those of the shoulder girdle, is applying a cold spray and stretching the muscle.[60] Pain is attributed to spasm in the shortened muscle,[60] but often the actual length of the muscle is not assessed before applying stretching techniques. Lengthened muscles can also become painful and should not be stretched. For example, when a muscle is subjected to injurious tension by lifting a heavy object, it can become strained. If the muscle remains under continuous tension, it will become elongated and painful. When the postural alignment examination indicates a muscle is elongated, then strain, rather than shortness, is considered the likely cause of pain.

Strain is a minor form of a tear in which the filaments of the muscle have been stretched or stressed beyond their physiologic limit resulting in disruption of the Z-lines to which the actin filaments attach (Figure 2-13). Disruptions that alter the alignment of the myofilaments interfere with the tension-generating ability of these contractile elements.[35] The consequence is muscular weakness and, in many cases, pain when the muscle is palpated or when resistance is applied during contraction of the muscle.

If a muscle is strained, the reparative process occurs more readily when the muscle is not subjected to strong resistance or to constant tension. For most muscles the anatomic limits imposed by joints to which the muscles attach help maintain the fibers at their appropriate resting length. Postural muscles of the shoulder and hip can become excessively stretched. For example, if the upper trapezius muscle is strained, weight of the shoulder girdle is excessive for the muscle, the shoulder's pull on the muscle causes it to elongate, and the muscle is unable to heal. Frequently, strained muscles are painful because they are actually under continuous tension, even when they appear to be at rest. The discomfort is often reduced when the muscle is supported at its normal resting length, the passive tension is reduced, and the patient is instructed to relax the muscle, thereby eliminating any voluntary or involuntary contractile activity. As long as the patient avoids excessive loads on the muscle, it should heal within 3 to 4 weeks.

The typical findings with manual muscle testing of a strained muscle is its inability to support the tested extremity against gravity when positioned at the end of its range. Further, the muscle is unable to maintain its tension at any point in the range when resistance is applied throughout the range, and pain is elicited. Clearly the tension-generating capacity of the muscle is impaired. If the strain is severe, the motion of the joint upon which the muscle is acting will also show quality of movement and range-of-motion impairment.

Case Presentation 2

History. A 32-year-old woman, whose job requires her to load food trays on a conveyor belt at shoulder height, has a sudden and severe onset of pain between the vertebral border of the right scapula and thoracic spine. The pain began after she attempted to lift a filing cabinet at work. She is seen immediately by a physician who refers her to a physical therapist, prescribing heat to the affected area and shoulder exercises three times a week. After 1 week, the patient returns to light duty at

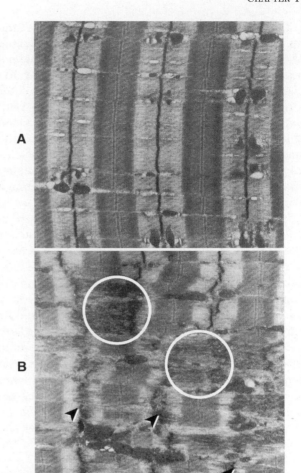

Figure 2-13

Micrograph showing normal striation pattern and Z-disks perpendicular to the long myofibrillar axis *(A)* and various disrupted regions *(B)*. Streaming and smearing of the X-disk material *(arrowheads)* and extension of the Z-disks into adjacent A-bands *(circled areas)* are shown. (From Lieber RL, Friden JO, McKee-Woodbum TG: Muscle damage induced by eccentric contractions of twenty-five percent strain, *J Appl Physiol* 70:2498, 1991.)

work, but 6 weeks later she still complains of severe pain and she is unable to return to her normal job. A magnetic resonance image of her thoracic spine does not indicate an abnormality.

Symptoms. She is referred to a second physical therapy clinic. During her initial visit the patient is observed to be approximately 60 pounds overweight, with large arms and breasts and deep indentations on the tops of her shoulders from the pressure of her bra straps. Her facial expression and the manner in which she holds her right arm close to her body with her elbow flexed indicate that she is still in pain. She rates her pain as 6 to 8 on a scale of 10 when attempting any type of shoulder motion and 4 to 5 out of 10 with her arm at rest. (The 10 rating is the most severe.)

Muscle Length and Strength. An examination indicates that the right scapula is greatly abducted and tilted anteriorly (Figure 2-14, *A*). Her scapula is manually positioned in the correct alignment, and her arm and forearm are supported by the physical therapist. After she is instructed to relax the musculature of her right shoulder girdle, she reports her pain has subsided (Figure 2-14, *B*). A manual muscle test indicates the strength of all components of her trapezius muscle as weak, graded 3−/5. Weakness and pain limit her ability to move through the normal range of motion even in a gravity-lessened position.

Tape (Leukotape P with cover roll underwrap) is applied to the posterior aspect of the right shoulder girdle to support and maintain the scapula in a neutral position and to reduce some of the strain on the trapezius muscle by decreasing the abduction and depression of the scapula. The case report written by Host demonstrates that scapular position can be altered by the application of tape to the posterior shoulder girdle.[28]

Her bra straps are taped together, bringing them closer to her neck to reduce the downward pull on the lateral aspect of her shoulders. She is also instructed to support her arms on pillows whenever she sits and to support her right arm with her left arm to reduce the downward pull on her shoulder girdle whenever she stands. All shoulder exercises are eliminated for the next 5 days (Figure 2-14, *C*).

Outcome. On her second visit 4 days later, the patient reports a significant decrease in pain. She has kept her shoulder taped for 2 days. Her skin does not show signs of irritation, and she indicates that the extra support has eliminated her pain at rest. As a result, the tape was reapplied. On her third visit 1 week later, the patient no longer complains of pain at rest, and she can perform 160 degrees of shoulder flexion without pain in the gravity-lessened side-lying position with her arm supported on pillows. In this position the scapula rotates upwardly and adducts during shoulder flexion, in contrast to the limited scapular motion observed during the same movement performed in the standing position. Her shoulder girdle is taped to support the scapula in the neutral position relative to abduction or adduction, elevation or depression, and rotation. The tape remains in place for 2 additional days. She has been taped three times over a 2-week period.

She continues to support her arm passively to reduce the downward pull on her shoulder while sitting and standing. The gradual progression of her exercise program is as follows:

1. Gravity-lessened side-lying shoulder flexion
2. Shoulder flexion facing a wall with her elbow flexed and hand gliding up the wall
3. Shoulder flexion with the elbow extended

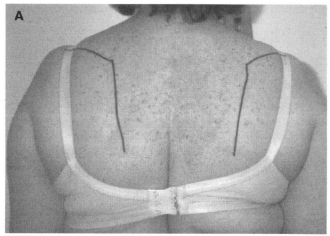

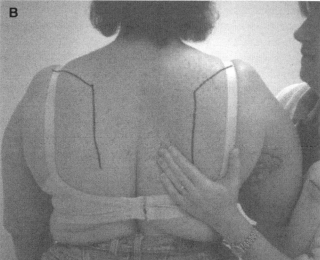

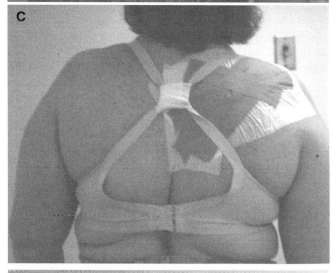

Figure 2-14

Strain of right thoracoscapular muscles. *A,* Right scapula was abducted and tilted anteriorly. *B,* Right shoulder was passively supported in the correct alignment to alleviate the strain on the scapular adductor muscles. When the patient relaxed the muscles, her pain was alleviated. *C,* Bra straps were taped together to bring the straps closer to the neck and to reduce downward pull on the lateral aspect of the shoulder.

4. Shoulder flexion and abduction while lifting light weights

Eight visits during 6 weeks after her initial visit to the second department, she is able to lift a 30-pound tray to shoulder level and has returned to full duty on her job.

Clinical relevance

The patient with a painful condition of the shoulder girdle should be examined for postural indicators of excessive muscle length. The patient with depressed shoulders could be at risk for muscle strain. Muscle spasms and pain can be present when the muscle is long and strained, not only when the muscle is short. Therefore stretching is not always the optimal intervention to alleviate muscle spasm or pain. Stretching and placing excessive force demands on the muscle is contraindicated if it is strained. When strain is suggested, a useful assessment method is supporting the muscle passively in a shortened position and noting the effect on the symptoms. If eliminating the stretch imposed on the muscle reduces the symptoms, the tentative diagnosis of strain is supported.

Observations of the movement characteristics of the shoulder girdle are also indicators of whether the affected muscle is producing the correct movement of the segments it controls. Manual muscle testing of both an atrophied and strained muscle will demonstrate weakness throughout the range, but strained muscles are also usually painful to palpation and when contracted maximally. The length of the muscle and the presence of pain are guides as to whether the muscle is merely weak from atrophy or weak from strain.

Management of muscle strain requires some form of muscular support to alleviate the strain and tension and facilitate the healing process before beginning a slowly progressive exercise program. The load on the muscle should be reduced while the muscle is weak to allow the affected muscle to move correctly the joint segments to which it is attached. The load is then progressively increased as the muscle strength improves and the correct movement of the joint segment is achieved.

Lengthened Muscle Secondary to Anatomic Adaptation—the Addition of Sarcomeres

Numerous investigators have demonstrated that when a muscle is maintained in a position of elongation (usually by casting), additional sarcomeres are added in series within the muscle cell. A study by Williams and Goldspink[60,72] demonstrates that when such adaptation of the anatomic length occurs, the muscle's length tension curve is shifted to the right because of the addition of sarcomeres in series.[71] However, with both mus-

cles in the same shortened position, the control muscle develops greater tension than the lengthened muscle (Figure 2-15).

When both the lengthened and control muscles are tested in the same shortened position, the difference in tension between the two (active-insufficiency) can be explained by the existence of greater overlap of actin and myosin filaments in the lengthened muscle. The muscle that generates the greatest tension at its longest length generates the least tension when tested at a shortened length. When the lengthened muscle (increased number of sarcomeres in series) is placed in a shortened position, the myofilaments in each sarcomere are excessively overlapped (Figure 2-16, *position A*) and thus cannot develop maximal tension. Although such anatomic adaptations have not been histologically demonstrated in human beings, a study comparing right and left hip abductor muscle strength at various muscle lengths supports this interpretation of the hypothesis of length-associated changes.[46]

Typically, the result of manual muscle testing of a lengthened (sarcomeres added in series) muscle indicates that it cannot support the joint segment in the shortened test position. The muscle can, however, tolerate strong pressure after it is allowed to lengthen slightly (a change of 10 to 15 degrees in a joint angle). A clinical example is seen in the individual with a habitual posture of adducted scapulae. Manual muscle testing of the serratus anterior muscle with the ad-

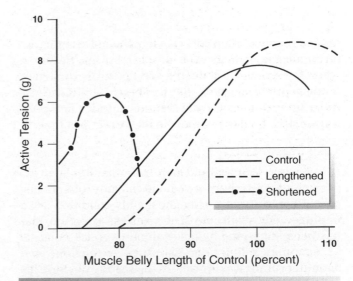

Figure 2-15

Anatomic muscle length adaptation. Lengthened muscle develops greater peak tension at a longer length. The same muscle in a shortened position develops less tension than the control muscle in a normal position. (Modified from Gossman, Sahrmann SA, Rose SJ: Review of length-associated changes in muscle. Experimental evidence and clinical implications, *Phys Ther* 62(12):1799, 1982.)

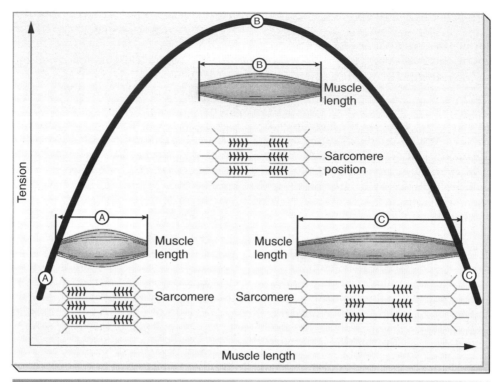

Figure 2-16

The length-tension relationship. The maximal strength that a muscle can develop is directly related to the initial length of its fibers. As a short initial length, the filaments in each sarcomere are already overlapped, limiting the tension that the muscle can develop (*position A*). Maximal tension can be generated only when the muscle is at an optimal length (*position B*). When the thick and thin myofilaments are too far apart, the lack of the overlap of the filaments prevents the generation of tension (*position C*). (From Thibodeau GA, Patton KT: *Anatomy & physiology*, 4e, St Louis, 1999, Mosby.)

ducted scapula (Figure 2-17) (a lengthened serratus anterior muscle) indicates the muscle is strong. However, when the scapula is abducted and upwardly rotated to its appropriate muscle testing position (a shortened serratus anterior muscle), the serratus anterior muscle is too weak to hold the scapula in its correct position.

Case Presentation 3

History. A 50-year-old male swimmer has been experiencing right shoulder pain in the anterolateral aspect. His physician has diagnosed his condition as an impingement syndrome. The exercise program that has been suggested by his swimming coach consists of scapular adduction, shoulder extension, and shoulder rotation exercises. In the resting position his scapulae are adducted with the vertebral borders of each scapula measuring 2 1/4 inches from the vertebral spine. (Approximately 3 inches is considered normal.) The muscle definition of the rhomboid muscles is more prominent than that of the other thoracoscapular muscles.

Symptoms. Right shoulder flexion range measures 170 degrees and is associated with pain at the acromion from 150 to 160 degrees of flexion. Scapular abduction and upward rotation is decreased during shoulder flexion. At the completion of flexion, the inferior angle of the scapula is still on the posterior aspect of the thorax and has not abducted and upwardly rotated enough to reach the midaxillary line. When the scapula is passively abducted and upwardly rotated by the therapist during active shoulder flexion, full range of motion is achieved and the patient does not experience pain.

Muscle Length and Strength. Muscle testing of the serratus anterior muscle indicates that in the abducted position, passively positioned by the physical therapist before instructing the patient to "hold," the muscle does not support the extremity against gravity in the test position. After the scapula is allowed to adduct slightly, the patient can hold the test position and tolerate maximum resistance.

Outcomes. The therapeutic exercise program designed for this patient teaches him to abduct and up-

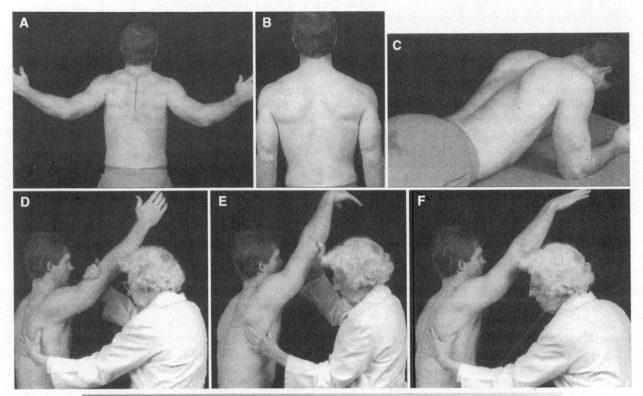

Figure 2-17

A, This subject has routinely performed both bench presses and shoulder adduction exercises with heavy weights, including seated rowing and bent over rowing. The rhomboid muscles have become over-developed. *B,* The abnormal position of scapular adduction is indicative of a lengthened serratus anterior. *C,* In a prone position and resting on the forearms, there is winging of the scapulae. The serratus is unable to hold the scapula against the thorax. *D,* When the shoulder is flexed to position the scapula for the serratus test, the scapula does not move to the normal position of abduction. However, the serratus tests strong in this position. *E,* The scapula is brought forward to the normal position of abduction by the examiner. *F,* The serratus anterior cannot hold the scapula abducted and upwardly rotated when the examiner releases the arm and the subject attempts to hold it in position. (From Kendall FP, McCreary EK, Provance PG: *Muscles: testing and function,* 4e, 1993, Williams & Wilkins.)

wardly rotate his right scapula in the gravity-lessened prone and side-lying positions, while avoiding maximal glenohumeral joint ranges of 150 to 160 degrees until the pattern of correct scapular motion is established. The goal is to have the scapula abduct and upwardly rotate so that the inferior angle of the scapula reaches the midaxillary line by the end of the range-of-shoulder flexion. Within 3 weeks of initiating his therapeutic exercise program, the patient no longer experiences shoulder pain; he has full range-of-shoulder motion and has resumed his swimming.

Clinical relevance

Many postural changes are associated with increased muscle length. When the length has been acquired by the addition of sarcomeres, as suggested by animal studies, the muscle can generate as much if not more tension than a normal length muscle when con-

tracting at its longer resting length. Manual muscle testing of individuals with postural impairments, such as forward shoulders or unilateral hip adduction (apparent leg-length discrepancy), indicates that many of these individuals cannot maintain the test position when maximum resistance is applied. However, when the joint position is changed 10 to 15 degrees to allow the muscle to elongate, maximum resistance can be applied and the muscle can maintain the test position.

This clinical finding suggests that such a muscle is not weak because of compromised contractile capacity, but it has undergone a maladaptive length change. Because the lengthened muscle is associated with joint malalignment evident in postural changes such as forward shoulders or postural hip adduction, correction is indicated. Even more importantly, the change in the length of the muscle also changes the movement of the joint controlled by the muscle.

The strategy for correction is to improve the muscle's performance at a shorter more normal length. To achieve this outcome the patient must work the muscle at a shorter length; to do so, the load imposed on the muscle must be reduced. For example, the patient may need to perform hip abduction in the side-lying position with his knee flexed to reduce the length of the lever that he will be lifting. For the same reason, shoulder flexion in the standing position may need to be performed with the elbows flexed to reduce the length of the lever that is being moved. Because the muscle is not injured or atrophied, special protective measures are unnecessary.

The goals of the treatment are to (1) change the resting length of the muscle, correcting the alignment of the segment to which it attaches, and (2) improve the control of the muscle and by its action enable the affected joints to move through their optimal range. When the lower and middle trapezius muscles are elongated and the scapula does not adduct during the last phase of shoulder flexion, correction of this action is an important part of the program.

Because length-adapted muscles can be strong, increasing the contractile capacity of the muscle is not the focus or an effective intervention. The focus is restoring ideal muscle length, because it is a necessary component of optimal control of the PICR, of optimal kinematics during movement, and thus of preventing or correcting musculoskeletal pain.

Shortened Muscle Caused by Anatomic Adaptation—the Loss of Sarcomeres

Stretching muscles is a common intervention performed by physical therapists because limited joint motion is a factor in musculoskeletal pain problems. Numerous articles have been written describing the best methods of stretching muscles. The muscles used most often in these studies are the hamstrings. Questions of clinical importance that concern muscle shortness include:

1. How much shortness of a muscle is necessary to affect joint and movement behavior?
2. Under what conditions of performance is shortness a factor?
3. What is the anatomic source of the shortness? In other words, is 10 degrees[30] of shortness in the hamstring muscles clinically important? What components of the muscle are producing this limitation?

Most clinicians agree that 45 degrees of shortness in the hamstrings is clinically important. However, changes in muscle length to this extent must involve different anatomic structures than changes from 5 to 10 degrees of a muscle whose effective excursion is 170 degrees. (This calculation is based on the shortest length of the muscle, the knee flexed with the hip extended to the longest length of the muscle, and the knee extended and the hip flexed to 80 degrees.) Certainly most individuals do not need the maximal excursion of the hamstring muscles for their daily or sporting activities; as a result, a deficit of 10 degrees of hamstring muscle excursion is relatively inconsequential.

In contrast, 10 degrees of shortness of the iliopsoas muscle can have an important consequence. Ten degrees of shortness of the iliopsoas muscle prevents hip extension beyond the neutral position. Because hip extension is a required component of normal gait, such a limitation can contribute to a musculoskeletal pain syndrome. The most important issue concerning muscle shortness is not the degree of loss but the percentage of loss of overall muscle excursion and the consequences of such losses on joint behavior during functional activities.

Studies have reported a rapid (i.e., 2- to 4-week time frame) loss of sarcomeres, primarily in series, in muscles immobilized in shortened positions.[60,62,71,72] With the loss of sarcomeres, the active length-tension curve of the shortened muscle shifts to the left of the normal length muscle (see Figure 2-15). When a muscle has shortened to the extent that the total number of sarcomeres in series in a fiber is reduced, physiologic correction requires that the sarcomere number be increased. Furthermore, because muscle cells are the most elastic components of muscle, they are the component most easily affected by stretching.

Performing vigorous passive muscle stretching exercises with the intent of achieving a great improvement in joint range of motion in a short period (e.g., 15 to 20 minutes) can disrupt the alignment of the filaments, actually damaging the muscle. Stretching a markedly shortened muscle should be achieved by prolonged elongation with low loads, with immobilization by casting the joint so that the muscle is maintained in a lengthened position or by using the dynamic splint. The percentage of overall change in muscle length that will result in a loss of sarcomeres has not yet been determined, as opposed to the loss of range of motion associated with changes in muscle length from other alterations in the series or parallel elastic components. Less than 10% to 15% of muscle shortness of its overall excursion is caused by short-time–dependent changes in muscle tissues (e.g., creep properties); thus length increases are achieved relatively rapidly. In contrast, muscle length changes of greater magnitude are caused by more permanent structural changes in muscle and support tissues with an actual loss of sarcomeres and perhaps a "laying down" of shorter collagen fibers. When length adaptations are the result of structural changes, different methods of intervention with a longer time course are required.

In many situations, individuals believe their muscles need stretching, not because their joint range of motion is limited but because the muscle cannot be rapidly passively elongated. The individual describes a "stiff" or "tight" feeling. Usually this tightness is not a function of overall muscle excursion; more likely it is a function of muscle stiffness.

The plasticity or mutability characteristic of muscles—adding or losing sarcomeres—has significant clinical implications. A physiologic stimulus for muscle length adaptation is the amount of passive tension applied to the muscle for a prolonged period. When the tension exceeds a certain level, the number of sarcomeres is increased. When the tension falls below a certain level, the number of sarcomeres is decreased. The adaptation in the number of sarcomeres is necessary to maintain the relationship of the overlap between the actin and myosin filaments (see Figure 2-16). Anatomic and kinesiologic relationships suggest that for most joint segments, antagonistic muscles become elongated when muscles around the joint become shortened.

Traditionally, emphasis is placed on stretching muscles that have shortened, but equal emphasis has not been placed on correcting muscles that have lengthened. The lengthened muscle does not automatically adapt to a shorter length when its antagonist is stretched for brief periods. A therapeutic exercise program that stretches the short muscle, such as the hamstring muscles, does not concurrently shorten the lengthened muscle, such as the lumbar back extensors.

The most effective intervention is to shorten the elongated muscle while simultaneously stretching the shortened muscle. This approach is especially important when the lengthened muscle controls the joint that becomes a site of compensatory motion as a result of the limited motion caused by short muscles. For example, during forward bending of the trunk, lumbar flexion can be a compensatory motion for limited hip flexion when the hamstring muscles are short. The most effective intervention is to address the length changes of all the muscles around a joint, not only the shortened muscle. Therefore if the lumbar spine flexes excessively (greater than 20 degrees), the back extensor muscles should be shortened along with stretching the hamstring muscles.

An effective method for correcting anatomic length adaptation is to contract the lengthened muscle while it is in a shortened position and to simultaneously stretch the shortened muscle. The therapeutic exercises that address both problems of the last example are (1) actively extend the knee while sitting to stretch the hamstring muscles, and concurrently (2) actively contract the back extensor muscles to maintain slight back extension and shorten the back extensor muscles. The hamstring muscles are considered markedly short when they lack 40

degrees of full range-of-active knee extension. A patient with this condition is instructed to sit erect while maintaining a slight contraction of the back extensor muscles with the heel resting on a footstool and the knee extended enough to place a slight but continuous stretch on the hamstrings. This position is maintained for as long as possible, preferably 20 to 30 minutes, and repeated at least six times throughout the day. The goals of these therapeutic exercises are to (1) shorten the elongated back extensor muscles, (2) stretch the shortened hamstring muscles, and (3) prevent compensatory lumbar flexion, which contributes to the lengthening of the back extensors. The presence of compensatory motion can interfere with maintaining the length of the hamstring muscles.

Case Presentation 4

History. A 34-year-old male distance runner who averages 50 to 60 miles per week is referred to physical therapy for treatment of low back pain. He works as a salesman, which requires that he spend most of his day driving to meet various clients. His low back pain has increased during the day, but he does not have pain when running.

Symptoms. The examination indicates a flat lumbar spine in standing. During forward bending, marked lumbar flexion is observed, during which the end range of lumbar flexion is 30 degrees and the end range of hip flexion is 65 degrees. His hamstring muscles are short, supported by the finding that his hips flex only 60 degrees during straight-leg raising. When driving, he sits with his lumbar spine in a flexed position. He drives with his car seat pushed as far back as possible, which requires maximum knee extension. Because of the shortness of his hamstring muscles, his hip flexion is only 65 degrees and thus his lumbar spine is forced into a flexed position.

Muscle Length and Strength. The patient is instructed in a program of hamstring muscle stretching that requires him to sit in a straight-back chair with his hips positioned at 90 degrees and his heel placed on a foot stool that places a slight but continuous stretch on his hamstring muscles. He is asked to maintain this position for as long as possible. He is also instructed to perform isometric back extension by pushing his thoracic spine against the chair back for ten repetitions at least five to six times a day while actively extending his knee. The patient is also instructed to move his car seat forward so that he does not have to maximally extend his knee, allowing him to sit with his hips at a 90-degree angle.

Outcome. His back pain subsides as soon as he avoids the position of lumbar flexion. Over a period of 4 weeks the range of his straight-leg raise improves 10 degrees, and during standing forward bending he no longer demonstrates excessive lumbar flexion. The patient has learned to limit his lumbar motion to the point of reversing the lumbar curve but not allowing his lumbar spine to go into excessive flexion.

Clinical relevance

Several factors must be considered when determining the clinical importance and the management of muscle shortness. The physical therapist must address the following questions:

1. Does the muscle shortness actually affect the range of motion of the joint that is used during functional or sporting activities?
2. Which anatomic structures are involved in the change (i.e., a loss of sarcomeres, the short time-dependent deformation, an elongation of series elastic elements)?
3. Is the patient's pain the result of the effect of a shortened or lengthened muscle?
4. Is it the actual degree of muscle excursion or the rate of excursion that causes the patient to feel a tightness?

Often shortened muscles that limit the excursion of a joint are associated with the development of excessive motion at another joint. Simultaneously restoring the ideal length to the lengthened muscles that cross the joint with excessive motion and the shortened muscles that cross the joint with limited motion are both necessary for the most effective outcome.

Dissociated Length Changes in Synergistic Muscles

Traditionally, synergistic muscles that perform a specific joint motion are thought to undergo similar structural changes in length, but careful testing often indicates that this is not necessarily the case. For example, not all the hip flexors are shortened when there is a limitation of hip extension. Typically, the length of the hamstring muscles is tested as a group by examining the degree of hip flexion during the straight-leg raise.[32] However, the different hip flexors and hamstring muscles contribute to movements other than flexion or extension. Consequently, one of the muscles can become shortened, whereas one of its synergists can retain its normal length or become lengthened. The most common compensatory movement direction is into rotation. In the case of the hip flexors, abduction is also a compensatory movement direction.

When testing hip flexor length, the hip is allowed to abduct or rotate medially at the limit of the excursion into hip extension, which then permits the hip to extend

another 10 degrees, the shortened muscle is the TFL, not the iliopsoas muscle. In fact, specific testing of hip flexor length often indicates that the iliopsoas muscle is lengthened when the TFL is shortened. Similarly, when testing the length of the hamstring muscles, if care is taken to prevent hip medial rotation while in the sitting position (the hip joint is flexed to 80 degrees), the terminal knee position is 15 degrees of flexion. If the hip is allowed to rotate medially and the knee flexion decreases, it is an indication that the medial hamstring muscles, not the lateral hamstring muscles, are shortened (Figure 2-18). Table 2-1 illustrates examples of common length imbalances in synergistic muscles.

The difference in the length of two synergistic muscles is a contributing factor to compensatory motion and the development of movement impairment syndromes. Most often the compensatory motion is into rotation. Care in assessing the muscle length, examining the postural alignment, and observing the specific motion of the joints controlled by the muscle are necessary to identify the dissociated length change impairments of synergistic muscles.

Muscle and Soft-Tissue Stiffness

Stiffness, which is defined as the change in tension per unit of change in length,[59] is discussed because this characteristic of muscle and other soft tissues is believed to be a major contributor to movement patterns and movement impairment syndromes. When passive motion of a joint is assessed, all the tissues crossing the joint contribute to the resistance, which can be referred to as joint

Table 2-1   Length Imbalances in Synergistic Muscles

MUSCLE MOVEMENT	SHORT MUSCLE	LONG MUSCLE
Scapular elevators and adductors	Levator scapulae	Upper trapezius
Scapular adductors	Rhomboids	Lower trapezius
Glenohumeral medial rotators	Pectoralis major	Subscapularis
Trunk flexors that tilt the pelvis in a posterior direction	Rectus abdominis	External oblique abdominal
Hip flexors	TFL	Iliopsoas
Hip abductors	TFL	Posterior gluteus medius
Hip extensors and knee flexors	Medial hamstrings	Lateral hamstrings
Ankle dorsiflexors	Extensor digitorum longus	Tibialis anterior

TFL, Tensor fascia lata.

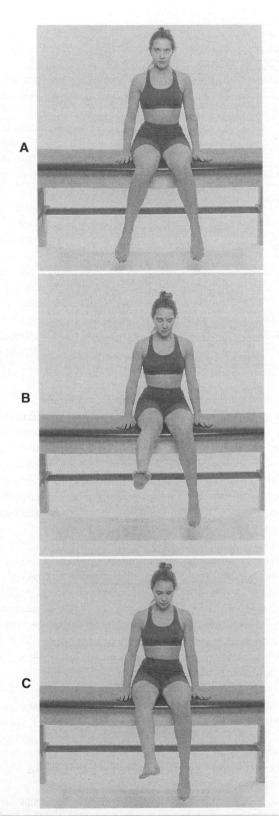

Figure 2-18

A, Sitting position with a resting alignment of hip medial rotation.
B, During knee extension, the degree of hip medial rotation increases.
C, Laterally rotated hip and decreased knee extension.

stiffness. When the range of motion of a joint is limited, it is also described as stiff. In this text, limited range of motion is not considered as a problem of stiffness.

Another concept of stiffness is the tension developed by a combination of active contraction and passive resistance. A variety of studies[6,8,22,69] have examined stiffness under both passive and active conditions. Under active conditions, stiffness refers to the total tension developed when muscles are stretched when actively contracting. For the purposes of this text, stiffness refers to the resistance present during the passive elongation of muscle and connective tissue, not during active muscle contraction or at the end of the range of motion. Stiffness, as discussed in this text, is primarily attributed to muscle, because the assessment is made during examinations of muscle length.

Stiffness is a characteristic of muscles, and muscles have been described as having properties that are similar to springs.[6,11,69] Thus the resistance that is felt when a muscle is passively elongated can be considered analogous to the resistance associated with elongating a spring (Figure 2-19). Components of muscle, which have been identified as contributing to the resistance to stretching, are the extracellular and intracellular series elastic structures. The current information suggests that the primary contributor to intracellular resistance to passive stretching is titin, a large connective tissue protein[34,68] (Figure 2-20). To a lesser extent, the weak binding of the cross bridges of the myosin filaments contribute to intracellular resistance.[54] There are six titin proteins for each myosin filament. Therefore increasing the number of myosin filaments affects the stiffness of the muscle because of the concomitant increase in the number of titin proteins.

Another contribution to muscle stiffness is *thixotropy,* which is the property of a substance that, when static for a period of time, becomes stiff and resists flow. It is defined as the property of various gels that become fluid when disturbed (i.e., by shaking).[42] Thixotropy is attributed to weak binding of the cross bridges, and it is considered a source of resistance to passive stretching but a minor contributor to the total passive resistance.

Hypertrophy is known to increase the number of contractile proteins and connective tissue proteins.[4] The increase in these proteins suggests a concurrent increase in the stiffness of the muscle because of both increased connective tissue proteins, such as titin, and increased contractile elements. Chleboun and colleagues have shown that the cross-sectional area of muscle is correlated with the stiffness of the muscle through the range as it is elongated, rather than at the end of its range.[9] Conversely, atrophy or loss of con-

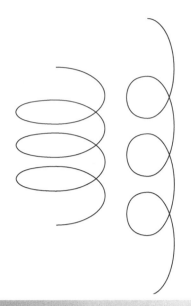

Figure 2-19

Springs illustrating differing levels of stiffness, as would be seen in muscles.

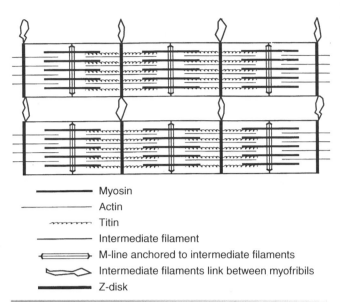

Myosin

Actin

Titin

Intermediate filament

M-line anchored to intermediate filaments

Intermediate filaments link between myofribils

Z-disk

Figure 2-20

Picture from skeletal muscle APTA. (From Friden J, Lieber RL: The structural and mechanical basis of exercise-induced muscle injury, *Med Sci Sports Exerc* 24:521, 1992.)

tractile elements decreases the through-the-range stiffness because of the reduction in both connective tissue proteins and the number of cross bridges.

Variation in the stiffness of muscles and joints can be a factor in the development of compensatory motion in contiguous joints and can contribute to musculoskeletal pain syndromes. For example, in the sitting position when the hamstring muscles are placed on stretch, the lumbar spine will flex to a greater range than when the hamstring muscles are not stretched as much. During forward bending this increased lumbar flexion range is not evident. The rate of forward bending is not examined in this study.[66] Thomas demonstrates that during the forward reach test, typically men will bend their lumbar spine, whereas women will flex their hips during the initial phase.[63] Men generally have shorter and stiffer hamstring muscles than women. This fact is consistent with the hypothesis that flexible tissues stretch more readily than less flexible tissues. The passive stiffness of the hamstring muscles is found to be significantly greater in the patient with low back pain than in control subjects.[61] The length of the hamstring muscles is not found to be significantly different between the two groups. These investigators did not suggest a possible explanation for this finding.

This text hypothesizes that motion occurs earlier at the joint with the lesser degree of stiffness, in this case the lumbar spine, rather than at the stiffer joint, which in this case is the hip joint. This does not mean that the range of lumbar spine motion is greater when the ham-

string muscles are taut. It suggests that motion will occur earlier at the more flexible segment in situations where motion involves both joints. During forward bending, the demands for maximum motion will cause the joint to move through its full range of motion. A possible long-term consequence, if this movement pattern is continually repeated, is that the flexibility of the lumbar spine will increase, predisposing the spine to move into flexion whenever flexion should be occurring at the hip joint.

When joints with common movement directions are in series and one of the joints is more flexible than the others, the flexible joint is particularly susceptible to movement. When movement occurs at this joint when it should remain stable, it is called *compensatory relative flexibility*, a phenomenon that is discussed later. This concept is best understood if the multiple segments of the human body are believed to be controlled by a series of springs. The muscles of the body are similar to a series of springs of differing extensibility, and the intersegmental differences in the extensibility of these springs contribute to compensatory motions, particularly of the spine.

Compensatory Relative Flexibility

CLINICAL OBSERVATIONS. Hypertrophy increases the stiffness of muscles through the range of motion.[9] Because of the intersegmental variations in the springlike behavior of muscles, a reasonable hypothesis is that increased stiffness of one muscle group can cause compensatory movement at an adjoining joint that is controlled by muscles or joints with less stiffness. A common clinical observation is that when passively testing the length of a muscle, movement of a contiguous joint occurs long before the muscle is fully elongated. The movement of the contiguous joint is a compensatory motion. For example, if the lumbar spine is particularly flexible in the extension direction and the latissimus dorsi muscle is relatively stiffer, the lumbar spine will extend when the patient performs shoulder flexion, even before reaching the end of the length of the latissimus dorsi muscle.

Under optimal conditions when the therapist passively flexes the knee with the patient lying prone, which stretches the rectus femoris muscle, there should not be movement of the pelvis and spine except possibly near the end of the knee flexion range of 115 to 125 degrees. If movement of the pelvis and spine occurs between 45 and 115 degrees of knee flexion, it may be that segments of the spine are more flexible than the rectus femoris muscle is extensible. As discussed later, this phenomenon does not necessarily mean that the rectus femoris muscle is short; but it implies that it is stiffer than the support provided to the pelvis and spine and therefore the stiffness produces lumbar extension.

When a patient performs active knee flexion, there are automatic stabilizing responses that can affect the movement of the pelvis and spine. For example, during active knee flexion in the prone position, the contraction of the hamstring muscles will tilt the pelvis posteriorly. However, to stabilize and limit the movement of the pelvis, the hip flexors and back extensor muscles should contract. This stabilizing action of the muscles can either be excessive or insufficient. (Alterations of this stabilization pattern are discussed under the section on motor control impairments.) The examples given in Figure 2-21 demonstrate different combinations of muscle stiffness and length impairments and their role in compensatory movements of the pelvis and spine.

The pelvis and lumbar spine are in the same correct alignment in the starting position. During either active and passive knee flexions, the following observations can be made:

1. *Normal length of the rectus femoris muscle.* The knee is flexed without lumbopelvic movement.
2. *Short rectus femoris.* Without lumbopelvic compensation, the knee is flexed without movement of the pelvis or lumbar spine, but knee flexion stops at 90 degrees, indicating short quadriceps muscles.
3. *Stiff and short rectus femoris muscle with lumbopelvic compensation.* The knee is flexed and the pelvis tilts anteriorly. The lumbar extension increases at 60 degrees of knee flexion, but the knee flexes to 135 degrees. When the therapist sta-

bilizes the pelvis, the knee flexion stops at 90 degrees.
4. *Stiffness, not shortness, of rectus femoris muscle with lumbopelvic compensation.* The knee is flexed and the pelvis is tilted anteriorly. The lumbar extension increases at 60 degrees of knee flexion, but the knee is flexed to 135 degrees. When the therapist stabilizes the pelvis, the knee still flexes to 135 degrees.
5. *Stiffness of rectus femoris muscle with automatic lumbopelvic stabilization.* During passive motion, but not active knee flexion, the compensatory lumbar extension motion is observed.
6. *Deficient lumbopelvic counter stabilization.* At the initiation of knee flexion, the pelvis is tilted posteriorly and the lumbar spine slightly reduces its curve.

Explanation of Figure 2-21

1. *Optimal balance of muscle stiffness and joint stability.* The rectus femoris muscle is stretched without compensatory lumbopelvic motion. Therefore the stiffness of the anterior supporting structures of the spine and the passive stiffness of the abdominal muscles are greater than or equal to the stiffness of the rectus femoris muscle.
2. *Shortness of rectus femoris muscle with counterbalancing stiffness of spinal structures and abdominal muscles.* Because the knee flexes to only 90 degrees, the rectus femoris muscle is short and the muscle excursion does not reach the expected standard. However, lumbopelvic compensatory motion is not evident even though the rectus femoris muscle is short. It is not stiffer than the anterior supporting structures of the lumbar spine and the passive extensibility of the abdominal muscles.
3. *Shortness of rectus femoris muscle with compensatory lumbopelvic motion* (Position 3A). With knee flexion, compensatory anterior pelvic tilt and lumbar extension occurs, even before the muscle reaches the limit of its excursion. The pelvic tilt increases as the knee flexion range increases (Position 3B). When the pelvis is stabilized, which prevents anterior pelvic tilt, the knee flexion is limited to 90 degrees (Position 3C). In contrast to the situation in Position 2, the shortness of the rectus femoris muscle is associated with compensatory anterior pelvic tilt. Thus not only is the rectus femoris shortened, but its stiffness is also greater than the stiffness of the anterior supporting structures of the lumbar spine and the abdominal muscles. An important implication is that when the rec-

tus femoris muscle is stretched to improve its overall length, the through-the-range stiffness remains. Therefore knee flexion elicits anterior pelvic tilt as long as the rectus femoris muscle is relatively stiffer than the structures preventing the anterior pelvic tilt or the lumbar extension. This phenomenon occurs even though the rectus femoris muscle is able to fully elongate. Correcting the faulty, compensatory pattern requires increasing the stiffness of the abdominal muscles and anterior supporting structures of the spine, in addition to stretching the rectus femoris muscle. It is possible that the compensatory motion occurs only when the rectus femoris muscle reaches the end of its excursion. At this point the resistance is particularly high and thus causes the compensatory motion of the pelvis. In this condition, increasing the length of the rectus femoris muscle eliminates the motion of the pelvis. This condition is not common.

4. *Compensatory motion without muscle shortness.* The knee flexes to 135 degrees (Position 4), but early in the range there is an associated anterior pelvic tilt and lumbar extension. When the pelvis is stabilized, the knee still flexes to 135 degrees. Clearly the compensatory motion is not associated with a short muscle. The most reasonable explanation is that the anterior supporting structures of the spine and the abdominal muscles are not as stiff as the rectus femoris muscle that has normal length. The relative degree of through-the-range stiffness of the rectus femoris versus the anterior trunk muscles and the anterior supporting structures of the spine is the key factor in determining the movement pattern and in creating the compensatory motion. The compensatory motion occurred long before the muscle reached the end of its range. Correction requires increasing the stiffness of the anterior trunk muscles.

5. *Compensatory motion with passive flexion controlled by active muscle contraction.* When the knee is passively flexed, the stiffness of the rectus femoris muscle is greater than the stiffness of the anterior supporting structures of the spine and the abdominal muscles, which causes compensatory anterior pelvic tilt and lumbar extension (Position 5A). When the hamstring muscles actively contract to flex the knee, the compensatory motion is eliminated (Position 5B). Possible explanations are that the posterior pelvic tilt elicited by hamstring contraction is sufficient to counteract the stiffness of the rectus femoris. Another explanation is that the abdominal muscles contract enough to counterbalance the anterior pelvic tilt and lumbar extension.

6. *Exaggerated posterior pelvic tilt.* In the normal joint stabilization pattern, the muscles that counteract the effect on joints (which are to remain stable) contract before the prime mover (Position 6). If they fail to do so or do not generate enough tension, the pelvis will posteriorly tilt. (Impairments in this control are discussed in the section on modulator elements.)

Clinical relevance

In the first five responses during knee flexion in the prone position, the pattern of motion can be explained best by the concept of the relative flexibility of structures, particularly when the knee flexion is performed passively by the examiner. This is true whether the pattern of motion is limited to one segment or associated with compensatory motions at other segments. The important implication is that correction of impaired movement patterns requires increasing the stiffness of the segments that demonstrates compensatory motion. The problem is not the lack of length of the muscle being stretched by the desired motion; rather, the problem is the relative stiffness of the muscle being stretched as compared with the stiffness of the muscles or supporting tissues at the site of the compensatory motion.

Teaching patients to perform the motion correctly in the test position is an effective way to reverse this compensatory pattern. The important issue is whether the subject can contract the abdominal muscles to prevent the compensatory motion. Exercise in the test position, such as knee flexion in the prone position while contracting the abdominal muscles, ensures that the motion is restricted to the segment that is supposed to move. The prescribed abdominal exercises require performance at the length necessary to prevent the compensatory motion. An abdominal muscle exercise program, such as the trunk curl sit-up or lower abdominal exercises (see Chapter 7), does not address the more critical factor, which is controlling the pelvis to prevent the compensatory motion.

An issue that has not been thoroughly studied is whether strengthening a muscle under one set of conditions automatically implies that its participation will generalize to other activities performed in different positions. This text proposes that training is relatively specific, and improving the contractile ability of a muscle does not ensure that its participation will become generalized to other activities. Therefore the desired muscle action should be practiced under the specific conditions in which it is to be used. When joints are arranged in series and they are the sites of compensatory movement, effective treatment requires simultaneous control of all the affected segments.

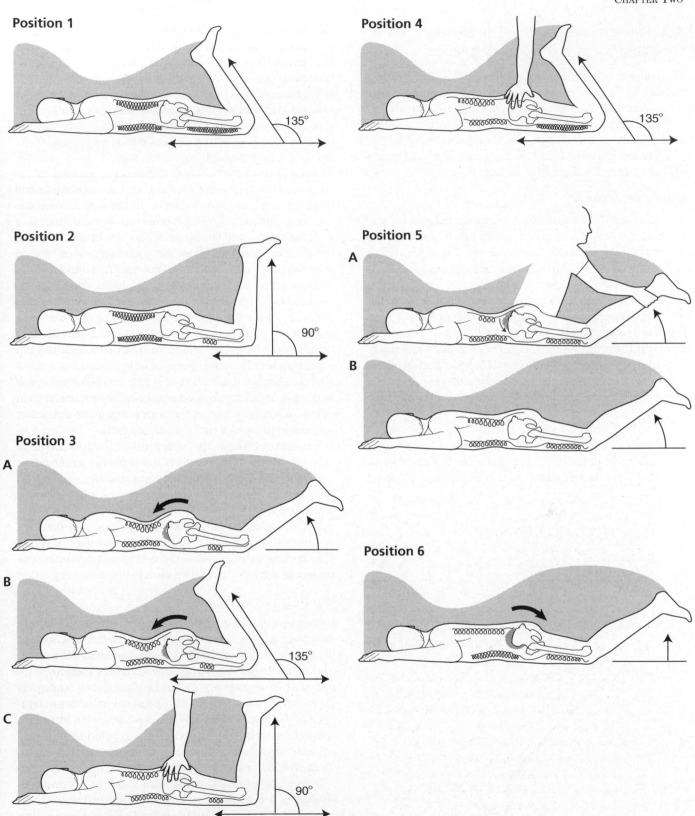

Position 1

135°

Position 2

90°

Position 3

A

B

135°

C

90°

Position 4

135°

Position 5

A

B

Position 6

Figure 2-21

Variations in lumbopelvic motion during knee flexion associated with differences in the stiffness of the abdominal and rectus femoris muscles. In the starting position of hip and knee extension, the pelvis and lumbar spine are in the same correct alignment as in position 1.

Base Element Impairments of the Skeletal System: Structural Variations in Joint Alignment

The following joint and bony structural variations contribute to musculoskeletal pain syndromes (Figure 2-22). Although the details of these variations and their relationships to pain are discussed in greater detail in later chapters, these faults are mentioned here to emphasize the importance of considering all components and their interrelationships in pain syndromes.

Hip Antetorsion

In this congenital condition the angle of the head and neck of the femur is rotated anteriorly, beyond that of the normal torsion with respect to the shaft. The result is a range of medial hip rotation that appears to be excessive, whereas the lateral rotation range appears to be limited. A study by Gelberman and associates shows that when the asymmetry between medial and lateral rotation is present, whether the hip is flexed or extended, structural antetorsion of the hip is present.[19] The hip is considered in antetorsion when the head and neck rotate more than 15 degrees anteriorly, with respect to the plane of the femoral condyles.

Case Presentation

History. A 22-year-old college student with radiologic evidence of arthritic changes in the lower two segments of the thoracic spine area is referred to physical

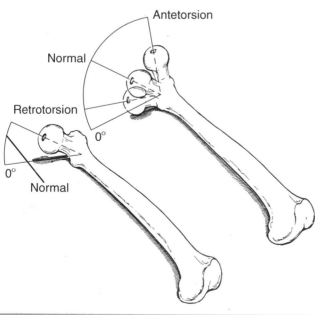

Figure 2-22

A representation of retrotorsion and antetorsion of the femoral neck. (From Malone TR, McPoil TG, Nitz AJ: *Orthopedic and sports physical therapy*, 3e, St Louis, 1997, Mosby.)

therapy for treatment of bilateral hip and low back pain. The severity of the pain in the hips and back has caused the patient to change colleges to reduce the walking distances to classes. Before experiencing the pain the patient was running 3 to 4 miles per day as part of a weight-control and fitness program. The patient complains of difficulty sleeping at night because of the pain. During examination the patient reports that the hip pain is decreased when the hips are flexed and medially rotated. The Craig test indicates that the neutral position of the hip joint is 35 degrees of medial rotation on the right and 35 degrees of medial rotation on the left, indicating she has a significant degree of hip antetorsion bilaterally.

Symptoms and Diagnosis. With correct alignment of the femurs in the hip joints, the alignment of her feet is pigeon-toed to an unacceptable extent. Therefore she walks with her feet pointed straight ahead, which causes her hips to be beyond the limit of their range into lateral rotation. Consequently, when she walks she has compensatory rotation in her spine because of the lack of lateral rotation in her hips. During normal gait the hip rotates laterally from shortly after stance phase to slightly after toe off.[29] When this rotation does not occur in the hip, it occurs as a compensatory rotation motion of the pelvis and then at the articulations of the spine. Running with her feet straight ahead further exaggerates this condition. The faulty alignment of the femoral head in the acetabulum is irritating the hip joint structures.

Outcome. Management requires the patient to greatly limit her weight bearing activity for 3 weeks and learn to walk with her feet in a partially pigeon-toed position, allowing the femoral head position to improve and the lateral rotation range to be available during gait. This management eliminates the hip and back pain. The patient is advised to avoid running.

Hip Retrotorsion

In this congenital condition, which is more common in men than in women, the angle of the head and neck of the femur rotates posteriorly with respect to the shaft. The result is that the range of medial rotation appears limited, but the lateral rotation range appears excessive. Hip retrotorsion can also be a cause of musculoskeletal pain of the hip and back. When a patient with hip retrotorsion forces the hip into a sustained position of medial rotation, the hip becomes painful because of faulty alignment. When a woman with a retroverted hip crosses her legs (thigh over thigh) while sitting, the result is excessive medial rotation, causing irritation of the anterior joint capsular tissues and hip pain. The excessive stretch of the hip lateral rotators from sitting with her legs crossed or sleeping on her side with the hip adducted and medially rotated further contributes to the faulty alignment and control of the hip joint.

With bilateral hip retrotorsion, the lack of hip medial rotation causes the lumbar spine to become the site of compensatory motion, particularly when work or recreational activities (e.g., golf) require rotational motions. Because it is socially acceptable for men to sit with their legs crossed by resting their ankle on the opposite thigh (hip abduction and lateral rotation), those with hip retrotorsion do not tend to develop hip pain problems. Further, the narrower pelvis of a man when lying on his side does not contribute to excessive hip adduction and medial rotation. Therefore when both sitting and sleeping in the side-lying position, men with hip retrotorsion are not at risk of assuming a faulty alignment of the hip as much as are women.

There are many other structural variations that contribute to musculoskeletal pain syndromes, the details of which are discussed in the chapter on lower extremity syndromes. Examples are (1) genu varum and valgum; (2) tibial torsion and tibial varum (sagittal and frontal planes); (3) supinated rigid foot; (4) short trunk and long extremities; (5) long trunk and short extremities; (6) small narrow upper body and large, wide lower body; and (7) wide shoulders.

Modular Element Impairments of the Nervous System

Impairments of the modulator element are extremely important. Unfortunately, the role of the nervous system as a contributing factor in musculoskeletal pain syndromes has not been addressed or even considered until recently. As therapists and other clinicians observe, many individuals with strong muscles develop pain syndromes. These syndromes need to be addressed through teaching the patient to control subtle movements by conscious effort rather than by increasing muscle bulk. The study by Hodges and Richardson shows that the recruitment of the transversus abdominis muscle is delayed in the patient with back pain, an example of a patient with a motor control problem.[26] Hides and colleagues have also shown that in the patient with low back pain, the multifidus muscle does not recover its bulk without a specific program of training.[24] This patient also has a motor control problem. The lack of extensive discussion reflects the limited information available, not the importance of this factor in movement impairment syndromes.

Altered Recruitment Patterns

Babyar reports that the patient with shoulder pain has excessive shoulder elevation during shoulder flexion to 90 degrees as compared with subjects without shoulder pain.[3] This excessive elevation is present even after the patient no longer experiences pain during this phase of the movement. Further, with verbal instructions the patient is able to correct his or her pattern of shoulder motion. The results of this study indicate that once a faulty movement pattern is established, the patient requires specific training to reestablish a more normal pattern.

Alterations in muscular strategies are also found during gait. A recent study by Mueller and associates shows that the patient with diabetes who has limited range of dorsiflexion and decreased power of push off uses a hip strategy for walking.[44] When a patient has weakness of the ankle plantar flexors muscles, the momentum generated by push off for the swing phase cannot be used; instead, the hip flexion phase tends to be exaggerated.

These variations of hip flexion versus ankle push-off strategies are seen in runners. Observations of runners who tend to keep their weight line posterior—closer to the rear than to the front of the foot—show they use the hip flexor strategy, which also involves an excessive use of the tibialis anterior muscle, leading to shin splints (Figure 2-23). In contrast, runners who keep their weight line forward can be observed to use more push off with their ankle plantar flexor muscles (Figure 2-24).

Altered Dominance in Recruitment Patterns of Synergistic Muscles

Alterations in the optimal recruitment of synergistic muscles can cause the action of a synergist to become more dominant than the action of other participating muscles. Alterations that can be clinically observed include consistent recruitment of either one muscle of a force-couple or of counterbalancing synergists. The result is a movement that is in the direction of the dominant synergist.

Dominance of the Upper Trapezius Muscle

The upper trapezius muscle, which is the upper component of the force-couple that controls the scapula, can be more dominant than the lower trapezius muscle. The trapezius muscle adducts and upwardly rotates the scapula, but the upper portion of the muscle elevates the shoulder while the lower portion depresses it. Excessive elevation of the shoulder, as reported in the study by Babyar,[3] is attributed to the dominance of the upper trapezius and a failure of the lower trapezius to counterbalance this action. As suggested by Babyar,[3] verbal directions that change the pattern are the most effective intervention.

The pattern of excessive elevation appears to be one that has become "learned" rather than an issue of muscle strength. Testing may indicate weakness of the lower trapezius muscle. However, treatment is not ade-

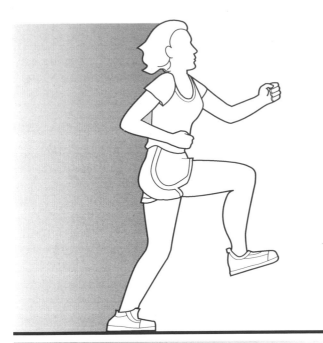

Figure 2-23

Runner pulling center of gravity, which contributes to excessive use of ankle dorsiflexion muscle.

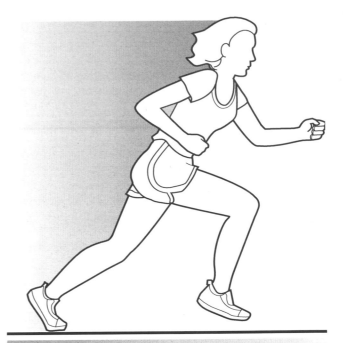

Figure 2-24

Runner chasing center of gravity allows ankle to plantarflex, thus alleviating the tonic activity of the dorsiflexion muscle.

quate when the patient is instructed with lower trapezius exercises alone. Instructing the patient in the correct performance of shoulder motion is essential, using a mirror to monitor the pattern of movement. Muscle recruitment and muscle contractile capacity are probably correlated, but strengthening will not necessarily change the pattern of recruitment. There is a greater likelihood that changing the pattern of recruitment will change the contractile capacity of the muscle and strength will be regained through correct usage.

Dominance of Hamstring Muscles Over Abdominal Muscles

The abdominal muscles and the hip extensor muscles have synergistic actions as a force-couple that tilts the pelvis posteriorly. When working properly the anterior abdominal muscles pull upward on the anterior pelvis, and the hamstring muscles pull downward on the ischial tuberosity of the pelvis, thus acting as a force-couple that tilts the pelvis posteriorly (Figure 2-25). The optimal relative contribution of these two synergists has not been described in the literature, but clinical observation suggests that there is considerable variation.

In the presence of weak abdominal muscles, the hamstring muscles are expected to exert the dominant effect on posterior pelvic tilt. Once this pattern is established, the hamstring action is constantly reinforced while the abdominal muscle action is reduced. The imbalance in action contributes to an imbalance in strength, with the hamstring muscles testing strong and the abdominal muscles testing weak.

Straight-leg raising in the supine position requires the synergy of the abdominal and the contralateral hip extensor muscles to counteract the pelvic anterior tilting action of the hip flexor muscles. Clinical observations suggest that the individual with weak abdominal muscles uses the contralateral hip extensor muscles to stabilize the pelvis during the straight-leg raise to a greater extent than the individual who has strong abdominal muscles.

To assess the interaction of the hamstring and abdominal muscles, electromyographic (EMG) activity was recorded during active straight-leg raising (hip flexion with knee extension) in the supine position. The study showed that the relative participation of these two synergists can vary, depending on the subject. If the patient's preferred pattern was hamstring muscular activity and if he or she was instructed to reduce the amount of right hip extension during left straight-leg raising, the abdominal muscle activity increased significantly.[40] The results of this study confirm what is inferred from the anatomy—a decrease in activity of one muscle of a force-couple is accompanied by an increase in the activity of the other. This type of habitual alteration in the reciprocal participation contributes to

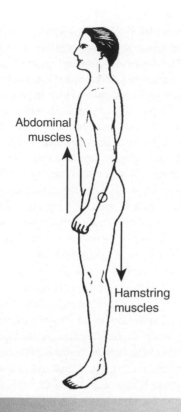

Figure 2-25

Counterbalancing force-couples of the trunk and hip girdles muscles. The abdominal muscles pull upward on the anterior pelvis, and the hamstring muscles pull downward on the ischial tuberosity of the pelvis, acting as a force-couple to rotate the pelvis posteriorly and flatten the lumbar spine. The back extensor muscles pull upward on the pelvis and the hip flexor muscles pull downward on the pelvis, acting as a force-couple to rotate the pelvis anteriorly and extend the lumbar spine. (From Soderberg G: *Kinesiology,* Philadelphia, 1986, Williams & Wilkins.)

muscle imbalances by reinforcing the demands on the stronger muscle and minimizing the demands on the weaker muscle.

Dominance of Hamstring Muscles Over Gluteus Maximus Muscle

The pattern of excessive dominance of one of the synergists of a muscular force-couple can lead to an impairment of the dominant muscle, such as an overuse syndrome. For example, the individual with an exaggerated swayback posture who stands in hip joint extension has diminished contour of the gluteal muscles, suggesting poor development of this muscle group. The swayback position of the upper back with the sway-forward position of the pelvis, combined with posterior pelvic tilt and hip joint extension, causes the line of gravity to fall markedly posterior to the hip joints. This type of posture minimizes the role of the hip extensors in maintaining the upright position of the trunk and is used by a patient with paraparesis when walking. This patient lacks hip ex-

tensor musculature but is able to maintain an upright position with the use of lower extremity braces and the swayback posture. Using gravity to create a hip extension movement will also cause the hip extensors to atrophy, particularly the gluteal muscles.

When an individual with a swayback posture performs hip extension in the prone position, the timing and magnitude of muscle participation, as inferred by changes in the muscle contour, suggest that the hamstring muscles are active before the gluteus maximus muscle. Performing a manual muscle test on the gluteus maximus muscle usually confirms that the muscle is weak. This pattern is the reverse of that observed in the individual with a lordotic posture. This observation suggests that the timing of recruitment can vary between synergists and that it can be reflected in a decrease in the strength of the less dominant muscle.

The variability in EMG onset of activity of the hip extensor muscles during hip extension performed in the prone position has been reported.[53] In the Pierce study the onset of gluteus maximus muscular activity follows the activity of the hamstrings by 2 seconds in one patient (Figure 2-26). The investigators did not relate the pattern of recruitment to the patient's posture or to the muscle size. A reasonable hypothesis is that when one muscle of a synergistic pair is the prime mover and is generating the greatest amount of tension for a specific action, the muscle will be susceptible to an overuse syndrome, such as hamstring muscle strain or iliotibial band fasciitis.

The hamstring muscles, acting as hip extensors and knee flexors, are particularly active during sports that involve running. The hamstring muscles are extremely susceptible to an overuse syndrome when they are dominant because of inadequate participation of the abdominal, gluteus maximus, or even rectus femoris muscles, as well as the lateral rotators of the hip. Therefore when assessing the factors that contribute to an overuse syndrome, one of the rules is to determine whether one or more of the synergists of the strained muscle are also weak. When the synergist is weak, the muscle strain is probably the result of excessive demands. The nondominant synergist should be tested for weakness, and the movement pattern should be carefully observed. Positive findings for weakness are consistent with inadequate participation of the nondominant synergist.

Other Examples of Altered Dominance in Synergistic Muscles

The altered recruitment patterns of specific muscles are similar to the altered muscle dominance patterns described in the previous section that discussed base element impairments. Altered recruitment patterns con-

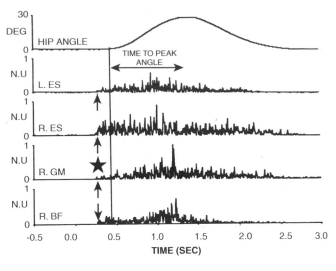

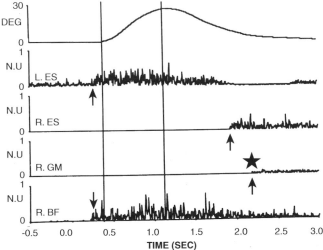

Figure 2-26

Variability at timing of hip extensor EMG activity during hip extension in the prone position. In some individuals the onset of the EMG of the gluteus maximus (GM) is much later than the onset of the EMG of the hamstring muscles (BF). (From Pierce MN, Lee WY: Muscle firing order during active prone hip extension, *JOSPT* 12:2, 1990.)

tribute to changes in muscle dominance in length and strength. This situation is analogous to the "chicken and egg" dilemma of which came first. Although there is no answer to the question, changes in recruitment pattern, muscle length, and muscle strength are relatively concurrent. The most effective remediation requires addressing all three impairments. The following are additional examples of muscles that demonstrate altered recruitment patterns:

1. The TFL and rectus femoris muscles are more dominant than the iliopsoas muscle in the action of hip flexion. In this situation the patient usually demonstrates excessive hip medial rotation. The patient usually has a swayback posture with a lengthened iliopsoas muscle and a shortened TFL muscle during single-leg stance.

2. The TFL, anterior gluteus medius, and gluteus minimus muscles are more dominant than the posterior gluteus medius muscle in the action of hip abduction. During manual muscle testing of the posterior gluteus medius, the patient substitutes by medial rotation and flexion of the hip.

3. The hamstring muscles are more dominant than the quadriceps muscles for the action of knee extension. In walking or running, once the foot is fixed by contact with the ground, the hip extension action of the hamstring muscles contributes to extension of the knee. Hip extension to assist in knee extension is commonly used by the patient who has weakness of the quadriceps muscles as a result of poliomyelitis. To reinforce the knee extension action, the patient often flexes the trunk slightly to use gravity to further contribute to the knee extension movement. A similar movement pattern is seen in the runner who uses the hamstring muscles for knee extension control. He or she demonstrates a pattern of bringing the knee backward to the body rather than bringing the body up to the knee as when climbing stairs (Figure 2-27) or when standing from a sitting position (Figure 2-28).

4. The extensor digitorum longus muscle is more dominant than the anterior tibialis muscle for the action of ankle dorsiflexion. During active dorsiflexion the patient demonstrates extension of the toes as the initial movement instead of ankle motion.

5. The rectus abdominis muscles are more dominant than the external oblique abdominal muscles for the action of posterior pelvic tilt. This situation is often accompanied by a depression of the chest. When this patient performs exercises for the lower abdominal (external oblique) muscles, he or she will have difficulty contracting the oblique muscles as indicated by palpation and will instead readily contract the rectus abdominis muscle with an associated slight trunk flexion or a depression of the chest.

6. The pectoralis major muscle is more dominant than the subscapularis muscle for the action of humeral medial rotation. In this movement pattern the range of humeral medial rotation from 50 to 70 degrees is often limited. When testing the medial rotation range of motion, palpation and observation of the head of the humerus indicates that it glides anteriorly. The excessive flexibility of the humeral head into anterior glide is further exaggerated by the contraction of the pectoralis

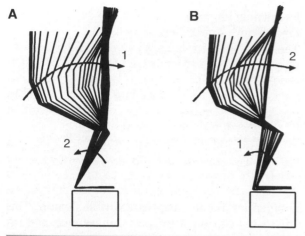

Figure 2-27

Two strategies for controlling the relationship of the trunk and knee during stepping up a step. *A,* Subject steps up by bringing the trunk toward the leg, which maintains a relatively stationary position as the body moves toward a vertical position over the foot. *B,* Subject steps by bringing the leg back toward his trunk as the body moves toward a vertical position over the foot. (Courtesy of Amy Bastian, PhD, PT.)

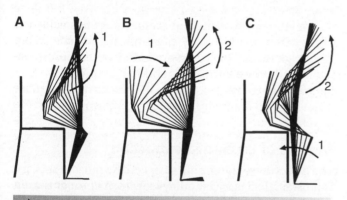

Figure 2-28

Sit to stand using three different strategies. *A,* The subject starts by sitting on the edge of the chair and then directly comes to a vertical position. *B,* The subject is sitting back in the chair and starts the motion by leaning forward, flexing the hips and then extending the back and hips to come to an erect position. *C,* The subject is sitting on the edge of the chair but brings the knees back toward the chair (toward the body) and then comes to the erect position with the knees partially extended. (Courtesy of Amy Bastian, PhD, PT.)

major. In contrast, when the subscapularis is the prime mover, its action contributes to posterior glide, not anterior glide, of the humeral head. The best test of the performance of the subscapularis is performed in the prone position with the shoulder abducted and in 70 degrees of medial rotation. To perform this test, the range of motion must be available. When the range of 60 to 70 degrees of humeral medial rotation is available and a manual muscle test of medial rotation is performed in the prone position, the muscles will test weak.

This result is attributable to excessive length or weakness of the subscapularis muscle. If the subscapularis is not participating optimally, the pectoralis major is often dominant.

Clinical relevance

The availability of multiple muscular strategies to create a specific joint moment has many advantages. The variety of strategies available enables the individual to respond to the demands of different activities to ensure that the loss of one muscle does not eliminate the control of the joint. However, the efficiency of recruitment patterns suggests that most often a preferred pattern is established. Therefore the patient has to be retrained during functional performance. The treatment program cannot be limited to strengthening exercises for the strained muscle. Instead, the patient is taught to reduce the amount of participation of the injured muscle in the action and increase the degree of participation of its synergists.

Recruitment and Relative Flexibility

The role of muscle stiffness as a contributing factor to compensatory movements is described in the preceding section on base element impairments. When muscle stiffness is the primary factor, the compensatory motion occurs when the muscle is passively stretched. However, when the compensatory motion occurs during the active contraction but not with the passive stretch of a muscle, the problem is primarily one of motor control.

Exaggerated Anterior Pelvic Tilt with Lumbar Extension During Active Knee Flexion

The most likely contributing factors are (1) excessive flexibility of the movement of the lumbar spine into the direction of extension, and (2) contraction of the hip flexor or paraspinal muscles to prevent posterior tilting associated with hamstring muscle contraction (Figure 2-29). However, because of the excessive flexibility of the lumbar spine, the contraction of the stabilizing muscles causes rather than prevents motion. A reinforcing cycle of activity is established, which continues to contribute to the excessive flexibility of the lumbar spine into the direction of extension. The patient must learn to minimize the magnitude of the stabilizing activity of the muscle to allow the lumbar spine to increase its stiffness.

Exaggerated Posterior Pelvic Tilt During Active Knee Flexion

In the normal joint stabilization pattern, muscles contract before the prime mover to counteract the effect on the joints of the action of the prime mover (Figure 2-30). To prevent posterior pelvic tilt, for example, the back extensor or hip flexor muscles should slightly contract

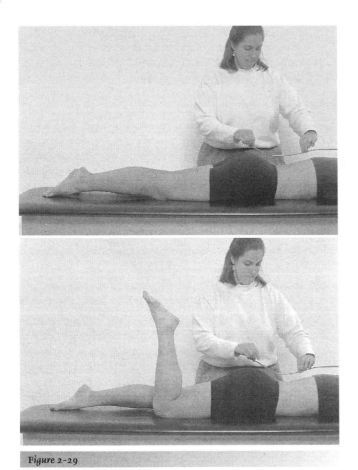

Figure 2-29

Exaggerated anterior pelvic tilt with lumbar extension during active knee flexion. Anterior pelvic tilt is caused by activity of the back extensor and hip flexor muscles plus excessive lumbar extension mobility.

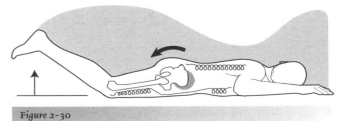

Figure 2-30

Exaggerated posterior pelvic tilt during active knee flexion. Contraction of the hamstring muscles to flex the knee posteriorly tilts the pelvis, which is not counteracted by back extensor and hip flexor activity.

before the hamstring muscles flex the knee. When the counterbalancing activity is delayed or when insufficient contraction prevents the movement of the segment to which the proximal end of the muscle is attached, there is inappropriate motion.

In the case of knee flexion performed in the prone position, the pelvis tilts posteriorly and the lumbar spine flexes slightly. This is another example of a relative flexibility problem; however, the mechanism is faulty joint stabilization and not one of compensatory motion. The contributing factor is excessive mobility of the segment that should remain stable or a motor control problem of appropriate timing or recruitment of stabilizing muscles.

Wrist Flexion Occurring During Finger Extension

Another example of a stabilizing muscle that causes movement rather than prevents motion is observed at the wrist (Figure 2-31, *A* and *B*). When asked to perform finger extension, many individuals demonstrate a concurrent small degree of wrist flexion. This type of movement pattern occurs most frequently in the individual

whose activities require repetitive wrist flexion. The repetitive wrist flexion decreases the stiffness and increases the flexibility of the flexion movement. In the normal pattern the fingers extend and the wrist flexors contract to prevent wrist extension. If, however, there is excessive wrist flexibility into flexion, the wrist flexes rather than remains neutral. As a result of this wrist flexion movement, the position of the flexed joint and the anterior position of the flexor tendons reduce the carpal tunnel space, which can result in carpal tunnel syndrome.

A study by Hodges and Richardson finds evidence of the alteration in timing of stabilizing muscles. This study reports that the transversus abdominis muscle, ordinarily the lowest threshold abdominal stabilizer of the lumbar spine during extremity motion, is delayed in its onset in the patient with low back pain when he or she flexes the hip.[26]

Patterns of Eccentric Contraction

The area where the timing of eccentric muscle activity is most critical is the shoulder girdle. As proper timing and magnitude of recruitment of the thoracoscapular and scapulohumeral muscles are essential to the initiation and performance of optimal shoulder motion, so is the termination of activity. When winging of the scapula occurs during the return from but not during shoulder flexion, the explanation indicates a condition other than weakness of the serratus anterior muscle (Figure 2-32, *A-C*).

Greater muscle tension is required for a concentric contraction than for an eccentric contraction against a given load.[36] Thus weakness of the serratus anterior muscle is more evident during the flexion motion than it is during the return from flexion motion. The most likely explanation is that the deltoid and supraspinatus muscles are not elongating or ceasing activity as rapidly as the serratus anterior muscle. This pattern can be a contributing factor in shoulder impingement syndromes. (The scapular winging syndrome is included in the chapter that discusses shoulder impairment syndromes.)

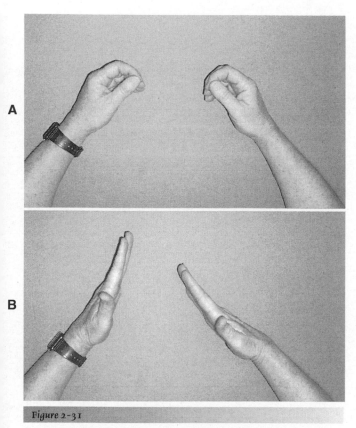

Figure 2-31

Variations in wrist behavior during finger extension. *A*, Neutral position of wrist with fingers relaxed. *B*, During finger extension, the left wrist stays neutral, but the right wrist flexes.

Several studies demonstrate that pain in a joint that is controlled by muscle (or pain in the muscle itself) can impede volitional efforts to contract the muscle.[2,15] A reasonable assumption is that when the patient learns to use different muscle strategies to produce movement at the affected joint, these strategies will continue to be used even when the pain is no longer present. The patient who has had knee surgery often uses hip extension with their foot fixed to assist with knee extension. In part, hip extensors are used because it is difficult to activate the quadriceps muscles. However, when this muscle strategy becomes a pattern of knee control, specific retraining is necessary to restore the normal pattern.

Biomechanical Element Impairments

The important role of the biomechanical element in movement necessitates its inclusion in the models, even though it is not a system of the body. The biomechanical element is an interface between motor control and musculoskeletal function that affects the pattern of muscle use and the shape of bones and joints. Possibly, because

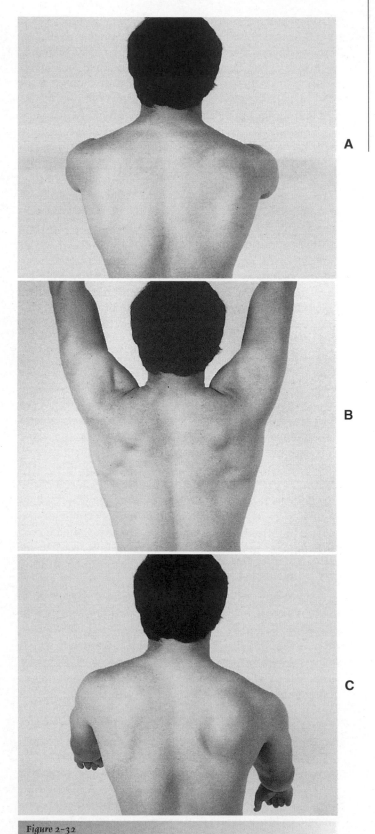

Figure 2-32

Scapular winging with return from flexion. *A*, Starting position. *B*, Shoulder flexion (no winging of scapula is noted). *C*, Return from shoulder flexion (winging of scapula is noted).

of the intrinsic relationship between musculoskeletal function and biomechanics, there is danger of redundancy in discussing biomechanics as a separate element. However, recognition of the role of biomechanics and how it contributes to movement impairment syndromes also provides additional directions and options for intervention that may otherwise be overlooked.

Biomechanics is defined as the science dealing with the forces, external and internal, that affect the body.[58] Mechanics consists of two main aspects of study of the forces that act on the body, dynamics and statics. *Dynamics*, which encompasses the study of kinematics and kinetics, is the aspect of biomechanics that is discussed in greatest detail by kinesiologists. *Kinematics* is the description of the motions of the body, whereas *kinetics* is the description of the forces that produce motion or maintain equilibrium. However, *statics*, which is the force that acts on the body at rest or in equilibrium, also affects tissues as described in the following text.

Statics: Effects of Gravitational Forces

Gravitational Forces Affecting Muscle Use
Therapists traditionally consider the effect of gravity when testing or devising exercise programs for muscle strengthening. Besides the effect of gravity on muscles during specific exercises, there is also the effect induced by changes in postural alignment. One of the most common examples is found in the individual with an exaggerated swayback posture. As discussed previously, the line of gravity is shifted significantly posterior of the hip joint in this posture. Because the swayback alignment decreases the demands on the hip extensors, the gluteal muscles of the individual with the swayback posture appear underdeveloped and usually test weak (Figure 2-33). Thus static forces contribute to atrophy of muscles.

Static forces can also increase the activity of muscles and change the interaction between agonists and antagonists. For example, occasionally tall, slender individuals stand in a forward leaning posture,[33] which causes the line of gravity to fall farther toward the front of their feet. The consequence is greater demand on the soleus muscle and less demand on the anterior tibialis muscle. In the forward leaning posture, the line of gravity is shifted toward the front of the foot, thereby minimizing the action of the tibialis anterior muscle (Figure 2-34).

In contrast, the individual who has a rigid foot with a high instep and whose line of gravity is more toward the rear of the foot tends to use the tibialis anterior muscle to bring the body forward. This individual has a greater tendency to develop anterior shin splints than does the individual with a normal foot alignment (Figure 2-35). The individual who leans forward has a

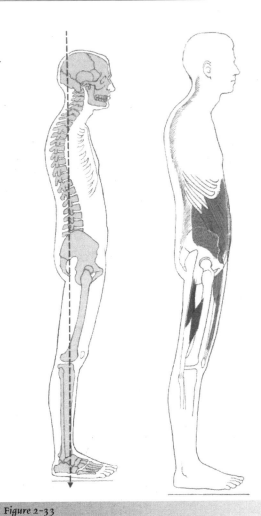

Figure 2-33

Swayback alignment in posture. (From Kendall FP, McCreary EK, Provance PG: *Muscles: testing and function,* 4e, 1993, Williams & Wilkins.)

tendency to develop metatarsalgia because of greater pressure on the metatarsal heads than if he or she did not lean forward.

Alterations of Gravitational Forces Acting on Joints and Bones
The static forces imposed on bone can affect their longitudinal shape, as well as the shape of joint surfaces. Studies document alterations in the shape of vertebrae because of the forces associated with scoliosis.[14] The forces resulting from altered vertebral alignment cause remodeling of the articular surfaces. Mechanical loads and the stresses and strains on bones affect their shape, whether by deterioration or exostosis.[18,47]

Another example related to faulty posture is found in the individual with genu recurvatum. The x-ray comparison of a normally aligned knee and the knee of an individual who stands with the knees in hyperextension illustrates several faults (Figure 2-36). As described by Kendall, a bowing of the tibia and fibula in the sagittal

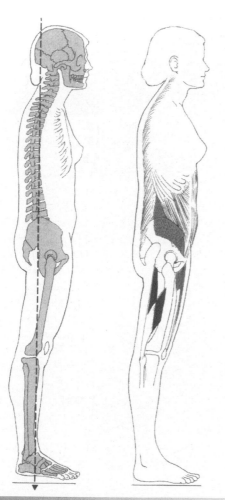

Figure 2-34

Flat back posture with slight forward lean. (From Kendall FP, McCreary EK, Provance PG: *Muscles: testing and function,* 4e, 1993, Williams & Wilkins.)

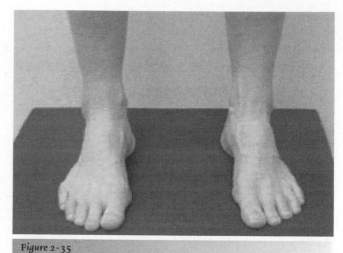

Figure 2-35

Rigid foot with high instep.

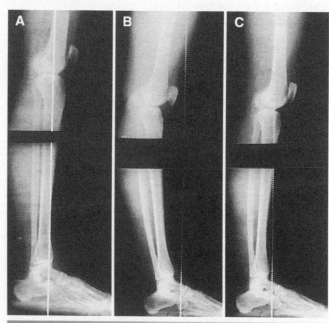

Figure 2-36

X-rays of the knees of two subjects. *A,* Subject has stood in good alignment throughout life. *B,* Another subject has stood with the knees hyperextended since childhood. *C,* Same subject in B stands with the knees in the neutral position. (From Kendall FP, McCreary EK, Provance PG: *Muscles: testing and function,* 4e, 1993, Williams & Wilkins.)

plane is a fault that is evident in the individual who has had hyperextension of the knee all his or her life.[32] However, careful examination of this individual indicates the presence of several other faults. They include (1) the downward sloping of the anterior articular surface of the tibia (see Figure 2-36, *C*), instead of a more horizontal orientation (see Figure 2-36, *A*); (2) the displacement of the femur anterior to the tibia, which is evident in the corrected knee alignment position (see Figure 2-36, *C*), instead of the anterior surface of both bones in the same vertical plane (see Figure 2-36, *A*); and (3) the inferior position of the patella (see Figure 2-36, *B, C*), which may be the result of diminished activity in the quadriceps muscles because of the hyperextended knee position. Consistent with Wolff's law, the anomalies of the tibia and fibula are induced by the forces associated with the hyperextended knee posture.[5]

Observation of a malalignment associated with hyperextended knees indicates that the anterior and posterior cruciate ligaments are placed under different de-

grees of stress. When the knee is hyperextended, the anterior cruciate ligament is in a shortened position with inconsistent stress; this malalignment can lead to a weakening of the ligament. The opposite condition is associated with the posterior cruciate ligament. Factors that predispose the knee to injury during pivot shift activities are (1) the oblique shape of the articular surface of the tibia with the anterior surface lower than the posterior, and (2) the weakness caused by reduced constant stress on the anterior cruciate ligament. Loudon reports the prevalence of hyperextended knees in the individual with anterior cruciate ligament deficiency.[38]

Another example of malalignment contributing to the further deterioration of a joint is the presence of genu varum. Varus of the knee joint occurs during a single leg stance when the line of gravity does not shift enough laterally to be close to the knee (Figure 2-37). This malalignment occurs because the varus moment (the perpendicular distance from the medial aspect of the knee to the line of gravity) at the knee is greater than that for a normally aligned knee. This larger varus moment further contributes to the varus deformity of the knee and consequently results in increased stress and a deterioration of the medial condyle of the tibia.

Dynamics: The Relationship Between Motion and the Forces Producing Motion

Kinetics: Description of the Forces Producing Motion

Deviations in alignment of weight-bearing joints contribute to the development of moments that increase the degree of the joint malalignment. For example, during the stance phase of gait (i.e., the hip medially rotates and the knee hyperextends), the result is a varus alignment of the knee joint. If, while weight bearing on the extremity, the weight line does not shift laterally, the varus force on the knee is greater than that on a normally aligned knee. The greater varus force further contributes to increasing the varus alignment of the knee.

Kinematics: Description of the Motions of the Body

The pattern of joint movement, considering both osteokinematic and arthrokinematic contributions, is the principal factor in the movement system balance (MSB) approach to musculoskeletal pain syndromes. The kinematic impairment, believed to be the most important contributing factor to the development of a pain syndrome, is that a joint develops a *directional susceptibility to movement* (DSM), which is a compensatory movement in a specific direction or a stress applied in a specific direction. The site of the compensatory movement is believed to be the site of pain.

Many of the movement impairment syndromes described in this text arise from faults in the arthrokinematics (accessory joint movements). One example is the femoral anterior glide syndrome in which the hip joint is in postural extension or hyperextension. Because of the development of shortness or stiffness of the posterior structures of the hip joint, the head of the femur does not follow the normal pattern of gliding posteriorly during hip flexion; as a result, the anterior joint capsular structures are impinged and painful. This con-

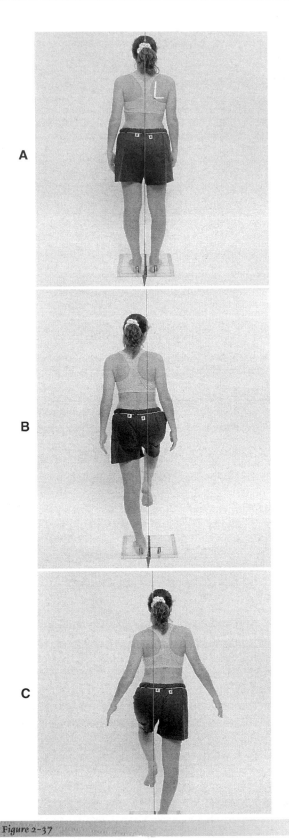

Figure 2-37

Marked varus of the knee joint during a single leg stance.
A, Starting position. *B,* Normal alignment during single leg stance. *C,* Marked varus moment that is present when the line of gravity does not shift laterally enough to be close to the knee.

dition is analogous to the preimpingement dynamics described at the shoulder.[30]

Assessing and restoring accessory motions is a major emphasis of the techniques of manual therapy, which are most often used as passive interventions. Although passive mobility of a joint is important, the active control of joint motion is considered most important. Muscle activity is one of the factors controlling the arthrokinematics. Impairments of muscle performance is a major contributing factor to impairments of accessory motions, and thus the correction of muscle performance is also a means of correcting the accessory motion impairments.

Observations and measurements of osteokinematics, the movement of joints in relation to one another, are parts of the standard assessments performed by the physical therapist. Deficits in the range of motion are most frequently used to assess the patient with a musculoskeletal pain syndrome. The loss of joint range of motion is the result of a loss of muscle length and from changes in capsular tissues and changes in the joint itself, which can also restrict the range of motion. Many texts describe methods of treating deficits in joint motions.

In the syndromes described in this text, the effect of changes in muscle length, strength, stiffness, and performance is especially emphasized. Some of the syndromes are classified by their osteokinematics, such as the hip extension and hip abduction syndromes. In these syndromes the condition is a muscle strain or a soft-tissue problem attributable to impairments in muscle performance. The reason for using physiologic movements as diagnostic categories for muscle and soft-tissue strains is to emphasize the dynamic nature of the presumed cause.

A major tenet of the MSB approach is that alterations in muscle performance (as depicted in the kinesiopathologic model) are the causative factors of painful conditions. Consequently, intervention requires assessing these factors and correcting those that are impaired. The emphasis on the multiple factors contributing to the development of a muscle strain is also intended to alert the clinician that a treatment program that only involves rest, modalities to alleviate inflammation, and strengthening exercises is not adequate for long-term correction and prevention of reinjury. Time will tell whether these categories are as useful as they are believed to be.

The movement impairment syndromes of the spine are named according to osteokinematic movements, even though these syndromes are impairments in arthrokinematics and not only muscle or soft-tissue strains. At this time it is not possible to decipher clinically arthrokinematic faults of the spine. Therefore the diagnostic categories involving the back are named for the major motions of flexion, extension, and rotation. (The details of these diagnoses are discussed in the chapter on movement impairment syndromes of the lumbar spine.)

Kinematics and Impairments of Joint Function

Arthrokinematics, the movement of joint surfaces in relation to one another, is not easily observed, but therapists have developed systems of assessment by passive displacement. One of the methods used to depict the arthrokinematics of a joint is the analysis of the PICR (see Figure 2-1). Frankel[17] has shown that in the presence of meniscal tears, the PICR is faulty (Figure 2-38). There is normal rolling and gliding between the femur and tibia through the range-of-knee motion (Figure 2-39, *A*). In contrast, when the PICR is abnormal, there can be compression at some points in the range and distraction at other points in the range-of-knee flexion and extension (Figure 2-39, *B*).

Although the PICR is abnormal when joint pathologic conditions are present, abnormal movement has also been documented before evidence of degeneration.[20,69] When radiologic examination indicates that degeneration has taken place, usually motion is restricted from fibrosis.

Other studies have also documented deviations of the PICR when joint structures are damaged. This situation creates a vicious cycle, because deviations in the PICR mean that the joint surfaces are not moving opti-

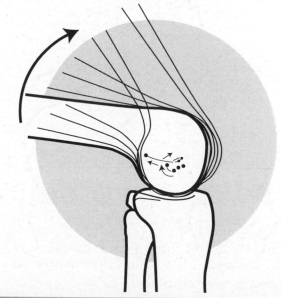

Figure 2-38

Abnormal instant center pathway for a 35-year-old man with a bucket-handle derangement. The instant center jump at full extension of the knee. (Adapted from Frankel et al: Biomechanics of internal derangement of the knee: pathomechanics as determined by analysis of the instant center of motion, *J Bone Joint Surg* 53A:945, 1971.)

mally in relation to one another, thus furthering the microtrauma to the joint. Currently, radiologic methods that are neither practical nor physiologic are the primary means of assessing the PICR. However, noninvasive methods are under development, which can be used during physiologic conditions, offering practical ways of using the PICR to assess accessory joint motions for both diagnosis and treatment.[27,39]

One method of depicting how faults in the PICR contribute to microtrauma at a joint is the model of stress, which provides a schematic representation of how stress affects several biological tissues (Figure 2-40).

Almost all musculoskeletal pain syndromes are considered mechanical disorders as compared with disease-based disorders. Therefore the ultimate cause of tissue irritation is a biomechanical impairment. The syndromes described in this text are termed movement impairment syndromes in recognition of the biomechanical basis of the underlying cause. Therefore biomechanical impairments are described in each of the syndromes.

Kinesiopathologic Model Applied to Patellofemoral Joint Dysfunction

Muscular Component Impairments
- Short or stiff tensor fascia lata–iliotibial band (TFL-ITB) or gluteus maximus muscle–iliotibial band
- Insufficient performance of vastus medialis oblique muscle
- Insufficient performance of posterior gluteus medius muscle contributing to dominant TFL activity
- Insufficient performance of iliopsoas muscle contributing to dominant TFL activity

Motor Control Impairments
- Dominant TFL-ITB activity as evidenced by excessive hip medial rotation during knee extension in the sitting position or during the stance phase of gait
- Dominant hamstring versus quadriceps activity during running, sitting-to-standing movement, and climbing stairs
- Altered force couple action of the vastus medialis oblique (VMO) and TFL muscles

Biomechanical Impairment
- Faulty alignment of patella in trochlear notch of the femur; patella positioned inferiorly, tilted inferiorly, and rotated laterally and superiorly
- Faulty PICR of patella during knee motion

A

B

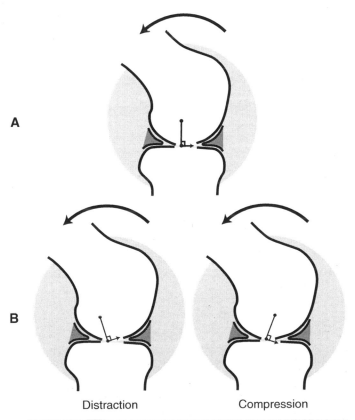

Distraction   Compression

Figure 2-39

A, Optimal PICR with normal gliding between the femur and tibia through the range-of-knee motion. *B,* Abnormal PICR resulting in compression and distraction during knee flexion. (Modified from Nordin M, Frankel VH: *Basic biomechanics of the musculoskeletal system,* 2e, Philadelphia, 1989, Lea & Febiger.)

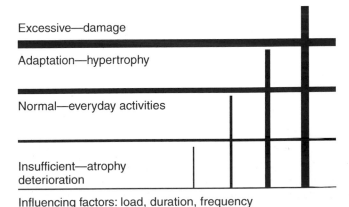

Excessive—damage

Adaptation—hypertrophy

Normal—everyday activities

Insufficient—atrophy deterioration

Influencing factors: load, duration, frequency

Figure 2-40

Tissue response to stress. Muscle, bone, and cartilage need normal range of stress to maintain an optimal level of physiologic properties. These tissue adapt to slight increases in stress by forms of hypertrophy. These tissues deteriorate when stress is below normal or above the adaptive range. (Courtesy of SA Sahrmann and MJ Mueller.)

Multiple Impairments of the Components of Movement

Case Presentation

History. A 35-year-old, highly competitive female marathon runner is experiencing pain on the posterolateral aspect of her right knee in the area lateral to the insertion of the biceps femoris muscle. The pain has been present for 6 weeks. Approximately 2 weeks before her consultation, she received ultrasound treatments to the painful area with minimal change in her symptoms. She does not have pain when walking, but her running is limited to 3 to 5 miles because of the onset of her symptoms. She rates her symptoms as a 3 to 5 on a scale of 10. The examination of her lower extremity indicates a varus alignment of the right knee. She has bilateral tibial varum. Closer examination of the right knee indicates that the femur is rotated medially with respect to the tibia, and the tibia appears to be displaced posterolaterally in relation to the femur, even in the sitting position with her knee flexed (Figure 2-41, *A-F*).

Symptoms. During a single leg stance on the right and when walking, the degree of varus of her right knee increases. This is attributable in part to the increase in medial rotation of the femur during the stance phase. The right biceps femoris muscle also appears to be particularly hypertrophied and prominent when viewed from the lateral aspect. The only positive finding with muscle length and manual muscle testing is a grade of 4+/5 of the right hip lateral rotators.

Muscle Length and Strength. Based on the observation of increased hip medial rotation during stance, the patient is asked to contract the muscles in her gluteal area to maintain hip lateral rotation during a single leg stance. The active contraction keeps the femur aligned with the tibia and decreases the previously observed varus alignment at the knee. She practices contracting her hip lateral rotators while standing for 5 minutes and then practices the same correction while walking. Her gait training session lasts 25 minutes.

Because of the lack of other specific muscle impairments, she is not instructed in any specific exercises. Her previously established program of stretching is considered adequate. The patient never returns for treatment because she left within 4 days for a series of 10-kilometer races in another country. The patient did contact the therapist by telephone and mail to indicate that she has not experienced any knee pain during her competition. She is also able to train intensively throughout the summer without developing significant knee pain. She indicates that when she feels any discomfort in her knee, she contracts her gluteal muscles to eliminate the problem.

Diagnosis. The movement impairment is excessive femoral medial rotation with respect to the tibia. Medial rotation is the DSM. Thus the site of greatest relative flexibility is the knee joint. The muscular impairment is weakness of the hip lateral rotators, but the most important observations are the posterolateral displacement of the tibia, the medial rotation of the femur, and the prominence of the right biceps femoris muscle.

These observations suggest a motor control impairment of recruitment patterns. The patient appears to be using the biceps femoris muscle as the primary lateral rotator of the hip instead of the intrinsic hip lateral rotators—the gemelli, obturators, piriformis, and quadratus femoris muscles. The obvious problem with the biceps femoris muscle becoming the dominant muscle is that it attaches to the ischial tuberosity proximally and to the tibia distally, except for the short head of the muscle. Therefore it does not directly control the rotation of the femur. In contrast, the six intrinsic hip lateral rotator muscles attach to the greater trochanter of the femur and thus provide the optimal control of the femur.

The biomechanical element impairments are malalignments of the knee, specifically, the varus, rotation, and posterolateral glide. During weight bearing the moments that are created by these impairments add to the malalignments. This type of analysis and intervention exemplifies the difference between addressing the source of the pain, which is the irritated structures on the posterolateral aspect of the knee, and addressing the cause of the problem. The cause is the movement impairment of tibial posterolateral glide.

Summary. As discussed, impairment in muscular, motor control, and biomechanical components all contribute to the cause; thus for optimal correction, all these factors must be addressed. In this case the intervention is simple and straightforward. The patient merely has to learn to activate the correct muscles at the correct time.

Support Element Impairments

The cardiopulmonary, metabolic, and endocrine systems are important to movement, but discussion of impairments in these systems and their relationship to musculoskeletal pain is beyond the scope of this text. Vital signs and respiratory rate should be routine components of the physical therapy examination. Oxygen consumption or response to exercise is needed to prescribe an appropriate aerobic exercise program. Screening examinations should always include the identification of potential systemic diseases that mimic musculoskeletal pain. A variety of books are available that address these issues and should be consulted for further information about appropriate examination techniques.

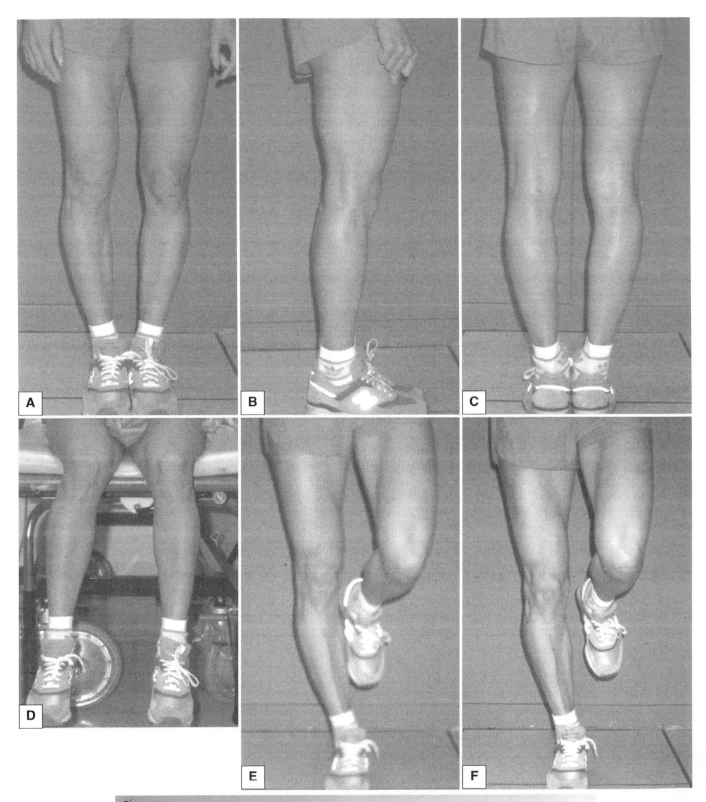

Figure 2-41

A, Varus alignment of right knee, bilateral tibial varum. *B,* Prominent biceps femoris muscle. *C,* Marked medial rotation of femur in relation to tibia, posterolateral displacement of the tibia. *D,* Medial rotation of femur, posterolateral displacement of tibia. *E,* Increased varus and medial rotation of femur during single-leg stance. *F,* Decreased medial rotation of the femur when activating the pelvic girdle lateral rotator muscles during single-leg stance.

Summary

The impairments in the components of the movement system discussed in this chapter highlight the factors that contribute to movement impairment syndromes. When examining a patient for musculoskeletal pain syndromes, all component impairments and their contributions to the pain syndrome need to be identified and corrected. The mechanical stress on tissues arising from movement impairments is the cause of a wide variety of tissue injuries. The various tissue conditions that are implicated in musculoskeletal pain syndromes are degenerative changes in cartilage and joints, ligament strains, joint inflammation, myofascial strains, myofascial tears, tendonitis, bursitis, neuropathic pain from entrapment, and compression and adhesions, to give just a few examples.

The approach advocated in this text suggests that identifying the mechanical cause is a more important step in correcting the problem and alleviating the pain than identifying the painful tissues, unless the tissue degeneration or strain is severe. Identifying and correcting impairments is an effective form of treatment, whereas alleviating local inflammation with physical agents is not. The latter does not address the cause but instead is directed at the tissue source of the pain. Even when the treatment for inflammation decreases pain, the relief is only temporary unless there is an associated change in movement patterns to prevent the return of the mechanical problem.

References

1. *American heritage dictionary*, Boston, 1985, Houghton Mifflin.
2. Arvidsson I, Eriksson E, Knutsson E, Arner S: Reduction of pain inhibition on voluntary muscle activation by epidural analgesia, *Orthopedics* 10:1415, 1986.
3. Babyar SR: Excessive scapular motion in individuals recovering from painful and stiff shoulders: causes and treatment strategies, *Phys Ther* 76:226, 1996.
4. Baldwin KM et al: Biochemical properties of overloaded fast-twitch skeletal muscle, *J Appl Physiol* 52:467, 1982.
5. Bassett CL: Effect of force on skeletal tissues. In Downey RC, Darling RC, editors: *Physiological basis of rehabilitative medicine*, Philadelphia, 1971, WB Saunders.
6. Blanpied P, Smidt GL: Human plantarflexor stiffness to multiple single-stretch trials, *J Biomech* 25:29, 1992.
7. Bohannon RW, Smith MB: Assessment of strength deficits in eight hemiparetic upper extremity muscle groups of stroke patients, *Phys Ther* 67:522, 1987.
8. Chesworth BM, Padfield BJ, Helewa A, Stitt, LW: A comparison of hip mobility in patients with low back pain and matched healthy subjects, *Physiother Can* 46:267, 1994.
9. Chleboun G, Howell JN, Conatser RR, Giesey JJ: The relationship between elbow flexor volume and angular stiffness at the elbow, *Clin Biomech* 12:383, 1997.
10. Claus H, Bullock-Saxon J: *An investigation of lumbar and pelvic sagittal posture comparing road cyclists with control subjects*, Brisbane, Australia, 1996, Proceedings of the 1996 National Physiotherapy Congress.
11. Cummings GS: Comparison of muscle to other soft tissue in limiting elbow extension, *JOSPT* 5:170, 1984.
12. DeFabio R, Badke MB: Relationship of sensory organization to balance function in patients with hemiplegia, *Phys Ther* 70:543, 1990.
13. Dewald JP et al: Abnormal muscle coactivation patterns during isometric torque generation at the elbow and shoulder in hemiparetic subjects, *Brain* 118:495, 1995.
14. Enneking WF, Harrington P: Pathologic changes in scoliosis, *J Bone Joint Surg (Am)* 51:165, 1969.
15. Fahrer H et al: Knee effusion and reflex inhibition of the quadriceps, *J Bone Joint Surg* 70B:635, 1988.
16. Fowler P: Shoulder problems in overhead-overuse sports: swimmer problems, *Am J Sports Med* 7:141, 1979.
17. Frankel VH et al: Biomechanics of internal derangement of the knee: pathomechanics as determined by analysis of the instant center of motion, *J Bone Joint Surg* 53A:945, 1971.
18. Frost HM: *Orthopaedic biomechanics*, Springfield, IL, 1973, Charles C. Thomas.
19. Gelberman RH et al: Femoral anteversion: a clinical assessment of idiopathic intoeing gait in children, *J Bone Joint Surg (Br)* 69B:75, 1987.
20. Gertzbein SD et al: Centrode patterns and segmental instability in degenerative disc disease, *Spine* 3:257, 1985.
21. Halar EM, Stolov WC: Gastrocnemius muscle belly and tendon length in stroke patients and able-bodied persons, *Arch Phys Med Rehabil* 59:476, 1978.
22. Hayes KC, Hatze H: Passive visco-elastic properties of the structures spanning the human elbow joint, *Eur J Appl Physiol* 37:265, 1977.
23. Hebert R: Preventing and treating stiff joints. In Crosbie J, McConnell J, editors: *Key issues in musculoskeletal physiotherapy*, Sydney, 1993, Butterworth-Heinemann.
24. Hides JA et al: Evidence of lumbar multifidus muscle wasting ipsilateral to symptoms in patients with acute/subacute low back pain, *Spine* 19:165, 1994.
25. Hislop H: The not-so-impossible dream, *Phys Ther* 55:1069, 1975.
26. Hodges PW, Richardson C: Inefficient muscular stabilization of the lumbar spine associated with low back pain, *Spine* 21:2540, 1996.
27. Hollman J, Deusinger RH: Videographic determination of instantaneous center of rotation using a hinge joint model, *J Orthop Sports Phys Ther* 29:463, 1999.
28. Host HH: Scapular taping in the treatment of anterior shoulder impingement, *Phys Ther* 75:803, 1995.
29. Inman VT, Ralston HJ, Todd F: *Human walking*, Baltimore, 1981, Williams & Wilkins.
30. Jobe FW et al: *Operative techniques in upper extremity sports injuries*, St Louis, 1996, Mosby.
31. Jobe FW: Shoulder problems in overhead-overuse sports: thrower problems, *Am J Sports Med* 7:139, 1979.
32. Kendall FP, McCreary FP, Provance PG: *Muscles: testing and function*, ed 4, Baltimore, 1993, Williams & Wilkins.
33. Kendall HO, Kendall FP, Boynton DA: *Posture and pain*, Malabar, Fla, 1952, Robert E. Krieger.
34. Labeit S: Titins: giant proteins in charge of muscle ultrastructure and elasticity, *Science* 276:1112, 1995.
35. Lieber RL, Friden JO, McKee-Woodburn TG: Muscle damage induced by eccentric contractions of twenty-five percent, *J Appl Physiol* 70:2498, 1991.
36. Lieber RL: *Skeletal muscle structure and function*, Baltimore, 1992, Williams & Wilkins.
37. Light KE, Nuzik S, Personius W: Low-load prolonged stretch vs high-load brief stretch in treating knee contractures, *Phys Ther* 64:330, 1984.

38. Loudon J, Jenkins W, Loudon KL: The relationship between static posture and ACL injury in female athletes, *JOSPT* 24:91, 1996.

39. Loudon J: *Reliability and validity of PICR, movement science*, St Louis, 1993, Washington University.

40. Mayhew T, Norton BJ, Sahrmann SA: Electromyographic study of the relationship between hamstring and abdominal muscles during a unilateral straight-leg raise, *Phys Ther* 63:1769, 1983.

41. McGill SM, Brown S: Creep response of the lumbar spine to prolonged full flexion, *Clinical Biomech* 7:43, 1992.

42. *Merriam-Webster's collegiate dictionary*, ed 10, Springfield, Mass, 1994, Merriam-Webster.

43. Moritani H, Devries HA: Neural factors versus hypertrophy in the time course of muscle strength gain, *Am J Phys Med* 58:115, 1979.

44. Mueller MJ et al: Differences in the gait characteristics of patients with diabetes and peripheral neuropathy compared with age-matched controls, *Phys Ther* 74:1027, 1994.

45. Nagi SZ: Some conceptual issues in disability and rehabilitation. In Sussman MB, editor: *Sociology and rehabilitation*, Washington, DC, 1965, American Sociological Association.

46. Neumann DA, Soderberg GL: Comparison of maximal isometric hip abductor muscle torques between sides, *Phys Ther* 68:496, 1988.

47. Nordin M, Frankel VH: *Basic biomechanics of the musculoskeletal system*, ed 2, Philadelphia, 1989, Lea & Febiger.

48. Nordin M, Frankel VH: Biomechanics of the knee. In Nordin M, Frankel VH, editors: *Basic biomechanics of the musculoskeletal system*, ed 2, Philadelphia, 1989, Lea & Febiger.

49. Norkin CC, Levangie PK: *Joint structure and function: a comprehensive analysis*, ed 2, Philadelphia, 1992, FA Davis.

50. Noyes FR: Functional properties of knee ligaments and alterations induced by immobilization, *Clin Orthop* 123:210, 1977.

51. Olney SJ, Richards C: Hemiparetic gait following stroke: part I: characteristics, *Gait & Posture* 4:136, 1996.

52. Pearcy MJ: Twisting mobility of the human back in flexed postures, *Spine* 18:114, 1993.

53. Pierce MN, Lee WY: Muscle firing order during active prone hip extension, *JOSPT* 12:2, 1990.

54. Proske U, Morgan DL, Gregory JE: Thixotropy in skeletal muscle and in muscle spindles: a review, *Prog Neurobiol* 41:705, 1993.

55. Sahrmann SA, Norton BJ: The relationship between spasticity and voluntary movement in the upper motor neuron syndrome, *Ann Neurol* 2:460, 1977.

56. Seligman JV, Gertzbein SD, Tile M, Kapasouri A: Computer analysis of spinal segment motion in degenerative disc disease with and without axial loading, *Spine* 9:566, 1984.

57. Sinkjaer T, Magnussen I: Passive, intrinsic and reflex-mediated stiffness in the ankle extensors of hemiparetic patients, *Brain* 117:355, 1994.

58. *Stedman's concise medical dictionary*, Baltimore, 1998, Williams & Wilkins.

59. Sternheim MM, Kane JW: *Elastic properties of materials, General Physics*, Toronto, 1986, John Wiley & Sons.

60. Tabary JC et al: Physiological and structural changes in the cat's soleus muscle due to immobilization at different lengths by plaster casts. *J Physiol* 224(1):231, 1972.

61. Tafazzoli T, Lamontagne M: Mechanical behaviour of hamstring muscles in low-back pain patients and control subjects, *Clin Biomech* 11:16, 1995.

62. Tardieu C et al: Adaptation of sarcomere numbers to the length imposed on muscle. In Guba FMG, Takacs O, editors: *Mechanism of muscle adaptation to functional requirements*, Elmsford, NY, 1981, Pergamon Press.

63. Thomas JS, Corocos DM, Hasan Z: The influence of gender on spine, hip, knee, and ankle motions during a reaching task, *J Mot Behav* 30:98, 1998.

64. Tipton CM, James SL, Mergner W, Tcheng T: Influence of exercise on strength of medial collateral ligaments of dogs, *Am J Physiol* 218(3):894, 1970.

65. Travell JG, Simons DG: *Myofascial pain and dysfunction: the trigger point manual*, Baltimore, 1983, Williams & Wilkins.

66. van Wingerden JP, Vleeming A, Stam HJ, Stoeckart R: *Interaction of spine and legs: influence of hamstring tension on lumbopelvic rhythm*, San Diego, 1996, The Second Interdisciplinary World Congress on Low Back Pain.

67. Viidik A: The effect of training on the tensile strength of isolated rabbit tendons, *Scand J Plast Reconstr Surg* 1:141, 1967.

68. Wang K et al: Viscoelasticity of the sarcomere matrix of skeletal muscles, *Biophys J* 64:1161, 1993.

69. Wiegner AW, Watts RL: Elastic properties of muscle measured at the elbow in man: I. normal controls, *J Neurol Neurosurg Psych* 49:1171, 1986.

70. Wilder DG, Pope MH, Frymoyer JW: The biomechanics of lumbar disc herniation and the effect of overload and instability, *J Spinal Disord* 1:16, 1988.

71. Williams P, Goldspink G: Changes in sarcomere length and physiologic properties in immobilized muscle, *J Anat* 127:459, 1978.

72. Williams P, Goldspink G: The effect of immobilization on the longitudinal growth of striated muscle fibers, *J Anat* 116:45, 1973.

73. Zatisiorsky VM: *Kinematics of human motion*, Champaign, Ill, 1998, Human Kinetics.

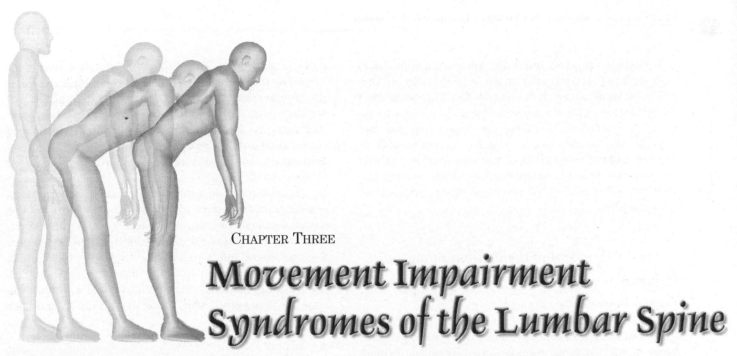

Movement Impairment Syndromes of the Lumbar Spine

Chapter Highlights

Normal Alignment of the Lumbar Spine
Motions of the Lumbar Spine
Muscular Actions of the Lumbar Spine
Movement Impairment Syndromes of the Low Back

Chapter Objectives

After consideration of the information presented in this chapter, the reader will be able to:

1. Describe the standards for ideal alignment and identify structural variations of the spine and pelvis.
2. Describe the standards for the normal ranges of the motions of the spine.
3. Identify the contributions of each abdominal muscle to the movements and to the stability of the trunk and pelvis and prescribe appropriate exercises.
4. Understand the characteristics of each movement impairment syndrome of the low back.
5. Perform an examination of the patient with low back pain, consider the contributing factors, and establish a diagnosis.
6. Develop and instruct the patient in a diagnosis-specific intervention program of exercise and modification of life activities, which contributed to formation of the movement impairment syndrome.

Introduction

A majority of spinal dysfunction is the result of cumulative microtrauma caused by *impairments in alignment, in stabilization, and in movement patterns* of the spine. In the properly functioning spine, the balanced isometric support and control provided by the trunk muscles prevent these impairments. *When dysfunction occurs, the major objective is the identification of the direction of the alignment, stress, or movement of the spine that consistently elicits or increases the patient's symptoms.* Reproducible motions of the spine or extremities can produce the symptoms that elicit stress or movement. The site of the symptoms is particularly susceptible to movement because it becomes more flexible than the other sites at which motion also occurs. This susceptibility to movement further exaggerates the flexibility of the site because it is repeatedly subjected to motion.

Most movements involve the participation of multiple segments, and the relative contribution of each segment is a function of its mechanical characteristics. Movement follows the principles of mechanics. Among those principles is the law of physics, which states that *movement takes place along the path of least resistance.* When a system is multisegmented, as in the case of the human movement system, the greatest degree of motion occurs at the most flexible segment.

Thus most spine dysfunctions occur because of excessive relative flexibility, particularly at specific segments, rather than at the segment of reduced flexibility. The reduced flexibility of some segments invariably contributes to compensatory motion at the most flexible segments. Although a specific problem exists in the vertebral column (e.g., facet hypertrophy, disk degeneration, spondylolisthesis, nerve impingement, bulging disk), correction of the impairment performance of trunk muscles helps reduce the abnormal stresses that led to the problem. Once the appropriate trunk muscle control and lower extremity muscle flexibility are achieved, most often back pain subsides without direct treatment to the spine itself. After the correction is made, the spine is no longer subjected to the traumatic stresses.

The keys to preventing and alleviating spinal dysfunction are (1) to have the trunk muscles hold the vertebral column and pelvis in their optimal alignments and (2) to prevent unnecessary movement. To achieve these goals, the muscles must be the correct length and strength and be able to produce the correct pattern of activity. During movement of the extremities, optimal isometric contraction of the trunk muscles is needed to appropriately stabilize the proximal attachments of the limb muscles.

Normal Alignment of the Lumbar Spine

Standing

Normal Position

A forward convex curve of the lumbar spine is the normal or neutral position. A study of 14- to 15-year-old adolescents, using an estimation of vertebral bodies from the external profile of the spine in the sagittal plane, calculates the lumbar curve from the vertebral centroid curve. Male adolescents have a curve of 25.6 degrees, and female adolescents have a curve of 30.8 degrees.[45] The curvatures calculated from vertebral centroids located on the bodies of the vertebrae are expected to differ from those observed from external landmarks, such as the spinous processes (Figures 3-1 and 3-2). Inclinometers and flexible rulers can be used to measure external lumbar curves. Because two different methods are used to calculate the curve obtained by these devices, there is some variation in the reported values. The study by Youdas uses a flexible ruler to measure the lumbar curve of five men and five women with a mean age of 25 years. This study reports values ranging from 21 to 49 degrees and a mean value of approximately 34 degrees using both tangent and trigonometric methods to calculate the curves[59] (Figure 3-3). Thus a general assumption can be made—the lumbar curve in young individuals ranges from 25 to 30 degrees. Ohlen and colleagues use an inclinometer as their measurement device. Their study reports that the thoracic curve ranges from 30 to 33 degrees.[41] Loebl also uses an inclinometer to measure the thoracic spine. He reports similar values of 32 to 37 degrees for the individual younger than 40 years and values of 40 to 41 degrees for the individual older than 60 years.[29]

Impairments

Acquired impairments in the sagittal plane are either a decreased lumbar curvature resulting in a flat back or an increased lumbar curvature resulting in a lordosis. Judging the depth of the lumbar curve is not always easy. The reference for the ideal curve is provided in Figure 3-4, and an example of good lumbopelvic align-

ment is shown in Figure 3-5. The lumbar curve is affected by the tilt of the pelvis. A correlational between the lumbar curve and pelvic tilt has not been shown, nor should one be expected for both statistical and anatomical reasons. However, as demonstrated, tilting the pelvis anteriorly increases the lumbar curve, whereas tilting the pelvis posteriorly decreases the lumbar curve (Figure 3-6 on page 55).

Lumbopelvic alignment is often used for clinical assessment of the patient with lower quarter pain, but the measures used for this assessment can be misleading. Typically, the following three different measures are used to assess lumbopelvic alignment: (1) the lumbar curve, (2) the deviation from the horizontal line between the posterior superior iliac spine (PSIS) and anterior superior iliac spine (ASIS), and (3) the hip joint angle.

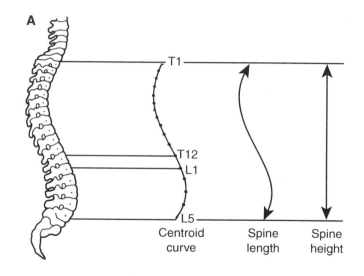

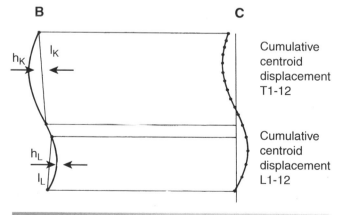

Figure 3-1

Shape of the spine. Calculation of the measurement variables: *A*, Spine length and height. *B*, Kyphotic and lordotic angles and spine depth. Kyphotic angle = 4 × arctan (2 × h_k/l_k); lordotic angle = 4 arctan (2 × h_L/l_L); spine depth = $h_k + h_L$. *C*, Cumulative centroid displacements of the thoracic and lumbar regions. (From Pearsall DJ, Reid JG: Line of gravity relative to upright vertebral posture, *Clin Biomech* 7:80, 1992.)

Examples of each measure can vary because of factors other than acquired impairments in lumbopelvic alignment. For example, a man often has structural variations in the curvature of his lumbar spine in the standing position. When the iliac crest is obviously higher than his belt line, he will consistently have a flat lumbar spine (Figure 3-7 on page 56). This patient is not standing in a posterior pelvic tilt because his PSIS is not lower than his ASIS and his hips are not in extension, which would be the finding if his flat lumbar spine had been an acquired impairment of posterior pelvic tilt. Often this patient also has retrotorsion of the hips.

When the patient has a flat lumbar spine, the flexibility of the hips becomes particularly important. During forward bending, the individual with a flat lumbar spine must immediately flex the hips to avoid excessive flexion of the spine (Figure 3-8 on page 56). A tall man with relatively greater pelvic height to overall height is more prone to low back pain than the tall man who does not have a tall pelvis.[36]

Structural factors can also influence the measurement of the line between the PSIS and ASIS. In women the structure of the pelvis can vary dramatically. In some the ASIS is notably lower than the PSIS; however, the

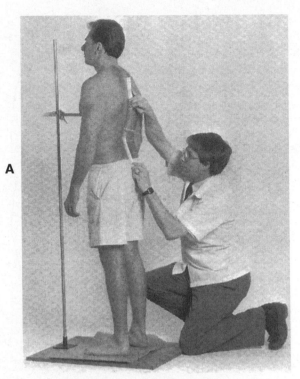

A

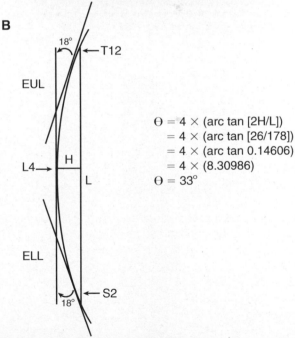

B

$$\Theta = 4 \times (\text{arc tan } [2H/L])$$
$$= 4 \times (\text{arc tan } [26/178])$$
$$= 4 \times (\text{arc tan } 0.14606)$$
$$= 4 \times (8.30986)$$
$$\Theta = 33°$$

Figure 3-3

Procedure for measuring the sagittal mobility of the lumbar spine when the subject is standing. *A*, The subject stands on a wooden platform, and an adjustable dowel is mounted to a vertical rod and positioned so that it lightly touches the subject's xiphoid process. The tester carefully molds the flexible curve to the midline contour of the subject's lumbar spine. Twist ties attach to the curve project horizontally and mark the location of spinous processes of T12, L4, and S2. *B*, The contour of the lumbar spine obtained from the flexible curve is carefully traced by the tester onto a poster board. (From Youdas JW, Suman VJ, Garrett TR: Reliability of measurements of lumbar spine sagittal mobility obtained with the flexible curve, *JOSPT* 21(1):13, 1995.)

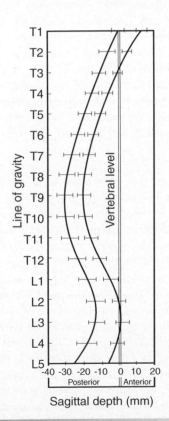

Figure 3-2

Relation of the male and female average vertebral centroid curves to the main line of gravity. (From Pearsall DJ, Reid JG: Line of gravity relative to upright vertebral posture, *Clin Biomech* 7:80, 1992.)

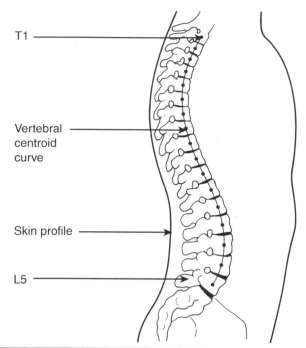

T1

Vertebral
centroid
curve

Skin profile

L5

Figure 3-4

Normal spinal curve. Relation of the vertebral column to the line of gravity. (From Pearsall DJ, Reid JG: Line of gravity relative to upright vertebral posture, *Clin Biomech* 7:80, 1992.)

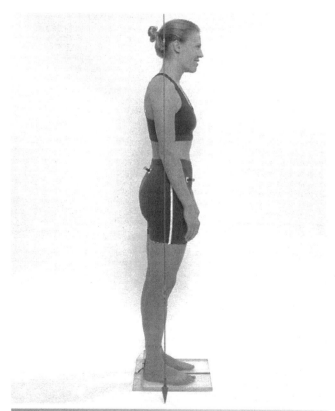

Figure 3-5

Ideal lumbopelvic alignment.

pelvis is not tilted anteriorly, the hip is not flexed, and the lumbar spine is not lordotic (Figure 3-9 on page 57). The hip joint angle is affected by the knee joint angle and by the pelvic tilt. When the knees are hyperextended, the hip joint is extended even though the pelvic tilt may be ideal (Figure 3-10 on page 57). Thus the assessment of lumbopelvic alignment should be based on a positive finding of two out of the three measurements.

Symmetry of the lumbar paraspinal area is another alignment impairment that is particularly important in the patient with low back pain. A side-to-side difference of $1/2$ inch or greater, which a trained therapist can reliably detect, is one of the tests used for the rotation category.[54] Asymmetry can be attributed to either postural rotation of the lumbar spine to one side or to unilateral hypertrophy of the paraspinal muscles. (The movement tests that differentiate these two conditions are described in the section on motions of the lumbar spine.)

Sitting

Normal Position

In the normal sitting position, the pelvis posteriorly tilts relative to the standing position. As a result, the lumbar spine reverses its anterior curve and becomes flat (Figure 3-11 on page 58). When the spine becomes flat, increased pressure is exerted on the disks because the pressure is reduced on the facet joints, as compared with the pressure exerted on the disks in the standing position.[39] If the inward curvature of the lumbar spine is increased while the patient is in a sitting position, the pressure on the disks decreases, but it is not as low as when the patient is in a standing position.

Impairments

Additional factors that affect the load on the lumbar spine include the line of gravity and the activity of the iliopsoas muscle. When sitting the lumbar spine is flat, the line of gravity is anterior to the spine and it increases the load on the spine. The more forward the line of gravity relative to the spine and the larger the shoulders, the greater the load on the spine. When a person does not use the backrest of the chair but uses hip flexor muscular activity to maintain an alignment of the spine and pelvis, additional compressive force and anterior shear forces are placed on the spine. A further exaggeration of anterior pull on the spine during sitting is found in the individual who sits on the end of the chair, which requires the use of the hip flexor muscles to hold him or her in hip flexion. When sitting in a standard chair, the feet of the individual who is shorter than 5 feet, 4 inches in height do not touch the ground; thus there is an anterior pull on the pelvis and spine from the unsupported position of the lower extremities.

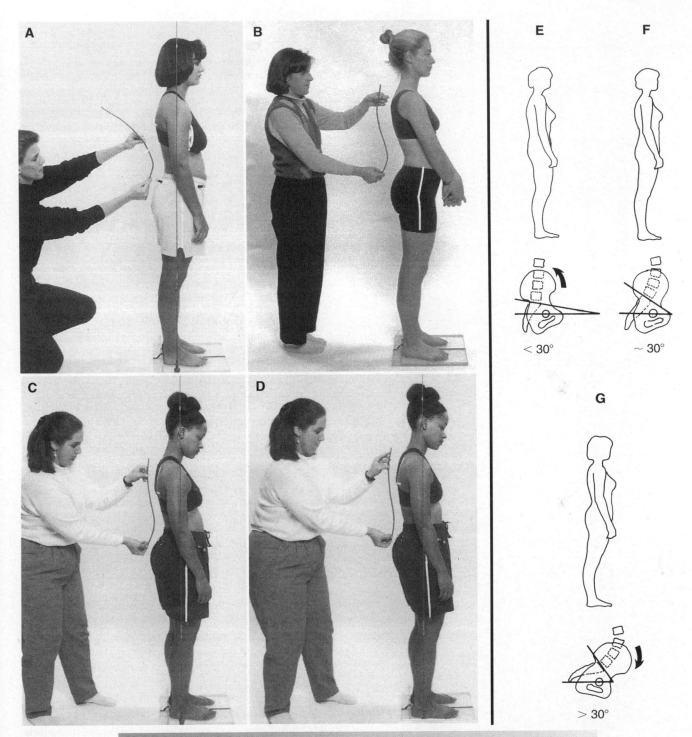

Figure 3-6

Faulty pelvic alignment as a result of: *A,* weak and long abdominal muscles. *B,* Short and stiff hip flexors. *C,* Apparent anterior tilt. *D,* Posterior tilt. Effect of pelvic tilting on the inclination of the base of the sacrum to the transverse plane (sacral angle) during upright standing. *E,* Tilting the pelvis backward reduces the sacral angle and flattens the lumbar spine. *F,* During relaxed standing the sacral angle is about 30 degrees. *G,* Tilting the pelvis forward increases the sacral angle and accentuates the lumbar spine. (Parts E, F, G from Nordin M, Frankel VH: *Basic biomechanics of the musculoskeletal system,* 2 ed, Philadelphia, 1989, Lea & Febiger.)

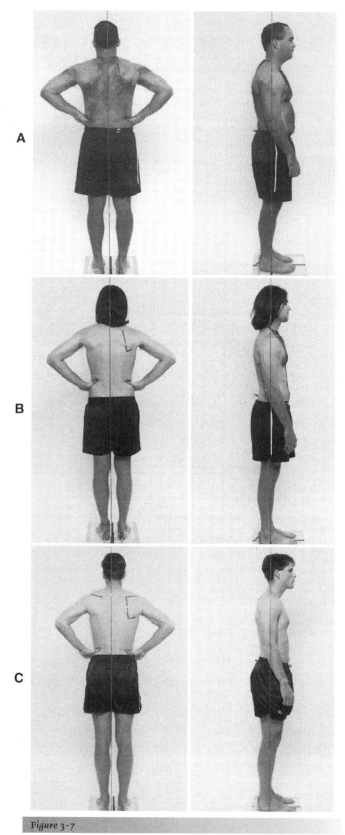

Figure 3-7

Posterior and side view examples of men with variations in the heights of their iliac crests. *A,* Slightly high iliac crests as judged by the differences between the top of the iliac crests and the beltline. *B,* High iliac crests. *C,* Iliac crests level with beltline.

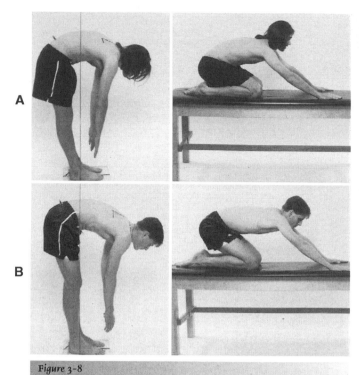

Figure 3-8

Variations in lumbar spine motion during forward bending and quadruped rocking. *A,* Limited hip flexion with excessive lumbar flexion. *B,* Good hip flexion with optimal lumbar flexion.

Another subtle yet common impairment is the tendency for a person to sit leaning to one side, often leaning onto an arm rest that is too low for the trunk height or the length of the arms. This position of lateral flexion can contribute to back pain, particularly in the individual whose lumbar spinal movement is isolated to only one or two lower segments of the lumbar spine.

A markedly kyphotic thoracic spine will cause the patient to sit in lumbar extension. When a patient has pain sitting in this position, the hips can slide forward to flatten the lumbar spine. Also, a firm pillow can be placed behind the lumbar spine to provide vertical support for the thoracic spine while decreasing the extension moment on the lumbar spine. The pillow should not contribute to the inward lumbar curve.

A tall man who has long tibias often sits with his knees higher than his hips, which contributes to lumbar flexion. He needs to adjust the chair so that his hips and knees are in the same horizontal plane. If the chair does not adjust, he should use a pillow in the seat of the chair to raise the height from the floor. A man who has a large abdomen also tends to sit in lumbar flexion. He should use a seat that is higher in the back than in the front so that his hips are not placed in greater than 90 degrees of flexion.

In summary, sitting impairments include a number of alignment faults other than lumbar flexion. Ideally,

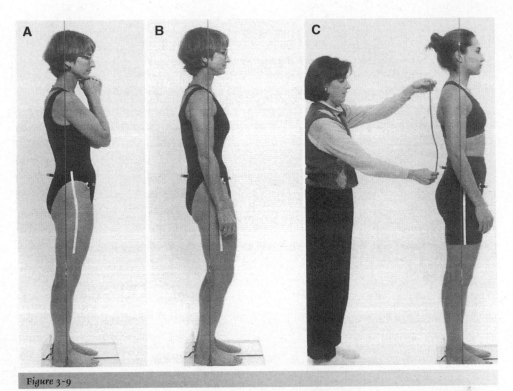

Figure 3-9

Two examples of women with a low anterior superior iliac spine (ASIS) in relation to posterior iliac spine (PSIS). *A,* Relaxed standing, ASIS is much lower than PSIS. *B,* Posteriorly tilting the pelvis to align ASIS and PSIS, eliminates the lumbar curve. *C,* Normal lumbar curve.

the patient should sit all the way back in the chair to use the back support. The shoulders should be in line with the lumbar spine, and the hips should be at a 90-degree angle with the knees in the same horizontal plane as the hips. If the feet do not reach the floor, they should rest on a footstool. The patient should not lean to one side. Accommodation must be made for structural variations such as long tibias, short legs, large abdomen, large buttocks, and thoracic kyphosis. A patient may magnify his or her complaints by simply contracting the proximal thigh muscles while sitting. For example, a woman may hold her knees together when sitting, another individual may subconsciously arch the back when tense, and another may contract the hamstring muscles, which can tilt the pelvis posteriorly.

Motions of the Lumbar Spine

Path of the Instant Center of Rotation

As with movement of the limb joints, the motion between the surfaces of the adjacent bones of the spine are analyzed by determining the path of the instant center of rotation (PICR). The location of the PICR has been determined for the different motions of the spine and is shown in Figure 3-12. For flexion and extension, the axis of rotation lies in the posterior half of the disk.

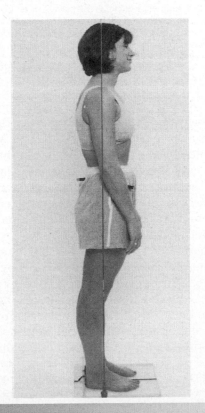

Figure 3-10

Woman with hyperextended knees causing the hip joint to become hyperextended, but the pelvic tilt remains ideal.

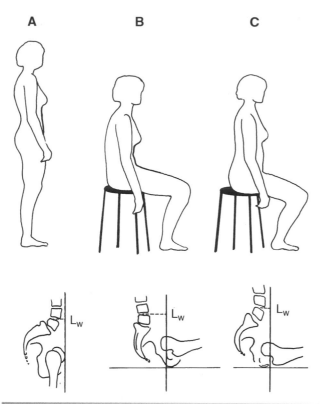

Figure 3-11

Compared with relaxed upright standing *(A)*, the line of gravity for the upper body (already ventral to the lumbar spine) shifts further ventrally during relaxed unsupported sitting as the pelvis is tilted backward and the lumbar lordosis flattens *(B)*. This shift creates a longer lever arm (L_W) for the force exerted by the weight of the upper body. During erect sitting, the backward pelvic tilt is reduced and the lever arm is shortened *(C)*, but it remains slightly longer than during relaxed upright standing. (From Nordin M, Frankel VH: *Basic biomechanics of the musculoskeletal system*, 2 ed, Philadelphia, 1989, Lea & Febiger.)

The location of the PICR is used to calculate the moment exerted by muscle fascicles on the lumbar spine.[2] The degree of flexibility of the spine suggests that changes in the vertebral alignment may affect the location of the PICR and therefore affect the moments exerted by the different muscles. Such changes have not been reported, but the possibility exists. These changes may have important clinical implications.

The alteration in the action of the sternocleidomastoid muscle from a cervical flexor (i.e., when the intrinsic neck flexors are contracting) to a cervical extensor (i.e., when the intrinsic neck flexors are not contracting) is one example of how changes in the alignment and stabilizing function of a synergistic muscle have important clinical consequences. An alteration in the PICR is associated with degeneration of the disks (Figure 3-13); this finding should be considered when developing exercise programs for the patient with low back pain. As discussed in Chapter 2, the alteration in the PICR is associated with changes in the surface motion of the two articulating segments, causing compres-

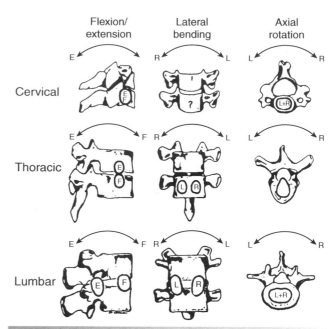

Figure 3-12

Approximate locations of instantaneous axes of rotation (IAR) in the three regions of the spine undergoing rotation in the three traditional planes. *E,* Approximate location of IARs in extending from neutral position; *F,* IARs in flexion from neutral position; *L,* IARs in left lateral bending or left axial rotation; *R,* IARs in right lateral bending (left or right axial rotation). (From White AA III, Panjabi MM: *Clinical biomechanics of the spine,* Philadelphia, 1978, JB Lippincott.)

sion or distraction to occur during the motion. Compression or distraction may be a source of continued trauma to the joint. In the presence of disk degeneration, the patient should be instructed to perform exercises that limit the motion of the spine, rather than promote increased movement.

Flexion: Forward Bending

Normal

Forward bending from a standing position is the motion that is most commonly used in daily activities. During the forward bending motion, the initial motion is the posterior sway of the pelvis as the hips flex, which allows the center of gravity to remain within the base of support. As the hips start to flex, the lumbar spine begins to reverse its inward curve and, on completion of the reversal of the lumbar curve, the rest of the motion is hip flexion.

Woolsey and Norton have analyzed the studies in which the lumbar range of motion is measured with an inclinometer.[58] Based on their analysis, the mean *range of motion* of lumbar flexion is 56.6 degrees.[58] The lumbar spine should not complete more than 50% of its motion into flexion before hip flexion is initiated.[40] At the completion of flexion there should be a straightening or flattening of the lumbar spine. The straight spine is described as flat rather than flexed.[27]

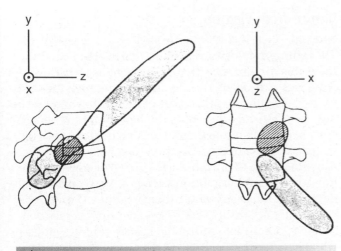

Figure 3-13

Changes in the location of the instantaneous axes of rotation in the lumbar spine motion segment, with and without degenerative disk disease in flexion *(left)* and right lateral bending *(right)*. (From Rolander SD: Motion of the lumbar spine with special reference to the stabilizing effect of posterior fusion, *Acta Orthop Scand* 90:1, 1966.)

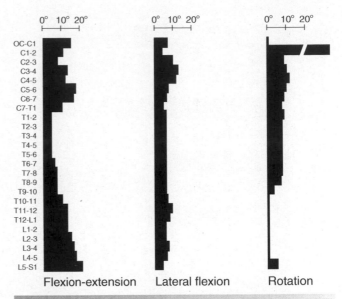

Flexion-extension   Lateral flexion   Rotation

Figure 3-14

A composite of representative values for type and range of motion at different levels of the spine. (Adapted from White AA III, Panjabi MM: *Clinical biomechanics of the spine,* Philadelphia, 1978, JB Lippincott.)

The *final degrees of lumbar flexion* is even more important than the range of motion of the lumbar spine. Studies using inclinometers positioned over L1 (with the appropriate subtraction of the number of degrees of hip flexion) indicate an average final flexed position between 20 and 25 degrees.[10] The final degree of lumbar flexion curvature is a more important value than the range of motion, because initial alignment is a major factor in the range-of-motion measurement. The range-of-motion value is based on the lumbar spine aligned at the starting position in approximately 20 to 30 degrees of extension. Consequently, when the range of motion is 50 degrees, the lumbar spine reaches a maximum flexion curvature of 20 degrees. In the patient with a flat back, a lumbar alignment in standing of 0 degrees and the same total range of motion of 50 degrees are both dangerous. There are two important questions to ask.

1. Is the lumbar spine reversing its curve and becoming flat?
2. Is the lumbar spine flexing beyond the optimal anatomic limits and therefore excessively stretching the posterior supporting tissues?

In addition to the issues of total range of motion of the lumbar spine and maximal degree of lumbar flexion is the motion of each vertebral segment. White and Panjabi report the flexion-extension range between the vertebral segments is approximately 4 degrees in the upper thoracic spine, 6 degrees in the midthoracic spine, and 12 degrees in the lower thoracic spine. The motion between the vertebral segments in the upper lumbar spine is approximately 12 degrees, and then it increases approximately 1 degree for each lower segment, reaching

the maximum range of motion of 20 degrees between L5 and S1[56] (Figure 3-14).

In maximum flexion, the erector spinae muscles become inactive, and thus the stress is on the passive elements of the muscles and ligaments.[14] Approximately 20 minutes of stretching at the end of flexion increases the range by 5 degrees, which is attributed to the creep properties of the soft tissues. Approximately 50% of the original stiffness is recovered within 2 minutes after resuming normal alignment. However, longer than 30 minutes is required to recover the normal amount of soft-tissue stiffness.[31] These findings support the concept that sustained positions can alter the properties of soft tissues and can become contributing factors to altered alignment.

Impairments

A final flexed position greater than 25 to 30 degrees is excessive lumbar flexion. Also considered an impairment is lumbar flexion greater than 50% of its total range before any amount of hip flexion is observed. Esola and associates report that subjects with low back pain move more in the lumbar spine than at the hips during the 30- to 60-degree phase of forward bending.[12] Another factor contributing to mechanical low back pain is the failure of all segments to maintain their contribution to motion. When failing to do so, the consequence of such failure is that the other segments move more than their optimal range of motion (Figure 3-15). Because of these compensatory motions, exercises must be carefully performed, ensuring against some segments becoming hypermobile while others remain hypomobile. Based on

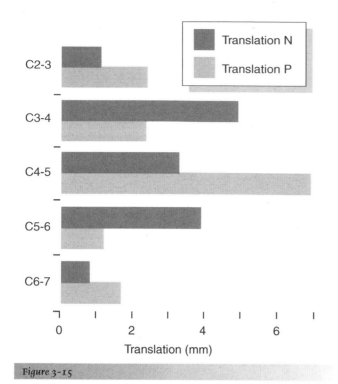

Figure 3-15

Ranges of sagittal plane translation for flexion-extension motion. Restricted motion at C5-6 is associated with excessive motion at C4-5. *N*, Normal; *P*, Pathologic. (From Singer KP, Fitzgerald D, Milne N: Neck retraction exercises and cervical disk disease. In Singer KP, editor: *Integrating approaches.* Proceedings of the Eighth Biennial Conference of the Manipulative Physiotherapists Association of Australia, 1993, Perth Western Australia.)

the concept of relative flexibility, which proposes that the least stiff segment moves more readily than stiffer segments, developing a program that improves the mobility of restricted segments in the multisegmental spine is a challenge. Even when the stiffest segment is passively moved, for that movement to occur during activity, the segment has to move as easily as the most flexible segment. Alignments at the end of the forward bending motion are illustrated in Figure 3-16.

Typically, men tend to flex more readily in the lumbar spine, and women flex more easily in the hips. In a study by Thomas and associates,[51] subjects in a standing position are asked to perform two reaching tasks using two different target heights. Men move more in the spine than in the hips (spine/hip ratio is 1:20) and women move more in the hips than the spine (spine/hip ratio is 0:20). These ratios are not end-range motions, but they demonstrate that initial movement patterns vary and can be sex specific. The report of these movement patterns supports the belief that patients need to be retrained to move correctly and that these sites of movement are not determined by reaching the limits of a muscle's length.

Return from Flexion

Normal

The return from forward bending can also be a factor in the patient's pain. As with forward bending, a variety of strategies are used. During the return from forward bending, ideally the initial part of the motion should be hip extension, and then both the hips and spine should concurrently continue their extension motions until the patient is in the upright position (see Figure 2-12). Because the range of hip motion is 70 to 80 degrees and the range of the lumbar motion averages between 30 to 50 degrees, the hips move more than the spine. The motions should be smooth and relatively concurrent versus consecutive, other than during the initiation of the motion with hip extension.

Impairments

With the motion initiated at the lumbar spine or immediately after a short period of hip extension, the return from forward bending is an impairment found in some patients who have pain caused by extension (see Figure 2-12). This type of motion increases the compressive forces on the spine.[34] When a patient with low back pain demonstrates this type of motion, he or she often performs daily activities with only a few degrees of repeated lumbar flexion and extension motions. The movements are confined to the lumbar spine instead of the hip joints, which should be the site of motion.

Another type of impairment associated with the return from forward bending is exaggerated forward sway of the hips and ankles, which reduces the load on the hip. This type of return from forward bending is primarily found in the individual with a swayback posture who has weak hip extensors.

Extension

Normal

Extension of the lumbar spine is an increase in the anterior curve. According to Kendall, the range is highly variable; consequently, a standard for reference measurement is difficult to establish.[27] The reported value for the maximum lumbar extension curve is approximately 50 degrees.[59] When considering functional activities, there is not a demand for a large range of motion into extension.

Impairments

The problems arising from impairments of the lumbar spine stem more from excessive extension stresses that are focused on one or two spinal segments than from the lack of range of motion. The back extensor muscles, which restrain lumbar flexion, are located on the posterior aspect of the spine. In contrast, the abdominal muscles, which restrain lumbar extension, are located on

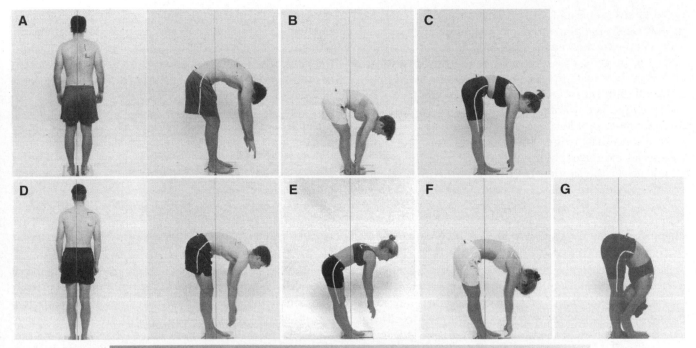

Figure 3-16

Examples of different alignments at the end of forward bending. *A,* Body proportions of long trunk relative to length of lower body. Hips shift backward, range-of-hip flexion is limited, knees are slightly flexed and lower thoracic spine flexion is slightly excessive. This forward bending pattern is necessary to keep the center of gravity in the base of support. *B,* Hips are shifted backward and knees are slightly flexed, which allows the center of gravity to remain centered in base of support even though the trunk is long. *C,* Normal hip flexion, lumbar spine is flat, just reversing its curve, excessive thoracic flexion. *D,* Body proportions of short trunk relative to length of lower body cause normal hip flexion range of motion with slightly increased lumbar flexion. *E,* Marked backward shifting of hips with sway from ankle, limited hip and trunk flexion is demonstrated. This pattern is consistent with shortness of the gastrocnemius muscles and a stiff spine. *F,* Reversal of the lumbar curve so that the lumbar spine is flat with excessive thoracic flexion. *G,* Excessive hip flexion flexibility.

the anterior surface of the abdomen. The location of the abdominal muscles is much further away from the site of the motion than that of the back extensor muscles. Studies on the spinal motion segment and the adjoining vertebrae and interposed disk have shown that the spinous processes, disks, and apophyseal joints are primary restraints to hyperextension.[1] Hyperextension, like hyperflexion, damages the interspinous ligaments and can cause sudden disk prolapse and long-term structural damage to the disks.[1] Although the anterior longitudinal ligament is not considered strong enough to resist large extension forces,[52] anatomically it should contribute to the prevention of an extension alignment of the lumbar spine. As the disks degenerate, the anterior longitudinal ligament is no longer pulled as taut as when the disks are at full height, thus compromising the extension restraint from this ligament. Spinal stenosis is relatively common in the individual older than the age of 65 and is another example of a problem associated with lumbar extension. Even without structural changes in the spine, extension movements significantly decrease the central canal area and the midsagittal and

subarticular sagittal diameters, whereas flexion has the opposite effect.[23] These findings support the concept of dynamic stenosis, in addition to the well-accepted concept of static stenosis caused by degenerative and hypertrophic structural changes.

The repeated hyperextension performed by gymnasts is cited as a cause of low back pain[41,42] and spondylolysis.[24] Active back extension, in particular, and, to a lesser extent, simultaneous shoulder and hip extension performed in the quadruped position cause high levels of compression forces.[5] When the abdominal muscles are taut, limiting the excursion of the thoracic spine, the extension movement primarily occurs in the lower lumbar spinal segments rather than throughout all of the lumbar segments.

Rotation

Normal

The overall range of lumbar rotation is calculated to be approximately 13 degrees. The rotation between each vertebral segment from T10 to L5 is 2 degrees. The greatest rotational range is between L5 and S1, which is 5 degrees (see Figure 3-14). The vertical orientation in the transverse plane and the 45-degree angle orientation in the frontal plane of the facet joints are the reasons for limiting the rotational range in the lumbar spine.[56] In contrast, greater range of rotation at the lumbosacral joint is possible because of the oblique orientation of its facet joints.[30] The thoracic spine, not the lumbar spine, should be the site of the greatest amount of rotation of the trunk. When an individual practices rotational exercises, he or she should be directed to "think about the motion occurring in the area of the chest" and not the waist.

Impairments

Stiffness or shortness of the oblique abdominal muscles restricts the rotational motion (Figure 3-17). Some patients with low back pain have asymmetry in the appearance of the lumbar paraspinal muscles, which can be reliably detected if the side-by-side difference is $1/2$ inch or greater.[54] Asymmetry is attributed to either a postural rotation of the lumbar spine to one side or a greater bulk of the paraspinal muscles on one side. When differential muscle development causes the asymmetry, lateral flexion to the side opposite the larger muscle is more limited than lateral flexion toward the same side. The reason for this asymmetry in motion is the greater stiffness of the larger muscle. If the paraspinal asymmetry is the result of postural rotation, the lateral flexion movement pattern is restricted range of motion to the same side as the asymmetry and normal range of motion to the opposite side.

Studies by Pearcy show that the greatest amount of rotation occurs when an individual is in a sitting position and the lumbar spine is flexed and the supporting tissues are relaxed.[43,44] Rotational ranges of $3 1/2$ degrees have been shown to tear the annulus of the disk.[43,44] Based on clinical observations, one of the greatest contributors to excessive rotation of the lumbar spine is repetitive rotational motion while sitting at a desk. Many individuals rotate the trunk to get to a computer, to answer the telephone, to open file drawers, or to reach an adjacent counter. In the sitting position the lumbosacral junction is most vulnerable to repeated stretching by the rotational activities. Sports, such as golf, racquetball, and squash, are the most common contributors to excessive rotation of the lumbar spine, particularly because the feet are planted during the motion. Tennis and volleyball do not contribute as much to rotational problems because the feet are not fixed at the time of rotation and the whole body is used in the follow-through motion.

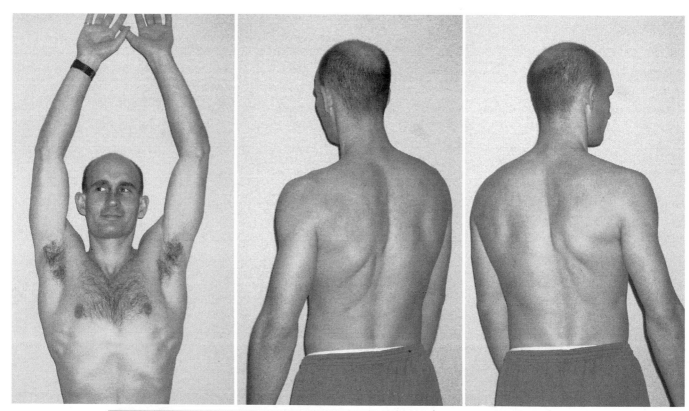

Figure 3-17

Shortness of the abdominal muscles, the external oblique muscles on one side, and the internal oblique muscles on the other side limit the range of motion of trunk rotation. The asymmetry and the subcostal angle are demonstrated.

Rotation of the pelvis precipitating rotation at the lumbosacral joints is another factor. When muscles such as the tensor fascia lata (TFL) or other hip flexors become short, the restraint for hip extension imposed by these muscles often causes compensatory pelvic rotation during the stance phase of gait. The rotation of the pelvis causes motion to occur at the lumbosacral junction and not throughout the thoracic spine, as should occur during gait. Unilateral shortness of the TFL muscle can be a particularly important contributor to excessive pelvic rotation because of its hip medial rotation and flexion action. When the TFL is short, it can act as a major source of restraint to both hip extension and lateral rotation during the stance phase of gait.

Lateral Flexion or Side Bending

Normal

The range of motion of lateral flexion or side-bending range is reported to be greatest (8 to 9 degrees) in the lower thoracic segments because they are not restricted by the ribs. The average degrees of lateral flexion for the other thoracic segments and for the lumbar vertebrae is 6, except for the lumbosacral segment, which has only 3 degrees of lateral flexion.[56] Lateral flexion is associated with rotation of the lumbar vertebrae toward the convexity of the curve. With lateral flexion occurring to the right, the rotation of the lumbar vertebrae is to the left. In the thoracic spine, the coupled motion causes rotation of the vertebrae toward the side of the concavity.[57] Based on 6 degrees of motion at each lumbar segment, the total motion from L1 to S1 is 27 degrees. Although limited by the ribs, the thoracic lateral flexion has a potential greater than 75 degrees, depending on the number of vertebral segments of the thoracic spine, participating in the motion.

The greater excursion of the thoracic spine compared with the lumbar spine raises the question of the usefulness of the assessment in which the excursion of the fingers along the side of the leg is used as an indication of lumbar lateral flexion motion. Because more than three fourths of the motion originates from the thoracic spine, it seems questionable to assume that any limitation of motion is secondary to restriction of the lumbar spine. What may be more useful than the excursion of the hand are observations of the shape of the curve and the axis of motion of the lumbar spine. During an optimal pattern of lateral flexion, the lumbar spinal segments bend and form a smooth curve.

Impairments

Because the motions of rotation and lateral flexion are coupled, impairments of the alignment or the motion of one of these movements affects the other. For example, if the lumbar spine is malaligned causing it to be rotated to one side, lateral flexion to that side is limited. If the spine rotates to the right posturally, the lateral flexion motion is limited because the spine is unable to rotate to the left as necessary for the side-bending motion. In contrast, lateral flexion to the left is performed without restriction because the spine is already rotated to the right.

Another sign of lateral flexion impairment is evident when, during the motion, the lumbar spine appears straight with an axis of rotation at only one segment rather than a relatively smooth curve throughout the entire lumbar spine. Most often this type of motion occurs at the lower lumbar segments in the individual who has well-developed lumbar paraspinal muscles. One explanation is that the stiffness of the hypertrophied paraspinal muscles restricts the excursion of these muscles; consequently, motion occurs at the interface of the musculotendinous junction, which is at approximately L4-5 and S1. Support of this hypothesis is found when resistance is applied to the lateral trunk at the level of the lower lumbar segments on the side to which the lateral flexion is performed. With support preventing the motion at the lowest lumbar segments, the lumbar spine demonstrates a lateral curve rather than a straight line. The explanation is that the paraspinal muscles are stiffer than the musculotendinous junction. Rather than allow the motion to occur at the site of least resistance, blocking this site forces the paraspinal muscles to stretch, allowing motion to occur at the other lumbar segments (Figure 3-18, *A* and *B*). Some patients are unable to flex laterally when motion is prevented at the lumbosacral junction (Figure 3-18, *C-F*).

Translation Motion

Normal

Translation occurs as part of the complex motions of the spine that accompany flexion, extension, rotation, and lateral flexion. As with rotation motions, translation motions involve shear forces, which are often the most damaging to tissues.

Impairments

Instabilities are most often associated with impairments of translation motions. Spondylolisthesis, which is a forward slipping of one vertebra in relation to another, is an exaggeration of translation motion in the sagittal plane. Anterior shear forces that are generated by the psoas muscle contribute to excessive translation motion of the vertebrae. Excessive translation motion contributes to spinal stenosis.

Compression

Although compression is not a motion of the lumbar spine, compression forces are altered by muscle position and contraction, as well as during changes in position and during activities such as carrying objects. When the disk is normal, the vertebral body or endplate

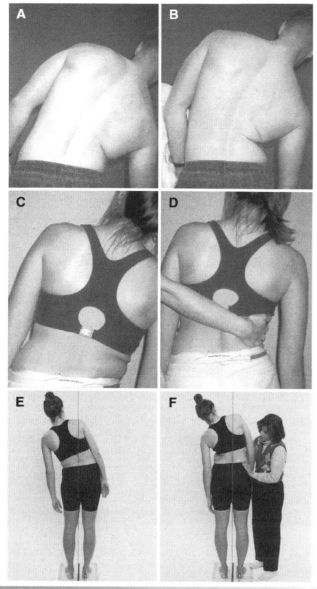

Figure 3-18

The effect of stiffness or shortness of the paraspinal muscles on the range and pattern of lateral flexion of the trunk. *A,* Young man with well-developed erector spinae muscles is shown. When side bending, the axis of motion is at the low lumbar spine at the level of the iliac crest. *B,* When the therapist provides stabilization on the lateral side of the thorax at the level of the iliac crest during side bending, the entire lumbar spine appears to have a smooth curve. The change in the curve indicates that the erector spinae are stiff but not short. Movement at the lowest lumbar segment is because this path offers the least resistance for lateral flexion. *C,* Young woman with low back pain is depicted. When side bending to the left, the motion is restricted to the lumbar spine at the level of the iliac crest. The rest of her spine remains straight. *D,* When stabilized at the level of the iliac crest, subject is unable to side bend, indicating that her erector spinae muscles are short. *E,* The same woman 4 months later no longer has back pain as long as she is careful. Side bending is still characterized by movement at the lowest lumbar segment and now occurs primarily in the thoracic spine. *F,* When stabilized the subject is able to side bend by moving the thoracic rather than the lumbar spine. She can also move in the thoracic spine without lumbar spine stabilization. By limiting her motion to the thoracic spine, the subject eliminates the back pain.

will fracture before the disk is damaged[11]; however, when the disk is degenerated or damaged, compression is an important contributing factor to the patient's symptoms. For example, a patient may have radiating symptoms when sitting but not when recumbent, standing, or walking. Further, when he or she sits in lumbar extension, the symptoms are often eliminated. Sitting with an increased curve decreases the compression on the disk because part of the force is distributed to the facet joints (Figure 3-19). The facet joints share 30% of the total load when the spine is hyperextended.[28] Compression is less when the patient is recumbent, standing, and walking than when sitting. Walking at a fast rate can increase the compressive load to 2.5 times the body weight on the spine at L3-4, whereas walking at a slow rate keeps the compressive load close to body weight.[6]

Summary

The alignment of the spine affects the forces on the spine and the degree of muscular activity. The movements of the spine are complex and multidirectional, even when motion seems to be occurring in a specific direction. Because movements of the spine involve multiple segments, it becomes difficult to both assess the dysfunction and develop exercise programs that will ensure optimal participation of each segment in the motion. As stated by Nordin, "Restriction of motion of one part of the spine causes increased motion of another part

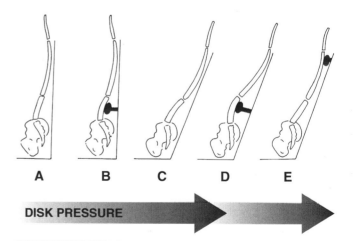

DISK PRESSURE

Figure 3-19

Change in pressure on the lumbar spine in different sitting positions. *A,* Backrest inclination is 90 degrees, and disk pressure is at a maximum. *B,* Lumbar support decreased disk pressure. *C,* Backward inclination of the backrest to 110 degrees but with no lumbar support produces less disk pressure. *D,* Lumbar support with this degree of backrest inclination further decreases the pressure. *E,* Shifting the support to the thoracic region pushes the upper body forward, moving the lumbar spine toward kyphosis and increasing disk pressure. (Adapted from Andersson GBJ, Ortengren R, Nachemson A, Elfstrom C: Lumbar disc pressure and myoelectric back muscle activity during sitting. I. Studies on an experimental chair, *Scand J Rehab Med* 6:104, 1974.)

of the spine."[39] It is difficult to develop exercise programs that will provide stability of the spine, prevent compensatory motions, and improve the strength and control of the trunk musculature without causing undesirable compressive or shear forces or without contributing to malalignment of the spine. Correction of subtle malalignments, compensatory motions, or stress imposed on the spine, particularly when localized to a few segments by daily activities, is the key to remediation of mechanical low back pain. Therefore the therapist must become proficient at observing the subtle deviations in movement patterns at specific segments and must not simply focus on overall excursions of motion.

Muscular Actions of the Lumbar Spine

Back Muscles

Latissimus Dorsi

The latissimus dorsi is the most superficial of the back muscles and has a broad attachment through the thoracolumbar fascia from the lower six thoracic spinous processes, all of the lumbar spinous processes and sacrum, and the iliac crest. The fibers then converge superiorly and laterally to attach to the humerus (Figure 3-20). The thoracolumbar fascial attachment of the latissimus dorsi muscle provides the mechanism for this muscle to affect the lumbopelvic alignment. Contraction of the latissimus dorsi muscle creates an extension force on the spine and tilts the pelvis anteriorly. If the muscle is short, the back extends as a compensatory movement when shoulder flexion stretches the muscle to the limits of its length. Consistent with the concept of relative flexibility, if the latissimus dorsi is stiffer than the abdominal muscles, which limit lumbar extension, the back extends when the latissimus dorsi stretches, even when the muscle is not short. In the patient with low back pain that occurs with extension, the shortness or stiffness of this muscle contributes to pain when he or she reaches over head.

Erector Spinae

The muscles that make up the erector spinae group are the iliocostalis, which is situated the most lateral, the longissimus, and the spinalis, which is situated the most medial of the group (Figure 3-21). Bogduk and Macintosh provide useful insights into the actions of the erector spinae muscles. Their studies describe the superficial and deep divisions of this group, and they provide a detailed analysis of the variations in forces generated by these two divisions.[2]

SUPERFICIAL GROUP. The lateral iliocostalis muscles and the medial longissimus group make up the superficial division. These muscles attach to the thora-

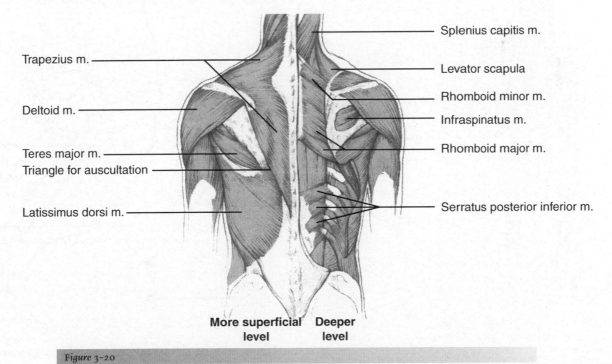

Trapezius m.

Deltoid m.

Teres major m.

Triangle for auscultation

Latissimus dorsi m.

Splenius capitis m.

Levator scapula

Rhomboid minor m.

Infraspinatus m.

Rhomboid major m.

Serratus posterior inferior m.

More superficial level   **Deeper level**

Figure 3-20

Superficial back muscles. On the left are the more superficial back muscles, including latissimus dorsi and trapezius muscles. On the right, slightly deeper muscles are found, including the serratus posterior inferior and oblique muscles of the abdominal wall. (From Mathers et al: *Clinical anatomy principles,* St Louis, 1996, Mosby.)

columbar fascia and insert cranially into the ribs. As discussed by Porterfield and DeRosa, the muscle bulk of these superficial erector spinae muscles is lateral to the spinous processes and is found only in the mid-to-upper lumbar spine.[46] The superficial group runs superiorly and posteriorly from the pelvis to the ribs. Therefore they are pulled taut when the pelvis tilts anteriorly or when the spine shifts backward or rotates to the same side. These muscles have an optimal lever arm for producing extension of the lumbar spine, even though they do not attach to the lumbar spine. According to the study by Bogduk, between 40% and 80% of the total extensor moment on the lumbar spine is exerted by the superficial fibers of the iliocostalis and longissimus muscles, whose fibers attach at the thoracic level and only to the erector spinae aponeurosis. More specifically, the thoracic erector spinae muscles contribute 50% of the extensor moment, influencing L4-5, and 70%

to 80% of the extensor moment affects the upper lumbar spine.[2] Contraction of these muscles also produces anterior pelvic tilt.

DEEP GROUP. The deep division originates from the ilium and deep surface of the thoracolumbar fascia, and it inserts into the transverse processes of the lower lumbar vertebrae. The course of the muscle fibers is superior, medial, and anterior; as a result, the major forces produced by contracting the deep group is compression and posterior shear or, perhaps more accurately, the prevention of anterior shear (Figure 3-22). Because the bellies of these muscles lay close to the spinous processes, they can be palpated through the thoracolumbar fascia. Tension in these muscles is important in counterbalancing the anterior shear forces generated by the iliopsoas muscles or the translation motion during activities such as forward bending.[46] According to Bogduk, when the patient is in the upright posture, the lumbar back extensors produce a posterior shear on L1-4 and an anterior shear on L5.[2] Bogduk believes that extension exercises performed in any position can be injurious when compression contributes to the patient's

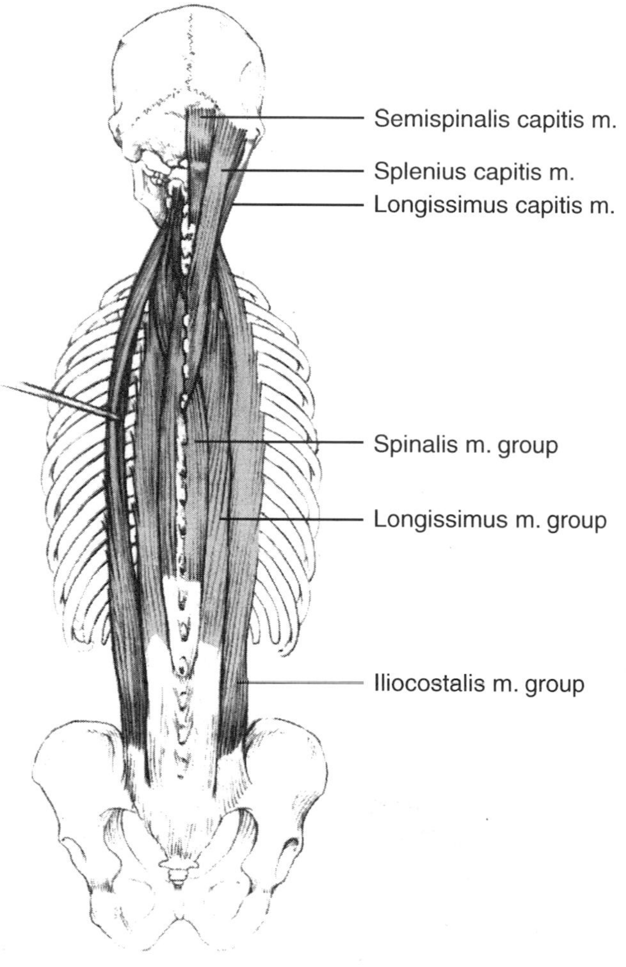

Semispinalis capitis m.

Splenius capitis m.

Longissimus capitis m.

Spinalis m. group

Longissimus m. group

Iliocostalis m. group

Figure 3-21

The large longitudinal set of muscles of the back, located between the midline and angles of ribs, are the erector spinae. (From Mathers et al: *Clinical anatomy principles,* St Louis, 1996, Mosby.)

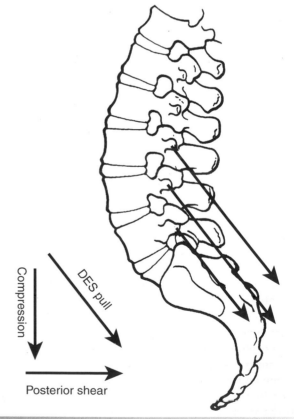

Figure 3-22

Line of pull is caused by the orientation of the deep erector spinae muscle. Since it attaches close to the axis of lumbar motion, it provides a dynamic posterior shear force and a compression force. (From Porterfield JA, Derosa C: *Mechanical low back pain: perspectives in functional anatomy,* Philadelphia, 1998, WB Saunders.)

condition and particularly when translatory instability of the lumbar spine is present. Based on Bogduk's studies, McGill also advises against extension motions performed at the end of the range.[34]

Multifidus

Although the multifidus is classified as a transversospinal muscle, its designation does not consider the fact that it originates from the dorsal surface of the sacrum, the sacrotuberous ligament, the erector spinae aponeurosis, the posterior superior iliac spine, and the posterior sacroiliac ligaments (Figure 3-23). The multifidus muscle covers the surface of sacrum and then runs superiorly and medially to attach to the spinous processes of the sacral and lumbar vertebrae. The multifidus fills the channels between the sacrum and ilium and between the lumbar spinous and transverse processes.[46] Thus when there is prominence of soft tissue along the paraspinal area, it is primarily the muscle bulk of the multifidus. The normal bulk of this muscle makes it virtually impossible to palpate the transverse processes of the lumbar vertebrae.

Because of its attachment to the spinous processes, the multifidus has a longer lever arm for producing extension than do the erector spinae muscles that attach to the transverse processes. The most important action of the multifidus is controlling the flexion and anterior shear of the spine during forward bending via its eccentric contraction. The multifidus is not an important contributor to rotation, but its activity during rotation counterbalances the flexion forces generated by the abdominal muscles, which are the primary rotators of the trunk.[46] Similar to other back extensor muscles, the multifidus exerts a compressive force on the lumbar spine, which contributes to the stability of the spine. Hide and colleagues report that the patient who, after the first episode of unilateral low back pain, has atrophy of the multifidus on the symptomatic side requires a program of exercises designed to recover muscle bulk.[19] When compression contributes to patient's symptoms, contraction of the back extensors accentuates the problem.

Interspinales and Intertransversarii

As suggested by their names, the interspinales and intertransversarii are small muscles that run between the spinous and transverse processes of the vertebrae. The interspinales are believed to contribute to extension, and the intertransversarii affect extension and lateral flexion. Because these muscles are small, their contributions to these motions are limited. Of greater significance is the proprioceptive role of these muscles, which have four to seven times the number of muscle spindles as the multifidus.[38]

Quadratus Lumborum

Although the quadratus lumborum muscle (Figure 3-24) is significantly smaller than the back extensors, its attachments suggest that the quadratus lumborum plays an important role in lumbopelvic motion, especially in stabilizing the spine—a belief that is shared by McGill.[32] One portion of the quadratus attaches to both the iliac crest and transverse processes, whereas another portion runs from the iliac crest to the ribs. The quadratus lumborum is optimally situated to provide control of lat-

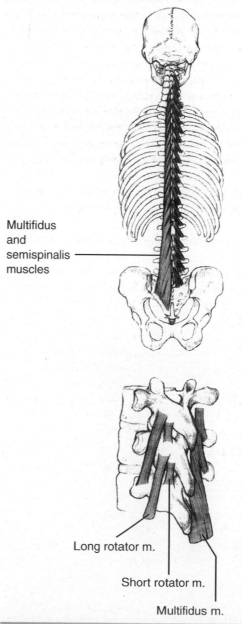

Multifidus and semispinalis muscles

Long rotator m.

Short rotator m.

Multifidus m.

Figure 3-23

Transversospinal muscles. Deep to erector spinae is the transversospinal group of muscles. (From Mathers et al: *Clinical anatomy principles,* St Louis, 1996, Mosby.)

eral flexion to the contralateral side via its eccentric contraction and to provide control of the return from lateral flexion via its concentric contraction. The muscle is also positioned to play a role in the rotation that occurs between the pelvis and spine during walking.

Iliopsoas

The iliopsoas muscle originates on the anterior surfaces of the transverse processes of all the lumbar vertebrae, the sides of the vertebral bodies, and the intervertebral disks of the last thoracic and all lumbar vertebrae[27] (see Figure 3-24). The action of the iliopsoas is to flex the hip. When the proximal attachments are stabilized, the thigh is moved to the chest. When the distal attachment is fixed, the hip is flexed by moving the spine and pelvis toward the thigh. Based on his anatomic studies, Bogduk does not believe the attachment of the psoas muscle has a long enough lever to act as a prime flexor of the lumbar spine. His analysis indicates that in the erect posture the psoas exerts an extensor moment on the upper lumbar spine and a flexor moment on the lower segments. These moments are exaggerated when the spine is extended, whereas all moments on the lumbar segments tend to be flexion when the spine is flexed.[3] The forces that have substantial magnitude are those of anterior shear and compression.[3]

Studies by Santaguida show that the psoas can flex laterally and, by compression, stabilize the lumbar spine.[48] Juker and colleagues' electromyographic (EMG) studies of the iliopsoas and abdominal muscles during a variety of exercises provide useful information to guide the development of programs for the patient with low back dysfunction. Among the important points of the study are the following:

1. The iliopsoas participates as strongly during sit-up exercises performed with the hips and knees flexed as when they are extended.
2. The psoas muscle is activated during push-up exercises, but abdominal muscular activity is minimal.
3. The rectus abdominis muscle is more strongly activated than the oblique muscles during curl-up exercises.
4. Maximum activity of the psoas occurs with resisted hip flexion.
5. Cross-curl exercises activate the oblique muscles only slightly and not significantly more than curl-up exercises do.[25]

The clinical implications of these studies are to minimize iliopsoas activity in the exercise program when compression and anterior shear are the sources of the patient's pain. Compression and anterior shear also need to be minimized when extension is the cause of pain. The patient must be taught to alter significantly their daily activities. Considerations include teaching the patient to (1) slide the lower extremity by pushing the foot along the bed and not lifting the lower extremity off the bed when supine, (2) roll without lifting the lower extremity, (3) use the hand to flex the hip passively when side lying, and (4) use the hand to lift the lower extremity when getting into a car. Any exercise that uses the hip flexors should be avoided. Juker's studies also indicate that there is activity of the psoas muscle when the patient sits without support.[25]

Many patients prefer to lie supine with the hips and knees supported in the flexed position (Figure 3-25). This position is consistent with a reduction of compression and anterior shear forces exerted by the psoas muscle and thus reduces symptoms. The straight-leg raise used for nerve tension signs is also affected by iliopsoas activity. When a patient tests positive for nerve tension when contracting his or her hip flexor muscles, the symptoms are often alleviated once the therapist supports the weight of the patient's lower extremity while instructing the patient to totally relax his or her musculature. This finding suggests that the problem is the effect of shear or compression on the spine and not a true entrapment of the nerve. Even in the quadruped position when rocking backward toward the heels, contraction of the hip flexor muscles can contribute to symptoms. This becomes evident when the patient is instructed to rock backward by pushing with his or her hands rather than by flexing the hips. With this change in the production of the movement, symptoms are diminished or alleviated.

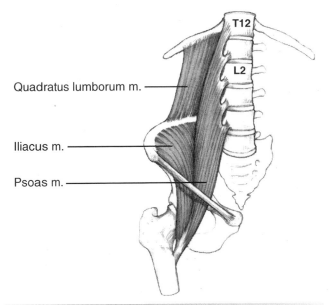

Quadratus lumborum m.

Iliacus m.

Psoas m.

T12

L2

Figure 3-24

Iliopsoas muscle. The iliacus and psoas major have different origins but unite distally to form a common insertion into the lesser trochanter of the femur. (From Mathers et al: *Clinical anatomy principles*, St Louis, 1996, Mosby.)

In summary, any stress created by the iliopsoas muscle, even with minimal activity, can be an important contributor to the symptoms of the patient with low back dysfunction. Therefore the therapist needs to examine carefully the contribution that the activity or the stretch of this muscle is having on patient's symptoms and provide appropriate instruction to counteract the effects of psoas activity by abdominal contraction or recommend changes in the movement patterns.

Abdominal Muscles

Strengthening the abdominal muscles has interested the general public and those involved in rehabilitation. This interest is attributable, in part, to the appearance of the sought-after flat abdomen and, in part, to what is assumed to be protection of the spine. However, many people with strong abdominal muscles develop back pain with an over-zealous approach. Often the programs designed to strengthen abdominal muscles will, in fact, contribute to muscle imbalances and pain syndromes. The most important aspect of abdominal muscle performance is obtaining the control that is necessary to (1) appropriately stabilize the spine, (2) maintain optimal alignment and movement relationships between the pelvis and spine, and (3) prevent excessive stress and compensatory motions of the pelvis during movements of the extremities. In fact, Cholewicki and others report that only 2% to 3% of maximum voluntary activity of the abdominal muscles is necessary for stabilizing the spine during upright unloaded tasks.[7] Thus the selection and instruction of abdominal exercises for a patient with low back pain has to be based on an examination that not only assesses strength but also identifies the control that is needed and the direction and type of stresses that are contributing to the patient's symptoms.

Because of wide promotion in the media, many individuals perform various forms of curl (crunches), cross-curl (diagonal crunches), and sit-up exercises with the consequence of the rectus abdominis becoming the dominant abdominal muscle. The study by Juker and colleagues indicates that there is a greater percentage of rectus abdominis activity (68%) during the performance of sit-ups than there is external oblique activity (19%) or internal oblique activity (14%).[25] The dominance of the rectus abdominis often compromises the participation of the oblique abdominal muscles, particularly the external oblique. The primary disadvantage of improving the performance of the rectus abdominis and not the oblique muscles is that the rectus cannot produce or prevent rotation, and shortness or stiffness contributes to a thoracic kyphosis.

Although the EMG values reported by Juker suggest that the activity of external and internal oblique muscles are comparable during the sit-up, this study does not address the relative participation of these muscles during the different phases of the exercise. The anatomic arrangement of the muscles suggests that the internal oblique is the most active during the trunk-curl phase. The external oblique, though active, does not contribute to the actual trunk curl; rather, it contributes more to maintaining posterior pelvic tilt associated with the sit-up phase.

External Oblique

The origin of the anterior fibers of the external oblique is the external surface of ribs five through eight, and it inserts into the aponeurosis that terminates as the linea alba. The origin of the lateral fibers is the external surfaces of ribs nine through twelve; and the insertion is into the inguinal ligament, into the anterior superior iliac spine and pubic tubercle, and into the anterior half of the iliac crest (Figure 3-26). Consistent with the other abdominal muscles, the external obliques (lateral fibers), when acting bilaterally, flex the lumbar spine. The origin of this muscle from the rib cage and its insertion into the pelvis are consistent with the most effective action of this muscle, that is, the posterior tilt of the pelvis. As discussed by Kendall and colleagues, the external oblique is referred to as a lower abdominal muscle because its angle of pull controls the lower half of the body by tilting the pelvis posteriorly.[27] Acting with the contralateral internal oblique muscle, the external oblique produces rotation of the trunk. The lateral fibers can also tilt the pelvis laterally.

A

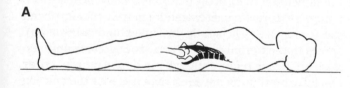

B

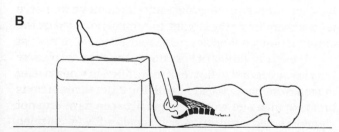

Figure 3-25

A, When a person assumes a supine position with legs straight, the pull of the vertebral portion of the psoas muscle produces anterior shear and compressive forces on the lumbar spine. *B,* When the hips and knees are bent and supported, the psoas muscle relaxes and the loads on the lumbar spine decrease. (Modified from Nordin M, Frankel VH: *Basic biomechanics of the musculoskeletal system,* 2 ed, Philadelphia, 1989, Lea & Febiger.)

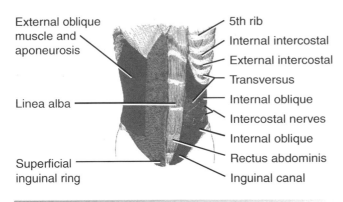

External oblique muscle and aponeurosis

Linea alba

Superficial inguinal ring

5th rib

Internal intercostal

External intercostal

Transversus

Internal oblique

Intercostal nerves

Internal oblique

Rectus abdominis

Inguinal canal

Figure 3-26

The abdominal muscles consist of the external obliques, which originate on the rib cage and insert into the pelvis and the aponeurosis of the rectus abdominis. The internal oblique muscles, whose fibers run perpendicular to the external obliques, originate on the pelvis and insert into the rib cage and the aponeurosis of the rectus abdominis. The rectus abdominis originates on the pelvis and inserts into the sternum. Deep to these muscles is the transversus muscle, whose fibers, as indicated by the name, run horizontally around the trunk. (From Jenkins DB: *Hollinshead's functional anatomy of the limbs and back,* 6 ed, Philadelphia, 1991, WB Saunders.)

During most daily activities, the primary role of the abdominal muscles is to provide isometric support and limit the degree of rotation of the trunk, which, as discussed, is restricted in the lumbar spine. A large percentage of low back problems occur because the abdominal muscles are not maintaining tight control over the rotation between the pelvis and the spine at the L5-S1 segment. Further, they are not preventing excessive anterior tilt of the pelvis or spine during activities that involve lower extremity musculature. In contrast, excessive abdominal muscle activity, shortness, or stiffness contributes to posterior pelvic tilt and lumbar flexion.

Because the external oblique muscle controls or prevents anterior pelvic tilt, as well as pelvic rotation when it acts with the contralateral internal oblique to control lateral pelvic tilt, an appropriate form of exercise is to challenge this control by moving the extremities. Before recommending an exercise that requires a strong contraction of the hip flexor muscles, the patient with low back pain should be able to lie supine with the hips and knees extended without symptoms. A reasonable hypothesis is that the anterior tilt of the pelvis, the extension of the spine, the anterior shear, or the compression associated with the hip flexor pull is the source of the pain; and this pull should be minimized. The abdominal muscles are the source to counteract this pull, but the program needs to be progressive, enabling abdominal muscular activity to prevent the alignment change or to control the stress that is inducing the symptoms. The exercise recommendations discussed in Chapter 7 outline a progressive program designed to im-

prove the performance of the external oblique muscle without excessive use of the hip flexors. Two important exercises for the patient with pain associated with lumbar extension are the following:

1. With the patient in the supine position with one hip and knee flexed, he or she slides the opposite extremity into extension and then extends the other lower extremity so that both lower extremities are extended.
2. With the patient in the standing position with the low back flat against the wall and with the hips and knees flexed, he or she tightens the external oblique muscles and then straightens the hips and knees while keeping the back flat.

The frequent performance of isometric contraction of the external oblique muscles while standing is an undervalued exercise that is effective and convenient. The trunk-curl and sit-up exercises are not effective exercises for the external oblique muscle. They enhance the participation of the rectus abdominis and internal oblique muscles, which interferes with the performance of the external oblique.

Another exercise that improves the performance of the lateral fibers of the oblique muscle is hip abduction in the side-lying position. The contraction of the hip abductors tilts the pelvis in a downward lateral direction, and the lateral abdominal muscles counteract the tilt. The patient must not abduct the contralateral hip for control of the pelvis to optimize the use of the lateral abdominal muscles. The interdigitation of the origin of the external oblique with the origins of the serratus anterior and latissimus dorsi muscles provides another avenue for inducing activity in the external oblique muscles. The patient performs upper extremity movements involving these muscles. The study by Juker and associates[25] shows that external oblique activity is greater during a push up, which requires activity in the serratus anterior and latissimus dorsi muscles, than it is with the curl exercise. Thus any resistive exercise that requires strong latissimus dorsi or serratus anterior activity is also a means to improve the isometric control provided by the external oblique muscles.

Based on clinical observations, the external oblique muscles are found to be weak more often in women than in men, which is consistent with the differences in body builds of men and women. Typically, men have broader shoulders and proportionately smaller lower extremities, whereas women have smaller upper bodies and proportionately larger lower extremities. Therefore greater demands are made on the external oblique muscles to control pelvic tilt in women than in men.

One sign of external oblique muscular weakness is a wide, greater than 90-degree, infrasternal angle. Zoeller and associates found the angle to be 83 degrees.[60]

The medial caudal oblique direction of the muscle fibers narrows the infrasternal angle when the muscle contracts. When the angle is excessively wide, the muscle may be stretched and lack normal stiffness. In contrast, when the infrasternal angle is markedly narrow, the external oblique muscle may be too short. To differentiate whether the angle is narrow because of structural variation rather than muscle shortness, the patient is instructed to flex the shoulders as far as possible and then take a deep breath. If there is no increase in the infrasternal angle, the muscle is likely to be too short.

Internal Oblique

The lower anterior fibers of the internal oblique muscles originate from the inguinal ligament and iliac crest near the anterior superior iliac spine, and they run transversely to insert into the crest of the pubis and linea alba. The upper anterior fibers originate from the anterior one third of the intermediate line of the iliac crest and run obliquely in a medial-oriented direction and upward to insert into the linea alba. The lateral fibers of the internal oblique originate from the middle one third of the intermediate line of the iliac crest and thoracolumbar fascia. They run in an oblique direction upwardly and medially to insert into the inferior borders of the lower three ribs and linea alba.[27] The anterior fibers support and compress the abdominal viscera and flex the vertebral column. Acting with the contralateral external oblique, the anterior fibers rotate the vertebral column. The lateral fibers flex the vertebral column and depress the thorax. Acting with the ipsilateral external oblique muscle, the lateral fibers flex the vertebral column laterally. Acting with the contralateral external oblique, they rotate the vertebral column.[27]

The internal oblique muscles are referred to as the upper abdominal muscles because of the direction of their line of pull, which is consistent with their most effective action, that is, the flexion of the upper half of the body. The trunk-curl exercise places greater demands on the internal oblique than on the external oblique. Because those teaching fitness frequently promote this exercise, the most common imbalance encountered in the individual who has performed abdominal exercises is an over development of the internal oblique and rectus abdominis muscles. A wide infrasternal angle may be the result of shortness of the internal oblique abdominal muscle.

Trunk-Curl Sit-Up Exercise

Recommending abdominal exercises that involve trunk flexion is too often a choice between an exercise that can be safely performed and one that is an optimal exercise for improving muscle performance. The safest trunk flexion exercise is the trunk curl with hips and knees flexed, especially for the individual who is participating in a class, who is not examined individually by a physical therapist, and who is not individually instructed. This recommendation is based on the belief that there is less chance of injury performing this exercise than there is with hip flexor muscular contraction without adequate counterbalancing abdominal muscular activity. Recommending and teaching the best exercise requires professional examination and instruction. An individual who performs a trunk-curl sit-up must be able to maintain the curl as he or she attempts to perform the sit-up component, which requires contraction of the hip flexors. Not only does the trunk curl sit-up require the abdominal muscles to maintain the trunk curl, but it also requires them to maintain the posterior pelvic tilt. The greatest demands are made on the abdominal muscles when the hip flexor action is initiated during the latter phase of the trunk curl at the start of hip flexion—the sit-up. Therefore limiting the exercise to the curl does not require maximum performance from the internal oblique muscle.

Kendall provides an excellent detailed analysis of the differences in performing the trunk-curl sit-up with the hips and knees extended versus the hips and knees flexed.[27] The study of Juker and associates[38] supports Kendall's assertion that the bent-knee sit-up does not eliminate iliopsoas activity. Because of the compression and anterior shear forces associated with contraction of the psoas muscle, proper determination of this exercise and proper instruction in exercise technique are essential to prevent injury to the spine. The most common error made in general instruction in the trunk curl is not matching the client's level of strength with the appropriate level of demand made by the exercise. Unfortunately, the prevailing belief is to instruct the client to perform the exercise at the hardest level at the beginning of the exercise program. Commercial promotions often demonstrate performance with the hands placed behind the head, which is the hardest level because the center of gravity is more superior than when the arms are at the sides or in front of the body. Placing the hands behind the head is also potentially dangerous, if the individual pulls or rotates the head too strongly, injuring the cervical spine or cervical arteries.

To design an optimal and safe exercise program that includes trunk-curl sit-ups, the following components should be assessed carefully:

1. How far can the patient curl? What is the passive flexibility of the patient's spine? Some individuals have stiff spines, others have flexible spines, and others fall between the two extremes. To determine the available range, the patient is placed in the supine position and the therapist passively curls the trunk to the point where the hips begin to flex.

2. Are the hip flexors short, and particularly is the iliopsoas muscle short? When the length of the hip flexor muscle does not allow enough posterior pelvic tilt to flatten the lumbar spine, the lumbar spine will remain in an inward curve, which contributes to the anterior shear forces on the lumbar vertebrae when the psoas muscle contracts.

3. When the patient initiates the trunk curl, does the pelvis tilt posteriorly? When the hip flexors are short, the pelvis is not able to tilt posteriorly. In another scenario, when the patient initiates the action with the hip flexors rather than with the abdominal muscles, the pelvis will not tilt posteriorly.

4. Can the patient curl to the limit of his or her spinal flexibility at the easiest level of the exercise, which is with the shoulders flexed and the elbows extended so that the arms are positioned in front of the thorax?

5. Does the patient curl to the same degree of trunk flexion when the level of the exercise is made more difficult by (a) folding the arms on the chest, and (b) placing the hands on top of the head? When the degree of trunk flexion is not maintained, the patient initiates the hip flexion sit-up phase too early and the abdominal muscles are not strong enough to perform at this level of the exercise.

6. Does the patient have a thoracic kyphosis? This exercise will contribute to the problem.

7. Does the patient maintain the curl at the initiation of the hip flexion phase? When the patient does not maintain the curl, the abdominal muscles are too weak to perform the exercise at the harder level and the anterior shear stress on the lumbar spine is exaggerated.

8. If the exercise is performed with the hips and knees flexed but the feet are not stabilized, the patient has to extend the hips to keep them from flexing during the hip flexion phase. When the hip flexors are contracting to curl the trunk, the only way the feet can stay on the supporting surface is by contracting the hip extensors. Juker and colleagues[38] found that when an individual pushes the feet into the ground during the sit-up, activity of the psoas muscle increases. To flex the hips, the psoas muscle has to contract more strongly to overcome the resistance from the active hip extension when the hips and knees are flexed rather than extended.

9. The trunk-curl sit-up is mechanically more difficult for men than it is for women because of the distribution of body mass.

10. When the trunk-curl sit-up is performed with the hips and knees flexed and the feet not stabilized, the axis of rotation is shifted to the lumbar spine, which can contribute to the development of excessive lumbar flexion. When the hips and knees are flexed, the patient has to reach a greater degree of hip flexion at the end of the sit-up than he or she must achieve when the hips and knees are extended. Because the patient has to increase the amount of hip extensor muscular activity, it becomes more difficult to flex the hips to achieve the vertical position of the pelvis. This problem is greater for men than it is for women.

11. When the feet are stabilized, does the patient initiate the hip flexion phase without completing the trunk-curl phase? The action of the hip flexors is enhanced when the feet are stabilized, thus enabling the muscle group to flex the hip with a straighter trunk when compared with a situation in which the distal attachment of the hip flexors is not stabilized.

12. The hands should not be positioned behind the head, because the patient may pull the head and neck into excessive flexion or rotate the head as a result of an asymmetrical pull of the hands. The hands should be on top of the head or at the side of the head to avoid the risk of injuring the neck.

13. The chin should be brought toward the Adam's apple, not to the chest. The action of cervical flexion should reverse the curve but not to the point of excessive flexion with the risk of anterior shear at the lowest cervical vertebra. The neck should not extend, which is the movement that occurs when the patient's face is aligned to look forward rather than downward (Figure 3-27). This method is frequently demonstrated on televised exercise programs and in many exercise videotapes. If the movement causes pain in the neck or down the arms, the exercise is contraindicated.

Diagonal curls should be performed with limited range involving only the thoracic spine; otherwise, diagonal curls are potentially harmful. Rotation of the lumbar spine is more dangerous than beneficial, and rotation of the pelvis and lower extremities to one side while the trunk remains either stable or is rotated to the opposite side is particularly dangerous. If the patient can rotate the hips (femur in the acetabulum) and not the pelvis, the exercise is acceptable. This form of the exercise promotes the stability of the pelvis and the flexibility of the hip joints, rather than contributing to excessive flexibility of the lower lumbar spine or pelvis in relation to the spine.

To improve the isometric performance of the abdominal muscles, the therapist instructs the patient in a supine position to use resistance to the arms while contracting the abdominal muscles. This is an effective and

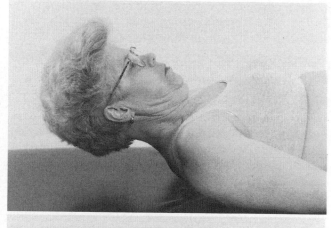

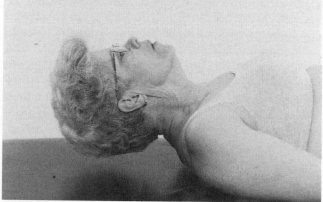

Figure 3-27

A, During the trunk curl, the cervical spine should also reverse its curve, as if the chin is moving toward the base of the neck. *B,* Incorrect movements include the head and chin remaining stationary or the cervical spine extending if the patient looks upward as the trunk curls.

safer strategy than curls and sit-ups. Many individuals develop strong abdominal muscles, even though they have not recently or have never performed trunk-curl or sit-up exercises. Proper use of the abdominal muscles during movements of the whole body and resistive exercises of the extremities are suitable stimuli for achieving adequate strength.

Also, some individuals have normal strength of both the internal and external oblique muscles and yet have poor control when these muscles have to work in a coordinated pattern to prevent rotation of the pelvis. The question of task specificity is applicable to all exercises. Does an exercise performed in one plane (e.g., the sagittal plane) or under one set of circumstances (e.g., lying supine) participate appropriately in a different circumstance (i.e., performing diagonal movements or performing exercises while standing erect).

Rectus Abdominis Muscle
The rectus abdominis muscle originates from the pubic crest and symphysis pubis. The fibers run vertically to insert onto the 5th, 6th, and 7th ribs and xiphoid process of the sternum.[27] The action of this muscle flexes the vertebral column and tilts the pelvis posteriorly, depending on which attachment is fixed. Because the rectus abdominis is contained in the sheath of the aponeurosis, which serves as the attachment for the other abdominal muscles, it is active when the other abdominal muscles are active. The study by Juker and colleagues indicate that during all flexion exercises, except for the isometric side support, there is a relatively high percentage of maximum voluntary activity in the rectus abdominis muscle.[25] As mentioned previously, shortness or stiffness of the rectus can contribute to a thoracic kyphosis. Dominance of the activity of the rectus abdominis over that of the oblique muscles can result in a compromise of the control of rotation.

Transversus Abdominis Muscle
The origin of the transversus abdominis muscle is the inner surfaces of the cartilage of the lower six ribs, the thoracolumbar fascia, the anterior three fourths of internal lip of the iliac crest, and the lateral one third of the inguinal ligament. The muscle fibers run transversely to insert into the linea alba, pubic crest, and pecten pubis.[27] The action of this muscle flattens the abdominal wall and compresses the abdominal viscera. Because the transversus abdominis muscle attaches to the thoracolumbar fascia, its contraction contributes to the stabilization of the lumbar spine.[13,33] The transversus muscle is the first abdominal muscle recruited for postural stabilization during movements of the upper or lower extremity in the erect position.[9,20] Hodges and associates suggest that the delayed onset of transversus activity plays a possible role in low back dysfunction in the patient with low back pain.[21] This delayed activity may cause inadequate stabilization of the lumbar spine during movements of the upper extremity. An effective method to activate the transversus muscle is instructing the patient to pull his or her navel toward the spine or attempt to narrow the waistline.[16]

Summary
Stabilizing the lumbar spine is an important part of a rehabilitation program for the patient with low back pain.[26] Some investigators and clinicians believe that control is the most important aspect of stabilization, which is related more to recruitment patterns and to timing and muscle endurance than it is to the strength achieved by nonspecific trunk flexion exercises. All abdominal muscles have a relatively unique role in providing the necessary level of stabilization, and the participation of these muscles needs to be balanced. The patient whose abdominal muscles test at 60% to 70% of normal strength has sufficient strength to perform most

daily activities safely. The focus of a program for this patient is the control of pelvic and trunk motion. For the patient whose abdominal muscle strength is below 60%, a program of exercises that progressively increases muscle strength is indicated. The challenge for the therapist is to devise a program that does not exert undesirable stresses on the lumbar spine. Unlike the neck muscles, there are no flexor muscles on the anterior surface of the spine. Consequently, the abdominal muscles are the only muscles that can prevent lumbar extension forces or stresses, as well as minimize anterior shear forces on the lumbar spine.

Movement Impairment Syndromes of the Low Back

The syndromes are named for the alignment, stress, or movement direction that most consistently produces pain. Not all patients have positive test findings for only one direction of movement, and some tests are more sensitive than they are specific. The intensity of the symptoms when movement is in a particular direction, the decrease of symptoms when movement is corrected, and the consistency of a movement direction that either increases or decreases the symptoms are all weighing factors in the tests that determine the appropriate diagnostic category (Box 3-1) (Chapter 3 Appendix).

Because of the variability of test results, *the examination is combinatorial rather than algorithmic.* Thus the therapist uses many tests to confirm or disconfirm a diagnosis, rather than using one test to serve as the key decision point. The purpose of an examination is to identify the diagnostic category and the contributing factors. For example, side bending is a test used to place the patient in a category, but testing the strength of the abdominal muscles is performed to identify a contributing factor, since weakness of the abdominal muscles is not specifically related to one diagnostic category.

In a study by Van Dillen and associates,[53] over 50% of the 169 patients tested are categorized as having an extension-rotation syndrome; the next largest group is categorized as having an extension syndrome. Patients

---

Box 3-1 Diagnostic Categories
(in order of observed frequency)

- Rotation-extension
- Extension
- Rotation
- Rotation-flexion
- Flexion

---

in this study have low back pain for a mean duration of 7 weeks. Most report previous episodes. Few are classified as having a flexion syndrome.

Lumbar Rotation-Extension Syndrome With or Without Radiating Symptoms

Symptoms and Pain

Degenerative conditions of the spine are caused by facet joint synovitis, hypermobility, progressive degeneration as a consequence of aging, or the repetitive trauma that is an inherent part of normal activity. Degenerative changes in the form of annular tears in the disks begin simultaneously with changes in the facet joint. A tear in the annulus leads to herniation. An enlargement of the facet joint occurs as the disk reabsorbs and spinal osteophytes form[22] (Figures 3-28 through 3-30). Consistent with the strategy used in the movement system balance (MSB) approach, the repetitive movements of normal activity that produce the trauma are identified, the contributing factors are eliminated, and the patient's movement patterns are altered. It is important to understand that the descriptions of the following specific pain problems detail pathologic dysfunctions at only one part of the joint. Changes in one part must be accompanied by changes in other parts of the motion segment because of their intimate relationship. Thus attempting to reduce undesirable stresses or movements is more effective than treating only one part of the motion segment in an exclusive manner. The specific pain problems or radiologic diagnoses that commonly coincide with the rotation-extension syndrome are the following:

1. Facet syndrome
2. Spinal stenosis
3. Spondylolisthesis
4. Spinal instability
5. Degenerative disk disease
6. Osteoarthritis of the lumbar spine
7. Herniated intervertebral disk

FACET SYNDROME. Commonly an early development in most degenerative conditions of the spine,[22] facet syndrome is a traumatic, degenerative, and inflammatory condition of the spinal articular joints that occurs after an irritation of its highly innervated joint capsular structures (Figure 3-31). Typically the complaints are an ache with prolonged inactivity, an improvement with an increase in activity, but perhaps a return of symptoms after activity. There can be transient sharp pains with sudden movements. The patient may report radiating symptoms, but they are not in a radicular pattern.[22]

SPINAL STENOSIS. Spinal stenosis is a narrowing of the spinal canal or the intervertebral foramen, which leads to vague and unusual symptoms (see Figures 3-28 through 3-30). This disorder is caused by the combination of disk degeneration, arthritis, and subluxation.[35]

Although more commonly found in the patient who is 65 years or older, some studies report this condition in patients as young as 40 years.[4,35] The classic characteristics of spinal stenosis are the presence of symptoms when standing or walking and almost immediate reduction of symptoms when sitting. The patient with spinal stenosis can usually stand and walk with minimal symptoms when they lean on a support to decrease the weight on the spine and increase the weight on the arms and upper torso (e.g., grocery cart).

SPONDYLOLISTHESIS. Spondylolisthesis is the forward slippage of one vertebra in relation to another. The patient with spondylolisthesis usually has back pain when maintaining one position and transient pain when changing positions. The most intense site of pain is usually in the back.

SPINAL INSTABILITY. Characteristically, the patient with spinal instability has pain with changes in position, but he or she cannot stay in one position for periods of time and tends to move frequently to achieve relief of the symptoms. Sitting is often worse than standing for symptom production.

DEGENERATIVE DISK DISEASE. For a disk to maintain its shock-absorbing properties, the nucleus must maintain normal hydration and the annulus fibrosus and vertebral end plate must be intact. When the water content of the nucleus diminishes and the gelatinous properties

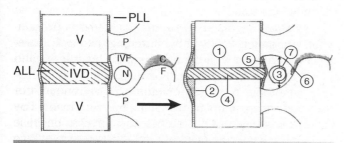

Figure 3-28

Sequence of degeneration—spondylosis. A normal functional unit *(left)*. Stages of degeneration *(right)*. *V,* Vertebra; *ALL,* anterior longitudinal ligament; *IVD,* intervertebral disk; *PLL,* posterior longitudinal ligament, *IVP,* intervertebral foramen; *P,* pedicle; *N,* nerve root; *C,* cartilage of the facet; *F,* facet; *1,* narrowing of the disk; *2,* formation of an osteophyte; *3,* narrowing of the foramen; *4,* sclerotic endplate changes; *5,* separation of the posterior longitudinal ligament from the vertebra; *6,* degenerative changes of the cartilage of the facet causing forminal stenosis; *7,* forminal stenosis leading to nerve root compression. (From Calliet R: *Low back pain syndrome,* 5 ed, Philadelphia, 1995, FA Davis.)

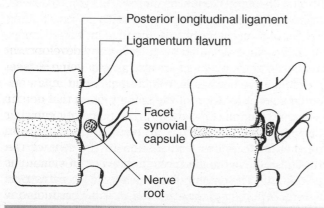

Figure 3-29

Invertebral foraminal nerve root impingement. A normal side view of the foramen and enclosed nerve root *(left)*. The degenerative changes, including osteophytes, thickened posterior longitudinal ligament, and facet changes that narrow the foramen *(right)*. (From Calliet R: *Low back pain syndrome,* 5 ed, Philadelphia, 1995, FA Davis.)

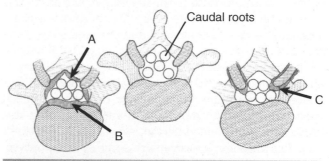

Figure 3-30

Spinal stenosis. The central figure depicts the caudal roots within a normal spinal canal. The left figure depicts total encroachment of the roots from hypertrophy of the lamina *(A)* and the posterior aspect of the vertebra *(B)*. The right figure shows encroachment of the root from hypertrophy of the facets *(C)*. (From Calliet R: *Low back pain syndrome,* 5 ed, Philadelphia, 1995, FA Davis.)

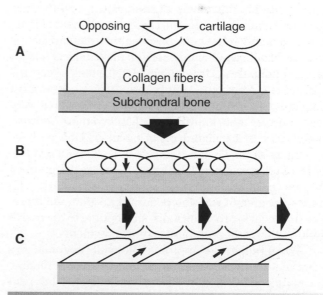

Figure 3-31

Shear deformation of cartilage. *A,* Opposing cartilages of a moving joint (facet) cause a curving deformation of the collagen fibers. *B,* This shearing force is augmented by compressive forces from gravity and muscular action. *C,* The shear effect has caused a degeneration of the collagen fibers. (From Calliet R: *Low back pain syndrome,* 5 ed, Philadelphia, 1995, FA Davis.)

are lost, the disk material becomes fibrocartilage; the fluid is no longer under pressure and does not function as a shock absorber. When the annulus remains intact, the mechanical stresses on the dysfunctional disk can cause back pain. The lumbosacral joint is the most frequent site of disk degeneration. A narrowing of the disk and the resulting change in the disk space contribute to segmental instability because the stabilizing ligaments are no longer taut. Pain is often worse when arising in the morning and may radiate into the lower extremities, although not along dermatomal pathways.

OSTEOARTHRITIS OF THE LUMBAR SPINE. The lumbar spine is a common site for degenerative changes in the patient older than 50 years of age. Osteoarthritis is characterized by the degeneration and thinning of the hyaline articular cartilage. When combined with thinning of the intervertebral disk, the joint space becomes narrow and irregular. The patient with osteoarthritis of the lumbar spine usually complains of pain and stiffness when arising in the morning or when remaining stationary for a prolonged period, especially with sitting. Usually symptoms improve with some activity, but extensive activity can increase symptoms. The patient may report radiating symptoms into the buttocks and the anterior thigh.[15]

HERNIATED INTERVERTEBRAL DISK. The rupture of the annulus fibrosis causes either herniation or prolapse of fragments or the entire nucleus into the spinal canal. Most often the extrusion is in a posterior or lateral direction. The nuclear material may push into the posterior longitudinal ligament or rupture through the ligament and extend directly into the spinal canal[15] (Figure 3-32). Saal and colleagues propose that pain arises not from mechanical pressure but from the chemical release of phospholipase A2 from the nucleus, which affects the nerve root.[47] A herniated intervertebral disk occurs most frequently in the patient between the ages of 25 and 50 years and in men more often than women. Approximately 90% of herniated disks occur at L4-5 with involvement of the L5 nerve root or at L5-S1 with involvement of S1 nerve root, probably because the greatest amount of motion occurs at these segments. The greatest degree of rotation occurs at L5-S1,[56] and therefore this level is probably more susceptible to excessive rotation than other lumbar vertebral segments.

When radiating symptoms follow dermatomal patterns, a neurologic examination is indicated. Screening for nonmechanical sources of musculoskeletal pain should be the first part of the examination for all patients. Discussion of such conditions and appropriate screening examinations are beyond the scope of this book, but excellent texts on the subject are *Differential Diagnosis in Physical Therapy* by Goodman and Snyder[18] and *Pathology, Implications for the Physical Therapist* by Goodman and Boissonnault.[17]

In the descriptions of the lumbar syndromes, a single bullet (•) designates the tests that identify the contributing factors and a double bullet (••) designates the tests for classification.

Movement Impairments

The causes of the patient's symptoms are extension and rotation motions, therefore the examination is designed to assess as many positions, stresses, or movements in these directions as possible. When the test motion causes pain or increases symptoms, the movement is corrected to confirm the movement effects and to support the validity of the test result.

STANDING POSITION. The following tests are performed with the patient in a standing position: (1) back against the wall, (2) forward bending, (3) return from forward bending, (4) lateral flexion, (5) rotation, and (6) single-leg stance.

•• *Back against the wall.* Pain that is present when standing is relieved by flattening the back, especially by standing with the lumbar spine against a wall.

• *Forward bending.* Forward bending may relieve symptoms. A translation motion or a stretch of the nerve may accompany forward bending. As a result, the forward bending motion can be considered a sensitive test but not a specific test.

•• *Return from forward bending.* Often the patient with this syndrome returns from forward bending by extending the lumbar spine early in the pattern, rather than moving through a smooth motion of extending the hips and gradually extending the back (see Figure 2-12). The symptoms should decrease when the patient changes the movement pattern, extending the hips and only gradually extending the back.

•• *Lateral flexion.* Because of the associated rotation with lateral flexion, an increase in symptoms with the side-bending motion is considered a positive finding for the rotation category. In addition to increased symptoms, the shape assumed by the spine and range of motion during the movement are also assessed. If the spine does not curve but bends from a single point, it is a potential sign of rotation of the spine toward the side of the lateral flexion (Figure 3-33). The range of motion to this side should be limited. To confirm the diagnosis, the therapist applies stabilization to the side of the trunk just above the iliac crest to prevent movement at the one site. The patient then repeats the lateral flexion pattern. When symptoms decrease, it is considered a positive test for rotation. The shape of the curve does not change when the spine is rotated, but the range of lateral flexion decreases. When stiffness of the muscles that are contralateral to the direction of the lateral flexion causes angulation of the movement, stabilization during the movement causes the shape of the spine to change from a sharp angle to a curve.

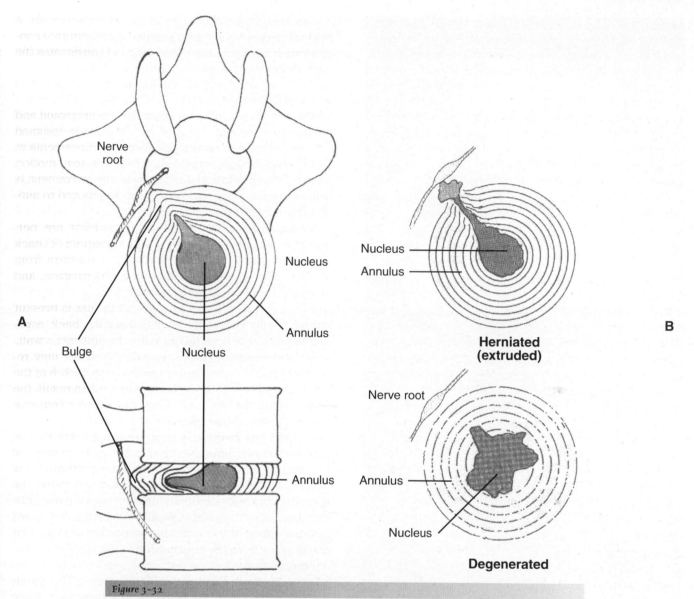

Nerve root

Nucleus

Annulus

Bulge   Nucleus

Annulus

A

Nucleus

Annulus

Herniated (extruded)

Nerve root

Annulus

Nucleus

Degenerated

B

Figure 3-32

Central disk herniation with annular bulge. *A,* The nucleus herniates externally through inner annular tears, forcing the outer annular fibers to bulge into the intervertebral foramen toward the nerve root *(top);* lateral view *(bottom). B,* Extrusion of the nucleus. The nucleus extrudes from the disk through the entire annular tear, termed a herniated nucleus or an extruded nucleus *(top).* The internal extrusion within an otherwise normal annulus causes the nucleus and inner annulus to degenerate *(bottom).* (From Calliet R: *Low back pain syndrome,* 5 ed, Philadelphia, 1995, FA Davis.)

• *Rotation.* The patient is asked to rotate to one side and then to the other while the therapist stabilizes the pelvis. Although most of the rotation motion takes place in the thoracic spine, a notably greater range to the side of suggested spinal rotation supports the clinical impression that the lumbar spine is rotated (Figure 3-34). The therapist should also determine whether the rotation is occurring in the lumbar spine.

• *Single-leg stance.* The patient is asked to stand on one leg while flexing the other hip to 90 degrees. The test is positive if there is rotation of the lumbar spine, pelvis (Figure 3-35), or hip adduction (hip drop).

SUPINE POSITION. The following tests are performed with the patient in a supine position: (1) hip flexor muscle length, (2) active hip and knee flexion, (3) hip abduction/lateral rotation from flexion, (4) passive hip flexion with knee extension, and (5) shoulder flexion to 180 degrees.

• *Hip flexor length.* The test is positive for compensatory motion when the pelvis tilts anteriorly or rotates while the hip is passively extended. A positive test of TFL or rectus femoris shortness without the pelvic motion is not strong support for the extension syndrome because of a lack of compensatory lumbopelvic motion.

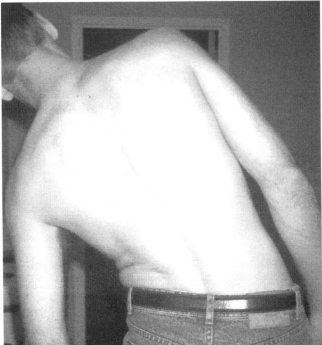

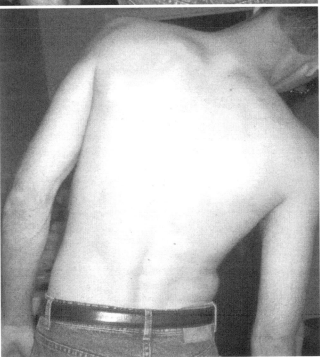

Figure 3-33

Asymmetric and impaired side bending. The subject is able to side bend to the left, but the movement appears to have a focal point of motion at the lumbosacral level with the rest of the lumbar spine remaining straight *(top)*. The side-bending range of motion to the right is limited, and very little change is demonstrated in the alignment of the lumbar spine *(bottom)*. The limited side bending to the right is consistent with the subject's lumbar spine already slightly rotated to the right. During side bending to the right, the subject's vertebrae should rotate to the left, but they cannot because he is rotated to the right. In contrast, if his lumbar vertebrae are already rotated to the right, he should be able to side bend farther to the left than he can to the right.

A positive test for shortness is one in which the knee held toward the chest and passive stabilization by the abdominal muscles, in combination, allow the hip to remain in flexion and do not cause the pelvis to tilt anteriorly or to rotate. This finding does not support a *directional susceptibility to movement* (DSM) of the lumbar extension-rotation syndrome, even though the hip flexors are short.

•• *Active hip and knee flexion.* Pelvic rotation that increases symptoms or has an excursion of more than 1/2 inch of rotation during the lower extremity motion supports the presence of lumbar rotation-extension syndrome. The pelvis rotates toward the side of the hip flexion. To confirm this positive finding, the therapist stabilizes the pelvis and assesses the effect on the symptoms.

•• *Hip abduction/lateral rotation from flexion.* As the knee moves laterally the pelvis rotates toward the moving lower limb during the first 50% of the motion. Symptoms may increase during this motion. Stabilizing the pelvis and assisting the limb as it moves laterally decreases symptoms. A decrease in symptoms is attributed to eliminating the rotation in the spine, eliminating the stress on the spine with the iliopsoas lengthening, or both.

• *Passive hip flexion with knee extended (straight-leg raise).* A positive test for neural tension is radicular pain into the leg before 60 degrees of hip flexion. When the patient reports symptoms, he or she is instructed to completely relax the lower extremity in the test position while the therapist supports the limb. Often the symptoms are eliminated, indicating that the cause of the radiating symptoms is the stress on the spine from the contraction of the hip flexors, not a tethered nerve.

• *Shoulder flexion to 180 degrees.* This movement can cause lumbar extension, and an increase in the low back symptoms.

SIDE-LYING POSITION. The following tests are performed with the patient in a side-lying position: (1) hip lateral rotation, (2) hip abduction with associated lateral pelvic tilt, and (3) hip adduction.

• *Hip lateral rotation.* The test is positive for rotation when the pelvis rotates and movement is not confined to the hip joint.

• *Hip abduction with associated lateral pelvic tilt.* The test is positive for rotation when the patient reports pain during the motion. The probable cause is lateral flexion stress on the spine from the contraction of either the iliopsoas or quadratus lumborum, both of which attach to the transverse processes of the lumbar vertebrae and laterally flex the spine.

• *Hip adduction.* The test is positive for rotation when there is pelvic tilt laterally, rather than isolated hip

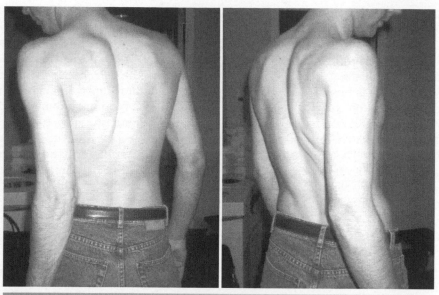

Figure 3-34

Asymmetric rotation. The patient has limited rotational range of motion to the left *(left)* and excessive rotation to the right *(right)*. The asymmetry in rotation is consistent with the asymmetry in side bending that suggests a static malalignment of the lumbar spine of being slightly rotated to the right.

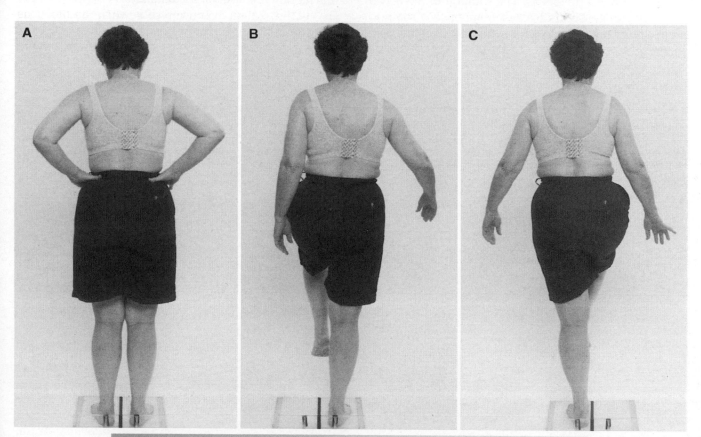

Figure 3-35

Rotation of lumbar spine during unilateral hip and flexion in the standing position. *A,* Lumbar spine is straight during two-legged standing. *B,* No change in lumbar alignment when standing on right leg and flexing left hip and knee. *C,* Rotation of lower lumbar spine when standing on left leg and flexing the right hip and knee.

adduction. The lateral pelvic tilt is accompanied by lateral flexion of the spine (Figure 3-36).

PRONE POSITION. The following tests are performed with the patient in a prone position: (1) knee flexion, (2) hip rotation, and (3) hip extension.

•• *Knee flexion.* The test is positive for lumbar rotation-extension syndrome when the pelvis tilts anteriorly with associated lumbar extension or the pelvis rotates, which can also be associated with an increase in symptoms. To confirm that the test is positive, the pelvis is stabilized and the therapist assesses the effect (on the symptoms) of knee flexion without movement of the pelvis. If the symptoms decrease, the positive test is confirmed.

•• *Hip rotation.* Rotation of the pelvis with rotation of the hip joint infers that rotation is also occurring in the spine. If symptoms increase, the spinal rotation is considered the source. To confirm this diagnosis, the pelvis is stabilized to prevent lumbopelvic motion and the therapist assesses the effect of hip rotation on the symptoms. A decrease in symptoms means they are the result of the spinal rotation produced by the compensatory rotation of the pelvis. The rotation of the pelvis is termed compensatory because lumbopelvic rotation is a means of compensating for insufficient hip rotation.

The compensatory rotation of the pelvis can occur with either hip medial or lateral rotation and with either one or both extremities. Most commonly, pelvic rotation occurs with lateral rotation. In some patients the rotation of the pelvis is always in one direction. Consequently, lateral hip rotation with one extremity produces pelvic motion, and medial hip rotation with the other extremity produces the same direction of pelvic motion.

•• *Hip extension.* The range into extension is limited to 10 degrees; as a result, the patient is instructed to limit the excursion. The spine is often observed to extend or rotate excessively. Determining excessive movement is most often based on the effect of hip extension on the spine, comparing one side with the other. The motion can also elicit symptoms, which is considered a positive test for lumbar rotation-extension syndrome. To confirm the role of extension or rotation, a pillow is placed under the patient's abdomen and the patient contracts the abdominal muscles while being instructed not to push the contralateral thigh into the table (i.e., to avoid hip flexion). Symptoms that are present during this motion are difficult to eliminate.

If the patient has symptoms when simply lying prone or if it is clear that extension is the diagnosis, the

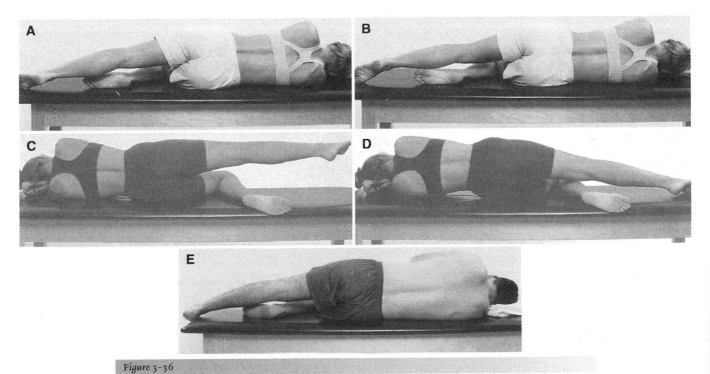

Figure 3-36

Variations in spinal alignment in side lying. *A,* Hip adduction is associated with lateral pelvic tilt and lateral flexion of the lumbar spine. *B,* If the lower extremity is slightly abducted, the pelvic tilt and lateral flexion of the lumbar spine are corrected. *C,* With a positive modified Ober test, the spine and pelvis are in neutral when the hip is abducted. The wide pelvis and narrow thorax of women contribute to lateral flexion of the spine in the side-lying position. *D,* When the hip adducts, the pelvis tilts laterally. Both the lumbar and thoracic spines laterally flex in this subject. *E,* When the trunk is long and broad and the pelvis is narrow (relative to the trunk), the spine is straight in the side-lying position.

test is not performed. If the patient has severe symptoms (> 6/10), this test should be omitted.

QUADRUPED POSITION. The following tests are performed with the patient in a quadruped position: (1) position effects, (2) rocking backward, (3) rocking forward, and (4) shoulder flexion.

• *Position effects.* Pain is usually minimal in the quadruped position and thus is most often used to alleviate the patient's symptoms. The suggested advantages of the quadruped position are the minimization of compression and the four-point support that allows the spine to assume a more optimal alignment than is possible under compression with the two-point support of standing.

•• *Rocking backward.* Symptoms usually decrease because of the slight increase in flexion. If the spine is rotated, the rotation may increase as the patient rocks backward. Often slight counter-pressure on the spine to the rotation while the patient rocks backward alleviates the symptoms.

In some patients the difference in the stiffness or range-of-flexion motion between the two hips is evident and contributes to rotational or lateral tilt of the pelvis and has, of course, an effect on the spine (Figures 3-37 and 3-38). Before repeating the rocking backward motion, the therapist should assess the role of hip flexi-

bility on the movement pattern. If the hip does not flex easily (i.e., the pelvis remains higher on the side that is being tested than on the opposite side), the hip is abducted, laterally rotated, or both. The patient should rock backward with symmetrical movement of the lumbopelvic area. If rocking backward causes symptoms in the patient whose tests strongly suggest an extension syndrome and in whom contraction of the hip flexors causes symptoms, he or she should be instructed to rock backward by pushing with the hands and not using the hip flexors. This strategy can reduce or eliminate the symptoms.

•• *Rocking forward.* Symptoms are often increased with the rocking forward motion. When the symptoms are severe and all other tests for extension are positive, this test is omitted. This motion is not to be used as an exercise.

•• *Shoulder flexion.* Rotation of the spine, so that one side is at least $\frac{1}{2}$ inch different in height than the other side during shoulder flexion, is a positive test for rotation. If symptoms increase, the patient is instructed to contract his abdominal muscles and the therapist may also manually assist by stabilizing the trunk to reduce the rotation; the effect on the symptoms is noted.

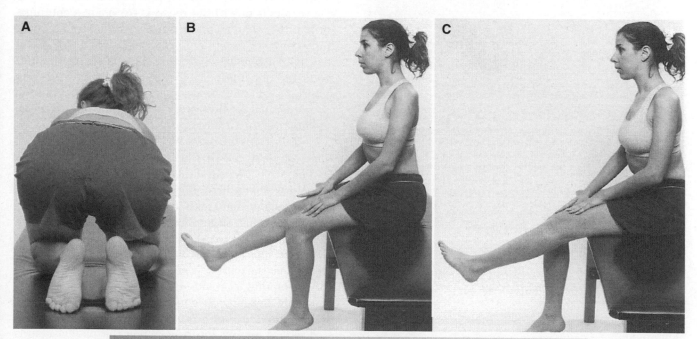

Figure 3-37

Rotation of the lumbar spine in the quadruped position and during knee extension. *A,* During rocking backward, the left hip flexes more than the right hip; as a result, the patient moves toward the left. The asymmetric hip flexion causes lumbopelvic rotation, as indicated by the asymmetric height of the left versus the right sides of the pelvis. The predisposition to lumbopelvic rotation is further illustrated during knee extension. *B,* During right knee extension, no rotation occurs. *C,* During left knee extension, the lumbopelvic area rotates counterclockwise, which confirms that the right hip extensor muscles are stiffer than the joints of the lumbopelvic area involved in rotation to the left. The pattern of joint rotation is the same during both backward quadruped rocking and knee extension.

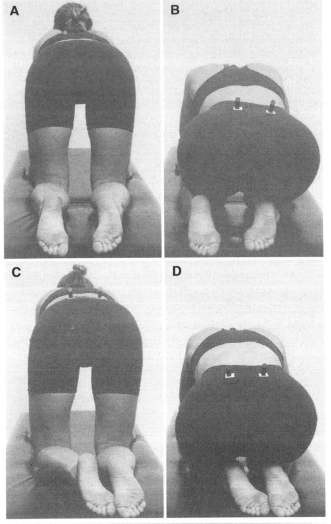

Figure 3-38

Variations in hip flexion flexibility contributing to lumbopelvic rotation. *A,* The pelvis is level in the starting position. *B,* During backward rocking, the right hip flexes more than the left, causing lumbopelvic rotation with the left side of the pelvis higher than the right. *C,* The left hip is laterally rotated. *D,* During backward rocking with the left hip laterally rotated, both hips flex equally, preventing compensatory lumbopelvic rotation. The left hip lateral rotator-extensors are stiffer than the spine. As a result, the lumbar spine rotates instead of the hip flexing, unless there is decreased stretch of the left hip muscles.

SITTING POSITION. The following tests are performed with the patient in a sitting position: (1) position effects and (2) knee extension.

•• *Position effects.* See the discussion under "Alignment."

•• *Knee extension.* The patient is asked to perform knee extension by sitting unsupported with the therapist placing his or her hand on the side of the lumbar spine of the knee that is to be extended. If the pelvis or spine rotates as the knee is extended, the test is positive for rotation. An increase in symptoms is not common unless there is a nerve tension sign. If symptoms increase, the patient is instructed to repeat the knee extension while the therapist stabilizes the spine and instructs the patient to halt the motion at the point the rotation is initiated.

WALKING

• *Gait.* During walking the pelvis often rotates excessively or lumbar extension is exaggerated during the stance phase to toe off. Normal rotation is 8 degrees around a central axis. Instructing the patient to contract the abdominal muscles and to place both hands on his or her iliac crests to eliminate the excessive motion should diminish the symptoms.

Alignment: Structural Variations and Acquired Impairments

STANDING POSITION. Alignment is not, nor is it anticipated to be, correlated with low back pain. Structural changes in vertebral alignment occur with aging, but these changes are not always clinically obvious. The patient with spinal stenosis usually has a flat lumbar spine, yet extension is a cause of the symptoms. In contrast, the patient with a lumbar lordosis, an abnormal exaggeration of the inward lumbar curve, can also have pain because of extension of the lumbar spine. Therefore alignment is a useful indicator, but it is not always correlated with pain. This variability in test results is one of the reasons for using a combinatorial rather than an algorithmic examination. As with the other tests, alignment provides a useful clue, but it may also be a negative finding. The following findings would be contributing factors to the rotation-extension syndrome: (1) lumbar lordosis, (2) thoracic kyphosis, (3) paraspinal asymmetry, and (4) hip joint, flexion, retrotorsion, or antetorsion.

• *Lumbar lordosis.* When the patient reports pain when standing and has an abnormal increase in the lumbar curve, these findings are positive for extension as a cause of pain. To confirm this diagnosis, the patient is instructed to stand with the back against a wall and to flatten the lumbar spine. The patient usually has to move the feet at least 6 to 12 inches forward of the wall, allowing the hips and knees to flex. The therapist must be certain that the patient is relaxing the back muscles and not attempting to stand straight. A decrease in symptoms indicates a positive test for extension.

• *Thoracic kyphosis.* A kyphosis can be associated with a lumbar lordosis. When the patient stands with the back against the wall, the shoulders and upper spine will be forward. The lumbar spine should be flat against the wall, to access whether flattening the lumbar spine reduces the symptoms.

•• *Paraspinal asymmetry.* When one side of the lumbar area is 1/2 inch larger than the other, it is considered positive for rotation. The postural asymmetry is then combined with the movement testing previously described to confirm a positive test of lumbar rotation.

• ***Hip joint.*** See Chapter 5 for the descriptions of antetorsion and retrotorsion.

SUPINE POSITION. When lying with hips and knees extended, pain is considered a positive test for lumbar rotation-extension syndrome. In the case of radiating symptoms, however, the stretch of the iliopsoas in this position can exert compression and anterior shear forces on the lumbar spine. Therefore this test is considered sensitive but not highly specific. Simply placing the hips and knees in flexion and requiring the patient to hold them in this position is not adequate for assessing the effect of reducing the extension stress. At times, the contraction of the hip flexors alone is sufficient to elicit symptoms. Therefore the patient's hips have to be passively supported in flexion, and the patient must completely relax all the lower extremity musculature. If the symptoms decrease, the test is positive for extension as a cause.

SIDE-LYING POSITION. In the side-lying position the lumbar spine can be in lateral flexion, particularly in the woman with broad hips. When symptoms are present, placing a towel with a few folds at the waist to support the spine in a level position decreases symptoms. Symptoms in this position are considered positive for rotation.

PRONE POSITION. Increased symptoms in this position are considered positive for extension. To confirm this diagnosis, a pillow is placed under the patient's abdomen to reduce the lumbar curve. If the symptoms are decreased, the test for extension is positive.

SITTING POSITION. An increase in symptoms associated with exaggerating the lumbar curve is a positive test for extension. To confirm this diagnosis, the patient is supported in the flat lumbar spine position. The patient with a marked thoracic kyphosis often maintains the spine in an extended alignment when sitting and may have symptoms because of this alignment. When the patient is short (e.g., under 5 feet, 4 inches tall), the feet may not touch the ground, which exerts an anterior tilt on the pelvis. The patient may be unaware that he or she is contracting the hip flexors or back extensors when sitting. Therefore the therapist needs to be sure the patient is completely relaxed and the back is supported in a flat alignment to assess the effect of extension stresses on the symptoms.

Relative Flexibility and Stiffness Impairments

The lumbar spine is excessively flexible into extension and rotation. The following factors contribute to the extension and rotation of the lumbar spine:

1. Hip flexors are stiffer than the abdominal muscles that tilt the pelvis posteriorly.

2. The hip abductor muscles are stiffer than the lateral abdominal muscles.

3. The TFL muscle is stiffer than the abdominal muscles that control rotation of the pelvis.

4. The latissimus dorsi muscle is stiffer than the abdominal muscles that tilt the pelvis posteriorly and flatten the lumbar spine.

Muscle and Recruitment Pattern Impairments

The therapist may observe impairment of recruitment patterns. During attempts of the patient to stand up straight, there may be more dominant recruitment of the back extensor muscles than the counterbalancing effects of the abdominal muscles. During attempts to return to standing from a leaning or bending forward position, there may be more dominant recruitment of the back extensor muscles than the hip extensors. During movements such as leaning forward when sitting or when sitting up from a recumbent position, there may be more dominant recruitment of the hip flexors than the abdominal muscles.

Impairments of muscle length and strength may also be observed. When neurologic signs are present, weakness may be present according to dermatomal involvement. Nonneurologic weaknesses may be present in the external oblique abdominal, rectus abdominis, transversus muscles, and posterior gluteus medius muscles. The TFL and rectus femoris muscles may be short or stiff.

Confirming Tests

Specific confirming tests are described under "Movement Impairments" in this chapter. Generally, reducing symptoms by decreasing the alignment, stress, or movement in the extension directions are the critical confirming tests.

Summary

In the patient with chronic back pain, rotation-extension is the most common cause of the symptoms. A series of tests are used to confirm this diagnosis. Not all patients test positive for all test items, but each scores a greater number of positive findings or the severity of symptoms is highest for the extension-rotation test items.

Treatment

The diagnosis is designed to direct the intervention. The primary strategy for an intervention program is eliminating the alignment, stress, or movement in the symptom-producing direction. The program does not emphasize movement in the opposite direction, except when the alignment impairment is excessive. For example, the patient with lordosis should decrease the curve by tilting the pelvis posteriorly and flattening the lumbar curve. *Most importantly, those daily activities and postures that contribute to stress or movement in the offending directions must be identified.*

Rotating the lumbar spine during activities (e.g., turning at the desk to reach a computer, the telephone, or a file drawer) is performed so frequently that few individuals realize that he or she is rotating while working. The patient often sits on the edge of the chair, which means he or she is using the hip flexors to maintain the position. The patient should sit back in the chair with the spine supported, producing a slight inward curve, and the hips and knees should be at the same height, and the feet should be on the floor. Leaning to one side or resting on one forearm is lateral flexion for tall individuals or for those who have a long trunk or proportionately short upper arms. Lateral flexion is associated with rotation, as well as with asymmetrical compression of the lumbar vertebrae.

Sports, such as racquetball, squash, and golf, involve rotation with the feet relatively fixed. Consequently, these sports are frequent contributors to rotational syndromes. Maintaining hip rotational flexibility is essential to minimize compensatory pelvic and lumbar rotation. Tennis and volleyball involve rotation; however, because the feet are not fixed and total body movement is more characteristic, the contribution to rotation is not exaggerated.

All the positive tests become the exercises that the patient must perform correctly. It is important that the patient understand that the focus of a corrective exercise program is to ensure that no symptoms are elicited while performing the exercises. Any exercise that increases the symptoms should be omitted until the next visit with the physical therapist.

STANDING POSITION. Standing with one hip adducted laterally flexes the spine and should be avoided. The patient should not sway the thoracic spine backward because of the extension moments or the increase in the curve of the lumbar spine that can result from this posture. The patient should contract the abdominal muscles isometrically, enough to exert tension to slightly tilt the pelvis posteriorly and to reduce the lumbar curve. If the patient reports pain when standing, he or she should stand with the lumbar spine against the wall, relaxing the back muscles.

SITTING POSITION. Sitting back in a straight back chair will relax hip and back muscles. The hips and knees should be at the same height. The trunk should be erect, not rotated or leaning to one side. Some patients are able to reduce the symptoms by pushing up on the seat of the chair or the arm rests, just enough to take the weight of the trunk off the spine.

ROLLING. While supine, depending on the severity of the symptoms, the patient should slide the heel along the bed to flex one hip and knee and then repeat with the other lower extremity. With both knees flexed, the patient should roll in one piece so that the arm and trunk are moving at the same time as the pelvis and lower extremities. The patient should not push down with the feet. To move to one side of the bed, the patient should be in the side-lying position and push backward with hands and legs. When the patient needs to move forward, he or she should pull on the edge of bed with the hands to move the upper body. If the pain is severe, the patient may have to use the hand to move the lower extremity forward to avoid the use of the hip flexors.

SITTING TO STANDING. The patient should move to the edge of the chair by pushing with the hands, avoiding any rotation of the hips from side to side. With the hips aligned over the knees, the patient should stand straight up, avoiding any motion that exaggerates back extension. It may be necessary to use armrests to push up from the chair. When sitting down, the patient may also need to lower his or her body using the hands, particularly if the thigh musculature is weak.

STAIR CLIMBING. The therapist needs to determine which phase of the stair climbing motion causes an increase in the patient's symptoms. The first phase of stair climbing is flexing the hip to place the foot on the stair. Contracting the abdominal muscles before lifting the foot may alleviate the pain; otherwise, the patient will have to ascend one step at a time. The second phase of stair climbing is raising the weight after the foot is on the step. One impairment that can be observed is back extension during this phase or inadequate hip extension that increases back extension. Instructing the patient to remain slightly forward and placing his or her weight on the handrail as he or she raises to the next step can prevent an increase in symptoms.

WALKING. The patient needs to walk slowly, which reduces the compression on the spine.[6] The patient has to limit pelvic rotation or anterior tilt, which often involves taking smaller steps than normal.

Case Presentation 1

History. For the past 5 months, a 63-year-old male executive who is employed at a large business firm has experienced severe pain in his back and left posterior thigh, extending into his leg. He is an active sportsman who regularly rides horses on his ranch. His radiologic studies indicate degenerative disk disease with spinal stenosis. Although surgery has been advised, he wants to try conservative intervention before agreeing to surgery.

Symptoms. His symptoms include pain when standing, which increases with walking. He rates the pain at a level of 6 to 7 on a scale of 10. He forces himself to walk in spite of the level of pain. The pain extends into his left groin area and down his posterior thigh into the posterolateral aspect of his leg. It subsides to a level of 2 to 3 on a scale of 10 when he sits. Although the patient has pain when recumbent, side lying is the most comfortable recumbent position.

Alignment Analysis. The patient is muscular with prominent back muscles. His upper back is swayed backward, although he does not have a posterior pelvic tilt. He has paraspinal asymmetry; his right side is more than 1 inch larger than his left, and his left hip is slightly higher than his right. He stands with hips abducted.

Movement Analysis. His symptoms increase when the patient is asked to place his feet together. This position causes the left iliac crest to be even higher than the right, as compared with pelvic alignment when his feet are apart. Five standing tests are performed: (1) forward bending, (2) lateral flexion, (3) rotation, (4) single-leg stance, and (5) standing with his back against the wall.

Forward bending. His symptoms decrease with forward bending, but they increase during the return movement. It is noted that his spine extends more rapidly than his hips during the return motion. When placing his hands on a table that is raised to a height where he can place his hands on it without bending, he performs forward bending by supporting his upper body on his hands and return movements. During the return motion, he is instructed to concentrate on extending his hips rather than his back. He has less pain when performing this movement as instructed.

Lateral flexion. Motion to his left side increases his pain, and the motion occurs at his lumbopelvic junction. Motion to his right side decreases pain, but he is unable to side bend far in this direction. His lumbar spine remains straight when movement occurs in the thoracic spine.

Rotation. When the patient is asked to rotate his spine, the range of motion to the right is notably greater than the range of motion to the left.

Single-leg stance. When asked to stand on his left leg, the left hip becomes adducted and he reports a slight increase in pain. During a right leg stance, symptoms associated with flexing the left hip increase, at which time lumbopelvic rotation to the right is evident.

Standing with back against the wall. His symptoms decrease when instructed to stand with his low back against the wall.

The following tests are performed with the patient in a supine position: (1) hip flexor length, (2) position effects, (3) hip abduction/lateral rotation from hip flexion, (4) passive hip and knee flexion, and (5) abdominal muscular strength.

Hip flexor length. Both the right and left TFL and rectus femoris muscles are short with a compensatory anterior pelvic tilt.

Position effects. The patient is unable to tolerate the hip and knee extended position. He cannot hold his left knee toward his chest (at 100 degrees of hip flexion)

and slide the right leg down toward hip extension without eliciting symptoms. On the left, he has to use his hands with a towel behind his thigh to flex his left hip and then lower the extremity back to the table, allowing it to extend. The right hip extends to neutral and the left hip extends to 30 degrees of complete extension. His symptoms increase when moving his left lower extremity.

Hip abduction/lateral rotation from hip flexion. Hip abduction/lateral rotation increases his symptoms, and there is an associated lumbopelvic rotation with greater motion with the motion of the left lower extremity than with that of the right.

Passive hip and knee flexion. There is resistance to passive hip and knee flexion at 100 degrees bilaterally.

Abdominal muscular strength. Abdominal muscular strength is not tested because of pain with active hip flexion motion.

The following additional tests are performed in four different positions: (1) side lying, (2) prone, (3) quadruped, and (4) sitting.

Side lying. The patient is more comfortable during the side-lying test when on his left side than on his right. When testing the strength of the posterior gluteus medius muscles, the left side is 3+/5 and the right 4+/5. During the test, it is noted that hip adduction from abduction is associated with lateral pelvic tilt. Hip lateral rotation is associated with lumbopelvic rotation.

Prone. When in the prone position, the patient's symptoms increase, but they are diminished with a pillow under his abdomen. The patient's symptoms increase when he initiates knee flexion, and there is anterior pelvic tilt and rotation observed with both right and left knee flexion. Hip rotation is not tested because the knee cannot be flexed to 90 degrees.

Quadruped. While in the starting quadruped test position, there is marked rotation of his lumbar spine toward the right. In the quadruped position, all symptoms are alleviated. Rocking backward causes the rotation to increase. The pelvis also rotates clockwise so that his pelvis appears higher on the right side than on the left.

Sitting. While sitting with his back against the back of the chair, he reports minimal symptoms. He does not report an increase in symptoms with the knee extension test, but the right hamstring muscles are short with knee extension −30 degrees of complete range of motion.

Muscle Length and Strength Analysis. When muscle length and strength are examined, the TFL and rectus femoris muscles are short bilaterally. The abdominal muscles are not able to control the motions of anterior pelvic tilt, rotation, or lateral pelvic tilt. The hamstring muscles are short, but they do not contribute to the pain. The gluteus maximus muscles are stiff, with the right muscle more stiff than the left.

Diagnosis. The patient's alignment and movement tests are clearly consistent with rotation and extension problems. His symptoms are alleviated when he flattens his lumbar spine, as evidenced by the report of decreased symptoms when the patient sits, when his hips are flexed, and when he is on his hands and knees. His symptoms increase with extension alignment and movements into extension. The diagnosis is lumbar rotation-extension syndrome.

Intervention. The primary focus of his intervention is to enable him to lie supine with his hips and knees extended. Until he can assume this supine position, he will be unable to stand free of symptoms.

From the hook-lying position, he is instructed to hold his left knee to his chest and slide the right leg into extension while contracting his abdominal muscles. With pillows under his right knee to support his hip in flexion, he is instructed to use a sheet under his left thigh, which he holds with both hands to act as an assist while sliding the hip and knee into extension and then bringing it back into flexion while contracting his abdominal muscles. With pillows under his right knee, he is asked to move his flexed left hip into abduction/lateral rotation while keeping his pelvis from rotating by contracting the abdominal muscles. This supine exercise is repeated on the contralateral side.

While in the side-lying position with a pillow between the knees to control medial rotation, the patient is instructed to rotate his hip laterally while keeping the pelvis stationary.

When in the prone position with a pillow under his abdomen, he is asked to contract his abdominal muscles and flex one knee and then the other knee while the therapist monitors his pelvis with his or her hands. He is asked to stop the motion with the onset of any pelvic tilting or at the onset of any symptoms.

From the quadruped position with his hips abducted and the right hip slightly rotated laterally, the patient is taught to rock backward, stopping at any increase in symptoms.

While in a sitting position, the patient performs knee extension and dorsiflexion.

When in a standing position with his back against the wall, the patient positions his feet far enough from the wall to allow his hips and knees to flex. From this position he is able to flatten his lumbar spine. The patient is then asked to contract his abdominal muscles and extend his hips and knees so that he slides up the wall. He is instructed to stop at onset of symptoms.

The patient is asked to modify some of his daily activities: He is instructed to sit back in his chair and avoid sitting on the edge of his chair, as he was accustomed to do at work. He is instructed to avoid rotating his trunk when sitting and reaching for articles on his desk. (His workspace and telephone were placed on a table behind his desk. He always turned to the right when answering the telephone.) The telephone is moved to his desk.

Outcome. The patient performs his exercises two times a day. Several times a day, he stands with his back to the wall to perform the recommended standing exercise. At the time of his second visit 1 week later, his symptoms when standing and walking are reduced to a level of 4 or 5 on a scale of 10. He diminishes the intensity of his pain to the level of 2 or 3 by standing with his back against the wall. When his symptoms are intense, he performs the rocking backward exercise, which eliminates his symptoms.

By his second visit 2 weeks later, he lies supine with his right hip and knee extended while his left hip and knee are flexed with his foot on the table. He extends his left hip to within 20 degrees of complete extension and he actively flexes his hip without symptoms by sliding his heel along the table. He does not have to hold his knee to his chest to decrease his symptoms. When prone, he flexes his knees to 100 degrees without an associated anterior pelvic tilt or pelvic rotation and without symptoms. At this point, he is instructed to begin hip rotation. Initially, hip lateral rotation causes pelvic rotation, which he is taught to control by contracting his abdominal muscles.

By his third visit 1 week later, he walks one block with symptoms that do not exceed a level of 2 to 3 on a scale of 10. With his back against the wall and with his hips and knees only slightly flexed, he stands without symptoms. There is a visible change in the contour of his spine; as a result, the rotation is greatly diminished and he no longer stands with his back swayed backward. He lies supine with his hips and knees extended bilaterally, though he has to contract actively his abdominal muscles to maintain this position without symptoms. Side-lying hip abduction and adduction are added to his program. Shoulder flexion while standing with his back against the wall is also added, but the range is limited because of a previous rotator cuff tear of his right shoulder.

For program modification, he continues to be seen by the therapist on a weekly basis for 8 weeks. At the end of this time, he walks for 1 mile without symptoms; he stands and performs all exercises without symptoms. The alignment of his spine continues to improve with the previous asymmetry only slightly evident at the time of his last visit. The patient is scheduled to play golf and is advised of the importance of rotating the hips, not the lumbar spine, when swinging his golf club. He is also advised to avoid playing competitively for the first few times on the golf course. The patient reports by telephone that he experiences some pain after playing golf, but he eliminates his symptoms by performing his exercises. He indicates that he will return to golf slowly.

Case Presentation 2

History. A 58-year-old male chief executive officer of his own business has pain down his left leg when standing and walking. When questioned about his work environment, the patient indicates that he works from two schedule boards that are situated behind his desk on the wall. There are three doors in his office, which allow staff to come from different directions, and his telephone is on the far edge of the left side of his desk. The schedule boards, office doors, and position of his telephone cause him to rotate in these directions many times a day. The patient is markedly overweight with a particularly large abdomen. To accommodate his abdomen and keep his feet well situated on the floor, he sits on the edge of his chair.

The patient has heart disease that is controlled by medication. He participates in a cardiac rehabilitation program, performing stretches that include the heel-cord stretch. To perform this stretch, the patient leans forward into the wall and extends his lumbar spine. He also performs pelvic rotation exercises in the hook-lying position.

He has had prior reconstructive surgery on his left knee, which is larger in appearance than the right, and the left knee is aligned in varus. The patient's pain problem has been diagnosed as degenerative knee joint disease with radiating symptoms into his thigh and leg. He has been scheduled for knee joint replacement surgery. A physician, who is a relative, has reviewed his spinal radiologic studies and believes there are findings compatible with spinal stenosis. He is referred to physical therapy for consultation to ascertain whether conservative management of his symptoms is a possibility.

Symptoms. The patient has immediate pain in his thigh and leg upon standing. His walking is limited to what he must do for work and self-care activities. When walking he rates his pain at a level of 6 to 7 on a scale of 10. When he tries to walk for long distances the pain increases to a level of 8 to 9. He has some symptoms when sitting, but he rates this pain at a level of only 1 to 2 on a scale of 10.

Alignment Analysis. There is a great increase in the lower lumbar curve and marked asymmetry of the paraspinal area with the left side approximately 3/4 of an inch larger than the right. He has a thoracic kyphosis. He is in slight anterior pelvic tilt. The iliac crests are level, and, as noted previously, the patient has varus of his left knee.

Movement Analysis. Five standing tests are performed: (1) forward bending, (2) lateral flexion, (3) spinal rotation, (4) single-leg stance, and (5) standing with back against the wall.

Forward bending. The patient's symptoms decrease with this motion, but returning from forward bending increases the symptoms.

Lateral flexion. Motion to the left increases his symptoms, and the movement is at the lower lumbar segments. Manually blocking the motion by supporting the patient at the waist decreases his symptoms during left side bending. No change in symptoms is noted with right side bending.

Spinal rotation. The range of motion to the left is greater than to the right.

Single-leg stance. Symptoms increase when the patient stands on either his left or right leg.

Standing with back against the wall. This position does not improve his symptoms.

The following tests are performed with the patient in a supine position: (1) hip flexor length, (2) position effects, (3) hip abduction/lateral rotation from flexion, and (4) lower abdominal muscular strength.

Hip flexor length. The TFL muscle is found to be short bilaterally, and there is immediate anterior pelvic tilt when passively lowering the hip into extension, which is observed on both sides.

Position effects. The patient needs pillows under his upper thoracic spine to accommodate his thoracic kyphosis. He is unable to lie with hips and knees extended because of symptoms in his left lower extremity. With his left knee held passively toward his chest, the patient can extend the right lower extremity. With his right knee held to his chest, he can extend the left lower extremity to within 20 degrees of complete hip extension without symptoms. The patient can slide his left lower extremity along the table, but he is not able to lift it from the table without initiating symptoms.

Hip abduction/lateral rotation from flexion. The patient performs this motion on his right side with no pelvic rotation. However, when he performs this movement with his left hip, there is pelvic rotation and some increase in symptoms.

Lower abdominal muscular strength. The lower abdominal muscles are not tested because of pain with active hip flexion. However, functionally the patient is unable to restrain anterior pelvic tilt or pelvic rotation, indicating a weakness of the abdominal muscles.

The following additional tests are performed in four positions: (1) side lying, (2) prone, (3) quadruped, and (4) sitting.

Side lying. Pelvic rotation occurs with hip lateral rotation on his left side but not on his right.

Prone. The patient tolerates the prone position, but only when a pillow is placed under his abdomen. When testing knee flexion, the patient's left knee flexes only to 90 degrees and there is compensatory pelvic rotation with both right and left knee flexion. Testing hip rotation is also associated with pelvic rotation, but this movement does not produce symptoms.

Quadruped. The patient cannot assume this position because of the pathologic condition of his knee.

Sitting. The patient is symptom free when sitting with his back against the back of a chair and with the muscles of his lower extremities relaxed. When testing knee extension, there are no symptoms produced; however, a slight hamstring shortness is evident.

Muscle Length and Strength Analysis. The hip flexors are stiff and short, and the abdominal muscles are weak.

Diagnosis. The patient's symptoms are related to the alignment of his spine and not associated with movements or weight bearing on his knee. The key alignment producing his symptoms is extension, but the rotation of his spine undoubtedly contributes to the narrowing of the intervertebral foramina. The weakness of his abdominal muscles and their lack of support for his spine when he contracts his hip flexors contribute to his problem. Flexing his lumbar spine in noncompression positions, such as leaning on a supporting surface or assuming the quadruped position, alleviates his symptoms. However, the quadruped position cannot be used because of his knee problem. The diagnosis is rotation-extension syndrome.

Intervention. The primary goals of the patient's program are to eliminate the rotational movements in his activities, decrease his rotational alignment, and improve the strength and decrease the length of his abdominal muscles.

When in a supine position, the patient performs heel slides, initially with one knee held to chest and then from the hook-lying position while contracting the abdominal muscles. He also performs hip abduction and lateral rotation. The patient cannot perform exercises in the side-lying position because of the pathologic condition of his knee joint. When in a prone position, he performs knee flexion. He is not able to tolerate exercises in the quadruped position. When in a sitting position, the patient performs knee extension. When standing, the patient is instructed to lean over his desk and stretch his spine by reaching forward while keeping his hips and knees flexed. This key exercise completely eliminates his symptoms. However, returning to the standing position remains difficult. He cannot simply straighten up because this motion extends his back. Instead, he is instructed to flex his hips and knees to a greater degree, so that they are moving under the desk; as a result, he is in a position similar to sitting. From this position he stands straight up by pushing slightly with his arms on the desktop. He maintains this position for short periods of time without any symptoms. The patient uses this standing exercise many times a day to alleviate his symptoms and to improve the alignment of his spine.

The patient has also rearranged his office, closing all but one door and moving his schedule boards so that they are in front of him. He no longer has to turn to see them.

Outcome. When the patient returns to the therapist after 1 week, he can stand momentarily without experiencing any symptoms. He can also stand with his back resting against the wall without symptoms. He can sit and he can move from a sitting to standing position without symptoms. By the end of the second week, the patient can lie supine for brief periods with his hips and knees extended.

With weekly visits to physical therapy, after 1 month the patient is able to walk for five or six blocks and he is able to stand for 15 to 20 minutes without symptoms. When he experiences pain, he alleviates it by standing with his back against the wall or leaning over the desk and returning to the upright position as instructed. The keys to his recovery are the changes in his office and movement patterns and the improved control of his abdominal muscles, which prevents the hip flexor pull on his spine.

After approximately $1^{1}/_{2}$ years, the patient returns to physical therapy for evaluation and treatment intervention for low back and leg pain. He has performed well with minimal symptoms and is always able to control his symptoms with his key exercises. Unfortunately, the patient has had another heart attack requiring bypass surgery. He has become quite invested in an exercise program and is now exercising six times a week, using weight training machines and performing water aerobics. Although the patient has lost a great amount of weight and has improved muscle definition (the most marked improvements are in the rectus abdominis and the back extensors), he is performing exercises that emphasize back extension or are performed with his back extended. The water aerobics, which involve repetitive hip flexion movements, are also contributing to his problem. A careful analysis is made of his exercise program. A recommendation for changing the performance of several exercises and an omission of some others is made. He is also instructed to resume the supine exercise of holding his knee to his chest while contracting his abdominal muscles and sliding his hip and knee into extension, using the change of the symptoms as a guide to determine the extent of the motion. With these recommendations, his back pain is eliminated and he is able to walk with only slight pain in his leg.

Lumbar Extension Syndrome

The lumbar extension syndrome with or without radiating symptoms is the second most common category of patients found in the study by Van Dillen and associates.[53] As previously discussed, the loss of disk height exaggerates the problems associated with narrowing of the intervertebral foramen, which is already narrowed by extension of the spine. This diagnosis is common in patients with chronic or repeated episodes of back pain, in individuals older than 60 years of age, and in women with very weak abdominal muscles.

Symptoms and Pain

Complaints range from pain in the lumbosacral area to radiating pain into the buttock, posterior thigh, lateral thigh, and/or foot. The medical problems or associated diagnoses are spinal stenosis, degenerative disk disease, spondylolisthesis, herniated disk, and osteoarthritis of the spine.

Alignment

The structural variations in alignment in patients with the extension syndrome include thoracic kyphosis, as found in the older individuals or younger persons with Scheuermann's disease, and which is most often associated with lumbar lordosis. The common acquired impairments of alignment are swayed upper back or anterior pelvic tilt and lumbar lordosis.

Movement Impairments

STANDING POSITION. The following tests are performed with the patient in a standing position: (1) forward bending and (2) return from forward bending.

•• *Forward bending.* This movement decreases symptoms, but when the patient has radiating pain, pain may increase during this test. In some patients, particularly those with a large abdomen or weak abdominal muscles, contracting the abdominal muscles and asking the therapist to support his or her abdomen during flexion may reduce the symptoms.

•• *Return from forward bending.* This movement increases symptoms when the patient extends the spine faster than he or she extends the hips. To confirm this diagnosis, the patient is instructed to return from forward bending by extending the hips while keeping the back from extending; the therapist notes the effect of this movement on the symptoms.

SUPINE POSITION. The following tests are performed with the patient in a supine position: (1) position effects, (2) hip and knee flexion, and (3) shoulder flexion.

•• *Position effects.* Compared with both hips and knees extended, symptoms decrease when a pillow is placed under the knees or when both knees are passively pulled to the chest.

• *Hip and knee flexion.* The initiation of this movement causes anterior pelvic tilt and may increase

symptoms. To confirm a positive test for extension, the patient contracts the abdominal muscles to prevent the tilt during the hip flexion movement, and the therapist notes the effect of this movement on the symptoms. A patient may have to use his or her hands to pull the knee to the chest to avoid any hip flexor muscle activity. A towel or sheet can be placed under the thigh, which the patient then holds with his or her hands to move the lower extremity.

• *Shoulder flexion.* Flexion of the shoulder to 180 degrees causes lumbar extension and may increase the symptoms.

PRONE POSITION. The following tests are performed with the patient in a prone position: (1) position effects, (2) knee flexion, and (3) hip extension.

•• *Position effects.* Symptoms increase in the prone position but decrease when a pillow is place under the abdomen.

•• *Knee flexion.* Initiation of this movement causes anterior pelvic tilt and may increase the symptoms. To confirm a positive test for lumbar extension, the therapist stabilizes the pelvis to prevent the anterior tilt and notes the effects on the symptoms.

•• *Hip extension.* This movement causes excessive lumbar extension and may increase the symptoms.

QUADRUPED POSITION. The following tests are performed with the patient in a quadruped position: (1) lumbar extension and flexion, (2) rocking forward, and (3) rocking backward.

• *Lumbar extension and flexion.* Allowing the lumbar spine to extend increases the symptoms, and flexing the lumbar spine decreases the symptoms.

•• *Rocking backward.* This movement decreases the symptoms. The patient may have to push with the hands to rock backward to avoid using the hip flexors.

•• *Rocking forward.* This movement causes an increase in the symptoms.

SITTING POSITION. The following tests are performed with the patient in a sitting position: (1) lumbar extension and (2) flat or flexed lumbar spine.

•• *Lumbar extension.* Arching the back by pulling the lumbar spine forward into extension increases the symptoms.

•• *Flat or flexed lumbar spine.* Instructing the patient to sit with the back flat and supported or slumped decreases the symptoms.

STANDING WITH BACK TO WALL. The flat lumbar spine test is performed with the patient in this position.

•• *Flat lumbar spine.* This movement decreases symptoms. The patient relaxes the back muscles and does not attempt to stand up straight. The patient's feet are far enough away from the wall to allow the lumbar spine to flatten against the wall. The patient also flexes the knees and hips.

GAIT. The lumbar extension test is performed while the patient is walking.

• *Lumbar extension.* When walking, there is excessive lumbar extension during the stance phase that increases symptoms. To confirm this diagnosis, the patient is asked to contract the abdominal muscles and take small steps. The therapist notes the effect of these movements on the symptoms.

Summary

Alignment, stresses, or motions that contribute to lumbar extension increase symptoms, whereas the prevention of these stresses or motions decreases symptoms.

Flexibility and Stiffness Impairments

The lumbar spine is more flexible into extension than either the counteracting tautness of the abdominal muscles that tilt the pelvis posteriorly or the anterior supporting structures of the spine that limit extension. The hip flexors are stiffer than the abdominal muscles that tilt the pelvis posteriorly. The latissimus dorsi muscle may also be stiffer than the abdominal muscles and contribute to excessive lumbar extension.

Muscle and Recruitment Pattern Impairments

The activity of the hip flexor muscles is more dominant than the abdominal muscles when, for example, the patient leans forward while in the sitting position. The activity of the back extensor muscles is more dominant than the activity of the hip extensors.

Impairments of muscle length and strength may also be observed. External oblique abdominal muscles may be weak or long. Hip flexor muscles, as well as lumbar paraspinal muscles, may be stiff or short, especially in the patient with a thoracic kyphosis. A weakened gluteus maximus may be present.

Confirming Tests

Flattening the lumbar spine decreases the symptoms. Eliminating hip flexor muscular activity, particularly the activity of the iliopsoas muscle, decreases the symptoms.

Summary

Structural changes in the lumbar spine, such as a loss of disk height or the formation of exostoses at the facet joints, reduce the tautness of the restraining ligaments and narrow the intervertebral foramen. Structural changes also alter the alignment of the facet joints. Control by the abdominal muscles is particularly important in preventing excessive lumbar extension, both at rest and during movements. The emphasis is on control,

which implies that the abdominal muscles are functioning optimally at the right length, which is not synonymous with generalized abdominal strengthening exercises. Excessive activity of the hip flexors, particularly the iliopsoas muscle, contributes to the extension problem. The patient needs to be aware of how daily activities contribute to the problem and how to use the abdominal muscles effectively.

Treatment

PRIMARY OBJECTIVES. The primary objectives of the program are to correct the lumbar lordosis, if present, and to improve the activity of the abdominal muscles to avoid the extension stresses that increase the patient's symptoms. Often there is an imbalance in the stiffness of the abdominal muscles as compared with that of the hip flexors. With such imbalance, stretch of the hip flexors causes anterior pelvic tilt and lumbar extension. A variety of postures, such as sitting at the edge of the chair, exaggerate lumbar extension. Examples of activities that contribute to lumbar extension are as basic as moving from a sitting to a standing position by arching the back or as basic as walking, especially when the patient has short hip flexor muscles and weak abdominal muscles. The most effective rehabilitation program identifies the impaired movement patterns and instructs the patient to correct these patterns, enabling the patient to almost constantly correct the causes of the pain.

CORRECTIVE EXERCISE PROGRAM

Supine exercises. Exercises that emphasize shortening and stiffening of the abdominal muscles while stretching the hip flexors are the most common intervention. These supine exercises may begin with heel slides and hip and knee extension from the hook-lying position and may progress to more challenging exercises for the external oblique muscles that are described in Chapter 7. When there is shortness of the lumbar back extensors, the patient may need to perform bilateral knee-to-chest exercises, but he or she has to avoid the pull of the hip flexors on the lumbar spine while performing this exercise. The exercise of hip abduction and lateral rotation from flexion improves the control of pelvic rotation by the abdominal muscles. If the patient has a kyphosis, shoulder flexion with the spine stabilized will help correct this postural impairment. Asking the patient to take a deep breath or to simply lift his or her chest while the arms are flexed over the head will help correct depressed chest alignment.

Side-lying exercises. Hip abduction improves the control of the pelvis by the lateral abdominal muscles. When the TFL, anterior gluteus medius, or gluteus minimus are short, improving the performance of the posterior gluteus medius is important to counterbalance the activity of these hip flexor muscles.

Prone exercises. Knee flexion and preventing anterior pelvic tilt by contracting the abdominal muscles improve the performance of the abdominal muscles and also stretch the rectus femoris and TFL muscles. Hip lateral rotation also helps stretch the TFL muscle. Hip extension is usually contraindicated when the patient has symptoms, because this movement increases lumbar extension.

Quadruped exercises. Instructing the patient to flex the lumbar spine in this position while rocking backward often decreases symptoms. If the patient has a thoracic kyphosis, this exercise allows the thoracic spine to straighten, which is a useful position in which to start correcting this alignment.

Sitting exercises. Correcting impairments of sitting alignment is a most important therapeutic measure. The patient uses the back of the chair, and he or she may need a footstool. If the patient has a kyphosis, the abdominal muscles are contracted to keep the lumbar spine flat and the shoulders are flexed while maintaining an erect thoracic spine to improve the performance of the thoracic paraspinal muscles.

Standing exercises. While standing against the wall with the lumbar spine flat and the knees and hips flexed, the abdominal muscles are contracted and the hips and knees are extended. This extremely effective exercise is the best for improving the control of the abdominal muscles while avoiding hip flexor muscular activity. Many patients get relief from symptoms by simply assuming this position. Performing shoulder flexion while contracting the abdominal muscles is also another exercise for improving alignment and the performance of the abdominal muscles.

CORRECTING POSTURAL HABITS AND MOVEMENT PATTERNS. After observing the sitting alignment and the sit-to-stand and walking patterns that can contribute to lumbar extension, the patient is taught how to correct these patterns. Another activity that contributes to symptoms is driving an automobile with a standard transmission that requires bilateral hip and knee flexion. The patient needs to minimize this motion, contracting the abdominal muscles when performing this motor pattern. The patient is instructed to rotate the right hip while pivoting on the heel to move from the gas pedal to the brake, instead of using active hip and knee flexion to perform the same function.

Case Presentation

History. A 32-year-old woman is referred to a physical therapist for evaluation and intervention of pain in her abdominal, pelvic, and low back areas. She was involved in a serious motor vehicle accident 6 years earlier. She sustained fractures of her pelvis that healed with some malalignment of her pelvis. She works as a doctor's assistant in a busy general medicine practice.

Her work activities involve a great deal of standing and bending during the day. Five days before her referral, she was involved in another automobile accident. She is now experiencing pain in her abdomen and pelvis. A radiologic examination reveals no new findings. The pelvic fractures from her previous accident are on the right side of her pelvis.

Symptoms. Her symptoms worsen when she tries to move, particularly when recumbent. Turning and changing positions in bed is painful. She feels best in the morning after arising but experiences increasing pain during the latter half of her workday. The patient has tenderness throughout her abdomen and pelvis. She rates her pain at 6 to 7 out of 10.

Alignment Analysis. The patient is slightly built with a marked increase in the lumbar curve in her lower spine. She is in anterior pelvic tilt. When standing, her left iliac crest is slightly higher than the right. She sits with most of her weight on her left buttock, and in a sitting position her right iliac crest appears to be lower than the left. Elevating her right ischial tuberosity makes her more uncomfortable, because she prefers to have most of the weight bearing on her left ischial tuberosity.

Movement Analysis. She experiences pain when standing, and she cannot tolerate standing with her back against the wall because of the marked tenderness over her sacrum. The following standing tests are performed: (1) forward bending, (2) lateral flexion, (3) rotation, and (4) single-leg stance.

Forward bending. This motion increases her pain. Supporting her body weight with her hands and arms on a table allows her to bend forward with less discomfort. She also reports pain with the return movement from forward bending.

Lateral flexion. This motion does not change her symptoms, and she has symmetrical C-curves with side bending to the left and right sides.

Rotation. These motions are symmetrical.

Single-leg stance. With flexion of either hip, this motion increases her back pain.

The following tests are performed with the patient in a supine position: (1) hip flexor length, (2) position effects, (3) hip abduction/lateral rotation from hip flexion, (4) abdominal muscle strength, and (5) hip and knee flexion.

Hip flexor length. While performing this test, her pelvis almost immediately moves into an anterior tilt when either hip is lowered into extension, even though the patient has completely relaxed her hip flexor muscles. She reports an increase in back pain when the hip is in 30 degrees of flexion. The right hip extends slightly less than the left.

Position effects. She reports increased symptoms when her hips and knees are extended. However, even when her hips and knees are flexed passively, she is uncomfortable because of the tenderness over her sacrum, which is quite prominent.

Hip abduction/lateral rotation from hip flexion. This motion causes pain in her hips with only the slightest of motion. Both the right and left hips are painful.

Abdominal muscular strength. The strength of the abdominal muscles is less than 1 out of 5.

Hip and knee flexion. Initiation of unilateral hip and knee flexion is almost immediately associated with pelvic rotation and an increase of symptoms. Stabilizing her pelvis decreases her symptoms.

The following additional tests are performed in five positions: (1) side lying, (2) prone, (3) quadruped, (4) sitting, and (5) stance phase of gait.

Side lying. The patient is more comfortable in this position than in the supine position. Although she has a broad pelvis, her symptoms are not improved by a support under her side at waist level. Hip movements are all painful.

Prone. The patient needs a pillow under her abdomen to tolerate this position. There are no changes in her symptoms and no pelvic motion when testing knee flexion in the prone position. She is not able to perform the movements to test hip rotation because of the pain in her hips.

Quadruped. The patient reports pain in her pelvis in the quadruped position, which increases with attempts to rock backward. She also feels pain in her lower abdomen in this position.

Sitting. The patient stands only 5 feet, 2 inches tall. Consequently, her feet do not touch the ground. When properly positioned, enabling her to use the backrest of the chair and a foot stool to support her feet, she is comfortable.

Stance phase of gait. When the patient walks, marked pelvic rotation is evident during the stance phase, bilaterally.

Muscle Length and Strength Analysis. The hip flexors are short, and the abdominal muscles are weak and painful to palpation.

Diagnosis. The patient has tenderness over her entire pelvic and abdominal areas. Her hip flexors are short, and she is in anterior pelvic tilt. Any movement that requires the use of her abdominal muscles increases her pain. The soreness and tenderness after the most recent automobile accident can be attributed to muscle strain, as well as to the additional stress on her pelvis and lumbar spine caused by her preexisting pelvic malalignment and lordosis. The diagnosis is abdominal muscle strain and lumbar extension syndrome without radiating symptoms.

Intervention. The primary recommendation is that she use lumbopelvic support. She is fitted with an elastic back brace that supports her abdominal muscles and her spine. She is also taught how to perform heel slides, but her discomfort in the supine position makes it difficult for her to perform these exercises. Because of her schedule, the patient does not return for intervention for 4 weeks. This is a reasonable period to wait for a return visit, because time is necessary for the muscle strain to subside. The elastic back brace gives her significant relief from pain.

Approximately 4 weeks after her first visit, she is reevaluated. She reports that the back brace has helped her and that she is able to function during the day and is more comfortable when standing. She no longer feels the same tenderness in her abdominal muscles, but she still experiences pain in her pelvis and low back. She rates her pain at 4 to 5 out of 10. When standing, a marked lordosis is obvious and the hip flexor length test supports shortness of her hip flexors, including her iliopsoas. She lacks 25 degrees of complete hip extension bilaterally. During the test, more anterior pelvic tilt is evident on the right side than on the left.

When in a supine position, the patient is taught to hold one knee to her chest, contract her abdominal muscles, and slide the other hip into extension. She is instructed to repeat this exercise with the contralateral extremity. With a pillow under her abdomen and lying in the prone position, the patient is instructed to contract her abdominal muscles and then flex her knee. When standing with her low back against the wall and her hips and knees flexed enough to allow her lumbar spine to flatten against the wall, she is instructed to extend her hips and knees while contracting her abdominal muscles. The therapist also observes that when the patient becomes uncomfortable while standing, she repeatedly extends her back. She is asked to avoid this movement and to stand with her lumbar spine against the wall for a brief period.

The patient returns 2 weeks later and reports that for 1 week she experienced an increase of tenderness in her anterior pelvic area, but now she feels better. She is sleeping better and is able to roll and turn without pain. She also tolerates a full day of activity without significant discomfort. Since she has switched her strategy of leaning back when uncomfortable to standing with her back supported against the wall, the pain diminishes more rapidly.

The patient can lie supine with her hips and knees extended with minimal discomfort, but she has to contract her abdominal muscles actively. Her hip flexor length test indicates that her hip flexors still lack 10 degrees of normal length. In the prone position, she is still unable to abduct her hip or perform more than 10 degrees of hip medial or lateral rotation without pain in the hip joints.

The slight increase of pain in the anterior pelvic area is attributed to the stretch of her hip flexors and the strengthening of her abdominal muscles. Her back pain is clearly related to the lordosis and increased extension movements of her lumbar spine. For her maintenance program she is instructed to continue performing her current exercises and hip abduction in the prone position with a pillow under her abdomen. She is asked to limit the range of motion to the onset of pain in her hips. A walking program is recommended during which she is to contract her abdominal and gluteal muscles on the side of the swing leg at heel strike. She is also instructed to place her hands on her pelvis while walking to monitor the motion and to limit rotational movements, which requires that she take smaller steps.

Outcome. Approximately 3 months after her initial visit, the patient is able to tolerate a full day of activity without pain. She performs all activities of daily living without difficulty or symptoms. She can lie supine with both hips and knees extended for prolonged periods. Her hip abduction motion has increased to 15 degrees bilaterally, and her hip rotation ranges are also 15 degrees.

Lumbar Rotation Syndrome

Although rotation is a common cause of pain, it is not common to find a patient that has a pure lumbar rotation syndrome. Because lateral flexion includes the rotation movement, there are some patients that experience increased symptoms with simply rotating or side bending movements. They fall into this category.

Symptoms and Pain

Symptoms are usually transient and occur with changes in position. The patient with lumbar rotation syndrome may also have difficulty sitting in one position for a prolonged period. He or she may have low level aching in the back. Radiologic diagnoses include degenerative disk disease, spondylolisthesis, osteoarthritis, spinal instability, and facet syndrome.

Alignment

The structural variations in alignment and body proportions that may be present in patients with the rotation syndrome include the following: (1) a broad pelvis with a narrow trunk, (2) a bony leg-length discrepancy, (3) hip antetorsion or retrotorsion, and (4) scoliosis. The acquired impairments in alignment are asymmetry between the right and left lumbothoracic paraspinal areas and apparent leg-length discrepancy.

Movement Impairments

STANDING POSITION. In the standing position the following tests should be performed: (1) forward bending, (2) lateral flexion, (3) rotation, and (4) single-leg standing.

•• **Forward bending.** Most often this movement does not cause pain. Some asymmetry in the lumbar spine may be evident in the fully flexed position. The return from forward bending may cause pain when the patient slightly rotates while returning to the upright position.

•• **Lateral flexion.** This movement can be asymmetric when comparing one side with the other. The lumbar spine has a single segment that is the axis of motion during lateral flexion, which may be associated with hypertrophy or stiffness of the paraspinal muscles (see Figure 3-19, *C-F*). Also, there may be an increase in symptoms with lateral flexion. To confirm the positive test for lumbar rotation, the patient is stabilized on the lateral side of the thorax at the level of the iliac crest on the side to which the patient is side bending. The therapist asks the patient to repeat the motion and notes any changes in symptoms, shape of the curve, or range of motion.

• **Rotation.** Rotation toward one side versus the other can be asymmetric.

• **Single-leg stance.** This position is associated with lateral trunk flexion (Figure 3-39) or with pelvic rotation.

SUPINE POSITION. The following tests are performed with the patient in a supine position: (1) hip flexor length, (2) position effects, (3) hip and knee flexion, (4) hip abduction/lateral rotation from flexion, and (5) lower abdominal muscular strength.

• **Hip flexor length.** Often the anterior pelvic tilt during the test is greater on one side than on the other.

•• **Position effects.** Symptoms may increase when hips and knees are extended. If the TFL muscle is short, flexing or abducting the hip will decrease the symptoms because the rotation of the pelvis is alleviated.

•• **Hip and knee flexion.** Since pelvic rotation may occur during active hip and knee flexion, this movement may increase symptoms. To confirm a positive test for lumbar rotation, the pelvis is stabilized and the therapist notes the effect on the symptoms.

•• **Hip abduction/lateral rotation from flexion.** This movement may cause pelvic rotation and an increase in symptoms. To confirm a positive test for lumbar rotation, the pelvis is stabilized and the motion is repeated. The therapist notes the effects of this motion on the symptoms.

• **Lower abdominal muscle strength.** Preventing lumbopelvic rotation by controlling the abdominal muscles is more important than abdominal muscular strength. Many patients have strong abdominal muscles, but they do not control the lumbopelvic rotation associated with movement of the lower extremities.

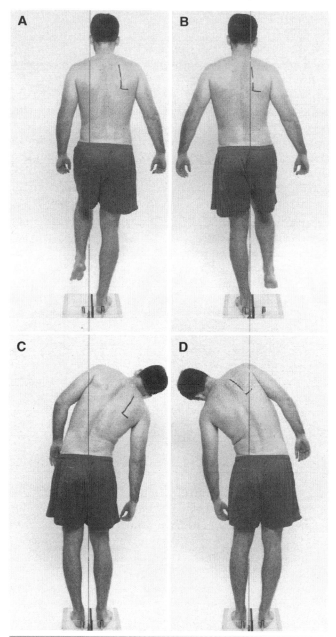

Figure 3-39

Lateral flexion flexibility during single-leg standing and side bending. *A,* Left hip and knee flexion while standing on the right lower extremity does not cause lumber spine moton. *B,* Right hip and knee flexion while standing on the left lower extremity causes thoracolumbar flexion. *C,* Side bending to the right is associated with minimal lateral shift of the pelvis. *D,* Side bending to the left is associated with lateral shift of the pelvis and a greater degree of thoracolumbar flexion than side bending to the right. The differences in the trunk motion during the two tasks suggests that lateral upper trunk flexion to the left is more flexible than to the right.

• **Rolling.** Symptoms may increase when the patient rolls onto his side and rotates his pelvis by pushing with the feet before turning the upper body. To confirm a positive test for lumbar rotation, the pa-tient is instructed to roll so that the trunk and pelvis move together. The therapist notes the effect on the symptoms.

Additional tests are performed in the following four positions: (1) side lying, (2) prone, (3) quadruped, and (4) sitting.

SIDE-LYING POSITION

• **Hip lateral rotation.** This movement may be as-sociated with pelvic rotation.

• **Hip abduction and adduction.** Either move-ment may be associated with a lateral pelvic tilt, which supports a positive test for lumbar rotation because lat-eral flexion of the lumbar spine is associated with rota-tion (Figure 3-40).

PRONE POSITION

•• **Knee flexion.** This movement may cause pelvic rotation and an increase in symptoms. To confirm a pos-itive test for lumbar rotation, the pelvis is stabilized and the motion is repeated. The therapist notes the effects of the knee flexion movement on the symptoms.

•• **Hip rotation.** This movement may be associ-ated with lumbopelvic rotation and an increase in the symptoms. To confirm a positive test for lumbar rota-tion, the pelvis is stabilized and the hip rotational mo-tion is repeated. The therapist notes the effects of the movement on the symptoms.

QUADRUPED POSITION

•• **Rocking backward.** The lumbar spine or pelvis rotates as the patient rocks backward. The pelvis may also tilt laterally. The symptoms may lessen because of the decrease in compression between the vertebral seg-ments.

•• **Shoulder flexion.** This movement may cause rotation of the lumbar spine.

SITTING POSITION

•• **Knee extension.** This movement may cause ro-tation of the pelvis and spine.

Summary

The primary problem is rotation of the spine. Rather than throughout the spine, the motion occurs at one or two segments. This tendency for excessive rotation may also occur during movements of the extremities.

Flexibility and Stiffness Impairments

The lumbar spine is more flexible into rotation and lat-eral flexion at the lower segments than it is at the upper segments and during the hip motions of adduction and rotation. The paraspinal muscles can be stiffer than the abdominal muscles, contributing to the lateral flexion occurring at only a couple of segments. The hip ab-ductors can be stiffer than the lateral abdominal mus-cles, contributing to lateral pelvic tilt and associated lateral flexion of the spine.

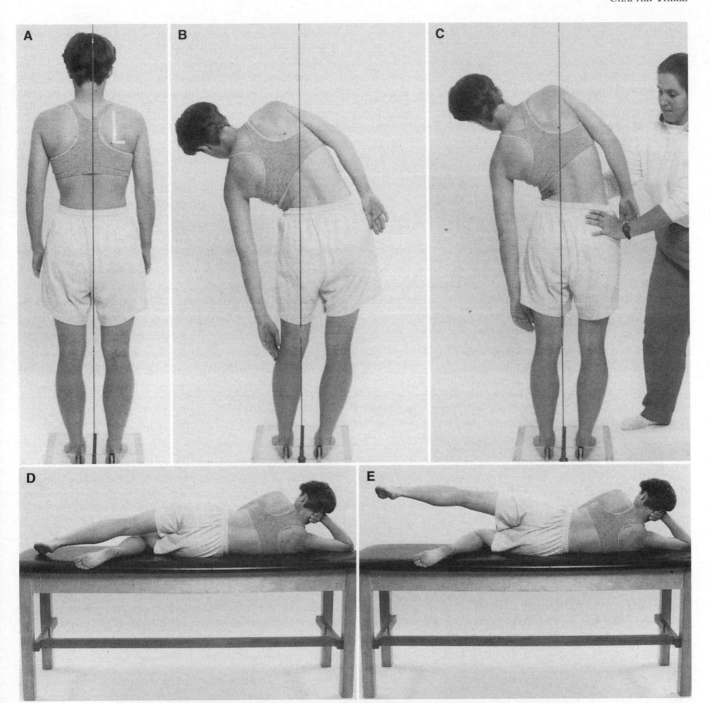

Figure 3-40

Relative flexibility of the lumbar spine during side bending. *A,* Neutral alignment of the lumbar spine is demonstrated during standing. *B,* During side bending, the movement appears to be occurring at the lowest lumbar segments. *C,* Blocking the motion at the most flexible site demonstrates that the rest of lumbar spine can side bend, as long as motion is blocked at the segment where it occurs most easily. *D,* When the patient is lying on her right side, the motion at the flexible lumbar segment is evident. *E,* When she abducts her hip while maintaining slight hip extension, the pelvis tilts laterally and the motion at the lumbopelvic segment is further increased.

Muscle and Recruitment Pattern Impairments

There is inadequate recruitment of the external oblique and the contralateral internal oblique to control rotation. Dominance of the activity of the rectus abdominis muscle may contribute to this recruitment pattern impairment. There may also be length and strength impairments. The TFL, hip abductor, and/or paraspinal muscles may be stiff or short.

Confirming Tests

Preventing the lumbar rotation or lateral flexion that occurs with trunk movements or during movements of the extremities decreases the patient's symptoms.

Summary

Rotational motions are usually a frequent part of the patient's activities. Although the thoracic spine has the greatest rotational range, in some patients the rotation involves the lumbar spine. As a result, the lowest lumbar segments become particularly flexible in the direction of rotation. Some muscles of the hips become stiffer than the abdominal muscles. The lack of control by the abdominal muscles contributes to the compensatory trunk rotation and lateral spine flexion. As a result, rotational motions that should be confined to the hips also involve the lumbar spine.

Treatment

PRIMARY OBJECTIVES. Preventing rotation in lumbar spine or the lumbopelvic articulation decreases the symptoms. This objective is best achieved by helping the patient identify the rotational movements that are performed during daily activities, such as rotating at a desk or leaning on one arm into lateral flexion. Although patients may rotate their chairs, they often do so by the momentum of turning their upper bodies. If patients participate in sports that involve rotation, maximizing the rotational flexibility of the hips to avoid compensatory motions in the lumbar spine is an essential part of the program. Correction of the rotation malalignment is achieved primarily by the rocking backward exercise using the quadruped position. Other exercises are designed to increase the stability provided by the abdominal muscles.

CORRECTIVE EXERCISE PROGRAM

Supine. The progression of exercises for the lower abdominal muscles (described in Chapter 7) is designed to improve the control and performance of the abdominal muscles. The exercise of hip abduction/lateral rotation from flexion and hip adduction/medial rotation will also improve the control of the abdominal muscles and teach the patient to prevent associated lumbopelvic rotation. Another exercise that improves the performance of the abdominal muscles is abduction of the shoulder on a diagonal of 135 degrees with a weight and then the return movement of shoulder adduction to 90 degrees.

Side lying. Performing hip lateral rotation to dissociate hip motion from lumbopelvic motion is helpful to the patient with the rotation syndrome. Additional exercises that improve the control of the lateral abdominal muscles include hip abduction and adduction performed without lateral pelvic tilt.

Prone. Knee flexion and hip lateral rotation without lumbopelvic rotation improve the extensibility of the hip and anterior thigh muscles and the performance of the abdominal muscles.

Quadruped. The patient should perform the rocking backward motion while preventing any rotation of the spine or hip joint. Another exercise that improves the control of the abdominal muscles is unilateral shoulder flexion while contracting the abdominal muscles, which prevents lumbar spine rotation.

Sitting. The patient should perform knee extension while preventing lumbopelvic rotation.

Standing. The most important exercise in the standing position is the performance of lateral flexion with a support at the lateral side of the trunk at the waist level to prevent any lateral shear or single axis motion in the lowest segments of the lumbar spine.

CORRECTING POSTURAL HABIT AND MOVEMENT PATTERNS. As previously mentioned, the most important aspect of an intervention program is to help the patient identify the myriad of ways he or she may be provoking symptoms by rotating the lumbar spine during daily activities, as well as during recreational or sporting activities. The strategy is preventing the rotation in the lumbar spine and limiting the rotation to the hip joints and the thoracic spine. However, the therapist must be certain that the motion is occurring in the upper thoracic spine. Many people sit while laterally flexed or slightly rotated without being aware they are assuming these postures. Crossing the legs or sitting on a leg can also rotate the spine. Short people are the most likely to sit on their legs because their feet do not touch the ground while using most chairs.

Case Presentation

History. A 26-year-old graduate student has developed back pain, primarily as the result of sitting in class for 5 to 6 hours a day. Her course of study requires this prolonged sitting for 5 days a week. The patient is quite active in sports and participates in intramural volleyball, Frisbee, basketball, and softball. She has experienced episodes of back pain in the past, but typically they have been of short duration and have not interfered with her sporting or studying activities or her ability to concentrate in class.

Symptoms. The symptoms are described as an aching in her lower back across the lumbopelvic area. When severe, she rates her pain at a level of 5 to 6 on a scale of 10. Her symptoms usually improve after sleeping at night. She prefers sleeping in a prone position. Most recently her discomfort has increased enough to awaken her at night when she turns.

Alignment Analysis. The patient's chest is slightly depressed. She stands with her upper back swayed back, but she is not in a posterior pelvic tilt. As a result, there is some increase in the extension of her lower lumbar curve. She is slender with good muscle development.

Movement Analysis. The following standing tests are performed: (1) forward bending and return from forward bending, (2) lateral flexion, (3) rotation, and (4) single-leg stance.

Forward bending and return from forward bending. Both movements are performed without any increase in symptoms. Her hip flexibility is good with 85 degrees of hip flexion, and her lumbar spine has a final flexion position of 15 degrees.

Lateral flexion. When the patient flexes to either side, the motion occurs only in the lowest of the lumbar segments and her spine remained perfectly straight without any curvature. The motion also increases her symptoms. When stabilized at the side of the thorax, she is unable to side bend. This finding is the same when she attempts motion to either side.

Rotation. The range is the same on both sides and does not elicit symptoms.

Single-leg stance. There is slight pelvic rotation toward the side of the stance leg with the trunk remaining in a constant position.

The following tests are performed with the patient in a supine position: (1) hip flexor length, (2) hip and knee flexion, and (3) hip abduction/lateral rotation from flexion.

Hip flexor length. There is normal length, and the movement is performed without compensatory motion. She does not experience symptoms with her hips and knees extended.

Hip and knee flexion. Passively, her hip flexibility is within normal limits. Actively, pelvic rotation of $1/2$ inch is evident with movement of either lower extremity with no change in symptoms.

Hip abduction/lateral rotation from flexion. There is slight pelvic rotation during the first 50% of the motion. There is more rotation with the right lower extremity motion than there is with the left.

The following tests are performed in four positions: (1) side lying, (2) prone, (3) quadruped, and (4) sitting.

Side lying. There is no pelvic rotation during either the hip lateral rotation test or the hip abduction and adduction test.

Prone. The prone position does not produce a change in symptoms. During the knee flexion test, there is no pelvic motion and no change in symptoms. There is slight pelvic rotation during hip lateral rotation, primarily during the last part of the range. This compensatory motion is present with hip rotation with both the right and left lower extremities.

Quadruped. There are no signs of rotation in the resting alignment. There is no change in alignment or in symptoms during the rocking backward test.

Sitting. Flexing or extending her spine does not change her symptoms. When she leans to one side, even slightly, the movement occurs at the lowest lumbar segment, as has been seen in the standing position during lateral flexion. There is no lumbar or pelvic motion during the knee extension test. Hamstring length is normal.

Muscle Length and Strength Analysis. The back extensor muscles are short, as derived from the patient's inability to flex the thorax laterally when motion is blocked at L4, L5, and S1. All other muscles are within normal limits for length and strength, except there is some evidence that the abdominal muscles do not prevent pelvic rotation during lower extremity movements.

Diagnosis. The only notable muscle impairment is a shortness of the patient's back extensor muscles. She also stands in a slightly exaggerated position of lumbar extension, but she does not have any symptoms that are produced by extension nor are her symptoms alleviated by lumbar flexion. The patient indicates that she has been working as a part-time waitress and has been carrying heavy trays. This activity, combined with her sports, had created a DSM of lumbar rotation. In this system, lateral spine flexion impairments are considered rotational impairments. When she sits in class, she has a habit of frequently shifting from one side to another. Her books are kept on the floor next to her chair; as a result, she frequently leans to one side to select a book or notebook. This repetitive motion irritates her lower spinal motion segments and probably creates a situation that has resulted in instability. The diagnosis is lumbar rotation syndrome.

Intervention. The primary objective of the program is to eliminate the subtle side-bending motions that the patient is performing. The exercises are selected on the basis that they will help her control the pelvis and prevent any rotational motions of the lower lumbar spine.

From the supine position, the patient is taught the movements of the active hip and knee flexion exercise in which she contracts her abdominal muscles to prevent pelvic rotation. She performs the hip abduction/lateral rotation exercise by contracting her abdominal muscles to prevent pelvic rotation. From the prone position she performs hip lateral rotation while contracting her abdominal muscles, again to prevent pelvic rotation. From a sitting position she is instructed to place her hand against her side, just above the iliac crest, and lean her shoulders without side bending her lumbar spine. She is asked to avoid any side-bending movements when sitting.

A standing exercise, along with these sitting recommendations, is considered the most important part of her exercise program. She places her hand at her side, just above the iliac crest, and leans to the side by tilting her shoulders without moving her lumbar spine. She also contracts her abdominal muscles by "thinking about pulling her navel toward her spine," and she does not allow her upper back to sway back. She is instructed to perform this exercise frequently during the day. There are no recommended side-lying or quadruped exercises.

Outcome. The patient has been away from the classroom setting for 6 weeks, and, as a result, the time she has spent in a sitting position is minimal. She is physically active during this interval and even participates in sports. When she is reexamined 6 weeks later, she performs all movements without compensatory lumbopelvic rotation. She is able to tilt her shoulders laterally while maintaining a constant position of her lumbar spine, which had not been previously possible. The patient indicates that she does not have any back pain, though she had a brief episode after falling while using a trampoline. After this incident the patient had a 4-month period of sitting approximately 6 hours a day, but she has not experienced any significant back pain. She reports that she has to be careful; as long as she does not lean to the side and continues to perform her standing lateral flexion exercise, she does not experience pain.

Lumbar Rotation-Flexion Syndrome

Studies by Pearcy show that when the patient is in a sitting position, the lumbar spine allows a greater degree of rotation than when he or she assumes an upright or a forward leaning position.[44] Therefore the individual who sits at a desk in a slumped position and then rotates to reach a computer, the telephone, or into a file drawer is at risk for developing lumbar rotation-flexion syndrome. Clinical practice suggests that the most likely candidates for pain associated with flexion are men, usually between the ages of 18 and 45 years. In part, this trend may be because men have less hip flexion flexibility, are taller than women, and have longer tibias, which cause them to sit in lumbar flexion when the chair is not properly adjusted. When a patient with long tibia bones stands from a sitting position, the spine rather than the hips is often flexed when leaning forward to initiate the movement of lifting the hips off the seat of the chair.

Symptoms and Pain

Back pain is present most often with sitting, bending, and twisting. Pain is often worst on rising in the morning and improves with moving or after a hot shower. The patient may also have radiating pain into the buttocks and lower extremities. Radiologic diagnoses include herniated disk, degenerative disk disease, osteoarthritis, and instability. The severity of the symptoms varies, depending on the acuity of the condition and the severity of the problem.

Movement Impairments

STANDING POSITION. A patient has fewer symptoms when in a standing position than when he or she is sitting. The following tests are performed with the patient in a standing position: (1) forward bending, (2) corrected forward bending, (3) lateral flexion, (4) rotation of the trunk, and (5) single-leg standing.

•• *Forward bending.* Most often the lumbar spine flexes more readily than the hips, the range of hip flexion may be limited, and in this scenario the symptoms may increase. The paraspinal area of the spine may appear to be asymmetric. Although many men have limited hip flexion during forward bending, shortness of the hamstring muscles is not always the primary reason. If a man is asked to support his upper body with his arms by placing his hands on an elevated table, he will likely achieve at least 75 to 80 degrees of hip flexion. Limited hip motion is the result of the influence the hamstrings exert to control the weight of the trunk, not because the muscles are short. Stretching the hamstring muscles is not a recommended method of changing the forward bending pattern. As previously mentioned, forward bending is considered a sensitive test, not a specific test.

•• *Corrected forward bending.* To confirm a positive test for lumbar flexion, the patient places his hands on a table and forward bends by flexing the hips, not the lumbar spine. The symptoms should decrease. The patient may also need to flex the knees when bending forward.

•• *Lateral flexion.* Symptoms may increase and the motion should be asymmetrical. To confirm a positive test for lateral flexion, the therapist provides support at the lateral side of the thorax to prevent the motion of one segment and notes the effect of the movement on the symptoms.

• *Rotation of trunk.* This movement is often asymmetric in the range of motion.

• *Single-leg stance.* There is often rotation in the lumbopelvic area with asymmetry noted from side to side.

SUPINE POSITION. The following tests are performed with the patient in a supine position: (1) hip flexor length,

(2) position effects, (3) hip and knee flexion, and (4) hip abduction/lateral rotation from flexion.

• *Hip flexor length.* Unilateral TFL muscular stiffness with compensatory lumbopelvic rotation is a relatively common finding in the patient with lumbar rotation-flexion syndrome.

• *Position effects.* The patient's symptoms do not usually increase with the hips and knees extended.

• *Hip and knee flexion.* Rotation of the pelvis with an increase in symptoms or rotation with more than $1/2$ inch of motion, usually asymmetric from side to side, is considered a positive finding for lumbar rotation. The range into hip flexion is less than 120 degrees or there is associated lumbar flexion during passive hip flexion. With bilateral hip flexion, there is increased symptoms and compensatory lumbar flexion.

•• *Hip abduction/lateral rotation from flexion.* There is increased symptoms or compensatory pelvic rotation of more than $1/2$ inch. To confirm a positive test for lumbar rotation, the pelvis is stabilized. The therapist notes the effects of the hip motion without pelvic movement on the symptoms.

SIDE-LYING POSITION. Positive results in the following tests support the finding of excessive lateral flexion of the lumbar spine and thus of a rotational DSM and are performed with the patient in a side-lying position: (1) hip lateral rotation and (2) hip abduction and adduction.

• *Hip lateral rotation.* This movement may be associated with pelvic rotation.

• *Hip abduction and adduction.* These movements may be associated with lateral pelvic tilt in rostral direction.

PRONE POSITION. The following tests are performed with the patient in a prone position: (1) position effects, (2) knee flexion, and (3) hip rotation.

• *Position effects.* Symptoms may decrease in this position.

•• *Knee flexion.* This movement may cause lumbopelvic rotation and result in an increase in symptoms. To confirm a positive test for lumbar rotation, the pelvis is stabilized and the knee flexion motion is repeated. The therapist notes the effects of the movement on the symptoms.

• *Hip rotation.* This movement may be associated with pelvic rotation and an increase in the symptoms. To confirm a positive test for lumbar rotation, the pelvis is stabilized and the motion is repeated. The therapist notes the effects of the movement on the symptoms.

QUADRUPED POSITION. The following tests are performed with the patient in a quadruped position: (1) position effects, (2) rocking backward, and (3) shoulder flexion.

• *Position effects.* Allowing the lumbar curve to increase and thereby reduce the degree of flexion may decrease the symptoms.

•• *Rocking backward.* The lumbar spine or pelvis may rotate while rocking backward, and the symptoms may increase. The pelvis may also tilt laterally.

•• *Shoulder flexion.* This movement may cause rotation of the lumbar spine.

SITTING POSITION. The following tests are performed with the patient in a sitting position: (1) position effects, (2) lumbar flexion, and (3) knee extension.

•• *Position effects.* Increasing the lumbar curve may decrease the symptoms.

•• *Lumbar flexion.* Flexion of the lumbar spine may increase the symptoms.

•• *Knee extension.* This movement may cause lumbar flexion and rotation of the pelvis and spine.

Summary

The motions of flexion and rotation are the primary causes of low back pain or radiating symptoms. Movements of the extremities contribute to the lumbopelvic rotation. Identifying the direction of the predominant rotational pattern is useful in determining which activities may be the primary contributor to the movement impairment. The other tests also help identify which movements of the extremities contribute to the problem.

Alignment: Structural Variations and Acquired Impairments

The flat lumbar spine is a structural variation more frequently observed in men, who normally have longer trunks in proportion to the lower body. Other structural variations are leg-length discrepancies and hip retrotorsion and antetorsion. Hip retrotorsion is found more frequently in men, and hip antetorsion is found more frequently in women.

Acquired impairments of alignment include the flat back with posterior pelvic tilt and hip joint extension, a swayback posture, a large abdomen, and an apparent leg-length discrepancy.

Flexibility and Stiffness Impairments

The lumbar spine is more flexible into flexion and rotation than the hamstring and gluteus maximus muscles are extensible. The hamstring muscles are stiffer than the back extensor muscles.

Muscle Recruitment Pattern Impairments

When standing in a swayback posture, the abdominal muscles, particularly the rectus abdominis, provide more trunk support than do the back extensor muscles. The rectus abdominis, TFL, and hamstring muscles may be short or stiff. The abdominal muscles have poor control of lumbopelvic rotation.

Confirming Tests

Preventing flexion and rotation of the lumbar spine decreases or eliminates the patient's symptoms. The method of confirming each test is described by the specific test.

Treatment

PRIMARY OBJECTIVES. The primary objective is to improve the control provided by the abdominal muscles, which prevents rotational motions of the lumbar spine without contributing to the lumbar flexion. The other muscles, whose performance needs to be improved, are the back extensors. The back extensor muscles need to be shortened or stiffened to (1) prevent compensatory lumbar flexion, (2) improve the motion of hip flexion, and (3) maintain the spine in a flat alignment when sitting. Because rotation is also a component of the patient's problem, correcting muscles that are short or stiff and contribute to rotation is another important aspect of the program. The patient also needs to know which activities, when performed, are causing incorrect movement patterns. For example, when an individual plays golf, he or she needs to ensure that the hips and thoracic spine are rotating, not the lumbar spine. When the patient has retroverted hips, he or she needs to stand with the hips slightly rotated laterally with the feet pointing outward, so that medial rotation range is available at the hips.

CORRECTIVE EXERCISE PROGRAM

Supine exercises. The patient performs active hip and knee flexion while preventing pelvic rotation by contracting the abdominal muscles. Placing a folded towel under the lumbar spine will help prevent lumbar flexion that can result from the contraction of the abdominal muscles. The patient should carefully grade the amount of the contraction. After completing the flexion motion, the patient should use the hands to pull the knee to the chest to stretch the short or stiff hip extensor muscles. Care should be taken not to flex the lumbar spine during this exercise. The patient should perform hip abduction–lateral rotation from flexion and prevent lumbopelvic rotation by contracting the abdominal muscles.

Side-lying exercises. The patient performs hip lateral rotation without lumbopelvic rotation, as well as hip abduction and adduction while preventing lateral pelvic tilt.

Prone exercises. The patient performs knee flexion and then hip rotation while preventing lumbopelvic rotation by contracting the abdominal muscles. To improve the performance of a weak gluteus maximus muscle and decrease the dominance of the hamstring muscles, the patient performs hip extension through a limited range. This exercise will also improve the performance of the back extensor muscles. The patient performs shoulder flexion from 90 to 180 degrees to improve the performance of the back extensor muscles.

Quadruped exercises. The patient performs a rocking backward motion while preventing lumbar flexion and increasing hip flexion without lumbar rotation.

Sitting exercises. The patient performs knee extension with the spine against a straight-back chair. The patient should slightly extend the back while extending the knee and preventing lumbopelvic flexion or rotation.

Standing exercises. The patient performs the forward bending movement with the axis of motion in the hip joints, allowing the knees to flex. The patient performs lateral flexion with support at the side of the thorax at the level of L4 and L5.

CORRECTING POSTURAL HABITS AND MOVEMENT PATTERNS. The patient sits erect with the lumbar spine flat and hips flexed to 90 degrees. The head and shoulders are in line with the hips and not forward of the spine, which creates a flexion moment on the spine. If the patient has long tibia bones, the seat should be raised so that the hips and knees are at the same level. While moving to a standing position, the patient moves to the edge of the chair and then maintains a straight position of the spine. The patient must not lean to one side when sitting or stand with one hip in adduction; both positions cause lateral flexion of the spine. If the patient participates in any rotational activities, such as racquetball or golf, he or she should modify the pattern of the swing.

Case Presentation

History. A 39-year-old cardiologist has had episodes of low back pain since college, but they have not interfered with his activities. The patient performs cardiac catheterizations, which he believes has contributed to his recent episodes of back pain. For the year before his referral to physical therapy, the pain episodes have increased in frequency and severity. The last episode, 1 month before his physical therapy consultation, had been severe enough to keep him from working. He had remained at home in bed for 3 days. The patient also plays golf and has tried to play at least once a week when weather permits.

Symptoms. The patient's pain is located in his lower back, with pain radiating into his left buttock. During his last episode, the pain had radiated down his left lower extremity. After approximately 3 days the radiating pain in his thigh and leg had ceased. No change has been found in his reflexes, muscle strength, or sensation in the right lower extremity. The patient has less pain when in a standing position than in a sitting position and has been most comfortable when walking. During his acute episode he had been most comfortable when lying on his back on the floor with his hips and knees supported in flexion. At the time of his examination, he had rated his pain at a level of 3 to 4 on a scale of 10 in the standing position. In the sitting position he had rated the intensity of this pain at a level of 6.

Alignment Analysis. The patient is 6 feet 2 inches tall with a slender build. He has a slight thoracic kyphosis, and his lumbar spine is flat. His iliac crests are 2 inches higher than his belt line, and he has a flat lumbar spine. His iliac crests are level, and no pelvic tilt or rotation is present. The left side of the lumbar paraspinal area is approximately $1/2$ inch larger than the right.

Alignment Analysis. The following standing tests are performed: (1) forward bending, (2) forward bending with hip flexion only and hand support of upper body, (3) lateral flexion, (4) rotation, and (5) single-leg stance.

Forward bending. This motion increases the symptoms in his spine. During the movement his lumbar spine flexes more rapidly than his hips. In the fully flexed position, the lumbar flexion is 20 degrees, and the hip flexion range is 65 degrees. During the return from forward bending, his symptoms decrease.

Forward bending with hip flexion only and hand support of upper body. When the patient flexes his knees and hips and reduces the degree of lumbar flexion motion, his symptoms do not increase as much as they did with the previous forward bending motion.

Lateral flexion. This motion increases his symptoms, particularly when side bending to the left. The range of side-bending motion toward the left is less than it is toward the right. Lateral stabilization at the iliac crest level decreases his symptoms.

Rotation. The range of motion is slightly greater rotating to the left than it is to the right.

Single-leg stance. With left hip flexion, his pelvis rotates toward the left. During right hip flexion, no lumbopelvic rotation is evident.

The following tests are performed with the patient in a supine position: (1) hip flexor length, (2) hip and knee flexion, (3) hip abduction/lateral rotation from flexion, and (4) abdominal muscular strength.

Hip flexor length. The TFL muscles are found to be short bilaterally. When hip abduction is prevented during the test, there is compensatory lumbopelvic rotation when testing the left lower extremity. The patient's symptoms decrease when recumbent. He is even more comfortable when a small pillow is placed under his left knee or his left hip is abducted.

Hip and knee flexion. When tested passively, there is resistance to hip flexion at 100 degrees on the left and 110 degrees on the right. When tested actively, there is pelvic rotation during the first 50% of the left hip flexion motion and no pelvic rotation during the right hip flexion motion.

Hip abduction/lateral rotation from flexion. There is no pelvic rotation observed with movement of either lower extremity. There is no change in symptoms with this motion.

The following additional tests are performed in four positions: (1) side lying, (2) prone, (3) quadruped, and (4) sitting.

Side lying. When testing hip lateral rotation, pelvic rotation is evident with movement of the left lower extremity but not with the right. When testing left hip abduction, there is lateral pelvic tilt and an increase in symptoms; when pelvic motion is restrained, the patient still has an increase in symptoms. There is no change in pelvic tilt during right hip abduction. When testing left hip adduction, there is an associated lateral pelvic tilt but no change in symptoms. No pelvic tilt occurs during right hip adduction.

Prone. The patient is comfortable in the prone position and his symptoms are minimal. When testing left knee flexion, the pelvis rotates counterclockwise without a change in symptoms. When the hip is abducted and the knee flexion is repeated, the pelvis does not rotate. There is no pelvic motion evident during right knee flexion. The pelvis rotates counterclockwise during left hip lateral rotation. No movement is evident during right hip lateral rotation. Lateral rotational range of motion is 50 degrees on the left and 55 degrees on the right. Although both the left and right hips rotate only 5 degrees medially, no pelvic motion occurs during hip medial rotation.

Quadruped. The lumbar spine is in slight flexion in the quadruped position. When rocking backward, the lumbar spine flexes during the initiation of the movement into hip flexion. At approximately 50% of the full excursion backward, the pelvis rotates counterclockwise and the hips shift toward the right. This change in pelvic alignment means that the right hip flexes more than the left. The left hip is abducted and slightly rotated laterally, and when the patient rocks backward the pelvis does not rotate and the hip flexion range is symmetrical.

Sitting. The patient's symptoms increase when he sits with his lumbar spine flexed. When the lumbar spine is extended his symptoms decrease. In the standard chair the patient's knees are higher than his hips. Lumbopelvic rotation and posterior pelvic tilt occur at −45 degrees of left knee extension, and the patient reports increased symptoms when the lumbopelvic motion occurs. During right knee extension to -35 degrees, his pelvis tilts posteriorly and the lumbar spine flexes with only a slight increase in symptoms. When the lumbopelvic motion is prevented, the knee extends to -45 degrees bilaterally. Assessment of hip rotational range of motion in the sitting position indicates that left hip lateral rotation is 50 degrees and right lateral rotation is 55 degrees. Medial rotational range is 5 degrees bilaterally. These findings are consistent with hip retrotorsion.

Muscle Length and Strength Analysis. The patient's external oblique muscles are tested at $3+/5$. The left posterior gluteus medius is tested at $4+/5$, and the right is tested at $5/5$. The gluteus maximus, hamstring, and both right and left TFL muscles are short.

Diagnosis. The patient's examination indicates that his lumbopelvic area is particularly susceptible to rotation to the left, or counterclockwise rotation, and that his lumbar spine flexes easily. Although his abdominal muscles generate enough tension to limit the rotation, there are contributing factors that are more dominant. A major contributing factor is the retrotorsion of his hips. As a right-handed golfer, his hips should rotate medially during the follow through of his golf swing. Because the structural variation of the hip prevents medial rotation, rotation at the lumbopelvic junction has become a compensatory motion. The shortness of the TFL muscles also exaggerates pelvic rotation during the stance phase of gait, particularly on his left side.

The left hip extensor muscles are stiffer than the right; therefore when the patient rocks backward while in the quadruped position, his right hip flexes more readily than his left. The stiffness of the left hip extensor muscles causes the lumbopelvic rotation and a shifting of the pelvis toward the right. By abducting and laterally rotating the left hip, the tension decreases on the posterior musculature. As a result, the patient can rock backward with symmetrical hip flexion range because the left hip is no longer stiffer than the right.

When taking a client's history, the patient sits on a stool that is lower than the seat of a chair. Typically, he crosses his right leg over his left and turns slightly to the left to make notes in the client's chart. When examining his recumbent clients, he leans over to use the stethoscope. When performing the cardiac catheterization procedure, he is required to wear a lead apron, lean forward, and slightly turn to the left. All these habits contribute to the lumbopelvic rotation and flexion. The diagnosis is lumbar rotation-flexion syndrome.

Intervention. While in the supine position, the patient places a towel that has been folded a few times under his lumbar spine. He performs active hip and knee flexion while contracting his abdominal muscles, but only enough to prevent pelvic rotation and without flattening his lumbar spine. At the end of the hip flexion range, he uses his hands to pull his knee toward his chest, limiting the motion-to-hip flexion and avoiding lumbar flexion. He performs hip abduction/lateral rotation from hip flexion while controlling pelvic rotation by contracting the abdominal muscles and avoiding lumbar flexion.

From the side-lying position, the patient performs hip lateral rotation without pelvic rotation. Hip abduction and adduction are not recommended because the patient's symptoms increase, even with stabilization. A possible explanation for the increased symptoms is lateral flexion of the lumbar spine from the contraction of the quadratus lumborum muscle as it assists in stabilizing the pelvis during the hip abduction motion.

When in a prone position, the patient performs knee flexion, stabilizing the pelvis by contracting the abdominal muscles and again avoiding an increase in the lumbar flexion. He performs hip lateral rotation with an emphasis on stabilizing the pelvis. This exercise helps stretch the TFL muscles.

While in the quadruped position, the patient rocks backward while maintaining a flat and unflexed lumbar spine, ensuring that the hips are flexed. The left hip is positioned so that it is slightly abducted and rotated laterally for the first few repetitions of the exercise; the hip joint then gradually assumes a neutral position in the frontal and transverse planes.

His chair is raised so that his hips and knees are at the same height. When sitting in a chair that cannot be raised, he places a pillow or wedge in the seat of the chair, and support is placed behind the entire lumbar spine. In this sitting position the patient performs knee extension without flexing his thigh, because contraction of his hip flexor muscles often increases his symptoms.

While in a standing position he performs forward bending movements while supporting his upper body. The main emphasis of this exercise is to teach the patient to move in the hips, not in the lumbar spine. Therefore he flexes both his hips and knees and leans forward a few degrees while supporting his upper body with his hands placed on a tall counter. There is no increase in symptoms when performing this exercise, and the patient is instructed to repeat it at least eight to ten times per day.

The patient is asked to modify some of his daily activities. He now sits on a straight back chair when taking a client's history, and writes on a desktop. He does not sit for longer than 30 minutes and stands for a few minutes before sitting down again. He flexes in the hips and knees when leaning forward during a client's examination. For his catheterization procedures, he is instructed to obtain a two-piece lead apron or tie the apron to his body with the strap around his pelvis. He leans forward at the hips and does not flex the lumbar spine. He slightly rotates the left hip laterally, so that the foot points laterally. This position provides hip medial rotation range and thus reduces the likelihood of rotation in the lumbar spine. When playing golf the patient stands with his feet pointing straight ahead but rotates the hips laterally, so that his feet point slightly laterally. He practices rotating the hips during the golf swing, rather than the lumbar spine. If necessary, he is advised to take lessons with a golf professional who can monitor his swing.

Outcome. The patient is extremely compliant with his program and makes the suggested modifications in his work and sport activities. He visits physical therapy four times over a 5-week period. By the second visit he correctly performs all his exercises and does so without symptoms. He flexes his hip 45 degrees while supporting his upper body with his hands without increasing his symptoms. After 5 weeks he can forward bend without hand support by flexing his hips to 75 degrees and simultaneously flexing his knees. He can sit in an erect posture for 1 hour without an increase in symptoms. If he experiences symptoms, he immediately relieves them by rocking backward in the quadruped position, making certain that he flexes in the hips, not in the lumbar spine.

Lumbar Flexion Syndrome

Lumbar flexion syndrome with and without radiating symptoms is more often found in men than women and in young individuals. Acutely herniated disk problems are most often associated with flexion.

Symptoms and Pain

A patient can experience back pain of varying degrees of severity and acuity, as well as varying degrees of radiating symptoms. Pain problems include herniated disk disease, lumbosacral strain, lumbago, and degenerative disk disease.

Movement Impairments

STANDING POSITION. The following tests are performed with the patient in a standing position: (1) position effects and (2) forward bending.

• *Position effects.* In the standing position the patient has less symptoms than when he or she is sitting.

•• *Forward bending.* The lumbar spine is often flat; it flexes more readily than the hips, and this movement increases the symptoms (Figure 3-41, *A* and *B*). To confirm a positive test for lumbar flexion, the patient performs forward bending with hip flexion only when the hands are on a raised table to support the body. The therapist notes the effect of this movement on the symptoms. If the patient has radicular symptoms, there may be an increase of symptoms, even with the corrected forward bending.

SUPINE POSITION. The following tests are performed with the patient in a supine position: (1) position effects, (2) hip and knee flexion, and (3) bilateral hip and knee flexion.

• *Position effects.* In the supine position the patient is often able to keep his hips and knees extended without increasing his symptoms. If compression contributes to his symptoms, he may need to flex his hips and knees.

•• *Hip and knee flexion.* At the end of this movement, passively pulling his knee to his chest may increase his symptoms because of the associated lumbar spine flexion.

•• *Bilateral hip and knee flexion.* At the end of this movement, passively pulling his knees to his chest may increase his symptoms because of the associated lumbar spine flexion.

PRONE POSITION. The following tests are performed with the patient in a prone position: (1) position effects and (2) knee flexion.

•• *Position effects.* The prone position may decrease symptoms.

• *Knee flexion.* At the initiation of this movement, there may be posterior pelvic tilt, but this finding is not common.

QUADRUPED POSITION. The following tests are performed with the patient in a quadruped position: (1) position effects and (2) rocking backward.

•• *Position effects.* In the quadruped position the lumbar spine is often flexed and the hips are in less than 90 degrees of flexion. When the patient allows his lumbar spine to flatten or assume a neutral alignment. often symptoms will decrease.

•• *Rocking backward.* When performing this movement, the lumbar spine flexes and the symptoms may increase (Figure 3-41, *C*). To confirm a positive test for lumbar flexion, the patient maintains a flat lumbar spine and rocks backward by flexing only at the hips. The therapist notes the effect of this motion on the symptoms.

SITTING POSITION. The following tests are performed with the patient in a sitting position: (1) position effects, (2) spine in flexion, (3) spine in extension, and (4) knee extension.

•• *Spine in flexion.* With the lumbar spine in flexion, there is an increase in the symptoms (Figure 3-41, *D*).

•• *Spine in extension.* With the lumbar spine in extension, there is a decrease in the symptoms.

•• *Knee extension.* This movement causes posterior pelvic tilt and lumbar flexion and may increase the symptoms (Figure 3-41, *E*). To confirm a positive test for lumbar flexion, the spine and pelvis is supported to prevent the flexion movement. The therapist notes the effect of preventing this motion on the symptoms.

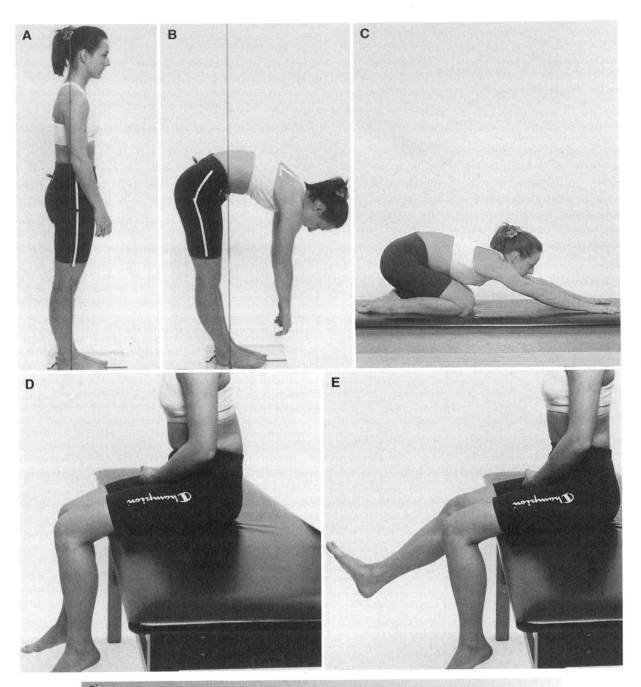

Figure 3-41

Excessive lumbar flexion flexibility. *A,* Flat lumbar spine is demonstrated while standing (marker at S2). *B,* Excessive lumbar flexion is shown during forward bending. *C,* Excessive lumbar flexion at the end of the backward movement is demonstrated in the quadruped position. The pull of the hamstring muscles or the weight of the upper trunk cannot be contributing to the lumbar flexion in this position. *D,* In the sitting position, the preferred alignment is lumbar flexion. *E,* Sitting with the hip in 90 degrees flexion, the knee extension is −20 degrees, thus her hamstring muscles are within 10 degrees of optimal length. The length of the hamstrings cannot be the cause of the limited hip flexion (60 degrees) during forward bending.

Summary

There are only a few movements of the extremities that impose flexion on the lumbar spine, whereas there are many movements of the extremities that impose rotation or extension motion on the spine. Major contributing factors that impose flexion on the lumbar spine include the following:

1. Sitting with the lumbar spine flexed with the head and shoulders forward of the spine
2. Having a structurally flat back
3. Developing excessive flexion flexibility of the lumbar spine, which causes forward leaning motions to occur more readily in the spine than in the hips

Because of the intimate relationship between the back extensor muscles and the spine, correcting the deficiency of back extensor muscular stiffness is easier than correcting the muscular stiffness deficiencies found in the other syndromes.

Alignment

The structural characteristics in alignment and body proportions that may be present in patients with the flexion syndrome include the following: (1) tall in height and having a long trunk relative to the lower body, (2) long tibias that cause the knees to be higher than the hips when sitting, and (3) a flat back without posterior pelvic tilt and usually high iliac crests. The acquired impairments in alignment are swayback posture and a flat back with posterior pelvic tilt.

Relative Flexibility and Stiffness Impairments

The lumbar spine is more flexible into flexion than the hips.

Muscle and Recruitment Pattern Impairments

The abdominal muscles may be recruited more readily than the hip flexors for leaning forward while in the sitting position. The hamstring and gluteus maximus muscles may be short and/or stiff. The back extensor muscles may be long and/or weak, whereas the abdominal muscles may be short and/or weak.

Confirming Tests

When the patient avoids the flexed alignment of his spine and learns to lean forward by moving the hips and not the lumbar spine, the symptoms will decrease.

Summary

Relatively few movements of the limbs contribute to patient symptoms. However, sitting and leaning forward are two contributing factors. Correcting these positions and motions can be difficult because they are involved in many daily activities.

Treatment

PRIMARY OBJECTIVES. The primary objective of the exercise program is to teach the patient to sit correctly and to move in the hips, not in the lumbar spine.

CORRECTIVE EXERCISE PROGRAM

Supine. The patient performs hip and knee flexion by passively pulling the knee to the chest with the hands, making certain not to flex the lumbar spine. If the rectus abdominis muscles have become short or stiff, the patient performs shoulder flexion to the maximum range and then lifts the chest to improve the length of the muscle.

Side lying. There are no specific exercises for this syndrome in the side-lying position.

Prone. The patient places the shoulders in flexion in the overhead position and flexes one shoulder at a time to improve the performance of the back extensor muscles. The patient places a pillow under the abdomen to bring the hips into slight flexion, and he or she performs unilateral hip extension to improve the performance of the back extensor muscles.

Quadruped. The patient allows the lumbar spine to become flat or slightly extended. The patient rocks backward, making certain the motion is hip flexion, not lumbar flexion.

Sitting. The patient sits and performs knee extension. Using the back of the chair as support, the patient performs isometric back extension. If the hamstring muscles are particularly short, the patient sits with his or her foot on a footstool, stretching the hamstring muscles for 15 to 20 minutes at a time. The patient leans forward, using hip flexion and not lumbar flexion, and performs the sit-to-stand motion without lumbar flexion.

Standing. The patient bends forward with motion occurring in the hips, not in the lumbar spine. The patient may need to flex the knees during this motion. He or she practices the squatting motion while avoiding lumbar flexion. If the rectus abdominis muscle is short or stiff, the patient stands with the back to the wall, shoulders flexed overhead, and chest lifted. Care is taken to avoid flattening the lumbar spine.

Correcting postural habits and movement patterns. The sitting posture and the movement pattern during leaning forward are two of the most important habits to correct. The patient may also perform bent-knee sit-up exercises, which should be eliminated.

Case Presentation

History. A 26-year-old male graduate student began experiencing back and left leg pain after a weight-training workout. While performing bilateral knee flexion in a prone position with a resistance of 200 pounds, he heard and felt a "pop" in his back and noted some back pain. Although he ceased the activity, he continued with the rest of his work out.

The patient works in a basic science laboratory, and he is taking a few classes. When he sits, he experiences a great deal of pain in his back and down his leg. He assumes he has strained his hamstring muscle and is performing stretches, such as forward bending. Although the stretches hurt while he is performing them, he feels better afterward.

The patient is referred for physical therapy consultation 2 months after the incident. He continues with his workouts but avoids the knee flexion exercise. The patient is committed to his strengthening program. He injured his left knee and had surgery the year before and can no longer run; consequently, the weight training is also his fitness program.

Symptoms. The patient is sleeping on the floor since the onset of his pain. He has been using a pillow under his hips and knees, and he experiences pain when he changes position. When in a sitting position, the patient rates his pain at a level of 7 to 8 on a scale of 10, both in his back and posterior thigh. When moving from sitting to a standing position, he also experiences an increase in pain. When in the standing position, his pain decreases to a level of 4 to 5 on a scale of 10. His ankle and knee jerks are normal, there is no weakness in the ankle or knee musculature, and his sensory tests are normal.

Alignment Analysis. The patient stands 5 feet, 10 inches tall. He has broad shoulders because of marked hypertrophy of the shoulder girdle muscles. He has good definition of the abdominal muscles. He has a slight thoracic kyphosis with depressed chest. His back is flat, but his iliac crests are at a belt-line level. He is in slight posterior pelvic tilt. The right previously injured knee is slightly flexed.

The following standing tests are performed: (1) forward bending, (2) lateral flexion, (3) rotation, and (4) single-leg stance.

Forward bending. The pain in his back and posterior thigh immediately increases. The symptoms decrease during the return motion. His symptoms increase with forward bending using hand support with only hip flexion.

Lateral flexion. This motion does not increase his symptoms.

Rotation. This motion is symmetrical with rotation to the right and to the left.

Single-leg stance. This motion is not associated with pelvic rotation, but it causes an increase in the symptoms with left hip flexion.

The following tests are performed with the patient in a supine position: (1) hip flexor length, (2) position effects, (3) hip abduction/lateral rotation from flexion, and (4) straight-leg raise.

Hip flexor length. There is no shortness and no compensatory pelvic motion.

Position effects. The patient has pain when he lies with his left hip and knee extended but not with his right hip extended.

Hip abduction/lateral rotation from flexion. There is no increase in symptoms or associated pelvic motion.

Straight-leg raise. The left posterior thigh pain is reproduced at 60 degrees of hip flexion. Pain decreases when the patient completely relaxes his hip flexion musculature.

The following additional tests are performed in four positions: (1) side lying, (2) prone, (3) quadruped, and (4) sitting.

Side lying. There is no increase in symptoms and no pelvic rotation with hip lateral rotation. With either hip abduction or adduction, there is no increase in symptoms and no lateral pelvic tilt.

Prone. The patient reports an increase in symptoms with some radiating pain into the lateral aspect of his leg, but placing a pillow under his abdomen relieves his symptoms. The knee flexion test produces a slight posterior pelvic tilt with no change in his symptoms. There is no pelvic rotation with the hip rotation test, but the patient reports a slight increase in symptoms with left hip medial rotation.

Quadruped. The lumbar spine is held in a flexed position, but there is no increase in symptoms when his spine is allowed to flatten. During the rocking backward test, there is an increase in symptoms with the hips flexed to 120 degrees.

Sitting. Slight flexion while sitting produces an almost immediate increase in symptoms. After placing support behind his lumbar spine and asking him to relax his hip muscles completely, the patient can sit comfortably for 10 minutes. When performing the knee extension test, the patient reports posterior thigh pain at −50 degrees of left knee extension. When he allows his thigh to rest on the chair, the knee extension range increases to −40 degrees. Right knee extension also increases the left posterior thigh pain.

Muscle Length and Strength Analysis. There is no muscle shortness, but the rectus abdominis muscle is stiff and contributes to the patient's thoracic kyphosis. There is no muscle weakness; however, his back extensor muscles are not as well defined as his abdominal muscles.

Diagnosis. The patient's symptoms are affected negatively by flexion, by an increase in the compression on his spine, and by the contraction of a left hip flexor, presumably the iliopsoas. Likewise, his symptoms are decreased by standing or lying recumbent or with a straight-leg raise, and the symptoms of the positive test are decreased by the relaxation of his hip flexor muscles. His symptoms increase with forward bending, but they do not increase with any rotation tests. The diagnosis is lumbar flexion with radiating symptoms along the sciatic nerve.

Intervention. The patient is taught an exercise that will help maintain the stability of his lumbar spine while moving his extremities and performing activities of daily living. Exercises that add to the compression forces on his spine are contraindicated. A regular exercise program is also important to the patient, and he intends to continue his upper body weight-training program. He is advised not to perform any exercises that involve lifting weights overhead or that cause an increase in his symptoms. The patient is also told that what he considers hamstring stretching is sciatica. He is advised to avoid all lumbar flexion motions and to limit the time he spends sitting. The patient performs a hip and knee extension exercise from the hook-lying position while contracting the abdominal muscles, stopping the motion at the onset of the symptoms. While also in a supine position, he performs hip abduction/lateral rotation from the hip flexed position. The patient performs hip abduction and adduction in a side-lying position. While assuming a prone position with a pillow under his abdomen, he performs knee flexion and hip rotation. When in the quadruped position, he is instructed to allow his lumbar spine to move toward the extended alignment and to stop the motion if he experiences any symptoms. While also in the quadruped position, he rocks backward to the point of the onset of symptoms, while limiting the motion to hip flexion and not allowing lumbar flexion. When sitting, he performs knee extension by sliding his left foot along the floor as far as possible to the onset of symptoms, avoiding lifting the thigh (flexing the hip). This exercise is performed with the right lower extremity, as well as the left. No exercises are recommended in the standing position because of the nerve tension sign and the increased compression associated with forward bending, which results in an increase in his symptoms.

Outcome. After 3 weeks of therapy, the patient no longer has symptoms when standing, but he still cannot sit for any period of time. He has a few transient episodes of sciatica in the right lower extremity. He is referred to an orthopedic surgeon who orders a magnetic resonance image (MRI) of his lower spine. The MRI indicates that the patient had a herniated disk at L4-5. He receives two epidural injections that improve his ability to sit for short periods. He does not experience any radiating symptoms, unless he sits for longer than 45 minutes. The MRI also indicates that he had some disk desiccation at L5-S1 and L3-4, which is attributed to his weight-training program.

The patient is seen every 2 weeks to monitor his program and his progress. Approximately 4 months after his initial physical therapy examination, he is able to rock backward in the quadruped position without symptoms. He can also lie prone with no symptoms, even without a pillow. His only remaining limitation is the inability to sit for longer than 45 minutes and to perform forward bending motions. His straight-leg raise test is negative, and he performs complete knee extension with either the right or left lower extremity without sciatica. He has started a program to improve the strength of his back extensor muscles. The initial exercise is unilateral shoulder flexion performed in the prone position with a pillow under his abdomen. He has to avoid any back extension in this position or tingling is elicited in his left foot. He also performs shoulder flexion in the quadruped position. Approximately 6 months after his initial visit, the patient is able to sit for 45 minutes. He still cannot bend forward unless his hands support his upper body. He has resumed his weight-training program, but he is using lighter weights and does not perform lifts with weights that exceed 50 pounds in either the standing or sitting position. Previously, he had been lifting 200-pound weights.

Sacroiliac Dysfunction

Sacroiliac (SI) dysfunction is not discussed as a diagnostic category in this text. Extensive information is available from practitioners who ascribe to dysfunction of the SI joint as a common cause of back pain. However, this text does not support this premise. Although many individuals have pain in the SI region, this text proposes that the pain does not arise from motion of the joint. Rather, pain in the SI region is the result of stress of the tissues that attach in this area. An exception to this belief can be found in a woman who is pregnant or who has recently given birth. Because of the hormonal changes in joint stability, this patient is susceptible to pain arising from SI joint dysfunction.

Extensive information is available on the limited movement of the joint—2 degrees or, at the most, less than 2 mm.[49,55] In fact, 76% of individuals older than 50 years of age have an ankylosed joint.[49] The ability to palpate a movement of less than 2 degrees or 2 mm is questionable. Studies that establish interrater reliability of the examinations recommended in this text indicate that after 6 months of practice, reliably discerning 1/2 inch or 250 mm of movement is exceedingly difficult, but possible.[54] It is difficult to understand on an anatomic basis the inference that movement tests of the SI joint with its excursion of 2 mm (e.g., standing flexion, supine long-sitting, and prone knee flexion) cause leg-length differences of 1/2 inch or more.[8] To support the premise of SI joint movement, the examiner has to palpate the change between the ilium and sacrum, not only the superior aspect of the sacrum. If joint hypermobility is believed to be the source of dysfunction, repeated manipulation furthers the mobility, rather than stabilizes the joint. The methods recommended for manipulation, particularly self-manipulation of the SI joint, cannot be considered to isolate the effect to the SI joint when many other joints that have greater flexibility are subjected to stress during the maneuver.

If the joint is indeed hypermobile, as possible with pregnancy, and susceptible to stresses that elicit pain, the principles for the movement impairment syndromes provided in this text are applicable for intervention. Stabilizing the joint, if necessary, with the use of appropriate external supports or taping, and a program that corrects soft-tissue impairments contributing to stress on this joint (e.g., a short or stiff TFL-iliotibial band [ITB], weak abdominal muscles) are effective means of correcting the dysfunction.

Compression

Differences in the compressive forces on the intervertebral disks in different positions were reported by Nachemson.[37] In addition, contraction of the psoas and the back extensor muscles also increases the compression forces on the spine. Compression force is the major factor if a patient's symptoms are alleviated or reduced when (1) recumbent, (2) standing rather than sitting, (3) sitting while supporting with the arms, or (4) sitting with the lumbar spine extended rather than flexed. Compression affects not only the disks but also the forces on the facet joints and ligaments. The effect of compression is not specific to any one category or diagnosis but must be considered as a contributing factor to the patient's movement impairment.

Additional Considerations

Additional considerations that can aid the diagnostic decision and development of an effective intervention program are the following:

• *Level of physical activity.* The patient who is sedentary is likely to have weak muscles that need to be strengthened, whereas the patient who is physically active needs to improve muscular control and the relative flexibility of different joint segments.

• *Job requirements.* The type of sustained posture or movement that a patient assumes or performs during the day is probably a major contributing factor to the characteristics of the movement impairment. For example, although a secretary spends most of the day sitting, she may frequently turn to use the computer or telephone or open a file drawer. The patient who performs a job that involves sustained physical activity needs to be thoroughly questioned about the nature of the positions and repetitive motions that are required.

• *Fitness activities and hobbies.* As job activities require sustained postures and repeated motions, so do fitness programs, sporting activities, and hobbies, such as painting and ceramics. Sports that require rotation, particularly with the feet fixed, such as racquetball, golf, and softball, are major contributors to rotational syndromes.

• *Household activities.* Vacuuming, sweeping, gardening, remodeling, or redecorating can involve rotation extension or motions, such as when working overhead while painting or hanging wallpaper. In contrast, bending, such as to paint low areas, suggest lumbar flexion. Sawing activities cause the patient to rotate or twist more than painting.

• *Physical characteristics.* Structural characteristics and body proportions that contribute to specific syndromes are described in the pertinent sections. However, the therapist should note various preferred postures and characteristics of body language that may contribute to a specific syndrome. Examples include the man with a large abdomen who slides his hips forward in his chair to accommodate his abdomen, or the short woman who sits in a rotated position on one hip so she can tuck her legs under her body in a side-sitting manner. Both postures contribute to the rotation syndrome. Another example is found in the woman who has a marked kyphosis or large buttocks. She sits with her lumbar spine in extension because she believes she is sitting in a straight alignment.

References

1. Adams MA, Dolan P, Hutton WC: The lumbar spine in backward bending, *Spine* 13:1019, 1988.
2. Bogduk N, Macintosh JE, Pearcy MJ: A universal model of the lumbar back muscles in the upright position, *Spine* 17:897, 1992.
3. Bogduk N, Pearcy MJ, Hadfield G: Anatomy and biomechanics of psoas major, *Clin Biomech* 7:109, 1992.
4. Bridwell KH: Lumbar spinal stenosis, diagnosis, management, and treatment, *Clin Geriatr Med* 10(4):677, 1994.
5. Callaghan JP, Gunning JL, McGill SM: The relationship between lumbar spine load and muscle activity during extensor exercises, *Phys Ther* 78:8, 1998.
6. Cappozzo A: Compressive loads in the lumbar vertebral column during normal level walking, *J Orthop Res* 1:292, 1984.
7. Cholewicki J, Panjabi M, Khachatryan A: Role of muscles in lumbar spine stability in maximum extension efforts, *Spine* 22:2207, 1997.
8. Cibulka MT, Koldehoff R: Clinical usefulness of a cluster of sacroiliac joint tests in patients with and without low back pain, *JOSPT* 29:83, 1999.
9. Cresswell AG, Oddsson L, Thorstensson A: The influence of sudden perturbations on trunk muscle activity and intraabdominal pressure while standing, *Exp Brain Res* 98:336, 1994.
10. Delitto RS, Woolsey NB, Sahrmann SA: Comparison of two noninvasive methods for measuring the lumbar spine excursion which occurs in forward bending, *Phys Ther* 67:743, 1987.
11. Eie N: Load capacity of the low back, *J Oslo City Hosp* 16:73, 1966.
12. Esola MA, McClure PW, Fitzgerald GK, Siegler S: Analysis of lumbar spine and hip motion during forward bending in subjects with and without a history of low back pain, *Spine* 21:71, 1996.
13. Farfan HF: *Mechanical disorders of the low back*, Philadelphia, 1973, Lea & Febiger.

14. Farfan HF: Muscular mechanism of the lumbar spine and the position of power and efficiency, *Orthop Clin North Am* 6:135, 1975.

15. Gartland JJ: *Fundamentals of orthopaedics*, Philadelphia, 1987, WB Saunders.

16. Goldman JM, Lehr RP, Millar AB, Silver JR: An electromyographic study of the abdominal muscles during postural and respiratory maneuvers, *J Neurol Neurosurg Psychiatry* 50:866, 1987.

17. Goodman CG, Boissonnault W: *Pathology: implications for the physical therapist*, Philadelphia, 1998, WB Saunders.

18. Goodman CG, Snyder TE: *Differential diagnosis in physical therapy*, Philadelphia, 1998, WB Saunders.

19. Hides JA, Richardson CA, Jull GA: Multifidus muscle recovery is not automatic after resolution of acute, first-episode low back pain, *Spine* 21:2763, 1996.

20. Hodges PW, Richardson CA: Contraction of the abdominal muscles associated with movement of the lower limb, *Phys Ther* 77:132, 1997.

21. Hodges PW, Richardson CA: Inefficient muscular stabilization of the lumbar spine associated with low back pain, *Spine* 21:2640, 1996.

22. Hresko MT: Thoracic and lumbosacral spine. In Steinberg GG, editor: *Orthopaedics in primary care*, ed 2, Baltimore, 1992, Williams & Wilkins.

23. Infusa A, An HS, Lim T, Hasegawa T, Haughton VM, Nowicki BH: Anatomic changes of the spinal canal and intervertebral foramen associated with flexion-extension movement, *Spine* 21:2412, 1996.

24. Jackson DW, Wiltse LL, Cirincione RJ: Spondylolysis in the female gymnast, *Clin Orthop* 11:68, 1976.

25. Juker D, McGill SM, Kropf P, Steffen T: Quantitative intramuscular myoelectric activity of lumbar portions of psoas and the abdominal wall during a wide variety of tasks, *Med Sci Sports Exerc* 30:301, 1998.

26. Jull GA, Richardson CA: Rehabilitation of active stabilization of the lumbar spine. In Twomey LT, Taylor JR, editors: *Physical therapy of the low back*, New York, 1994, Churchill-Livingstone.

27. Kendall FP, McCreary FK, Provance P: *Muscles testing and function*, Baltimore, 1993, Williams & Wilkins.

28. King AL, Prasad P, Ewing CL: Mechanism of spinal injury due to caudocephalad acceleration, *Orthop Clin North Am* 6:19, 1975.

29. Loebl WY: Measurement of spinal posture and range of spinal movement, *Ann Phys Med* 9:103, 1967.

30. Lumsden RM, Morris JM: An in vivo study of axial rotation and immobilization at the lumbosacral joint, *J Bone Joint Surg* 50A:1591, 1968.

31. McGill SM, Brown S: Creep response of the lumbar spine to prolonged full flexion, *Clin Biomech* 7:43, 1992.

32. McGill SM, Juker D, Kropf P: Quantitative intramuscular myoelectric activity of quadratus lumborum during a wide variety of tasks, *Clin Biomech* 11:170, 1996.

33. McGill SM, Norman RW: Low back biomechanics in industry: the prevention of injury through safer lifting. In Grabiner, editor: *Current issues in biomechanics*, Champaign, Ill, 1993, Human Kinetics.

34. McGill SM: Low back exercises: evidence for improving exercise regimens, *Phys Ther* 78:754, 1998.

35. Mercier LR: *Practical orthopedics*, St Louis, 1995, Mosby.

36. Merriam WF, Burwell RG, Mulholland RC, Pearson JC, Webb JK: A study revealing a tall pelvis in subjects with low back pain, *J Bone Joint Surg Br* 65:153, 1983.

37. Nachemson A: Toward a better understanding of back pain: a review of the mechanics of the lumbar disk, *Rheumatol Rehab* 14:129, 1975.

38. Nitz AJ, Peck D: Comparison of muscle spindle concentrations in large and small human epiaxial muscles acting in parallel combinations, *Am Surg* 62:273, 1986.

39. Nordin M, Frankel VH: *Basic biomechanics of the musculoskeletal system*, ed 2, Philadelphia, 1989, Lea & Febiger.

40. Norton BJ, Gauitierrez C, Schroeder B, Van Dillen L: Videographic* analysis of subjects with and without low back pain during forward bending, *Phys Ther* 76:529,1996.

41. Ohlen G, Wredmark T, Spangfort E: Spinal sagittal configuration and mobility related to low-back pain in the female gymnast, *Spine* 14:847, 1989.

42. Oseid S, Evjenth G, Evjenth O, Gunnari H, Meen D: Lower back trouble in young female gymnasts: frequency, symptoms and possible causes, *Bull Phys Educ* 10:25, 1974.

43. Pearcy MJ: Axial rotation and lateral bending in the number spine measured by three-dimensional radiography, *Spine* 9:582, 1984.

44. Pearcy MJ: Twisting mobility of the human back in flexed postures, *Spine* 18:114, 1993.

45. Pearsall DJ, Reid JG: Line of gravity relative to upright vertebral posture, *Clin Biomech* 7:80, 1992.

46. Porterfield JA, DeRosa C: Mechanical low back pain. In *Perspectives in functional anatomy*, ed 2, Philadelphia, 1998, WB Saunders.

47. Saal JS, Franson RC, Dobrou R, Saal JA, White AH, Goldthwaite N: High levels of inflammatory phospholipase A2 activity in lumbar disk herniations, *Spine* 15:674, 1990.

48. Santaguida P, McGill SM: The psoas major muscle: a three-dimensional geometric study, *J Biomech* 28:339, 1995.

49. Simon SR et al: Kinesiology. In Simon SR, editor: *Orthopedic basic science*, 1994, American Academy of Orthopaedic Surgeons.

50. Sturesson B, Selvick G, Uden A: Movement of the sacroiliac joints: a stereophotogrammetric analysis, *Spine* 21:218, 1989.

51. Thomas JS, Corcos DM, Hasan Z: The influence of gender on spine, hip, knee, and ankle motions during a reaching task, *J Mot Behav* 30:98, 1998.

52. Tkaczuk H: Tensile properties of human lumbar longitudinal ligaments, *Acta Orthop Scand Suppl* 115:1, 1968.

53. Van Dillen LR, Sahrmann SA, Norton BJ et al: Classification of patients with low back pain, *Phys Ther* (submitted 2001).

54. Van Dillen LR, Sahrmann SA, Norton BJ et al: Reliability of physical examination items used for classification of patients with low back pain, *Phys Ther* 78:979, 1998.

55. Vleeming A, van Wingerden JP, Snidjers CJ et al: Mobility of the SI joints in the elderly: kinematic and roentgenologic study, *Acta Orthop Scand* 7:170, 1992.

56. White AA, Panjabi MM: *Clinical biomechanics of the spine*, Philadelphia, 1978, JB Lippincott.

57. White AA: Analysis of the mechanics of thoracic spine in man: an experimental study of autopsy specimens, *Acta Orthop Scand Suppl* 127:1, 1969.

58. Woolsey NB, Norton BJ: Measurement of lumbar range of motion with an inclinometer, *Phys Ther* (submitted 2001).

59. Youdas JW, Suman VJ, Garrett TR: Reliability of measurements of lumbar spine sagittal mobility obtained with the flexible curve, *JOSPT* 21:13, 1995.

60. Zoeller R, Sahrmann S, Kuhnline M, Minor S: Changes in the infrasternal angle with abdominal contractions, *Phys Ther* 73:S104, 1993.

Chapter 3
Appendix

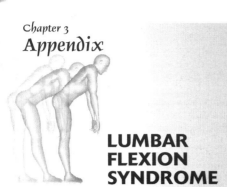

LUMBAR FLEXION SYNDROME

The primary dysfunction in this syndrome is that lumbar flexion motion is more flexible than hip flexion motion. Typically a flexion moment and compression are imposed on the spine when sitting. Lumbar flexion stress or motion causes symptoms in the low back or into the buttocks and/or lower extremity. This syndrome is found more commonly in younger individuals between the ages of 18 to 45 years, who are usually experiencing an acute pain episode. This syndrome is also more common in men than women, particularly tall men or those whose daily activities involve repeated forward bending. Most often, the back extensors are elongated and flexible while the hip extensors are short and stiff. This syndrome is most often associated with herniated disks, but it is less common than the lumbar rotation-flexion syndrome.

SYMPTOMS

- Symptoms are present or increase with positions or movements associated with lumbar flexion (e.g., sitting, driving, forward bending).
- Symptoms are absent or decrease in positions or movements of decreasing lumbar flexion (e.g., standing, walking).

KEY TESTS AND SIGNS

Standing position
FORWARD BENDING

- Greater relative flexibility of lumbar spine flexion than hip flexion flexibility
- Symptoms are present or increased

FORWARD BENDING (HIP FLEXION ONLY)

- Absent or decreased symptoms, relative to forward bending

Quadruped position

- *Preferred position:* Flexed lumbar spine
- *Rock back:* Greater flexibility of lumbar spine in flexion or longitudinal distraction than hip flexion flexibility (may or may not cause symptoms)

Sitting position

- *Preferred alignment:* Flexed lumbar spine
- Symptoms are present or increased, relative to sitting with lumbar spine in neutral or slightly arched inward
- *Knee extension:* Lumbar spine flexes

Supine position
HIP FLEXION AND KNEE FLEXED

- Symptoms are present or increased during final phase of hip flexion
- Lumbar spine flexes before 120 degrees of hip flexion
- Able to lie with hips and knees extended without increased symptoms
- Folded towel under lumbar spine decreases symptoms

ASSOCIATED SIGNS

(contributing factors)

Lumbar lordosis

Kyphosis in which an erect posture is obtained by exaggerating the lordosis (often observed in patients with osteoporosis)

Forward bending

Relative flexibility of hips flexion greater than the lumbar spine flexion flexibility

Limited range of lumbar flexion (lumbar spine does not reverse its curve)

Prone knee flexion

Anterior pelvic tilt and increased lumbar extension; may increase symptoms

Abdominal muscles

Weakness, excessive length, or inadequate stiffness of external oblique abdominal muscles

Short or stiff muscles

Hip flexors (one or two joints)

Lumbar paraspinal muscles

Body characteristics

Obesity with large abdomen

Large buttocks

DIFFERENTIAL MOVEMENT AND ASSOCIATED DIAGNOSES

Movement diagnosis

- Lumbar rotation-extension

Associated diagnoses

- Spinal stenosis
- Facet syndrome
- Degenerative disk disease
- Spondylolysis
- Osteoporosis

SCREENING FOR POTENTIAL MEDICAL DIAGNOSES REQUIRING REFERRAL

- Malignancy
- Inflammatory conditions (e.g., tuberculosis, osteomyelitis)
- Spinal cord compression
- Cauda equina disorder
- Fracture
- Osteoporosis
- Ankylosing spondylitis
- Spondylolisthesis
- Juvenile disk disease
- Scheuermann's disease

Chapter 3
Appendix

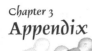

LUMBAR ROTATION SYNDROME

The primary dysfunction in this syndrome is that a segment of the lumbar spine rotates, side bends, glides, or translates more easily than other segments of the lumbar spine, the thoracic spine, or the hips. Rotation is broadly defined and includes movement directions other than flexion and extension. Spinal instabilities, which most often involve accessory motions, are included in this category because they are not clinically observable and therefore cannot be named for an accessory movement direction. In some patients, marked rotation of the lumbar spine is observable. In others, the rotation of the spine is not evident; rather, rotational motion of the pelvis, which must necessarily cause spinal motion or stress, is associated with lower extremity movement. In other patients, side-bending motions cause pain, but actual rotational alignment of the spine is not evident. No attempt is made to equate the side of rotation with the side of the symptoms.

SYMPTOMS

- Symptoms are often unilateral or greater on one side.
- Symptoms increase with rotation movements of the lumbar spine.

KEY TESTS AND SIGNS

Standing position
- *Alignment:* Paraspinal asymmetry
- *Side bending:* Symptoms are present or increase, relative to standing position
- *Motion:* Asymmetric

Supine position
HIP OR KNEE FLEXION
- Observe pelvic rotation

HIP ABDUCTION/LATERAL ROTATION FROM FLEXION
- Pelvis and lumbar spine rotates during the initial 50% of the lower extremity motion; lumbar spine is more flexible into rotation than the hip is into abduction/lateral rotation (lumbopelvic stiffness is insufficient to counter the eccentric control by the lower extremity musculature)
- Symptoms are present or increased, relative to starting position

Side-lying position
- Position may be painful
- Symptoms decreased with towel roll under waist
- *Hip lateral rotation:* Observe pelvic rotation
- *Hip adduction:* Observe lateral pelvic tilt

Prone position
- *Knee flexion:* Asymmetrical pelvic rotation
- *Hip and knee extension:* Asymmetric lateral rotation during hip extension
- *Hip rotation:* Prone lying; lumbopelvic rotation occurs during first 50% of hip rotation motion

Quadruped position
- *Alignment:* Observe asymmetry in lumbar spine region
- *Arm lift:* Rotation of spine

Sitting position
- *Knee extension:* Observe lumbopelvic rotation
- *Rocking backward:* Rotation of prominent lumbar segments may increase

ASSOCIATED SIGNS
(contributing factors)

- Activity requiring repeated movements of rotation (e.g., golf, tennis serve)

- Habit of rotating trunk and not entire body while sitting

- Habit of sitting on one foot, crossing legs, or leaning to one side

- Weakness, excessive length, or poor control of oblique abdominal muscles (external oblique on one side and contralateral internal oblique muscle)

- Asymmetric length of iliotibial band

- Apparent leg length discrepancy

DIFFERENTIAL MOVEMENT AND ASSOCIATED DIAGNOSES

Movement diagnoses

- Lumber rotation-flexion
- Lumbar rotation-extension

Associated diagnoses

- Spinal stenosis
- Facet syndrome
- Degenerative disk disease
- Spondylolysis
- Osteoporosis
- Scoliosis

SCREENING FOR POTENTIAL MEDICAL DIAGNOSES REQUIRING REFERRAL

- Malignancy
- Inflammatory conditions (e.g., tuberculosis or osteomyelitis)
- Spinal cord compression
- Cauda equina disorder
- Fracture
- Osteoporosis
- Ankylosing spondylitis
- Spondylolisthesis
- Juvenile disk
- Scheuermann's disease

Chapter 3
Appendix

LUMBAR ROTATION WITH FLEXION SYNDROME

The primary dysfunction is that a segment of the lumbar spine moves more easily in the direction of rotation-flexion than other segments of the lumbar spine, the thoracic spine, or the hips. Many of the descriptions of the flexion and rotation syndromes and their characteristics can be applied to this syndrome. This syndrome is more common than the pure flexion or pure rotation syndromes. Because a rotational component is so common, the therapist should always plan for this component in the treatment program.

SYMPTOMS

- Symptoms are often unilateral or greater on one side.
- Symptoms are present or increase with sitting-to-standing movement.

KEY TESTS AND SIGNS

Alignment

FORWARD BENDING

- Symptoms are present or increased, relative to standing; spinal asymmetry may be more evident

FORWARD BENDING (HIP FLEXION ONLY)

- Symptoms are decreased, relative to forward bending with lumbar flexion

Supine position

HIP ABDUCTION/LATERAL ROTATION FROM FLEXION

- Pelvis and lumbar spine rotate during initial 50% of the lower extremity motion
- Lumbar spine is more flexible into rotation than the hip is into abduction/lateral rotation (lumbopelvic stiffness is insufficient to counter the eccentric control by the lower extremity musculature)
- Symptoms are present or increased, relative to starting position
- Able to lie with hips and knees extended without increased symptoms
- Folded towel under lumbar spine decreases symptoms

ACTIVE HIP AND KNEE FLEXED

- Pelvic rotation observed during active hip flexion

Side-lying position

- Painful position, symptoms decrease with towel roll under waist
- *Hip lateral rotation:* Observe pelvic rotation
- *Hip adduction:* Observe lateral pelvic tilt

Prone position

- *Hip rotation:* Symptoms present or increased, relative to prone position
- Lumbopelvic rotation occurs during first 50% of hip rotation motion

Quadruped position

- *Alignment:* Preferred position is lumbar flexion with asymmetry
- *Rocking backward:* Observe lumbar rotation and pelvic tilt or rotation
- *Arm lift:* Rotation of spine present

Sitting position

- Symptoms present or increased with lumbar spine flexion, compared with neutral or extension positions
- Symptoms increases with knee extension if associated with pelvic or lumbar rotation

ASSOCIATED SIGNS
(contributing factors)

- Job or fitness activities requiring repeated unilateral limb movements or trunk rotation

- Apparent leg length discrepancy in standing alignment (postural or from leg-length discrepancy)

- Habit of rotating trunk and not entire body while sitting

- Habit of sitting on one foot or legs crossed

- Asymmetry of iliotibial band length from tensor fascia lata or gluteus maximus insertions

- *Prone knee flexion:* Pelvic rotation can be observed

- Oblique abdominal muscles do not provide adequate control of lumbopelvic rotation

DIFFERENTIAL MOVEMENT AND ASSOCIATED DIAGNOSES

Movement diagnoses
- Lumbar flexion syndrome
- Lumbar rotation syndrome

Associated diagnoses
- Bulging or herniated disk
- Scoliosis

SCREENING FOR POTENTIAL MEDICAL DIAGNOSES REQUIRING REFERRAL

- Malignancy
- Inflammatory conditions (e.g., tuberculosis or osteomyelitis)
- Spinal cord compression
- Cauda equina disorder
- Fracture
- Osteoporosis
- Ankylosing spondylitis
- Spondylolisthesis
- Juvenile disk
- Scheuermann's disease

Chapter 3
Appendix

LUMBAR ROTATION WITH EXTENSION SYNDROME

The primary dysfunction in this syndrome is that the position of stress or the movement into extension causes pain in the lumbar spine, buttocks, or lower extremities. This syndrome is the most prevalent in patients with low back pain. It is particularly common in patients with chronic and recurrent back pain, in individuals over 55 years of age, and in those who participate in rotational sports such as golf and racquetball. The degenerative changes in the spine, impairment of abdominal muscle control, rotational motion of daily activities, and rotational motions imposed on the lumbopelvic area by movements of the extremities all contribute to the prevalence of this syndrome. Many of the characteristics of extension and rotation syndromes can be applied to this syndrome.

SYMPTOMS

- Symptoms are often unilateral or greater on one side.
- Symptoms increase with extension and rotation movements of the lumbar spine.

KEY TESTS AND SIGNS

Standing position

- *Alignment:* Paraspinal asymmetry
- Increased symptoms when returning from forward bending
- *Side bending:* Symptoms present or increased, relative to standing
- Asymmetric motion during side bending and rotation of the trunk

Sitting position

- *Lumbar spine extension:* Symptoms present or increased, relative to neutral lumbar spine

Supine position

- *Hip and knee flexion:* Observe pelvic rotation
- *Hip abduction/lateral rotation from flexion:* Pelvis and lumbar spine rotates during the initial 50% of the lower extremity motion; lumbar spine is more flexible into rotation than the hip is into abduction/lateral rotation (lumbopelvic stiffness is insufficient to counter the eccentric control by the lower extremity musculature)
- Hips and knees extended increases symptoms
- *Hip flexion and abducted lateral rotation:* Symptoms present or increased, relative to starting position; relative flexibility in spine and hips

Side-lying position

- Position may be painful
- Decreased symptoms with towel roll under waist
- *Hip lateral rotation:* Observe pelvic rotation
- *Hip adduction:* Observe lateral pelvic tilt

Prone position

- *Knee flexion:* Symptoms present or increased, relative to prone position; observe asymmetric pelvic rotation
- *Hip extension with the knee extended:* Asymmetric lateral rotation of the lumbar spine during hip extension
- *Hip rotation:* Lumbopelvic rotation occurs during the first 50% of hip rotation

Quadruped position

- *Forward rocking:* Symptoms present or increased, relative to corrected starting position or rocking back
- *Backward rocking:* No symptoms or decreased symptoms, relative to rocking forward

ASSOCIATED SIGNS
(contributing factors)

- Activities requiring repeated movements of lumbar extension and rotation (e.g., golf, tennis serve)

- Habit of rotating trunk and not entire body while sitting

- Habit of sitting on one foot or crossing legs

- Poor control and performance of abdominal muscles in preventing lumbopelvic rotation and extension of the lumbar spine

- Asymmetric iliotibial band length

- Apparent leg-length discrepancy

DIFFERENTIAL MOVEMENT AND ASSOCIATED DIAGNOSES

Movement diagnoses

- Lumbar rotation-flexion
- Lumbar extension

Associated diagnoses

- Spinal stenosis
- Facet syndrome
- Degenerative disk disease
- Spondylolysis
- Osteoporosis
- Scoliosis

SCREENING FOR POTENTIAL MEDICAL DIAGNOSES REQUIRING REFERRAL

- Malignancy
- Inflammatory conditions (e.g., tuberculosis or osteomyelitis)
- Spinal cord compression
- Cauda equina disorder
- Fracture
- Osteoporosis
- Ankylosing spondylitis
- Spondylolisthesis
- Juvenile disk
- Scheuermann's disease

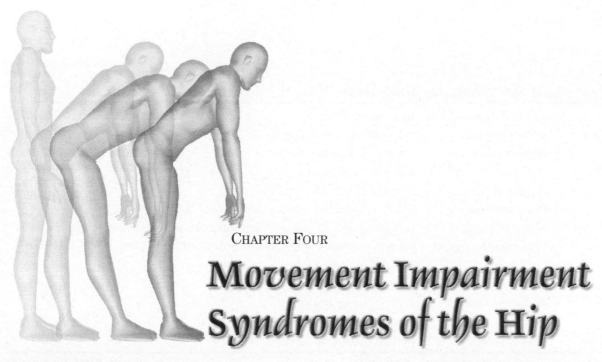

Movement Impairment Syndromes of the Hip

Chapter Highlights

Normal Alignment of the Hip
Motions of the Hip
Muscular Actions of the Hip
Movement Impairment Syndromes of the Hip

Chapter Objectives

After consideration of the information presented in this chapter, the reader will be able to:

1. Describe acquired postural impairments and structural variations of the lower extremity that contribute to movement impairment syndromes.
2. Identify the specific muscle actions related to movement impairments.
3. Recognize the differences between diagnoses named for physiologic movement and those named for accessory movements.
4. Identify the characteristics of each movement impairment syndrome of the hip.

In treating the patient with hip pain, the reader will be able to:

1. Perform an examination, consider the contributing factors, and establish a diagnosis.
2. Develop and instruct the patient in a diagnosis-specific treatment program and modification of the life activities, which contribute to the formation of the movement impairment syndrome.

Introduction

The majority of syndromes affecting the hip arise from impairments in the muscles attaching close to the proximal femur that control the alignment and motion of the femur in the acetabulum. Symptoms in the region of the hip joint can be referred from the low back or can be coincident with low back syndromes. Therefore careful analysis of hip joint movements and muscle control is essential to differentiate whether the syndrome is from the hip, from the spine, or from both the hip and spine. These possibilities must be considered during the examination.

The premise of this text is that painful sites arise, in part, because of differences in the relative flexibility of different segments, which are manifested by compensatory movements at intervening joints that have become particularly flexible. Subsequently, the pattern is continually reinforced and the joint develops a susceptibility to movement in the affected direction. This condition is referred to as a *joint's directional susceptibility to movement* (DSM). Even stiffness at the foot, as in the case of a rigid foot can have an effect on more proximal segments, such as the knee and hip. When the foot is rigid and does not dorsiflex during walking, compensatory motions, such as knee hyperextension or hip lateral rotation, can be a long-term result.

Two types of syndromes are discussed in this chapter. The first type is believed to arise from pain directly related to the hip joint. It is usually characterized by a movement impairment of an accessory motion of the femur. Thus these syndromes are identified by the name, femoral, and the offending accessory motion. The other type of syndrome is named for the physiologic motion that is painful because of musculotendinous dysfunction. This type of syndrome is identified by the name, hip, and impaired physiologic motion. Using the physiologic motion rather than the name of the muscle as the diagnosis for muscle dysfunction places the emphasis on correcting the pattern of muscular movement that performs the motion and not only on the palliative treatment of the painful muscle (Table 4-1).

Table 4-1 **Syndromes in Order of Frequency of Observation**

SYNDROME	ACCESSORY MOVEMENT	ASSOCIATED DIAGNOSES
Femoral anterior glide	Without rotation	Iliopsoas tendinopathy; bursitis
	With medial rotation	Iliopsoas tendinopathy; bursitis
	With lateral rotation	Adductor strain; iliopsoas tendinopathy; groin pull
Hip adduction	Without rotation	Gluteus medius strain; trochanteric bursitis
	With medial rotation	Lengthened piriformis syndrome; iliotibial band fascitis
Hip extension	With knee extension	Hamstring strain as a result of insufficient gluteus maximus or quadriceps participation
	With hip medial rotation	Hamstring strain as a result of insufficient intrinsic lateral rotator muscle participation
Femoral accessory		Early degenerative hip joint disease
Hypermobility		Labral tears
Femoral hypomobility	With superior glide	Degenerative hip joint disease
Hip lateral rotation		Shortened piriformis syndrome
Femoral lateral glide	Short axis distraction	Hip pain; popping hip; subluxation

Normal Alignment of the Hip

In the lower extremity, several structural variations can be predisposing factors to the development of muscle impairments and eventually to pain syndromes. Lower extremity structural variations can be difficult to distinguish from acquired impairments.

Pelvis

According to Kendall[11] the ideal alignment of the pelvis is present when the anterior superior iliac spine (ASIS) is in the same vertical plane as the symphysis pubis. The angular deviation between the horizontal plane and a line connecting the ASIS with the posterior superior iliac spine (PSIS) is a frequently used clinical assessment of pelvic tilt. A common belief is that this angle should be very small, usually less than 5 degrees. A study performed on cadaver pelves indicates that when the ASIS is in the same vertical plane as the symphysis pubis, the angle between the horizontal plane and the plane between the ASIS and the PSIS varies as much as 12 degrees.[2] Therefore the examiner should not expect a perfectly horizontal line between the ASIS and PSIS to be an indication of optimal alignment.

In some women the ASIS is much lower than the PSIS, but not because of an anterior pelvic tilt (Figure 4-1). Such extreme variation in the relationship between the ASIS and the PSIS has not been observed in men. The pelvic structural variation that has been reported in men is that of a tall pelvis. A tall pelvis is one in which the height of the pelvis, as measured from the ischial tuberosity to the peak of the iliac crest, is a greater percentage of the overall height than the av-

erage percentage.[3,13] Another structural variation that has been clinically observed is one in which a man's beltline is at least 1 inch lower than the top of his iliac crest, rather than just above it (Figure 4-2). Men with high iliac crests have flat backs that are not associated with posterior pelvic tilts. Therefore two fairly common structural variations can be misinterpreted as acquired postural impairments: (1) a low position of the ASIS in women, which can be interpreted as anterior pelvic tilt; and (2) a structurally flat back in men with high iliac crests in relation to their beltline, which is often incorrectly interpreted as an acquired alignment of lumbar flexion.

The hip joint angle is not always an accurate indication of pelvic tilt. This angle is affected by knee joint alignment and by pelvic alignment. When the knee is flexed the hip will be flexed, even if the pelvic tilt is neutral. When the knee is hyperextended the hip will be extended, even if the pelvic tilt is neutral (Figure 4-3) or slightly anterior.

Because of these potential sources of error when assessing pelvic tilt, the decision should be based on consistent findings in two of the three following determinations: (1) an increase or decrease in the normal depth of lumbar curve, (2) a marked deviation from the horizontal line between the ASIS and PSIS, and (3) an increase or decrease in the hip joint angle with neutral knee joint alignment. Another useful means of assessing the presence of an acquired postural impairment versus a structural variation is correcting the pelvic malalignment and observing whether the alignment of all affected segments is corrected.

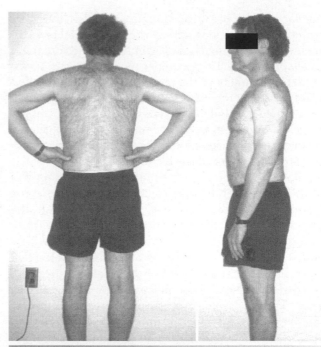

Figure 4-2

Tall pelvis with associated flat lumbar spine. This man has his hands on the top of his iliac crests *(left)*. The top of his iliac crests is more than 1 inch higher than his beltline. This man has a flat back *(right)*. This alignment is characteristic of men whose high iliac crests are notably higher than their beltlines.

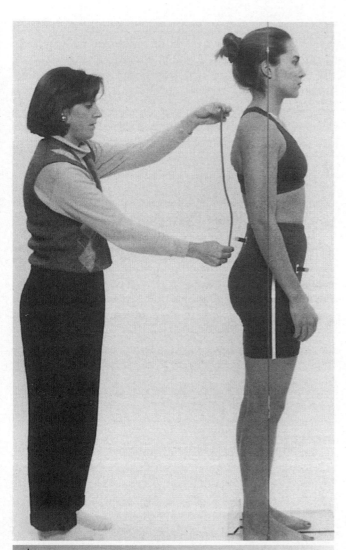

Figure 4-1

Structural variation of the female pelvis. Markers are placed on the anterior superior iliac spine (ASIS) and the posterior superior iliac spine (PSIS). Ideally, a line from the ASIS to the PSIS should deviate only 15 degrees from a horizontal line through the PSIS. In this case the ASIS is significantly lower than the PSIS, but the lumbar curve is not increased and the hip joint is in neutral (not flexed or extended).

When pelvic tilt is present, there should be corresponding changes in the alignment of the spine and hip joint. If correcting the pelvic alignment causes an undesirable change in the alignment of the spine or the hip joint, the impairment is probably structural, not acquired. For example, a structural variation is present when (1) the ASIS appears low in relation to the PSIS, and (2) when tilting the pelvis posteriorly causes the lumbar spine to lose its normal inward curve (see Figure 3-9).

Pelvic rotation around the vertical axis is often present in patients with hip pain. The examiner can assess pelvic rotation while he or she stands behind the patient

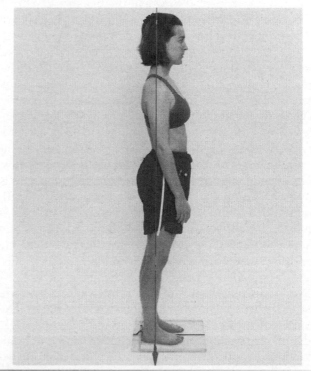

Figure 4-3

Hyperextended knees and hip joint angle. A slight anterior pelvic tilt is observed. Because her knees are hyperextended, the hips are not flexed but extended.

and places his or her fingers parallel to and on the ASIS. From this position, deviations from the frontal plane of the line between the left and right iliac spines are fairly readily perceived. The examiner must be certain to observe the alignment of the patient's feet to confirm that malalignment of the lower extremities is not the source of the pelvic rotation. If one foot is forward of the other, the pelvis may be rotated because of lower extremity alignment, not because of a pelvic rotation that is altering the alignment of the hip joints or spine.

Some patients who have unilateral hip antetorsion rotate the hip laterally to correct associated pigeon-toe alignment. Depending on the degree of antetorsion , the pelvis may also rotate toward the side of the hip with antetorsion. Because the pelvis is rotated, the spine will be rotated, and as a result these patients can develop low back pain. When the rotation of the pelvis is corrected, the new alignment can be perceived by the patient as being "wrong." Because of this misperception the patient needs oral and visual information about how to correct the malalignment and about the time required before the new position will seem normal.

Hip Joint

Hip flexion while standing erect can be present because of weakness or excessive length of the external oblique or rectus abdominis muscles. The hip flexor muscles can also be short or stiff. During gait the hip should extend 10 degrees.[8] However, when the hip flexor muscles are short or stiff in relation to the abdominal muscles, instead of the compensation being reflected in hip motion, there may be exaggerated anterior pelvic tilt and increased lumbar extension. Although great emphasis is placed on stretching hamstring muscles, little attention is given to maintaining the length of the hip flexor muscles or ensuring that the abdominal muscles are preventing anterior pelvic tilt. Every step taken during gait requires maximal excursion of the hip flexor muscles, but only minimal excursion of the hamstring muscles is required. Maintaining adequate hip flexor muscle length and optimal performance of the abdominal muscles is important in preventing increased lumbar lordosis and excessive anterior pelvic tilt, particularly under dynamic conditions such as walking and running.

Hip joint extension is a common postural fault evident in the individual who stands in swayback posture with posterior pelvic tilt and hyperextended knees. The combination of posterior pelvic tilt and knee hyperextension produces hyperextension of the hip joint. Standing in hip hyperextension (greater than 10 degrees) for prolonged periods can stretch the anterior joint capsule and place stress on the iliopsoas muscle and tendon. Activities that contribute to the development of hip hyperextension are distance running, ballet, modern dance, or any activity that includes the performance of "splits." The result of prolonged postural hip hyperextension is the development of the femoral anterior glide syndrome, which is described later in this chapter.

Hip joint lateral asymmetry or apparent leg-length discrepancy is a fairly common postural fault (Figure 4-4). In this postural alignment, the hip on the side of the high iliac crest is in adduction and the other hip is in abduction.[11] The difference between the heights of the iliac crests should be at least 1/2 inch to have clinical significance. Few individuals have true structural leg-length discrepancies in which either the femur or tibia is longer on one side. In individuals with structural differences, there is usually a history of congenital unilateral dislocation of the hip, a history of injury when they were younger that resulted in excessive bone growth, or a traumatic injury as an adult that caused a loss of bone length. An acute change in hip height in the patient with

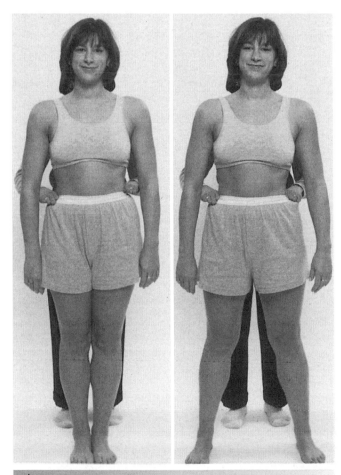

Figure 4-4

Apparent leg length discrepancy (iliac crest asymmetry). The left iliac crest is higher than the right iliac crest when the feet are together. Thus the right hip abductors are stiffer than the left hip abductors. Abduction of the hips levels the iliac crests because the abductors are not stretched.

low back pain and radiation into the hip may be the result of weakness of the hip abductor muscles. Hip adduction on one side and abduction on the other can contribute to hip pain, to back pain, and even to the occurrence of ankle sprain. When one iliac crest is high, the lateral pelvic tilt causes lateral lumbar flexion at the lowest segments. Lateral flexion is associated with spinal rotation, which is a common factor in low back pain (see Chapter 3).

The ankle may be affected by an apparent leg-length discrepancy in two ways. Usually on the side of the adducted hip (high iliac crest), the foot will tend to be supinated. During running or rapid changes in direction as required in sports, excessive length or weakness of the hip abductor muscles will allow the hip to move too far laterally over the foot when the foot is on the ground or allow the hip to adduct excessively during the swing phase of gait. The excessive hip adduction in both situations and the supinated position of the foot can contribute to inversion injuries of the ankle. The problem arises because the line of gravity falls medial to the hip and lateral to the ankle. Therefore a comprehensive program for the patient with inversion injuries of the ankle should include exercises for the hip abductor muscles, if these muscles are weak or long and the range of hip adduction is excessive.

Structural variations of the femur need to be assessed carefully as potential contributing factors to the pain problems of the hip and back. The limited range of hip rotation motion in one direction and the excessive range in the opposite direction can be associated with muscle shortness or weakness. Structural variations are relatively common and frequently contribute to the patient's problems. Knowledge of the presence of structural variations is also necessary for designing an accurate therapeutic exercise program. For example, the degree of lateral rotation in an exercise prescribed for the posterior gluteus medius (PGM) muscle has to be modified for the patient with hip antetorsion.

The neck of the femur and the transverse axis of the femoral condyles (see Figure 2-22) form the *angle of torsion* or *declination* in the frontal plane. The normal angle is approximately 14 degrees anterior in the average adult, but there can be variation. Antetorsion (anteversion) is a pathologic increase in the angle of torsion. Retrotorsion (retroversion) is a pathologic decrease in the angle of torsion.[15] At birth the angle of torsion is 30 to 35 degrees and the femoral head faces relatively anteriorly in the acetabulum. From birth to approximately 6 years of age the angle of torsion decreases and the orientation of the femoral head changes so that it faces more medially in the acetabulum. Children with antetorsion tend to prefer to sit in the W or "reverse tailor" position. Individuals with antetorsion that may be uni-

lateral or bilateral tend to be pigeon-toed unless tibial torsion is also present. In the W-sitting position the tibia is rotated laterally, and thus it may undergo rotational changes that compensate for the medial rotation of the femur. In the uncompensated position when the foot appears pigeon-toed, correcting the foot alignment rotates the hip laterally, causing the head of the femur to point anteriorly in the joint, which can then become a source of hip pain depending on the amount of rotation. Also, when correcting the foot position by rotating the hip laterally, the limit of hip lateral rotation range of motion may be reached. Consequently, the hip may be forced into excessive rotation, or pelvic rotation will be exaggerated during walking. During gait the hip normally rotates 10 degrees laterally from the midstance phase until the swing phase.[8]

The patient with antetorsion can appear to be in excessive hip medial rotation and may have genu valgus (knock-knees). If this patient continues to sit with the hip maximally rotated medially, hip pain can develop because of excessive medial rotation. If the patient forces the hip to rotate laterally by exerting pressure on the knees when sitting in the "tailor" or "cross-legged" position, hip pain can also develop because of pressure into the anterior joint structures by the femoral head. The physical therapist can provide a useful screening service by assessing the presence of antetorsion in young girls who are participating in ballet or any dance discipline that requires the ability to rotate the hips laterally so that the feet point 90 degrees laterally. If the antetorsion is not identified, young girls participating in ballet in which maximum hip lateral rotation is required can compensate with excessive rotation at the knee joint (Figure 4-5).

The patient with retrotorsion appears to have the feet turned out (i.e., duck walk or Charlie Chaplin gait). Correcting this foot alignment results in excessive hip medial rotation, causing the head of the femur to be directed more medially than when the head of the femur is in its optimal position. Clinical examples of hip retroversion causing groin pain were found in two professional women. Both of these women sat with their legs crossed with the hips in medial rotation. Their professions required them to spend most of their day sitting and talking with clients. They also participated in regular exercise programs, such as jogging and tennis. Their hip abductors, lateral rotators, and iliopsoas muscles were all stretched and weakened by the prolonged sitting in medial rotation. Correcting their sitting habits and the weakness of their hip abductor and lateral rotator muscles, as well as strengthening the iliopsoas muscle, alleviated their symptoms.

Retrotorsion can also contribute to low back pain if the patient participates in sports that require rotation

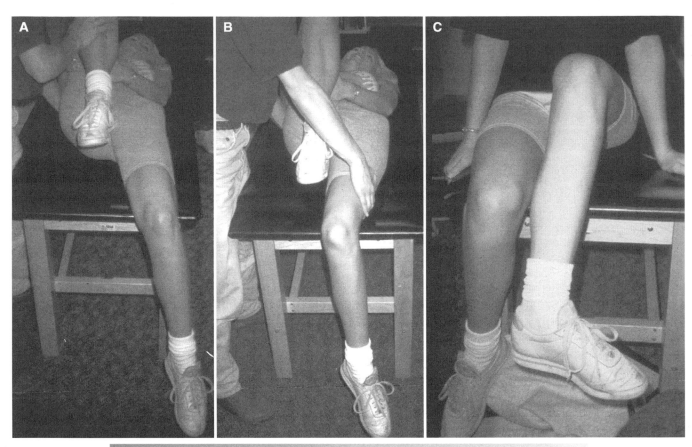

Figure 4-5

Excessive tibiofemoral rotation associated with hip antetorsion in an individual who has participated extensively in ballet. *A,* Hip extension of 10 degrees is only possible when the hip is abducted, indicating shortness of the tensor fascia lata–iliotibial band. *B,* When the hip is passively adducted, stretching the tensor fascia lata–iliotibial band, the tibia rotates laterally. *C,* Voluntary lateral tibial rotation indicates excessive range of motion.

with the feet relatively fixed, such as golf or racquetball. If the patient stands with the feet pointing straight ahead to hit a golf ball, he or she may reach the end of his or her hip medial rotation range and need to compensate with lumbar rotation because of the limited motion at the hips. To hit a golf ball correctly requires good hip medial rotational range.[17] If the patient has retroversion, he or she should stand with the feet pointing laterally so that more hip medial rotational range is available than if he or she stands with the feet pointing straight ahead and the need to compensate with excessive lumbar rotation is avoided. Walking with the foot turned laterally can contribute to hallus valgus if, during the stance phase, the patient brings his or her weight line over the medial aspect of the great toe, pushing it into a valgus-oriented direction.

The assessment of the angle of torsion needs to be performed carefully. Gelberman and colleagues[6] report that assessment of antetorsion should be performed in the prone position with the hip joint in neutral and in the sitting position with the hip flexed. In this prone position, hip medial and lateral rotation can be measured. If the medial rotational range seems excessive (i.e., greater than 50 degrees) and lateral rotation is limited (i.e., less than 15 degrees from the vertical), antetorsion is suggested (Figure 4-6). With the patient remaining in the prone position, the examiner can also perform the Craig test. The Craig test is performed by rotating the hip through the full ranges into medial and lateral rotation while palpating the greater trochanter and determining the position in the range at which the trochanter is the most prominently lateral (Figure 4-7). At this point of rotation, the femur is optimally situated in the acetabulum. If the angle is greater than 15 degrees in the direction of hip medial rotation when measured from the vertical and long axes of the tibia, the femur is considered to be in antetorsion. By performing this test the examiner will have an indication of the degree of antetorsion of the femur. One study reported that the Craig test is more reliable than radiologic techniques.[20]

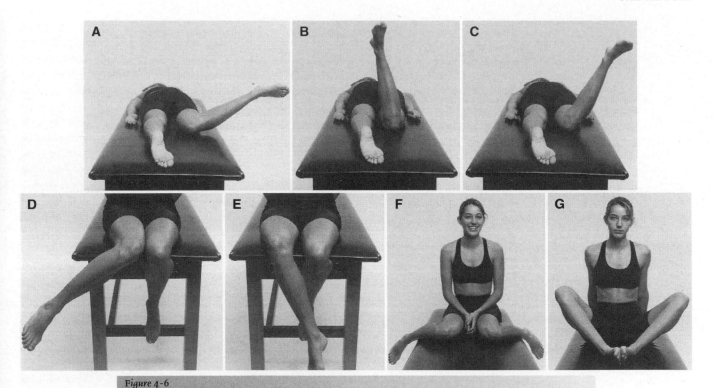

Figure 4-6

Effect of femoral antetorsion on hip rotation range of motion in the hip flexed and extended positions. *A,* In the hip extended position, medial rotation range of motion is excessive (65 degrees). *B,* The maximum degree of lateral rotation is limited (5 degrees). *C,* Craig's test is used to determine this subject's neutral hip rotation position (34 degrees). *D,* In the hip flexed positioned, medial rotation range is 60 degrees. *E,* Medial rotation range greatly exceeds lateral rotation range (25 degrees). *F,* Reverse tailor or W sitting is demonstrated. *G,* Limited hip lateral rotation interferes with the "Indian" sitting position.

In the prone position with the hip extended and in neutral abduction/adduction, shortness of the hip abductor/medial rotator muscles can limit the lateral rotational range (Figure 4-8). In the hip flexed position, muscles cannot limit the lateral rotational range. In the Gelberman study, the structural antetorsion of the hip (as verified by magnetic resonance imaging) was present when the asymmetry of medial rotational range of motion was much greater than the lateral rotational range in both the hip flexed and the hip extended positions.[6] In the case of retrotorsion, the range of lateral rotation should be greater than the range of medial rotation in both the flexed and extended positions of the hip. With the hip extended and the knee flexed, none of the musculature that limits medial rotation is taut, therefore the finding in this position should be valid (Figure 4-9). In the hip flexed position the gluteus maximus is pulled taut and can limit the medial rotational range of motion.

Tests of torsion are also important in prescribing hip abduction exercises because the exercise should be performed in the degrees of rotation that are appropriate for the patient's femoral configuration. Any patient with hip or back pain should be routinely assessed for the presence of torsional variations.

The *angle of inclination* needs to also be considered in the assessment. The neck of the femur forms an angle with the shaft in the frontal plane that varies during the life cycle, but it is approximately 125 degrees in the adult. At 3 weeks of age, the angle is 150 degrees.[18] In the adult, coxa valgum is present when the angle exceeds 130 degrees and coxa varum is present when the angle is less than 120 degrees (Figure 4-10).

Relationships between movement impairment syndromes of the hip and the angle of inclination have not been identified to date, but relationships between the contour of the thigh and the angle of inclination are suggested. In the presence of coxa vara, a reasonable assumption is that the greater trochanter may be particularly prominent and may be less flush with the lateral side of the pelvis. The patient with lateral prominence of the proximal thighs often believes there is excessive fat on the thighs, which may not be the case. In the side-lying position this patient is usually in marked lumbar lateral flexion because of the width of the pelvis and the exaggerated lateral prominence of the femur. In the side-lying position the same structural factors contribute to excessive hip medial rotation and adduction when the patient sleeps with the uppermost hip and knee flexed so that

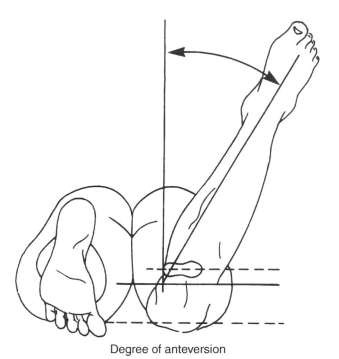

Degree of anteversion

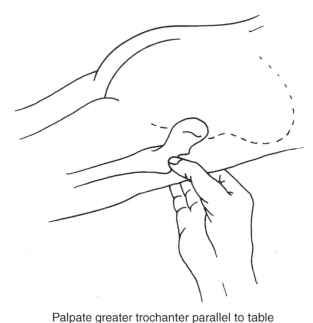

Palpate greater trochanter parallel to table

Figure 4-7

Craig's test. In the prone position, as the examiner rotates the hip, the most lateral prominence of the greater trochanter is determined, which is the neutral position of the femoral head in the acetabulum. (From Magee DJ: *Orthopedic physical assessment,* ed 3, Philadelphia, 1997, WB Saunders.)

the knee is resting against the bed. If the pelvis is wide the posterolateral hip muscles will be in a position of excessive stretch, which can lead to weakness. When the patient with weak abdominal muscles rolls from a supine to a side-lying position, the amount of trunk rotation can be greater than the rotation of the lower half of the body

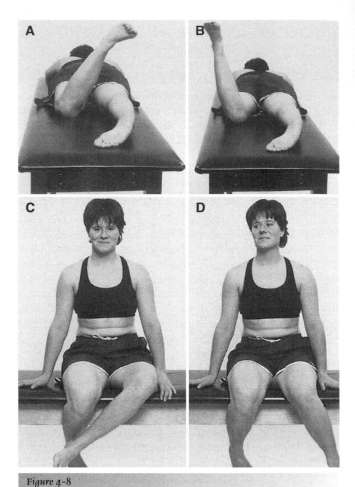

Figure 4-8

Hip lateral rotation limited by shortness of the tensor fascia lata–iliotibial band. *A,* In the hip extended (prone) position, hip lateral rotation is limited to 30 degrees. *B,* Medial rotation is limited to 20 degrees. *C,* In the hip flexed (sitting) position, hip lateral rotation is 50 degrees. *D,* Medial rotation is 25 degrees.

because the wider pelvis and hips have greater resistance to rotation than the narrower pelvis and hips. Clinically, an increased tendency of the tensor fascia lata–iliotibial band (TFL-ITB) to become short in the patient with this type of structure has been observed, possibly because the band remains positioned anterior to the greater trochanter rather than lateral over it.

It is recommended that this patient place a small pillow or folded towel under the waist when sleeping on his or her side and use a pillow between the knees in the side-lying position. The patient needs to practice log rolling and incorporate this motion into his or her daily routine, especially when moving in bed. Instructions in methods to restore or maintain the strength of the external and internal oblique abdominal muscles by frequent isometric contraction of these muscles are indicated as well. The patient should avoid sitting with the legs crossed to minimize the development of shortness of the TFL-ITB.

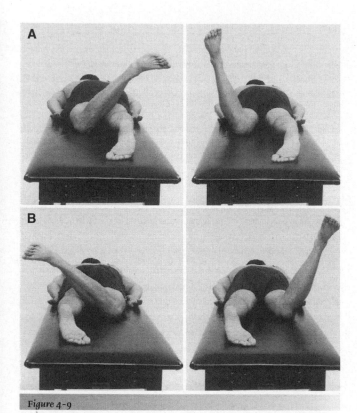

Figure 4-9

Hip retrotorsion. *A,* In the prone position, left hip lateral rotation range of motion of 50 degrees is less than normal *(left)* and the medial rotation range of motion is less than normal *(right)*. *B,* The right hip has the same pattern of excessive lateral *(left)* and limited medial range of motion *(right)*.

Knee Joint

Distinguishing structural variations from acquired faults at the knee can be challenging.

Sagittal Plane

In the sagittal plane, hyperextension and flexion can be acquired postural faults with hyperextension more common. In some patients the hyperextension is so exaggerated that even when attempting to stand correctly, the femur is anterior to the tibia rather than in the same plane (see Figure 2-36). With this degree of hyperextension, the posterior joint capsule is stretched, the anterior cruciate ligament is slacked, and the anterior articular surface of the tibia is altered by the compressive forces. In other patients the bowing of the tibia in the sagittal plane may suggest minimal genu recurvatum (Figure 4-11). In this condition the tibia is bowed, but the knee joint is not always in hyperextension. Careful examination is necessary to distinguish the presence of one or both of these malalignments. Postural knee flexion, particularly in the older individual, is usually a sign of degenerative knee joint disease.

Frontal Plane

In the frontal plane, genu valgum (knock-kneed) and genu varum (bowlegged) can be either structural or ac-

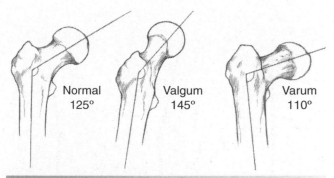

Figure 4-10

Angles of inclination. The femoral shaft and neck normally intersect at an angle of approximately 125 degrees. When this angle is abnormally large (about 145 degrees), the shaft of the femur is displaced laterally and coxa varum (bowleggedness) results. When the angle of the femoral shaft and neck is too small (about 110 degrees, the femoral shaft is displaced medially and coxa valgum (knock-kneedness) results. (From Mathers et al: *Clinical anatomy principles,* St Louis, 1996, Mosby.)

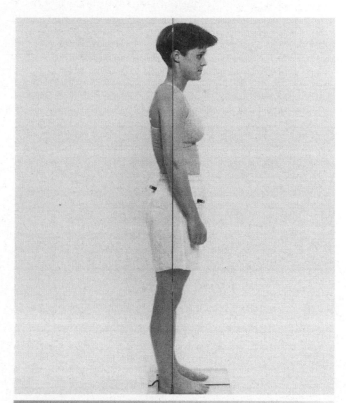

Figure 4-11

Tibial bowing in the sagittal plane. Side view illustrates bowing of the tibia, which can be mistaken for hyperextension of the knee joint. The knee joint is not hyperextended.

quired impairments (Figure 4-12). Although tibial varum, genu varum, and bowlegged are interchangeable terms,[22] clinically these often appear as different conditions. In some patients the bowing appears to be confined to the tibia, and in others the knee joint appears to be bowed. As shown in Figure 4-13 the right tibia appears bowed (tibial varum), but the knee joint appears to be relatively

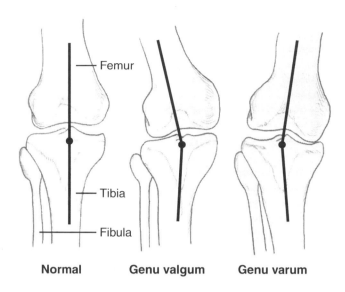

Femur

Tibia

Fibula

Normal   Genu valgum   Genu varum

Figure 4-12

Valgus and varus deformities at the knee joint. A valgus deformity is one in which the distal element of a joint (tibia) is deviated laterally (away from the midline). A varus deformity is one in which the distal element of a joint is deviated medially (toward the midline). (From Mathers et al: *Clinical anatomy principles,* St Louis, 1996, Mosby.)

well aligned. In contrast, the left knee appears to be bowed with a greater degree of tibial bowing. Standing on the left lower extremity increases the degree of varus, but standing on the right does not (Figure 4-14). Increased varus moment, such as that evident in the left lower extremity, can contribute to degenerative knee joint disease. Therefore radiologic analysis of the actual relationship of the femur to the tibia, as well as the shape of the tibia, is important to ascertain whether there are changes in the knee joint or simply a variation in the shape of the tibia. Exaggerated genu varum is most often an indication of degenerative knee joint disease (Figure 4-15). The patient with genu varum often walks with an antalgic gait, because this motion decreases the varus moment on the knee during the stance phase. When there is true genu varum at the knee joint and the patient does not shift his or her weight laterally during walking, the varum moment at the knee is increased, which can further contribute to the malalignment (see Figure 4-14). Hip medial rotation with knee hyperextension can give the appearance of genu varum (Figure 4-16).

Genu valgum appears to be a variation in the angulation of the femur rather than the tibia (Figure 4-17).

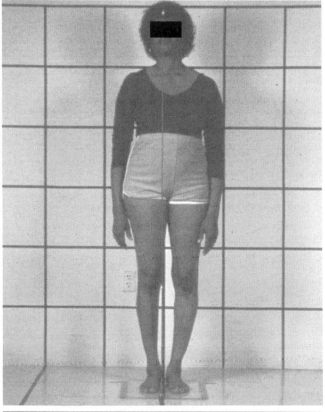

Figure 4-13

Tibial varum and genu varum. The right tibia is bowed in the frontal plane, but the knee is relatively well aligned. The left tibia and knee joint are bowed.

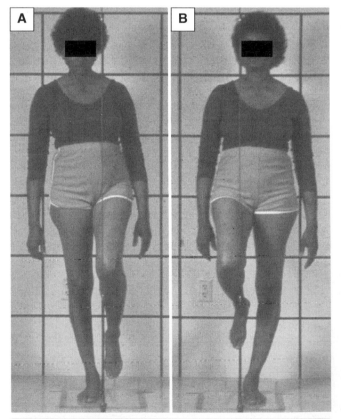

Figure 4-14

Increased genu varum during single-leg standing. *A,* Standing on the right leg does not increase the degrees of genu varum. *B,* Standing on the left leg does increase the degrees of varum.

Acquired postural impairments such as hip medial rotation can also give the appearance of genu valgum (see Figure 4-17). If the problem is an acquired fault, the foot should be pronated so that correction of the rotation also corrects the foot position. If the foot is neutral or supinated, the rotation is most likely structural (i.e., femoral antetorsion).

Tibial torsion, which is a structural rotation of the shaft of the tibia and not rotation of the entire tibia at the knee joint, is another structural variation (Figure 4-18). Tibial torsion is assessed with the knee flexed by determining the angle between the medial and lateral malleoli in relation to the horizontal plane. The normal angle is less than 20 to 25 degrees. Most often the torsion is in a lateral direction. If the foot is in the plane of the ankle, it will face laterally. Shortness of the iliotibial band (ITB) can contribute to lateral tibial rotation at the knee joint. If structural torsion is present and the ITB becomes short and the knee joint is flexible the pull of the band will laterally rotate the tibia (Figure 4-19). If the foot faces anteriorly, it is in inversion and the range into dorsiflexion may be limited because of this alignment (Figure 4-20, page 124).

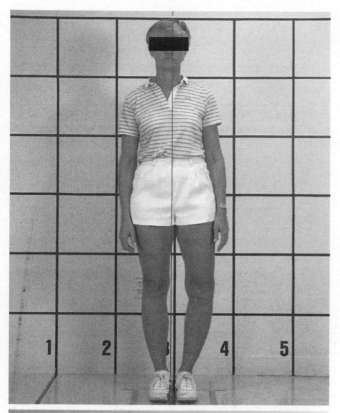

Figure 4-15

Genu varum and degenerative joint disease. This patient has diagnosed degenerative joint disease of her left knee with severe genu varum.

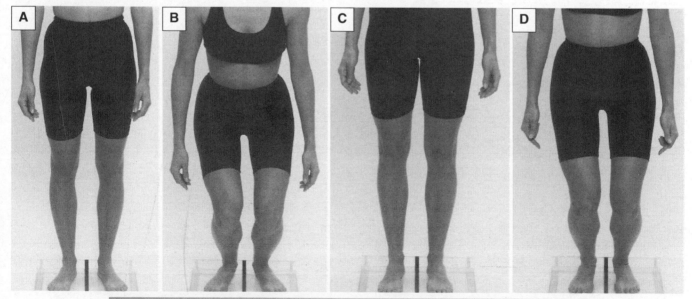

Figure 4-16

Acquired genu varum. *A,* Hip medial rotation and knee hyperextension cause genu varum. *B,* The feet are laterally rotated and pronated. Hip and knee flexion in this alignment contributes to foot pronation, and the path of the knee is medial to the big toe, which can contribute to hallux valgus. *C,* Correction of the hip medial rotation, knee hypertension, and lateral rotation of feet eliminates the genu valgum and foot pronation.
D, In the ideal alignment the path of the knee during hip and knee flexion is over the longitudinal axis of the foot, the second toe.

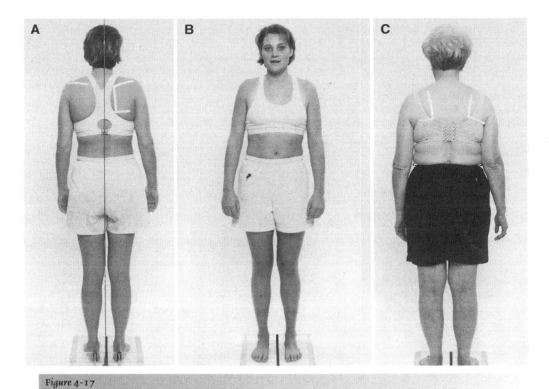

Figure 4-17

Genu valgum, structural and acquired. *A,* Back view of a young woman with structural genu valgum and supinated feet. *B,* Front view of the same woman, further illustrating supinated feet. *C,* Back view of an individual with hip medial rotation that has contributed to genu valgum and pronated feet.

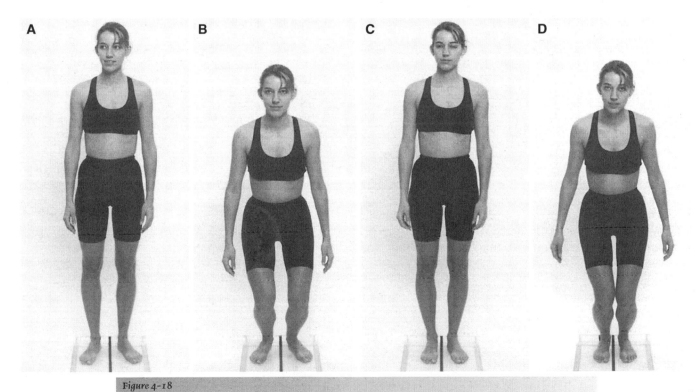

Figure 4-18

Tibial torsion. *A,* The knee is correctly aligned in the sagittal plane, but the feet are facing laterally as the result of tibial torsion. *B,* During hip and knee flexion with the feet laterally rotated the knee is correctly aligned. *C,* With the feet pointing forward, the knee becomes medially rotated. *D,* During flexion, the knee moves in a medial direction.

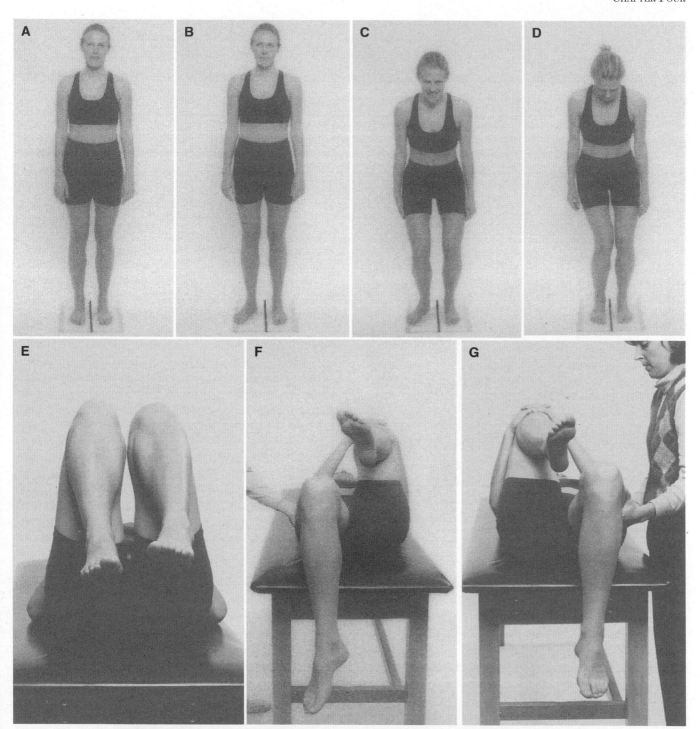

Figure 4-19

Unilateral tibial torsion exaggerated by short TFL-ITB. *A,* When the right tibia is laterally rotated, the knee faces anteriorly. *B,* During hip and knee flexion the knee alignment is correct. *C,* When the foot is corrected, the knee faces medially when standing. *D,* The foot also faces medially during hip and knee flexion. *E,* In the hip flexor length test position, the left tibia is laterally rotated. *F,* The lateral rotation increases as the TFL-ITB is stretched. *G,* The right tibia is not rotated in the resting position (shown in *D*) or with stretch of the band.

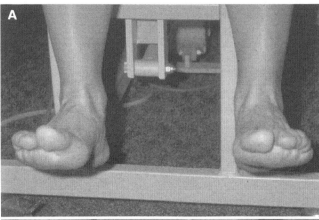

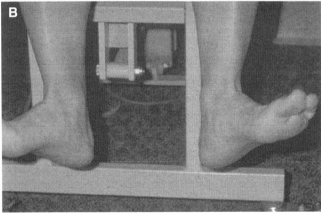

Figure 4-20

Tibial torsion and dorsiflexion range of motion. *A,* Tibial torsion is observed, but the foot is directed anteriorly. Thus the ankle is in inversion, which limits the dorsiflexion range of motion. *B,* When the foot is laterally rotated so that the ankle is in neutral, the dorsiflexion range of motion is increased.

Foot

When the foot is pronated, proximal forces primarily originating at the pelvis and hip contribute to the alignment fault. Most commonly, poor control of the hip lateral rotator muscles allows the hip to rotate medially and exert a pronatory stress on the foot. When the foot is supinated and rigid, the forces are directed up the closed kinetic chain rather than down. In this situation as in many others, the body follows the path of least resistance for motion. If the foot is stiff and does not adequately dorsiflex, the stress can be at the knee joint or at the hip joint if the knee is stable. Most often the knee joint is affected, causing either a rotation- or posterior-directed stress. Often tibial bowing in the sagittal plane can be observed in the patient with rigid feet or in the frontal plane if the foot is markedly supinated.

Motions of the Hip

Pelvic Girdle Motions

ANTERIOR PELVIC TILT. The ASIS is anterior to the vertical plane through the symphysis pubis.[11] Commonly used clinical indicators are when the ASIS is lower than the PSIS and the hip joint is flexed as indicated previously. The differences between the relative heights of the ASIS and PSIS should be greater than 15 degrees for clinical significance.

POSTERIOR PELVIC TILT. The ASIS is posterior to the vertical plane through the symphysis pubis.[11] When measuring the anterior and posterior pelvic tilt, the angle formed between the line connecting the posterior and anterior iliac spines and the horizontal plane varies by ±12 degrees in normal individuals.[2]

LATERAL PELVIC TILT. One iliac crest is higher than the other with differences of less than 1/2 inch considered within the normal range of variability.

ROTATION. The vertical plane through one ASIS is forward of the vertical plane through the other ASIS. Clockwise rotation occurs when the left ASIS is forward of the right. When the pelvis is rotated clockwise and the lower extremities appear to be facing anteriorly, the right hip joint is in postural medial rotation while the left hip joint is in lateral rotation. Often these faults of postural alignment are consistent with the differences in muscle stiffness or length. For example, in the alignment described, the right TFL may be short and the right posterior gluteus medius (PGM) muscle may be long, which is consistent with the postural alignment. On the left side, the PGM muscle or the hip lateral rotator muscles, the obturators, gemelli, and piriformis could be short or stiff.

Hip Joint Motions

HIP FLEXION. Movement occurs in an anterior direction around a coronal axis. The full range through flexion is approximately 125 degrees. During hip flexion there is slight posterior glide of the femoral head.

HIP EXTENSION. Movement occurs in a posterior direction around a coronal axis. The normal range is approximately 10 degrees. Normal standing alignment is 0 degrees of hip extension. During hip extension there is slight anterior glide of the femoral head. When the pelvis is tilted posteriorly enough to flatten the lumbar spine, the hip is in 10 degrees of extension in most individuals. When an individual stands with the knees hyperextended (genu recurvatum), the hip is extended. Therefore when the posterior tilt flattens the lumbar spine and the individual has hyperextended knees, the hip joint extension may approach 20 degrees (see Figures 2-34).

HIP MEDIAL ROTATION. Movement occurs around a longitudinal axis with the anterior surface of the thigh turning toward the midsagittal plane. The accessory motion is posterior glide. Normal range of motion is approximately 45 degrees, but this range is highly variable. Structural conditions affecting the range of motion include femoral antetorsion and retrotorsion, which have been discussed. Medial rotational range appears excessive in the individual with antetorsion of the hips, which, based on clinical experience, has a higher incidence in women than in men. The finding of hip antetorsion on one side only is common.

HIP LATERAL ROTATION. Movement occurs around a longitudinal axis with the anterior surface of the thigh moving away from the midsagittal plane. The accessory motion is anterior glide. Range of motion is approximately 45 degrees, but this range is highly variable. In the individual with hip retrotorsion, the range into lateral rotation appears to be excessive. This condition is found more often in men than in women.

·ABDUCTION. Movement occurs away from the midsagittal plane in the lateral direction. Normal range is approximately 45 degrees. During abduction, the femoral head should move inferiorly.

ADDUCTION. Movement occurs toward the midsagittal plane in the medial direction. Range is approximately 10 degrees. During adduction, the femoral head glides superiorly.

Hip Joint Accessory Motions

Although accessory motions of the hip joint are present, these are believed to be limited in range because of the depth of the acetabulum and the fibrocartilaginous acetabular labrum that deepens the acetabulum from less than one half to greater than one half of a sphere.

ANTERIOR GLIDE. Movement occurs in an anterior (ventral) direction. According to the convex-concave rule, anterior glide occurs with hip extension and lateral rotation.

POSTERIOR GLIDE. Movement occurs in a posterior (dorsal) direction with hip flexion and medial rotation.

SUPERIOR GLIDE. Movement occurs along the longitudinal axis in the cephalad direction. Superior glide occurs during hip adduction.

INFERIOR GLIDE (LONG AXIS DISTRACTION). Movement occurs along the longitudinal axis in the caudal direction with the hip in the resting position. Inferior glide occurs during hip abduction.

MEDIAL GLIDE. Compression occurs medially.

LATERAL GLIDE. Lateral- or short-axis distraction occurs.

Muscular Actions of the Hip

Anterior Trunk Muscles Affecting the Pelvis

The *external oblique abdominal muscle* tilts the pelvis posteriorly when acting bilaterally (see Figure 3-26). When contracting unilaterally and acting with the contralateral internal oblique muscle, the action is rotation of the trunk or pelvis. For example, acting together the left external oblique and right internal oblique muscles rotate the trunk counterclockwise or the pelvis clockwise.

Acting unilaterally, the lateral portion of the external oblique abdominal muscle moves the iliac crest on the same side cranially, causing a lateral tilt. This muscle commonly tests weak, particularly in women. Because of the critical role of the external oblique in tilting the pelvis posteriorly, flattening and supporting the lumbar spine, and controlling rotation, particularly with regard to preventing pelvic rotation, adequate performance is important. The external oblique muscle is often less dominant than the rectus abdominis muscle, which also tilts the pelvis posteriorly.[9] Therefore specific training for adequate participation is often necessary. Bilateral contraction of the external oblique muscles narrows the infrasternal angle and compresses the ribs and thus can reduce the tendency for the ribs to flare.

The *internal oblique abdominal muscle* when contracting bilaterally flexes the thorax and when acting unilaterally with the external oblique muscle performs rotation as described previously. When contracting unilaterally, the internal oblique will tilt the same side of the pelvis laterally, moving it cranially.

The *rectus abdominis muscle* flexes the thorax (curls the trunk) and tilts the pelvis posteriorly and is often more dominant than the internal and external oblique muscles.[21] If the rectus abdominis becomes dominant and the performance of the obliques is compromised, control of trunk or pelvic rotation is compromised because the rectus abdominis cannot control rotation. Because it attaches to the sternum, shortness or stiffness of this muscle contributes to a depressed chest and thoracic kyphosis (Figure 4-21).

The *transversus abdominis muscle* stiffens the spine and compresses the viscera. This abdominal muscle is another of those whose performance can be easily enhanced by a conscious effort to contract the muscle by "pulling the navel toward the spine."[7,19]

The *iliopsoas muscle* (see Figure 3-24) flexes the hip or tilts the pelvis anteriorly when the lower extremity is fixed. In the erect position, the iliopsoas muscle exerts a weak extension moment on the upper lumbar spine and a

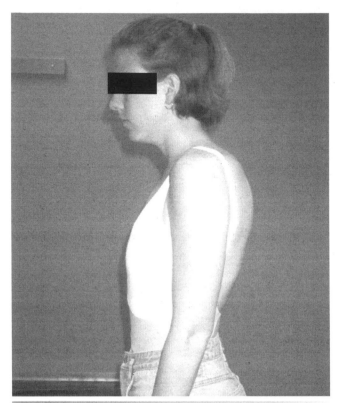

Figure 4-21

Short rectus abdominis. Depressed chest from shortness of the rectus abdominis.

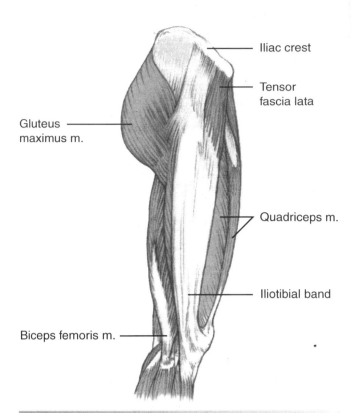

Iliac crest

Tensor fascia lata

Gluteus maximus m.

Quadriceps m.

Iliotibial band

Biceps femoris m.

Figure 4-22

Tensor fascia lata–iliotibial band. The TFL-ITB is a major contributor to impairments of the lower extremity. Its actions of abduction, flexion, and medial rotation of the hip are the most common motions of the hip joint. The attachment of the TFL-ITB to the patella and the lateral aspect of the tibia contribute to impairments of the patella and to lateral rotation of the tibia. (From Mathers et al: *Clinical anatomy principles,* St Louis, 1966, Mosby.)

flexion moment on the lower lumbar spine.[1] When the lumbar spine is flexed, the iliopsoas muscle exerts a flexion moment on all segments of the lumbar spine. According to the study by Bogduk and associates[3] the moments exerted on the lumbar spine are minimal. The major forces acting on the lumbar spine are compression and anterior shear forces. The lateral flexion moments exerted on the lumbar spine by the iliopsoas muscle are small.[3]

Because the iliopsoas muscle attaches to the anterior portion of the transverse processes of all lumbar vertebrae and intervertebral disks, it can contribute to mechanical dysfunction and often to a patient's symptoms. The iliopsoas muscle contributes to lateral rotation and abduction of the hip.

Posterior Muscles Affecting the Pelvis

When acting bilaterally the *erector spinae muscles* cause anterior pelvic tilt. When acting unilaterally these muscles cause lateral pelvic tilt (see Figure 3-21).

The *quadratus lumborum muscle* tilts the pelvis laterally; when the pelvis is fixed, it flexes the trunk laterally (see Figure 3-24). Because of its attachment to the transverse processes of lumbar vertebrae, the quadratus lumborum muscle contributes to lateral trunk flexion if it is short.

Anterior Muscles Affecting the Hip Joint

The *iliopsoas muscle* flexes and laterally rotates the hip joint slightly. The iliopsoas is the only muscle capable of flexing the hip at the end range of hip flexion.

The TFL-ITB flexes, rotates medially, and abducts the hip (Figure 4-22). When the knee is extended, the TFL-ITB can act to stabilize the knee, although it does not extend the knee.[10,16] In patients with a short ITB, during muscle length testing, if the hip is adducted from the hip extended and abducted position, the knee will extend from the passive tension of the band. When a patient sits without using the backrest on a chair, he or she is using the hip flexor muscles, which can include the TFL to maintain the hip flexion position. The lateral attachment of the TFL onto the tibial tuberosity can contribute to lateral tibial rotation if the knee is not stable. The lateral slips of the band attach to the patella and thus contributes to lateral glide of the patella.

The TFL commonly becomes short and stiff and is often mistaken for shortness of the iliopsoas muscle when, during hip flexor length testing, the hip is pre-

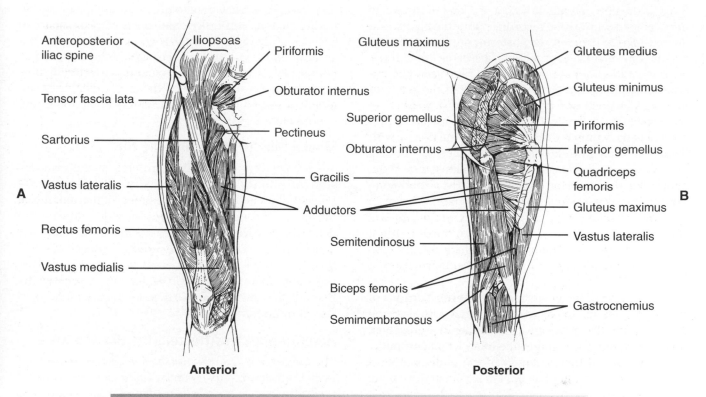

A, Anteroposterior iliac spine — Iliopsoas — Piriformis — Tensor fascia lata — Obturator internus — Sartorius — Pectineus — Vastus lateralis — Gracilis — Adductors — Rectus femoris — Vastus medialis

Anterior

Gluteus maximus — Gluteus medius — Gluteus minimus — Superior gemellus — Piriformis — Obturator internus — Inferior gemellus — Gracilis — Quadriceps femoris — Adductors — Gluteus maximus — Semitendinosus — Vastus lateralis — Biceps femoris — Semimembranosus — Gastrocnemius

Posterior

Figure 4-23

Muscles of the pelvis, hip, and thigh. *A,* Anterior view. *B,* Posterior view. (From Scuderi GR et al: *Sports medicine: principles of primary care,* St Louis, 1997, Mosby.)

vented from abducting. The TFL muscle tests strong when the iliopsoas or PGM muscle tests weak with the exception of when the TFL becomes strained. When the TFL becomes stiff or short and the lower extremity is fixed, its contraction can result in rotation of the pelvis because the TFL muscle is a medial rotator of the hip. If segments of the lumbar spine have become particularly flexible and easily rotate, the rotation of the pelvis will also cause rotation of the lumbar spine.

The *sartorius muscle* flexes, rotates laterally, and abducts the hip. It also flexes and rotates the knee medially (Figure 4-23).

The *rectus femoris muscle* flexes the hip and extends the knee.

Posterior Muscles Affecting the Hip

The *gluteus maximus muscle* extends and laterally rotates the hip (see Figure 4-23). The upper one half of the muscle abducts the hip; the lower one half adducts the hip. Approximately 80% of the gluteus maximus inserts into the ITB. Therefore this muscle exerts a strong influence on the band and can contribute to restricted hip adduction range. Shortness of this muscle can contribute to compensatory lumbar flexion when the individual is sitting with the hips flexed.

The gluteus maximus muscle can become atrophied, and its dominance as a hip extensor lessens, particularly in the individual who stands in a swayback posture, exaggerating the posterior distance of his or her weight line from the hip joint. Decreased activity in this muscle, particularly when combined with decreased performance of the other posterior muscles of the hip girdle, compromises the control of the femur in the acetabulum. The patient who stands in a posterior pelvic tilt and swayback posture will often walk with minimal use of the gluteus maximus muscle during the stance phase of gait. The patient with weak or absent hip extensor muscles can be taught to stand in the swayback posture because of the mechanical forces that contribute to the maintenance of hip extension. To avoid the mechanical effects that detract from the participation of the muscle, the patient with swayback posture needs to correct his or her alignment and actively contract the gluteus maximus muscle at heel strike to use the muscle effectively during gait.

The *posterior portion of the gluteus medius muscle* extends, abducts, and laterally rotates the hip (see Figure 4-23). This portion often becomes excessively lengthened or weak. Careful muscle testing allows the examiner to differentiate between the two conditions. If the patient cannot hold at the end of the range but is able to take strong resistance after the hip has adducted 10 to 15 degrees, the posterior portion of the gluteus medius muscle is probably excessively long. If the patient cannot hold at the end of the range and can tolerate only minimal resistance throughout the range of motion, the posterior portion is probably weak. The weakened muscle is usually associated with pain in the muscle belly, which is evident upon contraction or with palpation. If the muscle is long, the pain usually occurs during hip joint motions, because the pain source is the faulty control of the head of the femur in the acetabulum. This muscle is commonly affected by postural faults.

The *anterior portion of the gluteus medius muscle* abducts, medially rotates, and assists in flexion of the hip. This portion is usually strong, which further contributes to a tendency for excessive medial rotation of the hip.

Shortness of the posterior and anterior portions of the gluteus medius muscle is associated with postural hip abduction. The patient with his or her iliac crest high (postural adduction) on the side of an L4,5 neuropathy should be tested for weakness of the gluteus medius muscle. The lateral lumbar flexion associated with hip joint asymmetry can further contribute to the nerve root compression.

The *gluteus minimus muscle* abducts, rotates medially, and assists in flexion of the hip (Figure 4-24). The gluteus minimus is another muscle that contributes to the abduction-medial rotation tendency of the hip.

The *piriformis muscle* rotates laterally, extends, and abducts the hip when the hip is in flexion (see Figure 4-24). The length of this muscle needs to be considered carefully in the piriformis syndrome. Although the piriformis is commonly considered to be short when this syndrome is present, Kendall[11] reports that symptoms of this syndrome can also be found in the patient who has a lengthened piriformis muscle. In the clinical experience of the author of this text, this syndrome is found more frequently in the patient with a lengthened piriformis than in the patient with the shortened piriformis. The therapist must carefully examine the length of the muscle before planning intervention for the syndrome.

The *obturator internus and externus and superior and inferior gemelli muscles* are lateral rotators. They frequently become weak or stiff, but these muscles can also become excessively lengthened (see Figure 4-24). The obturator internus, superior and inferior gemelli, and piriformis muscles assist in abduction when the hip is flexed, whereas the obturator externus assists in the adduction of the hip. In the patient who stands in hip extension with the upper back in a swayback position, these muscles can become short or stiff

and can create resistance to posterior gliding of the hip during flexion. Stiffness or shortness can contribute to anterior groin pain, which is a symptom of the femoral anterior glide syndrome described in this chapter. The lateral rotator muscles are commonly affected by postural faults. Dysfunctions of these muscles are commonly observed in the patient with dysfunction of the central nervous system.

Medial Muscles Affecting the Hip

The *pectineus muscle* adducts, rotates medially, and assists in flexion of the hip (see Figure 4-23). The *gracilis muscle* adducts the hip and medially rotates and flexes the knee. The *adductor longus muscle* adducts and flexes the hip. The *adductor brevis muscle* adducts and flexes the hip. The *adductor magnus muscle* adducts the hip with the anterior fibers flexing the hip and the posterior fibers extending the hip. As discussed by Kendall, this muscle can participate in both medial and lateral rotation.[11]

Anterior Muscles Affecting the Hip and Knee

The *quadriceps femoris muscle* consists of four major muscle groups: *rectus femoris, vastus lateralis, vastus medialis,* and *vastus intermedius* (Figure 4-25). The rectus femoris muscle flexes the hip and extends the knee. The vasti arise from the anterior and posterior (linea aspera) surfaces of the femur. Because these muscles attach to the femur and tibia, they extend the knee and do not directly influence the hip joint. The vastus medialis oblique muscle has an important role in the medial glide of the patella.[12]

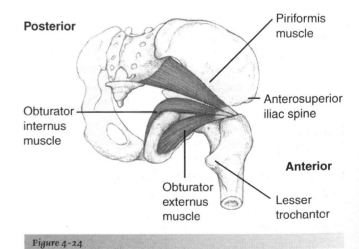

Posterior

Piriformis muscle

Obturator internus muscle

Anterosuperior iliac spine

Obturator externus muscle

Anterior

Lesser trochanter

Figure 4-24

Obturator internus and externus. These muscles are important rotators of the hip that also provide control of the femoral head in the acetabulum. Shortness or stiffness of the lateral rotator muscles is believed to contribute to the femoral anterior glide syndrome. (From Mathers et al: *Clinical anatomy principles,* St Louis,1996, Mosby.)

Posterior Muscles Affecting the Hip and Knee

The *semimembranosus* and *semitendinosus muscles* extend and rotate the hip medially and flex and rotate the knee medially (see Figure 4-23). This pair of muscles can become stiffer or shorter than its synergist, the biceps femoris muscle. This condition is seen in the individual who has excessive hip medial rotation. The imbalance is most evident during knee extension performed while in the sitting position. In the presence of shortness of the medial hamstrings, if the femur is allowed to rotate medially as the knee extends, the range of motion is close to normal. If the medial rotation of the femur is prevented as the knee extends, the range of motion is limited.

The *biceps femoris muscle* (see Figure 4-23) extends and rotates the hip laterally and flexes and rotates the knee laterally. The biceps femoris can become the dominant muscle for hip lateral rotation, the result of which is pain at the knee or the hip. The reason for this painful condition at the hip is that the biceps femoris muscle does not have attachments that extend from the pelvis to the femur. The short head of the biceps femoris muscle arises from the distal femur and inserts into the tibia. The distal origin of this muscle limits the effectiveness of its control on the proximal femur. If the knee is particularly flexible, contraction of the biceps femoris can contribute to lateral rotation of the tibia rather than just lateral rotation of the femur with the result being knee pain.

The hamstring muscles contribute to a number of motions of the lower extremity. Because of their multiple actions, as well as their requirements of extensibility, the hamstring muscles are frequently subject to strain. This strain can be attributed in part to their overuse when synergists are underused. An example of this problem is the dominant use of the hamstring muscles and the underuse of the gluteus maximus muscles. Runners with swayback posture, who have an atrophy and a weakness of the gluteus maximus muscles, can be predisposed to hamstring muscle strain (Figure 4-26). The hamstring muscles can also produce knee extension, substituting for the quadriceps muscles. When the foot is fixed by contact with the floor, hip extension also produces knee extension.

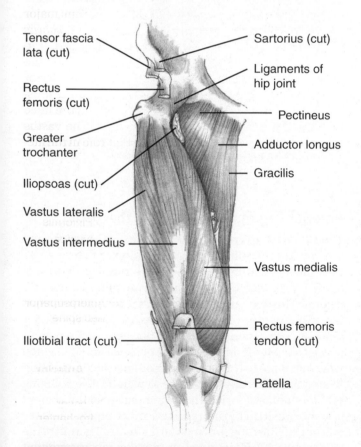

Tensor fascia lata (cut)

Sartorius (cut)

Ligaments of hip joint

Rectus femoris (cut)

Pectineus

Greater trochanter

Adductor longus

Gracilis

Iliopsoas (cut)

Vastus lateralis

Vastus intermedius

Vastus medialis

Iliotibial tract (cut)

Rectus femoris tendon (cut)

Patella

Figure 4-25

Rectus femoris and vastus lateralis, medius, and intermedius. The rectus femoris is a powerful flexor of the hip and participates in knee extension with the vasti. (From Reckling FW: *Orthopedic anatomy and surgical approaches*, ed 1, St Louis, 1990, Mosby.)

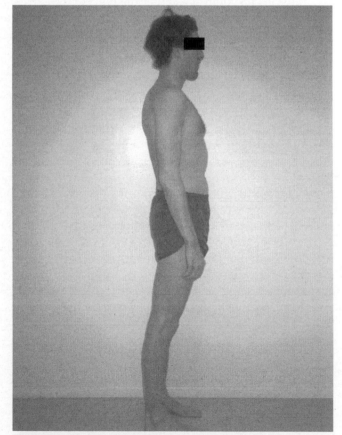

Figure 4-26

Swayback posture with posterior pelvic tilt and hip extension. Poor definition of gluteal musculature and well-developed hamstring muscles.

Discrepancies in the amount of participation of the medial versus the lateral hamstring muscles can also develop. For example, cyclists who keep their hip rotated medially while riding their bicycles tend to use the medial hamstring muscles more than the lateral hamstring muscles. The lateral hamstrings can become dominant lateral hip rotators and can diminish the activity of the intrinsic hip lateral rotators, obturators, gemelli, and piriformis muscles of the pelvic girdle. Observing the movement pattern and manual muscle testing are used to assess the presence of a change in dominance. For example, when a patient with persistent hamstring muscle strain has a swayback posture and poor definition of the gluteus maximus muscle, the results of the following tests are used to assess whether the hamstring muscles have become the dominant hip extensor:

- In the prone position at the initiation of hip extension, a visible change occurs in the contour of the hamstring muscles. The change in the contour of the gluteus maximus muscle, however, does not occur until the hip is almost completely extended.
- The manual muscle testing of the gluteus maximus muscle can confirm whether the muscle is weak or strong.

Posterior Leg Muscles Affecting the Knee and Ankle

The *gastrocnemius muscle* flexes the knee and plantar flexes the ankle (see Figure 4-23). Along with the soleus muscle (Figure 4-27), the gastrocnemius muscle is the primary plantar flexor of the ankle. However, in the individual involved in activities such as dance, this muscle may be weak. Weakness can also be found in the individual who has short heel cords and who uses the shortness to produce the force required for plantar flexion. To assess the presence of weakness, the therapist needs to provide resistance against plantar flexion at the ankle joint by holding at the calcaneus with the subtalar joint in neutral rather than at the metatarsal heads. When there is weakness of the gastrocnemius-soleus muscle group, the patient is unable to plantar flex the ankle to overcome the resistance applied by the therapist. The same patient generates a stronger plantar-flexion force against pressure applied at the level of the metatarsal heads. The explanation is that the patient is recruiting additional plantar flexors, such as the peroneus longus, tibialis posterior, flexor hallucis longus, and flexor digitorum longus muscles, to plantar flex the ankle and joints of the foot (Figure 4-28). To encourage use of the gastrocnemius-soleus group, the patient should "lift the heels" when performing plantar flexion rather than continuously repeating the faulty movement pattern of "going up on the toes."

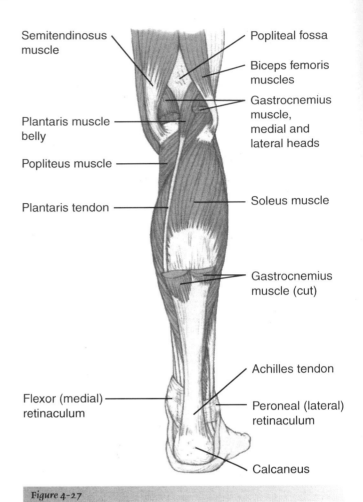

Figure 4-27

Soleus. The soleus muscle plantar flexes the ankle. (From Mathers et al: *Clinical anatomy principles,* St Louis, 1996, Mosby.)

Anterior Leg Muscles Affecting the Ankle

The *tibialis anterior muscle* dorsiflexes the ankle joint and inverts the foot at the subtalar joint (Figure 4-29). This muscle can be overused if the running pattern is one of prolonged dorsiflexion with minimal plantar flexion. This type of pattern occurs if the patient keeps his or her center of gravity somewhat posterior rather than anterior when jogging. For correction, the patient needs to push-off during the late phase of stance, which will contribute to a greater range-of-knee flexion and hip flexion and thus allow the foot to plantar flex, relaxing the dorsiflexors during the swing phase. If the patient does not push off during terminal stance phase, the knee and hip flexion ranges of motion decrease. Therefore the ankle must be maintained in dorsiflexion throughout swing phase to clear the foot. This type of repeated foot posture could lead to anterior shin splints, which is an overuse syndrome of the tibialis anterior. The pain is located on the anterolateral aspect of the tibia.

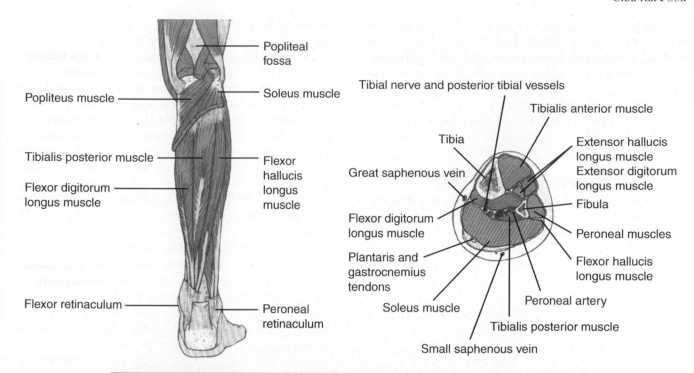

Figure 4-28

Deep calf muscles. The peroneus longus, plantar flexes and everts the ankle by exerting its actions on the foot. The tibialis posterior, flexor hallucis longus, and flexor digitorum longus plantar flex and evert the ankle. The tibialis posterior supports the longitudinal arch of the foot, and the other muscles flex the toes. Posterior shin splints is the result of a strain of one or all these muscles. The patient can substitute the action of these muscles for that of the gastrocnemius and soleus muscles. (From Mathers et al: *Clinical anatomy principles,* St Louis, 1996, Mosby.)

The tibialis anterior muscle is an antagonist of the peroneus longus muscle because it inverts the foot, whereas the peroneal muscles evert the subtalar joint. If the foot is pronated (everted) and the peroneus longus muscle is short, the foot will evert as it dorsiflexes rather than remain neutral with respect to inversion or eversion. This type of movement indicates the dominance of the peroneus longus muscle and contributes to excessive pronation of the foot. The patient should be instructed to dorsiflex and invert to stretch the peroneus longus muscle. The patient will often feel stretch along the lateral aspect of the leg while performing this exercise. The tibialis anterior muscle is also an antagonist of the peroneus longus muscle because the former dorsiflexes the ankle, whereas the latter plantar flexes the ankle.

The *extensor digitorum longus* muscle dorsiflexes the ankle and extends the toes. If the patient has hammer toes, the toe extensors and flexors are both short, whereas the lumbrical and interossei muscles are weak. A patient with hammer toes will dorsiflex the foot by contracting the toe extensors more strongly than the tibialis anterior muscle. This dominance of the toe extensors acting as ankle dorsiflexors is also evident when the

patient with hammer toes sits down or stands up. During these motions, the toes will extend because his or her center of gravity is too far posterior in relation to the feet and thus the patient will be pulling the body forward. Instead, the patient should have the weight line over the feet so that he or she is raising the body mass in the vertical direction more than pulling it forward. During the incorrect pattern the dorsiflexors and toe extensors muscles are used concentrically to pull the center of gravity forward or eccentrically to restrain the posterior movement of the center of gravity. If the patient keeps the center of gravity centered over the feet, the use of the plantar flexor muscles increases and the use of the toe extensor and ankle dorsiflexor muscles decreases. The patient needs to be instructed to keep his center of gravity over his feet as he or she comes up into a standing position from sitting and during the reverse motion. To accomplish this the patient moves to the front of the chair when standing up and sits close to the front of the chair when sitting down.

Hammer toes are associated with a prominence of the heads of the metatarsals. To correct this condition the patient needs to stretch both the flexor digitorum longus and the extensor digitorum longus muscles and to strengthen the lumbrical and interossei muscles by flexing the metatarsophalangeal (MTP) joints. When walking, the patient needs to press the toes, particularly at the MTP joint, into the floor or into the ground to distribute the pressure between the toes and the metatarsal heads rather than allowing the toes to extend and concentrate the pressure on the metatarsal heads.

The *peroneus tertius muscle* everts and weakly dorsiflexes the foot.

Lateral Leg Muscles Affecting the Foot

The *peroneus longus muscle* everts and plantar flexes the ankle (Figure 4-30). As discussed previously, this muscle pronates the foot and is often short in the individual with a pronated foot.

The *peroneus brevis muscle* everts and plantar flexes the foot.

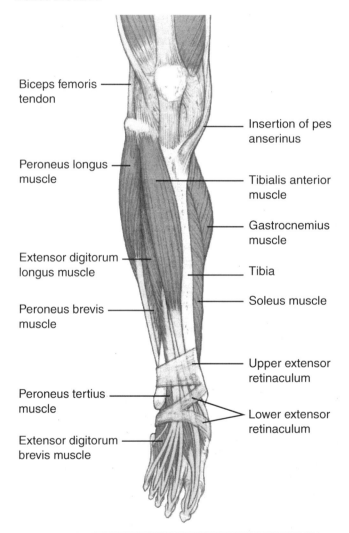

Figure 4-29

Tibialis anterior and extensor digitorum longus. The tibialis anterior dorsiflexes the ankle and everts the foot at the subtalar joint. The extensor digitorum longus dorsiflexes the ankle and extends the toes. (From Mathers et al: *Clinical anatomy principles,* St Louis, 1996, Mosby.)

Posterior Leg Muscles Affecting the Foot

The *soleus muscle* plantar flexes the foot.

The *tibialis posterior muscle* plantar flexes and inverts the foot and supports the longitudinal arch. When the foot is pronated, this muscle is stretched and when strained can become a source of posterior shin splints. In the patient with a rigid foot (i.e., a structurally high longitudinal arch), this muscle may be weak because the bony structure provides passive support and interferes with creating enough stress on the muscle to maintain its strength.

The *flexor digitorum longus muscle* plantar flexes the foot and flexes the interphalangeal (IP) and MP joints of the toes. This muscle along with the flexor digitorum brevis, lumbrical, and interossei muscles must counteract the extension of the toes at the MP produced by the extensor digitorum longus muscle. Optimizing performance of the flexor digitorum longus can help relieve the stress on the plantar fascia and thus strengthening exercises should be used when plantar fasciitis is present.

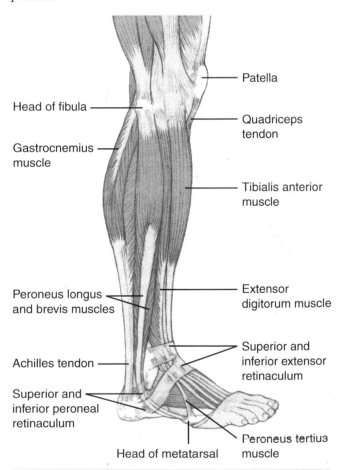

Figure 4-30

Peroneus longus and brevis. The peroneal muscles evert the ankle. The peroneus longus is a strong plantar flexor of the foot, whereas the peroneus brevis is a weak dorsiflexor. (From Mathers et al: *Clinical anatomy principles,* St Louis, 1996, Mosby.)

The *flexor hallucis longus muscle* plantar flexes the foot, flexes the big toe, and assists with inversion. Overuse of this muscle can contribute to posterior shin splints. Usually the pain is on the distal one third of the medial aspect of the tibia.

Muscles Attached to the Foot

The *extensor digitorum brevis muscle* extends the toes (see Figure 4-29). In the patient with hammer toes, this muscle is short. An effective way to stretch both the longus and brevis muscles is to instruct the patient to flex his or her toes when the foot is dorsiflexed and then maintain toe flexion while plantar flexing the ankle.

The *flexor digitorum brevis* muscle flexes the toes and reinforces the plantar fascia (Figure 4-31). This muscle is weak and short in the patient with hammer toes. It is also weak in the patient with plantar fasciitis. To strengthen this muscle and the flexor digitorum longus the patient is taught to provide resistance to toe flexion with his or her fingers. The patient also needs to be instructed to flex the toes when moving from a sitting to a standing position, from a standing to a sitting position, and during the push off phase of walking.

Muscle and Movement Impairments

Muscles that function as synergists for motion in one direction often have antagonistic actions for motion in another direction. For example, the TFL-ITB abducts,

flexes, and rotates the hip medially. The PGM muscle abducts, extends, and rotates the hip laterally. The TFL and PGM are synergists for frontal plane movement (hip abduction), but they are antagonists for sagittal and horizontal plane movements. If these muscles are balanced, hip abduction is performed without deviation in the sagittal or horizontal planes. If one of these muscles becomes dominant, during hip abduction the motion will also occur in the sagittal or horizontal plane consistent with the action of the dominant muscle. The less dominant muscle usually becomes excessively long or weak. Table 4-2 lists imbalances in the control of one joint.

The dominance is evident during muscle testing and during the observation of movement patterns. For example, during manual muscle testing of the PGM, the hip abductor medial rotator muscles are considered dominant when the patient flexes and rotates the hip medially rather than maintaining the correct position of the hip extension and lateral rotation. The PGM muscles often test weak or are unable to take resistance when the muscle is shortened maximally. During gait, the hip will excessively rotate medially at heel strike. These findings suggest dominance of hip abductor medial rotator muscles over the abductor lateral rotator muscles.

If the hamstring muscles are dominant during hip extension and knee extension, such as when climbing a stair, the knee moves back toward the body rather than remain relatively fixed as the thigh moves toward the

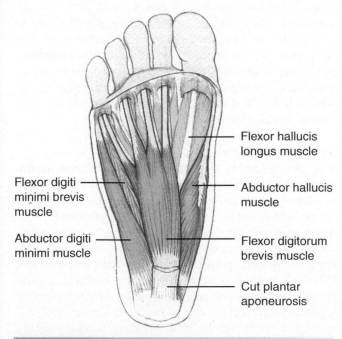

Figure 4-31

Flexor digitorum brevis. The flexor digitorum brevis attaches to the plantar fascia and flexes the proximal interphalangeal joint of the toes. (From Mathers et al: *Clinical anatomy principles,* St Louis, 1996, Mosby.)

Labels: Flexor hallucis longus muscle; Flexor digiti minimi brevis muscle; Abductor hallucis muscle; Abductor digiti minimi muscle; Flexor digitorum brevis muscle; Cut plantar aponeurosis

Table 4-2 Imbalances in the Control of One Joint

DOMINANT	LENGTHENED OR WEAKENED
TFL-ITB; AGM; gluteus minimus assisting in hip abduction with the medial rotation action becoming dominant	PGM
Hip adductors	Hip abductors
Hamstrings assisting in hip extension	Gluteus maximus
Hamstrings assisting in knee extension when foot is fixed	Quadriceps
Biceps femoris assisting in hip lateral rotation	Piriformis, gemelli, obturators, quadratus femoris
Semimembranosus and semitendinosus assisting in hip extension with the medial rotator action becoming dominant	Biceps femoris
TFL; rectus femoris assisting in hip flexion	Iliopsoas
Toe extensors assisting in ankle dorsiflexion	Tibialis anterior
Tibialis posterior; flexor digitorum longus; flexor hallucis longus; peroneus longus assisting in ankle plantar flexion	Gastrocnemius, soleus

AGM, Anterior gluteus medius; *PGM,* posterior gluteus medius; *TFL-ITB,* tensor fascia lata–iliotibial band.

tibia. The knee moves back toward the body because of the strong pull of the hamstring muscles, which causes hip extension. Because the foot is fixed, the hip extension also helps extend the knee. Weakness and fatigue of the quadriceps muscles are contributing factors to this change of dominance for knee control.

If the toe extensors are the dominant dorsiflexors of the ankle, when the patient is instructed to dorsiflex the ankle, the initial motion will be toe extension and the foot will tend to evert rather than to invert or remain in neutral. When this pattern is present, the patient often has reddened areas on the tops of the toes from contact with the tops of the shoes and the tops of the shoes have exaggerated creases. The patient may also have hammer toes. This patient tends to walk using the hip flexor strategy gait pattern during the swing phase as described in the text that follows.

Multisegmental movements also show changes in dominance patterns. For example, the normal and most ideal strategy for the swing phase of gait is one in which the primary source of momentum is from the plantar flexion moment that occurs during the push-off phase. This phase contributes to knee flexion, which stretches the rectus femoris, a hip flexor muscle. This stretching helps initiate hip flexor muscular activity during the swing phase of gait. Usually this type of gait pattern is associated with a larger excursion of the center of gravity anterior to the stance foot. The contrasting pattern is one in which the push off is greatly diminished and motion is generated at the hip for the swing phase. This gait pattern, which can be termed a *hip flexor strategy pattern*, is seen in the patient with weak plantar flexor muscles.[14] Patients with metatarsalgia have a similar gait pattern. The hip flexor strategy pattern is characterized by increased dorsiflexor muscular activity and decreased range-of-knee flexion. The line of gravity tends to remain closer to the stance foot and somewhat posterior compared with the push-off pattern. Patients with spastic diplegia, meningeal myelocele, and hemiplegia frequently use this type of gait pattern. The emphasis on flexor muscular activity can be a contributing factor to weakness of the hip extensors, shortness of the hip flexors, weakness of the plantar flexors, metatarsalgia, and hammer toes. Correction of these muscular and movement impairments requires specific exercises that improve the performance of the nondominant muscle and correction of the impaired movement patterns.

Movement Impairment Syndromes of the Hip

Consistent with the primary premise of this text, which is that compensatory joint motion in a specific direction is the cause of pain, syndromes of the hip are named for the direction of the movement most consistently associated with pain. As with the shoulder, pain related to the hip joint is usually associated with impairments of accessory movements. Pain that seems to arise from musculotendinous injury is associated with impairments of muscle participation and patterns of recruitment. As mentioned previously, the femoral syndromes are designated as such because the pain in these syndromes arises from joint structures. Syndromes of the hip are designated as such because the pain in these syndromes arises from musculotendinous injury.

Femoral Anterior Glide Syndrome

This section applies to the femoral anterior glide syndrome with and without medial rotation. The most common form of femoral anterior glide syndrome is with hip medial rotation. This syndrome occurs because of inadequate posterior glide of the femoral head during hip flexion, The hip flexion is accompanied by hip medial rotation. The anterior glide syndrome can also occur without the medial rotation component. Kinesiologic principles indicate that during flexion the femur should posteriorly glide, but in this syndrome the posterior glide is insufficient. The femoral anterior glide syndrome has many characteristics that are similar to the humeral anterior glide syndrome, which is a form of shoulder impingement. Just as shoulder impingement was initially believed to be bicipital tendonitis, this syndrome is often diagnosed as iliopsoas tendonitis. Although the iliopsoas tendon may be a source of symptoms, the cause of the tendinopathy is the pressure exerted by the femoral head against the anterior joint structures, which occurs when the postural alignment of the hip is hyperextension. This pressure combined with the diminished posterior glide of the femur during hip flexion causes the femur to impinge on the anterior tissues of the joint capsule.

Symptoms and Pain

Pain is present in the groin, particularly during hip flexion. It progresses to generalized hip pain, which may be the result of either joint inflammation from faulty movement of the femoral head in the acetabulum or inflammation of soft tissues surrounding the joint. Iliopsoas tendinopathy may also be present, as indicated by tenderness with palpation or pain with contraction. (The pain from iliopsoas contraction needs to be differentiated from the pain caused by impingement of capsular tissues at the end of the hip flexion range.) Active hip flexion should be avoided until inflammation subsides. Thus the patient should use his or her hand to flex the hip to more than 90 degrees. Stretching is contraindicated. (Refer to the discussion of iliopsoas tendinopathy later in this chapter.) Iliopsoas bursitis needs to be considered, but this condition is difficult to diagnose with certainty. Avascular necrosis, stress fractures of the lesser trochanter and medial aspect of the femur, and osteoarthritis can cause groin pain and should be considered. If pain is experienced during walking or during weight-bearing activities, the patient should be examined for these conditions. Activities that emphasize hip extension, such as running long distances and dancing, are often associated with the development of the femoral anterior glide syndrome. Postural hip extension is the primary contributing factor. This syndrome is most common in runners, because the exaggerated extension of the hip is part of the movement pattern of running. Dancers who excessively stretch the hip into extension and perform "splits" are also susceptible to this syndrome.

Movement Impairments

SUPINE POSITION. During hip flexion in the supine position, the femoral head does not glide posteriorly and most often it will rotate medially. When the hip is placed in lateral rotation, the knee is flexed and the hip is flexed passively; pressure exerted by the examiner at the inguinal crease in a posteroinferior direction prevents femoral anterior glide. The result is that the range of pain-free hip flexion is greater than when these pressures are not applied at the hip joint. Monitoring the axis of rotation during hip flexion by following the path of the greater trochanter during an active straight-leg raise confirms that the greater trochanter is moving in an anterior medial direction (Figure 4-32). During flexion of the normal hip, the greater trochanter maintains a relatively constant position. In contrast, during flexion of the affected hip the faulty path of the greater trochanter is often observed. If pressure is applied at the inguinal crease to maintain a constant axis of rotation while flexing the hip passively with the knee extended (i.e., passive straight-leg raises), the examiner feels resistance similar to a shortness of the hamstring muscles. If the pressure is removed the resistance is alleviated, but medial rotation or anterior movement of the greater trochanter can be palpated.

PRONE POSITION. Palpating the greater trochanter during hip extension in the prone position indicates whether its movement occurs anteriorly or medially, or whether it is maintaining a relatively constant position or is moving slightly posteriorly (Figure 4-33). One possible explanation for anterior movement of the greater trochanter is that if the hamstring muscles are the dominant hip extensor, only the distal portion of the femur moves posteriorly but not the proximal portion. This occurs because the proximal attachment of the hamstring muscles is the ischial tuberosity of the pelvis, and the distal attachments are on the tibia and fibula. Only the

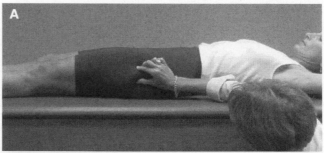

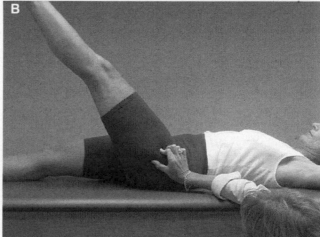

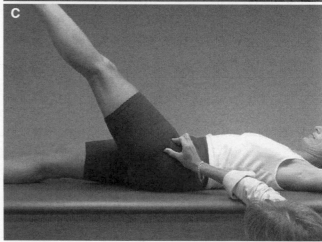

Figure 4-32

Impairment of the movement pattern of the greater trochanter during hip flexion. Instead of maintaining a relatively constant position during hip flexion, the greater trochanter moves in an anterior medial direction. *A,* Monitoring the greater trochanter in the starting position. *B,* Correct movement of the greater trochanter during hip flexion. *C,* Impaired movement because of anterior medial displacement of the greater trochanter associated with hip rotation during hip flexion.

short head of the biceps femoris attaches to the femur; because of the location of this attachment on the distal femur, its major action is knee flexion. The insertion of the hamstring muscles is to the tibia and fibula. During hip extension when the tension is being exerted on the tibia and fibula, the excessive flexibility of the anterior joint capsule allows the femoral head to glide anteriorly, particularly if the iliopsoas muscle is lengthened. Therefore the axis of rotation of the femur is displaced anteriorly, causing the proximal femur to move anteriorly while the distal femur moves posteriorly (see Figure 2-8). If the TFL is short, then the stretch on this muscle during hip extension can contribute to medial rotation of the femur, causing the greater trochanter to move in an anteromedial direction. The dominant action of the hamstring muscles versus the gluteus maximus muscle (a lateral rotator), combined with a shortness of the TFL muscle (a medial rotator), allows the femur to rotate medially during hip extension.

QUADRUPED POSITION. In the quadruped position the hips are flexed less than 90 degrees. As the patient rocks backward toward the heels, the affected hip does not flex as easily as the contralateral hip (see Figure 3-37). The restriction to hip flexion becomes evident when, in a completely flexed position, the pelvis on the affected side is higher than the other because of compensatory

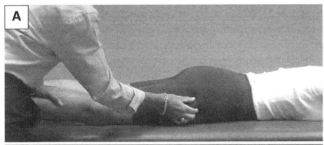
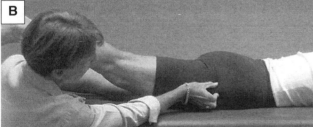
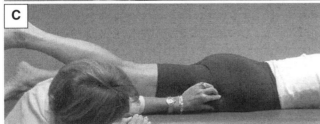

Figure 1-33

Impairment of the movement pattern of the greater trochanter during hip extension. Instead of maintaining a relatively constant position or moving in a slightly posterior direction during hip extension, the greater trochanter moves in an anterior or anterior medial direction. *A,* Starting position. *B,* Correct movement of the greater trochanter during hip extension. *C,* Anterior displacement of the greater trochanter during hip extension.

pelvic rotation. The restriction may also become evident when the pelvis moves laterally toward the unaffected side. Both impaired movement patterns indicate that the affected hip flexes less than the unaffected hip. If the affected hip is abducted or rotated laterally before the patient rocks backward, the hip flexion range of motion increases during the backward movement (see Figure 3-38). As the patient's movement pattern improves, the degree of hip flexion increases without abducting or rotating the hip laterally and symptoms decrease in intensity.

SITTING POSITION. In the sitting position, active knee extension is associated with hip medial rotation. If the hip is rotated laterally, the knee extension range is decreased or there is greater resistance to knee extension as evidenced by slower movement into extension.

Summary

The anterior joint capsule and its associated soft-tissue structures become stretched. The posterior structures become taut. In the anterior glide syndrome without medial rotation, the lateral rotator muscles become short in some cases. In the anterior glide syndrome with medial rotation, although the lateral rotators are stretched, they become taut as the hip medially rotates. Because the anterior joint capsule is stretched and the posterior structures are short and stiff, during hip flexion the femoral head does not glide posteriorly and the proximal femur exerts pressure against the anterior joint capsule. The result is a pinching of the anterior joint capsule structures. This impaired movement pattern can also contribute to iliopsoas bursitis and iliopsoas tendinopathy.

Alignment

STRUCTURAL VARIATIONS
1. Antetorsion (anteverted) hip
2. Genu valgus

ACQUIRED IMPAIRMENTS
1. Swayback posture
2. Posterior pelvic tilt
3. Poor definition of the gluteal musculature
4. Hip medial rotation
5. Hip extension
6. Hyperextended knees
7. Pronated foot

Relative Flexibility and Stiffness Impairments

The anterior glide of the femoral head is more flexible than the posterior glide, and the inferior glide is less flexible than the superior glide.

Muscle and Recruitment Pattern Impairments

The action of the TFL muscle is more dominant than that of the iliopsoas muscle. The TFL tests short on the affected side, despite the standing alignment examination that shows a flat back, hip extension, and hyperextended knees, all of which are consistent with excessive length of the iliopsoas muscle. When the hip is abducted during the hip flexor length test, the hip will often hyperextend. The iliopsoas muscle tests weak, and the TFL tests strong.

The action of the TFL muscle is more dominant than that of the PGM muscle. When the patient is in a single-leg stance, the hip rotates medially. During the PGM muscle test the hip rotates medially, which indicates that the TFL is dominant over the PGM.

The action of the hamstring muscles is more dominant than that of the gluteus maximus muscle. When the patient is in the prone position and performs hip extension, the hamstring muscle contraction is evident earlier than the gluteus maximus muscle contraction. The contour of the gluteus maximus muscle does not change until the hip is almost completely extended.

The action of the medial hamstring muscles is more dominant than that of the lateral hamstring muscles. When the patient is in a sitting position and performs knee extension, the hip rotates medially. When the hip is slightly rotated laterally, the knee extension range of motion is limited or is performed more slowly, which is indicative of resistance from the lateral hamstring muscles.

Impairments of muscle length and strength may also be observed. The iliopsoas muscle tests long and weak. Because the fibers of the iliopsoas muscle attach to the anterior joint capsule, contraction of this muscle is believed to keep the capsule from being pinched.[4] Therefore poor performance of the iliopsoas muscle can contribute to increased susceptibility of the capsule to impingement. The TFL muscle tests short, and the gluteus maximus or piriformis muscles test short and weak. The posterior hip joint structures are stiff or short or both, as indicated by resistance to hip flexion. The hamstring muscles also test short, particularly the medial hamstring muscles. The anterior hip joint structures are stretched, as indicated by excessive hip extension range of motion.

Confirming Tests

Active hip flexion causes pinching in the groin. When the hip flexor muscles remain completely relaxed, there is increased hip flexion range of motion without symptoms. The hip is rotated laterally, and the axis of rotation is maintained by posteroinferior pressure along the inguinal crease, preventing the anterior movement of the proximal femur. There is a faulty axis of rotation during

hip flexion, as indicated by a monitoring of the greater trochanter, and during hip extension, as indicated by monitoring of the greater trochanter. Repeated backward rocking in the quadruped position causes the range into hip flexion to increase.

Summary

An alteration of the path of the instant center of rotation (PICR) of the hip joint during hip flexion and often during extension typifies femoral anterior glide syndrome. The altered PICR during hip flexion, as indicated by a monitoring of the greater trochanter, is consistent with insufficient posterior glide and inappropriate medial rotation of the femoral head when there should be posterior and inferior glide and no rotation. Although the posterior structures of the hip are stiff, the hip medial rotation range of motion may be greater than the lateral rotation range of motion. A contributing factor is the failure of the hip flexor–lateral rotator muscles to counteract the hip flexor–medial rotator muscles.

Prolonged standing in hip extension can lead to hyperextension which causes excessive flexibility of the anterior hip joint structures. This flexibility, along with stiffness of both the hip extensor muscles and hip joint structures, creates a path of least resistance into anterior glide.

Intervention

PRIMARY OBJECTIVES. The primary objectives of an intervention program include the following:

1. Improve the posterior glide of the femur to correct impaired hip flexion motion
2. Reverse the altered hip flexor dominance by shortening the iliopsoas muscle so that the hip medial rotation produced by the TFL during hip flexion is appropriately counterbalanced
3. Correct the hip hyperextension and medial rotation if present

CORRECTIVE EXERCISE PROGRAM

Quadruped position. Rocking backward while in the quadruped position is the most important exercise and should be performed first. When performed correctly this exercise will stretch the hip extensor muscles and promote posterior and inferior gliding of the femoral head. The patient may need to push back with the hands if his or her groin is pinched from the contraction of the hip flexor muscles.

Supine position. Passive hip flexion is performed by the patient in the supine position to help restore the precise axis of rotation. If the thigh cannot be reached comfortably with the hands, the patient can use a towel behind the thigh to pull the knee toward the chest. It may be necessary to slightly rotate laterally and abduct the hip. The hip flexor muscles must remain relaxed.

Prone position. Knee flexion should be performed in the prone position, and the patient should prevent pelvic anterior tilt or rotation and hip joint abduction or rotation. Hip lateral rotation should be performed with the knee flexed to 90 degrees. This motion will stretch the ITB. Hip medial rotation performed with the knee flexed to 90 degrees will improve the extensibility of the hip lateral rotator muscles. Hip extension with the knee extended should not be performed unless the patient has a pillow under his or her abdomen to place the hip into flexion. This motion should be initiated while contracting the gluteus maximus muscle. To avoid stretching the anterior hip joint capsule, the hip should not extend past neutral. Hip extension with knee flexion must be performed in the same way to avoid stretching the anterior joint capsule.

Side-lying position. Hip abduction should be performed in the side-lying position with slight lateral rotation and extension of the hip to aid the recruitment of the PGM instead of the TFL muscle.

Sitting position. To increase the extensibility of the medial hamstring muscles, knee extension should be performed in the sitting position while maintaining the hip in a few degrees of lateral rotation. The patient should passively flex the hip by using his or her hands to lift the thigh to maximum flexion and then remove the hands from the thigh and actively hold the thigh in flexion. In this position the iliopsoas muscle is the only hip flexor that can hold the hip in this degree of flexion. If the patient can hold the hip in the end range of hip flexion and does not have pain, he or she can apply isometric resistance by pushing with his or her hand against the thigh.

Standing position. While standing on one leg the patient contracts the gluteal muscles to prevent hip medial rotation. The patient then bends forward using only hip flexion and then returns to a standing position by concentrating on contracting the gluteal muscles to produce hip extension, maintaining the contraction until he or she is upright.

CORRECTING POSTURAL HABIT PATTERNS. The patient performs a sit-to-stand movement without allowing the hips to rotate medially. The patient is instructed not to sit with his or her leg crossed or his or her thigh over the other thigh (i.e., hip flexion, medial rotation, adduction). If the patient must cross his or her leg, then he or she can sit with the lateral aspect of the leg on the opposite thigh (i.e., hip lateral rotation). The patient should not sleep with the hip rotated medially. It is important to correct the swayback standing alignment by instructing the patient to stand with his or her back to the wall, which can serve as a guide to the correct orientation for vertical alignment. The patient can also stand sideways to a mirror, and the therapist can teach correct alignment by instructing the patient to pull his or her hips backward.

Because new alignments feel unnatural, the patient needs to monitor alignment by using a mirror. The patient should be encouraged to contract the gluteus maximus muscle actively at heel strike when walking. Contraction will increase the participation of the gluteal muscles and decrease the dominance of the hamstring muscles.

Case Presentation 1

History. A 34-year-old female marathon runner is referred to physical therapy for evaluation and treatment. She has been running an average of 50 to 60 miles per week but is now unable to run because of hip pain. Both a computerized axial tomographic (CAT) scan and a bone scan of her hip joint detect no abnormalities, and she has received a cortisone injection in her right hip without relief of pain.

Symptoms. This patient has been experiencing pain in her right groin for 3 months, which has progressed to generalized pain deep in her hip joint. She had first noticed the pinching in the groin when in a squatting position.

Alignment Analysis. The patient stands with a slight degree of swayback with the hips extended, secondary to a posterior pelvic tilt and hyperextension of her knees. There is poor gluteal muscle definition, but hypertrophy of the musculature of her thighs is noted (Figure 4-34). Her right hip is slightly medially rotated, which is most obvious when viewing the patient from the back using the popliteal space and hamstring muscle insertions as reference points (Figure 4-35).

Movement Analysis

Standing. When in a standing position the patient achieves forward bending, primarily with lumbar flexion; also, there is limited hip flexion. While maintaining a relatively straight trunk, the return from forward bending is performed by swaying her hips and legs forward rather than by extending her hips.

Single-leg stance. Medial rotation of her hip and a slight lateral trunk flexion are noted when the patient stands on her right leg.

Supine. Active hip flexion in a supine position elicits pinching in the groin at 100 degrees of flexion. When her hip is flexed passively with slight lateral rotation and abduction, the flexion range reaches 120 degrees before symptoms are elicited.

Straight-leg raise. When the straight-leg raise movement is performed actively, the greater trochanter moves anteriorly and medially. When this movement is performed passively with pressure at the inguinal crease and the femur is placed in slight lateral rotation, the greater trochanter maintains a constant position. However, the examiner feels resistance to hip flexion that was not evident before the pressure was applied at the inguinal crease.

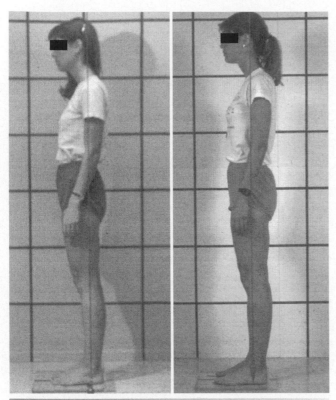

Figure 4-34

Side view of patient with femoral anterior glide syndrome with medial rotation before and after treatment. The patient stands in hip extension because of slight posterior tilt and hyperextended knees before treatment *(left)*. Postural alignment is corrected after treatment *(right)*.

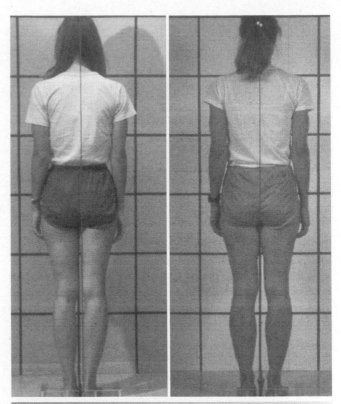

Figure 4-35

Posterior view of patient with femoral anterior glide syndrome with medial rotation. The medial rotation of her right femur can be observed by noting the position of the insertion of the hamstring tendons. Note poor definition of gluteal muscles before treatment (left). After treatment, the definition of the gluteal musculature is increased.

The following additional tests are performed in three different positions: (1) prone, (2) quadruped, and (3) sitting.

Prone. Contraction of the hamstring muscles precedes contraction of the gluteus maximus muscle when hip extension is performed in a prone position with the knee extended. The hip motion is almost complete before there is a visible change in the definition of the gluteus maximus muscle.

Quadruped. In the quadruped position the patient assumes an alignment of less than 90 degrees of hip flexion and the lumbar spine is in a flexed position. When rocking backward, the patient's lumbar spine flexes more easily than her hips, thus the lumbar spine flexes more than the hips.

Sitting. There is hip medial rotation and visible contraction of the TFL muscle during right knee extension. Associated hip rotation is not observed during left knee extension,.

Muscle Length and Strength Analysis. The right TFL muscle is short, and 15 degrees of hip abduction is required before the hip extends completely. The length of the left TFL muscle is normal. The right PGM tests weak, grading 4−/5, and the left PGM tests 4+/5. During the

testing of the right PGM, the hip flexes and rotates medially. The right and left gluteus maximus muscles test 4/5 and 4+/5, respectively. The right and left iliopsoas muscles test 4−/5 and 4+/5, respectively.

Diagnosis. Femoral anterior glide syndrome with medial rotation is the diagnosis.

Intervention. In the quadruped position the patient rocks backward, taking care to flex at the hips while restricting motion in the lumbar spine.

While in a supine position the patient is instructed to bring the knee passively to the chest with the hip slightly rotated laterally and abducted. She is asked to stop the movement at the onset of any pinching in the groin.

While in a side-lying position the patient performs hip abduction and lateral rotation with the knee slightly flexed.

While in a prone position, the patient is instructed to flex the knee. With the knee flexed to 90 degrees, the patient laterally rotates the hip. She places a pillow under the abdomen, fully flexes the knee, and then extends and slightly rotates the hip laterally by contracting the gluteus maximus muscle but limits the extension motion to neutral position of the hip.

While in a sitting position the patient performs knee extension while maintaining her hip in slight lateral rotation. She is instructed to avoid recruiting the TFL muscle. She is also asked to sit with her back against the back of a chair to support her upper body, which eliminates the requirement of active hip flexion and helps avoid TFL recruitment. The patient is asked to flex her hip passively to the end of the range, using both hands. She is instructed to stop the motion if she experiences any pinching. She holds her hip at the end of range with her hip flexor muscles and releases the hand support of her thigh.

While standing on the right leg only, the patient is asked to tighten her right gluteal muscles to prevent hip medial rotation. When standing on both feet she practices forward bending by flexing at the knees and hips, with the emphasis on hip flexion without lumbar flexion. She learns to return to a standing position by performing hip extension using the gluteal muscles.

When walking, the patient tightens the right gluteus maximus muscle at heel strike.

Outcome. The patient is examined six times over a 2½-month period. She initially performs six repetitions of each exercise twice a day but progresses to twenty repetitions by the end of 2 months. She is also asked to make a conscious effort to stand correctly and, when walking, to contract her gluteus maximus muscles at heel strike. She has also stopped the weight training exercises she had been performing for her quadriceps and hamstring muscles. Within 1 week she is able to rock backward and sit on her heels without hip pain. At the end of 2 weeks she is able to flex her hip to 125 degrees while in the supine position. As long as she passively performs the hip flexion within a range of 90 and 125 degrees using her hands, the patient does not experience pain. The strength of her right PGM muscle increases to a rating of 4/5. She is able to maintain correct alignment when standing and is able to avoid posterior pelvic tilt. When attempting to contract her iliopsoas muscle isometrically while in the sitting position with her hip maximally flexed, however, she experiences pain in her groin.

By the end of 1 month, she begins a program of easy jogging and walking for short distances. She is instructed to "push-off" with her ankle plantar flexor muscles and to keep her body weight slightly forward when jogging. At the end of 2 months she does not experience any pain during hip flexion in any position (e.g., when she performs the quadruped or supine exercises or when she squats or sits with her hip in maximum flexion). She is able to maintain an isometric contraction of the iliopsoas muscle without pain and is able to tolerate slight resistance. Both her right and left PGM muscles test normal (5/5). In the prone position she initiates hip ex-

tension with her gluteus maximus muscle and the greater trochanter is observed to rotate laterally. There is an obvious increase in the size and contour of her buttock muscles. She is able to jog for 5 miles at one time on alternate days. These changes have occurred even though the patient has not performed any resistive exercises with weights.

At the time of her last session, 2½ months after her initial visit, the patient is jogging 6 miles one day and 3 miles the next and has completed a 10-mile run without symptoms. She is instructed to maintain her exercise program as a post running routine, and she is asked to perform at least ten repetitions of each exercise.

After 1 year the patient indicates that she has successfully completed one marathon and is averaging 50 miles a week without hip problems.

Case Presentation 2

History. A 70-year-old woman is referred to physical therapy for severe right hip and leg pain that has become particularly troublesome when she walks or sits for any length of time. This hip and leg pain started 1 year earlier after a replacement of the femoral head but not the acetabulum. She has undergone intensive physical therapy, both as an inpatient and outpatient. The patient is 40 pounds heavier than her ideal weight and has diabetes with peripheral neuropathy. She uses one cane and has a pronounced antalgic gait.

Symptoms. The patient experiences pain when she lowers herself into the sitting position, when she actively flexes her hip, and when she slides her hip and knee into extension while lying in bed. The pain is located principally in her anterior groin, but it radiates into her medial thigh and down the posterior aspect of her leg. The goals of her previous physical therapy exercise program were to strengthen her hip flexor and abductor muscles and to have her walk without support.

Alignment Analysis. The patient has a thoracic kyphosis, a large abdomen, and stands with her pelvis aligned in anterior tilt with an increased curvature of the lower lumbar spine.

Movement Analysis

Standing-to-sitting. Posterior thigh and lateral leg pain decreases when the patient sits with back support. During the standing-to-sitting movement as pressure is exerted by the seat of the chair against her proximal thigh, pain is elicited in the anterior groin.

Sitting. When she extends her knee, her hip rotates medially and the patient experiences anterior thigh and groin pain. Palpation during knee extension, reveals a contraction of the TFL muscle. If the patient keeps her hip slightly rotated laterally, exerts minimal muscular effort, and does not lift her thigh at the same time, the pain is not reproduced when she extends her knee.

Supine. The patient is the most comfortable when her hips and knees are flexed and passively supported with pillows under the distal aspect of her thighs and behind her knees. During passive hip flexion, anterior deviation of the axis of rotation of the hip is noted. Active hip flexion, which is associated with hip medial rotation, elicits pain in the groin and along the posterior thigh and lateral aspect of the leg.

Muscle Length and Strength Analysis. The hip flexors are short and pull her into an anterior tilt, which is exaggerated because of her extremely weak abdominal muscles. The hamstring muscles are short, and muscle strength testing is not performed because of the severity of her pain and the obvious weakness of her abdominal and hip abductor muscles.

Summary. The patient's posterior thigh and leg pain originates from her spine. She has very weak abdominal muscles and is unable to contract these muscles isometrically. She has been performing many active hip flexion exercises without instruction to protect her spine from the anterior shear and compression forces associated with iliopsoas muscle contractions. Also, her abdominal muscles are too weak to counteract the anterior pelvic tilt that is produced by the contraction of the rectus femoris and TFL muscles.

The dominant hip flexor is her TFL muscle, which causes the medial rotation of the femur during hip flexion and during single-leg stance. The posterior soft tissues are stiff, and her hamstring muscles are short. Her groin pain is caused by an impingement of the femur on the anterior acetabulum. The surgeon reports that he replaced the head of the femur but not the acetabulum and now believes the impingement between these two structures is the source of her pain.

Her posterior thigh and leg pain during hip extension in the supine position is the result of increased lumbar extension, whereas the pain in the anterior thigh is caused by the stretch of her short hip flexor muscles. When pillows are placed under her upper back to accommodate the thoracic kyphosis and under her knees to flex her hips and knees and to flatten her lumbar spine, the patient is free of pain. However, she has to keep her hip flexor muscles relaxed to remain symptom free.

Diagnosis. The diagnosis is femoral anterior glide (anterior groin pain) and lumbar extension (posterior thigh pain) syndrome (see Chapter 3).

Intervention. From the hook-lying position the patient is instructed to hold her right knee toward her chest with her hands, to contract her abdominal muscles, and then to slide her left lower extremity into extension. She is instructed to stop the motion whenever she feels any increase in symptoms. To return to hip and knee flexion she is instructed to place pressure on her heel, bend her knee, and slide her foot up toward her hip in order to emphasize hamstring contraction and lessen hip flexor muscle contraction.

While in a sitting position the patient performs knee extension while maintaining a slight lateral rotation of the hip.

The patient is instructed to practice a sitting-to-standing motion with minimal assistance from her hands and to make an effort to contract her gluteal muscles as she stands up. She is encouraged to use her hands to sit down to minimize pressure against her thigh and to reduce her pain.

The patient is instructed to use two canes when walking, which eliminates her antalgic gait and side flexion. She is also taught to contract her gluteal muscles at heel strike and is encouraged to maintain the contraction of her abdominal muscles. Her pain is minimal when she walks as instructed.

Outcome. The patient is examined once a week for 4 weeks and then every other week for an additional 6 weeks. She shows steady improvement and can sit without experiencing pain in the anterior groin or posterior thigh regions. She is able to lie supine with both hips and knees extended and to actively flex her hip to 90 degrees without pain. She has progressed from using two canes to using one for minimal support. The patient is able to reach her left foot to apply cream, a major achievement. Although her hip flexion range is limited to 100 degrees of flexion, her surgeon has approved efforts to further increase the range of hip flexion. As a result, she eventually is able to reach her left foot through hip flexion, abduction, and lateral rotation.

Femoral Anterior Glide Syndrome With Lateral Rotation

Femoral anterior glide syndrome with lateral rotation is similar to the anterior glide syndrome with medial rotation, but it does not occur as frequently. A primary contributing factor is prolonged sitting with the leg crossed by placing the ankle on the opposite thigh, which is a position of maximum lateral hip rotation. This syndrome occurs more often in men than in women. Potentially, this syndrome may be more common than suggested by the clinical experience of the author of this text, because the symptoms of adductor strain are similar to those found with this syndrome. Activities such as ice-skating and ice hockey in which hip abduction and lateral rotation are the repeated motions can predispose participants to this syndrome with lateral rotation.

In the neutral position the head of the femur points slightly anteriorly. Therefore when the hip is stretched into lateral rotation, the head exerts pressure into the anterior joint capsule. In addition, the anterior joint capsule and its associated soft-tissue structures become stretched and the posterior structures, including the lateral rotator muscles, become short. If, during hip flexion, the anterior joint capsule is stretched and the posterior structures are short and stiff, the proximal femur will exert pressure against the anterior joint capsule and the posterior glide of the femoral head will become insufficient, particularly when the hip is rotated laterally. The result is a pinching of the structures of the anterior joint capsule. In this syndrome the pressure of the femoral head against the joint capsule may also occur when the hip rotates laterally and extends because these motions involve anterior glide, which stretches the capsule.

Symptoms and Pain

When the hip extends and rotates laterally, pain in the groin is usually worse in the weight-bearing position than it is in the recumbent position, although pain may also occur when the hip is flexed and rotated laterally. Pain is usually more medial in its location with this syndrome than it is with the femoral anterior glide syndrome with medial rotation. Minimal pain is present with hip flexion. Iliopsoas tendinopathy or bursitis and adductor tendinopathy are also symptoms of this syndrome.

Movement Impairments

Tests are performed in the following four positions: (1) standing, (2) supine, (3) prone, and (4) quadruped. While in a single-leg stance the hip rotates laterally. When the patient assumes a supine position the hip rotates laterally during hip flexion. From the prone position the hip rotates laterally and the greater trochanter moves posteriorly during hip extension. In the prone position, when the knee is passively flexed, the femur rotates laterally. In the quadruped position the patient assumes an alignment of less than 90 degrees of hip flexion.

Alignment

STRUCTURAL VARIATIONS

1. Femoral antetorsion. If the patient forces the hip into lateral rotation, the femoral head will exert pressure against the anterior aspect of the hip joint.

2. Tibial torsion. If the foot is rotated laterally, it can contribute to repeated lateral rotation of the hip during walking or to lateral rotation of the lower extremity when lying supine.

3. Rigid foot. Because the ankle does not dorsiflex easily, hip lateral rotation may be a compensatory motion that allows the patient to come over his or her foot during the stance phase of gait.

ACQUIRED IMPAIRMENTS

1. Posterior pelvic tilt

2. Hip joint extension

3. Knee hyperextension

4. Hip lateral rotation

Relative Flexibility and Stiffness Impairments

The accessory hip motion of anterior glide is more flexible than the accessory motion of posterior glide. This becomes evident to the examiner when passively flexing the patient's hip, and resistance is felt as the hip is flexed more than 90 degrees. In the quadruped position, as the patient rocks backward, the affected hip does not flex as much as the other hip. Hip motion into lateral rotation is more flexible than it is into medial rotation, as evidenced by the maintained position of lateral rotation and resistance to medial rotation. There is usually greater range of motion into lateral rotation than there is into medial rotation.

Muscle and Recruitment Pattern Impairments

The therapist may observe impairment of recruitment patterns. For example, the hip lateral rotator muscles are recruited more readily than the medial rotator muscles, and the hamstring muscles are dominant over the gluteus maximus muscles.

Impairments of muscle length and strength may also be observed. The hip lateral rotator muscles, as well as the hip extensors, the gluteus maximus, the hamstrings, and the piriformis muscles, may be short. The gluteus maximus, abductor medial rotator, and iliopsoas muscles are weak.

Confirming Tests

The pain present with hip extension and lateral rotation is decreased when the hip is rotated medially during hip extension. When hip extension is performed in the prone position, there may be excessive lateral rotation of the femur and the greater trochanter may appear to move posteriorly and laterally. When the knee is passively flexed in the prone position, the femur laterally rotates.

Summary

In the patient with femoral anterior glide syndrome with lateral rotation, the PICR of the hip joint deviates from the ideal pattern during hip extension. When the greater trochanter is monitored during extension, there is some posterolateral displacement and excessive lateral rotation. The muscular force couple of hip extensor medial rotators—semimembranous and semitendinous—are not counterbalancing the dominance of the hip extensor lateral rotators, biceps femoris, gluteus maximus, and piriformis muscles.

Intervention

PRIMARY OBJECTIVES. The primary purposes of an intervention program are to improve the posterior glide of the femoral head, decrease the dominance of the hip extensor lateral rotator muscles, and improve the participation of the hip medial rotator muscles.

CORRECTIVE EXERCISE PROGRAM

Supine position. While in the hook-lying position (i.e., hip and knee are flexed), the patient is instructed to adduct and rotate the hip medially and then reverse the movement into hip abduction and lateral rotation while limiting the excursion in a lateral direction. In some patients the movement into abduction and lateral rotation is not included in the exercise.

Prone position. While in the prone position, the patient is instructed to rotate the hip medially with the knee flexed to 90 degrees. The patient should avoid rotating the hip laterally, stopping at neutral.

Side-lying position. While in the side-lying position, the patient abducts the hip, maintaining a slight medial rotation and flexion of the hip.

Quadruped position. From the quadruped position, the patient rocks backward with an emphasis placed on limiting the motion to hip flexion and avoiding hip lateral rotation or abduction.

Sitting position. In the sitting position, the patient uses his or her hands to lift the thigh, so that the hip is in maximum flexion and then releases the hold on the thigh and uses the iliopsoas muscle to keep the hip flexed. Resistance can be applied to the thigh with the hand to improve the strength of the iliopsoas.

Standing position. While standing, the patient is instructed to limit forward bending to hip flexion with the knees flexed. The return movement from forward bending is performed with particular emphasis on using gluteal muscles without emphasizing a lateral rotation of the hip.

CORRECTING POSTURAL HABIT PATTERNS. While in the sitting position the patient is instructed to lean forward by flexing at the hips. He or she tries to limit how much flexion occurs in the spine. The patient is asked to avoid sitting with the legs crossed in a position where the lateral aspect of the leg is resting on the opposite thigh (i.e., hip lateral rotation, flexion, and abduction).

Case Presentation

History. A 46-year-old man reports right anterior hip pain that began when jogging. The pain is now evident when he walks. At the onset of his hip pain, which began approximately 4 months before his first visit to physical therapy, the patient was running 70 miles per week, both in the morning and evening. He has lost over 100 pounds since beginning his running program, but has been unable to run for 6 weeks before his first appointment. A consultation with an orthopedic specialist produced a magnetic resonance image (MRI) of his hip that showed no significant findings. Therefore no specific diagnosis has been made. The patient is an executive who spends most of his workday sitting at a desk. His only physical activity is jogging.

Symptoms. The patient has pain in the anteromedial aspect of his groin, which he reproduces by laterally rotating and extending his hip. The pain is more intense when he is in a weight-bearing position. He rates his baseline pain at 3 to 4 on a scale of 10, but the pain increases to a rating of 7 to 8 when jogging.

Alignment Analysis. The patient is less than 10% over his ideal body weight. He has a flat back and stands in posterior tilt and hip extension. His hips are rotated laterally and medial rotation is very limited. There is a slight degree of genu valgus. Lateral rotation provokes pain in his right hip, but not in his left.

Movement Analysis

Standing. When asked to bend forward, lumbar flexion occurs more readily than hip flexion. Maximum hip flexion is 70 degrees. When his gait is observed, it is noted that his hips excessively rotate laterally from midstance to push-off.

Prone. Knee flexion while in the prone position produces a slight rotation of the hip laterally. During hip extension there is lateral rotation of the proximal femur.

Quadruped. In the quadruped test position, his hips are held in 70 degrees of flexion. When he rocks backward his lumbar spine flexes, but his hip joints do not. When his hips are rotated laterally, the range into hip flexion without lumbar flexion increases.

Muscle Length and Strength Analysis. There is resistance to hip flexion at 90 degrees of hip flexion. This resistance to hip flexion increases when the hip is rotated medially, and it decreases when the hip is rotated laterally. The lateral rotational range of motion of the hip when performed in the prone position measures 50 degrees on the right side and 40 degrees on the left. During right hip lateral rotation, there is a wide arc of movement of the greater trochanter. His right hip does not rotate medially, and the medial rotational range of the left hip is 15 degrees. The strength of his hip abductor muscles is rated 5/5; the strength of his gluteus maximus muscles is rated 4−/5 on the right side and 4/5 on the left; the strength of his iliopsoas muscles is rated 4/5 on the right side and 5/5 on the left.

Diagnosis. The patient's alignment and movement tests are clearly consistent with femoral anterior glide syndrome with lateral rotation.

Intervention. The primary goals of intervention are to improve hip flexion and medial rotational range of motion and to decrease the resistance to posterior glide of the femoral head. Another goal is to improve the performance of the hip flexor and medial rotator muscles, such as the anterior gluteus medius and the gluteus minimus muscles.

While in the quadruped position, the patient is instructed to rock backward with an emphasis on hip flexion, avoiding lumbar flexion and hip lateral rotation.

In the supine position the patient is instructed to perform hip and knee flexion using his hands to pull his knee toward his chest, keeping the femur in neutral. With his hip and knee flexed, he performs hip adduction/medial rotation to stretch the hip abductor and lateral rotator muscles. While performing the reverse direction of this movement, he is instructed to limit hip abduction/lateral rotation to only 20 degrees beyond neutral.

From a side-lying position the patient performs hip abduction to 25 degrees with the hip slightly flexed and rotated medially.

While in a prone position the patient performs hip medial rotation with the hip extended and knee flexed to 90 degrees.

In a sitting position and with his pelvis vertical he is instructed to use his hands to lift his thigh passively into maximal hip flexion. He is then asked to release the hold his hands have on his thigh and use his iliopsoas muscle to maintain the hip flexion. When he is able to maintain the hip flexion, he applies resistance by pushing with his hand against his thigh into hip extension.

From a standing position he performs forward bending by limiting the motion to hip and knee flexion and returns to an upright position by actively contracting his gluteal muscles.

He is advised not to allow his feet to turn out more than a few degrees when walking.

Correcting Postural Habits. The patient is instructed not to sit with his legs crossed with the foot on the opposite thigh.

Outcome. The patient was examined five times over 6 weeks. By the third week he is jogging for 20 minutes every other day. By the beginning of the sixth week he is jogging for 40 minutes, 6 times a week, without symptoms. All symptoms are alleviated and no impairments are found, except his hip medial rotation remains limited. The patient is instructed to perform quadruped rocking after jogging and to limit his jogging frequency to one run on the first day followed by two runs on the next day, repeating this sequence throughout the week.

Hip Adduction Syndrome

Hip adduction syndrome can occur with or without excessive medial rotation. The only difference between the two conditions is the presence of excessive medial rotation in combination with excessive hip adduction. Only hip adduction with medial rotation, which is the most common of the two conditions, is discussed in this text.

In hip adduction with medial rotation, the PGM and lateral rotator muscles are long as the result of either a weakness or an increased length from the serial addition of sarcomeres. When there is excessive hip adduc-

tion, all hip abductor muscles are weak or lengthened. Hip adduction with medial rotation occurs more often in women than in men. Contributing factors to the development of this syndrome are a structurally wide pelvis and sleeping on the side, which allows the hip to adduct and rotate medially. The hip abductor muscles, posterolateral capsule, and lateral rotator muscles are all stretched. If the patient is a runner or participates in activities that involve hip medial rotation and increase the use of the hip flexor or medial rotator muscles, such as cycling, the imbalance between the flexor-medial rotator muscles and the extensor-lateral rotator muscles can be further exaggerated.

This syndrome is also associated with the piriformis syndrome. Freiberg,[5] who first described the piriformis syndrome, attributes the hip adduction syndrome to a shortened muscle. Kendall,[11] in contrast, attributes this syndrome to a stretched or lengthened muscle. If the patient's alignment while standing is hip medial rotation, adduction, and anterior pelvic tilt, the piriformis must be in a lengthened position. In this condition the patient may have sciatica from an entrapment of the nerve by the piriformis muscle. Hip adduction syndrome with medial rotation is also associated with ITB fascitis.

Symptoms and Pain

Pain in the areas of the gluteus medius muscle, which is superior and lateral to the greater trochanter, is found in this syndrome when the hip abductors are strained. Deep hip pain, trochanteric bursitis, and sciatica are also common. Pain along the lateral aspect of the thigh (e.g., ITB) that is characterized as an ache or burning sensation is often described when there is ITB fascitis. Some patients report the pain as a numbness; however, sensation is not impaired. The lateral thigh pain often wakes the patient at night or in early morning. The pain is greatest in the morning, diminishes after walking, but returns with fatigue.

Inflammation and fascial shortness may involve peroneal muscle fascia and entrap the peroneal nerve at the head of fibula, which produces symptoms along the peroneal nerve distribution. The examiner must assess whether the patient has a spinal source of radiation, because these symptoms are similar to an L4,5 radiculopathy. A spinal problem can initiate the syndrome, but inflammation of the ITB is a separate dysfunction that must also be addressed.

Key findings include tenderness to palpation along the ITB and nodules. Pain is usually reproduced by stretching the ITB or with adduction of the hip in a side-lying position. Occasionally, the symptoms can be produced by the exercise of hip abduction-lateral rotation in flexion, but the symptoms should diminish and the range of motion should increase with repetitions of the exercises. The TFL-ITB should test weak when ITB fascitis is present.

Movement Impairments

STANDING POSITION. While in a single-leg stance of the affected limb, there is hip adduction, hip medial rotation, or lateral trunk flexion over the stance leg.

WALKING. If there is weakness of the entire gluteus medius muscle there may be a gluteus medius limp. If the weakness is more severe, there may be lateral trunk flexion during the stance phase of the affected limb (i.e., antalgic gait). Because men have broader shoulders and narrower hips, the antalgic gait in men may not be as noticeable as it is in women. In patients with strong hip adductors, quadriceps, and hamstrings, there may not be a gluteus medius limp even if the hip abductors test weak.

Alignment

The structural variations found in patients with hip adduction syndrome include a broad pelvis and genu valgus. Acquired postural impairments include (1) apparent leg-length discrepancy caused by the adduction posture of the affected hip, causing the iliac crest to be in a higher position than the opposite iliac crest by more than $1/2$ inch, (2) hip medial rotation, and (3) a pronated foot.

Flexibility and Stiffness Impairments

Hip abductor lateral rotator muscles are more extensible than the hip abductor medial rotator muscles. The hip abductors of the affected side are more extensible than the hip abductors of the contralateral hip.

Muscle and Recruitment Pattern Impairments

Hip adductor muscles are more dominant than the hip abductor muscles. The sartorius may be used to abduct the hip when performing hip abduction in the side-lying position. In the side-lying position the patient may feel the muscular contraction along the distal medial aspect of the thigh when attempting to perform hip abduction. If medial rotation is an obvious component of the alignment and gait pattern, the TFL muscle may be recruited as the dominant hip abductor. The TFL-ITB may be participating in (1) stabilizing the knee in extension (particularly when the knee is hyperextended) and (2) hip abduction and flexion.

When assessing muscle length and strength, the PGM is long and/or weak in patients with this syndrome. The TFL muscle is short. Both the PGM and the TFL may test weak if they have become strained from overuse. The hip adductor muscles may be short, and the gluteus maximus and lateral rotator muscles are weak. The quadriceps muscles may also test weak, often in association with ITB fascitis.

Confirming Tests

Manual muscle testing (MMT) confirmed the presence of hip abductor muscle weakness and the patient had a positive Trendelenburg test and a gluteus medius limp. During single-leg stance the hip rotates medially. The hip lateral rotator muscles test weak. There is tenderness to palpation along the ITB, shortness or weakness of TFL-ITB, and pain when stretching the TFL-ITB. With entrapment of the sciatic nerve by the lengthened piriformis muscle, there is pain from the distal one third of the buttocks along the posterior thigh that usually stops at the knee but can extend farther distally.

Summary

The primary impairment in this syndrome is excessive hip adduction, which is the result of insufficient performance of the hip abductor muscles. In the patient with associated hip medial rotation the PGM and intrinsic hip lateral rotator muscles are lengthened or weak. In the patient with excessive hip adduction, there is insufficient activity in all of the hip abductor muscles. In the early stages of this syndrome the primary symptoms are pain in the strained gluteus medius muscle and either hip medial rotation or a slight hip drop during walking. In the severe stages of this syndrome the gluteus medius limp is obvious or the patient has an antalgic gait. If the patient has sciatic nerve entrapment from the piriformis, pain in the posterior thigh is present. The patient with sciatic entrapment usually has pain with palpation over the area of the piriformis muscle.

Intervention

PRIMARY OBJECTIVES. The primary objective of the intervention program is to improve the performance of the hip abductor and lateral rotator muscles, which may require alleviating strain, improving strength, or changing the length of the muscles. Because the abductor muscles are often long and weak, a systematic progression of exercises is necessary.

CORRECTIVE EXERCISE PROGRAM

Walking. When the hip abductor muscles are weak enough to cause an antalgic gait, the patient is instructed to use a cane to reduce the stress on the abductor muscles. The duration of walking should be limited.

Prone position. The initial exercises should be in the prone position so the patient does not lift the weight of the leg. The patient should perform hip abduction in this position because the hip extensor-abductor muscles are recruited more readily than the flexor abductor muscles. Another exercise is bilaterally contracting the gluteus maximus isometrically. Another exercise is performed when the hips are abducted slightly and rotated laterally with the knees flexed so that the medial sides of both feet are in contact with each other. In this position the patient performs isometric hip lateral rotation by pushing the feet together.

Side-lying position. While in a side-lying position, the hip lateral rotation/abduction exercise is performed. The selection of the degree of difficulty of the exercise is based on the therapist's examination. The therapist must be sure that the patient is evaluated for antetorsion of the femur to ensure that the instruction in this exercise does not require excessive hip lateral rotation.

Correcting postural habit and movement patterns. While standing, the patient must keep his or her weight equally distributed on both feet and should not stand in hip adduction on the affected extremity. The patient should avoid crossing his or her leg when sitting, and the duration of sitting should be limited. The patient should stand at least every 30 minutes and tighten the gluteal muscles. When moving from a sitting to a standing position and when moving in the reverse direction, the patient must not allow the knees to come together because this decreases the use of the hip abductor muscles and encourages the use of the hip medial rotator muscles. In the side-lying position the patient should use a pillow between the knees and not allow the affected extremity to be flexed, adducted, or rotated medially.

The treatment of ITB fascitis requires decreased use of the TFL-ITB, and increased use of the synergist muscles, such as the gluteus medius iliopsoas and the rectus femoris, is recommended. A progressive program of active exercises is necessary to improve the performance of the PGM and quadriceps muscles and the TFL-ITB. Taping along the band and ice applications are useful treatments for reducing the symptoms.

Supine position. If the TFL muscle is weak or strained, the patient should perform (1) hip abduction by sliding the lower extremity while maintaining the hip in slight medial rotation and (2) active hip and knee flexion exercises.

Side-lying position. In the side-lying position the patient should perform hip abductor exercises with the degree of difficulty appropriate for the degree of muscle weakness.

Prone position. In the prone position the patient should perform knee flexion while preventing pelvic tilt or rotation to stretch the rectus femoris and/or the TFL-ITB. The hip lateral rotation exercise can be used to stretch the ITB and improve the control by the lateral rotator muscles.

Sitting position. While in a sitting position the patient should perform knee extension while preventing hip medial rotation and flexion. The chair should have a backrest so that the patient does not use the hip flexors to maintain a sitting position.

Sitting-to-standing. The patient should practice going from the sitting to the standing position while avoiding hip adduction/medial rotation. He or she should be making a conscious effort to contract the gluteal muscles while coming to the standing position.

Single-leg stance. The patient should practice standing on one leg and making a conscious effort to contract the gluteal muscles to prevent medial rotation and adduction of the hip.

Walking. When walking, it may be necessary for the patient to use a cane to rest the ITB. The gluteal muscles should be contracted at the heel-strike phase of walking and then relaxed as the stance phase is completed.

Case Presentation 1

History. A 34-year-old woman has developed pain in the posterolateral aspect of her right buttock where the PGM muscle inserts. She is a social worker who spends most of her day sitting while counseling clients. The patient began a power-walking program approximately 6 months before the onset of her pain, walking 45 minutes every day. Approximately 1 month before experiencing the pain, she began a weight-training program. The patient is slightly overweight and has a small upper body with rather broad hips; she stands 5 feet 2 inches tall. The patient has taken dance lessons for many years, starting at age 6 and continuing through high school. She has a habit of standing on her right leg and allowing her right hip to adduct and rotate medially.

Symptoms. The patient rates her pain at 5 to 6 on a scale of 10 after walking three blocks. The pain diminishes after sitting for 1 hour. She is not able to sleep on her right side and is uncomfortable when lying on her left.

Alignment Analysis

Standing position. When assuming a standing position the patient exhibits a slight posterior tilt and her upper back is swayed. Her right iliac crest is 1/2 inch higher than her left. After standing for a few minutes she shifts her weight to the right lower extremity and allows her hip to adduct.

Side-lying position. In a resting side-lying position the patient's right hip assumes a position of pronounced hip adduction/medial rotation.

Movement Analysis

Standing position. When standing only on the right leg, the hip rotates medially and the trunk flexes to the right. When the patient stands only on the left leg, there is slight hip medial rotation but no hip drop or side flexion of the trunk. When the patient bends forward while in a standing position, her hips easily flex to 85 degrees.

Supine position. While in a supine position the patient's hip tends to adduct and rotate medially during active hip and knee flexion. The straight-leg raise test with the right extremity is performed with medial rotation, and the straight-leg test with the left is performed in neutral rotation.

Side-lying position. In a side-lying position, the patient performs right hip abduction with medial rotation and flexion. When she adducts to the starting position her right hip rotates medially, but her left hip does not.

Prone position. When the patient extends the right hip while lying in a prone position, the right hamstring muscles contract and the hip extends before an obvious change in the contour of the gluteus maximus. When extending the left hip while lying in a prone position, the hamstrings and gluteus maximus muscles change their contour simultaneously.

Quadruped position. When rocking backward while in the quadruped position, the pelvis drops toward the right, which indicates that the right hip flexes more easily than the left. This occurs because the right hip lateral rotators are weak and less stiff than the left hip lateral rotators.

Sitting position. While assuming a sitting position and extending the right knee, the hip rotates medially.

Sitting-to-standing position. While standing from a sitting position the patient's hips rotate medially and adduct, moving her knees toward one another.

Contributing Postural Habitual Patterns. The patient sits with her right thigh crossed over her left thigh. She sleeps most often on her left side with the right hip flexed, adducted, and rotated medially. During her power walking she emphasizes lateral motion of her pelvis, which causes hip adduction/medial rotation, similar to a race-walking style. Her weight-training program includes both resisted knee extension and hip abduction in the sitting position.

Muscle Length and Strength Analysis. The hip flexor length test indicates that her right TFL is short, and the hip medially rotates during the test. The abdominal muscles rate 3/5, and the PGM muscle rates 3+/5 with weakness throughout the range and with pain in the muscle. The left PGM muscle grades 4/5, and there is a tenderness with palpation in the right PGM muscle. The right and left gluteus maximus muscles grade 4−/5 and 4+/5, respectively; the right and left iliopsoas muscles grade 4/5 and 4+/5, respectively; the right and left hip lateral rotator muscles grade 4−/5 and 5/5, respectively, and the medial rotator muscles grade 5/5.

Diagnosis. The patient's alignment and movement tests are clearly consistent with hip adduction with medial rotation with strain of the PGM muscle.

Intervention. The primary emphasis of this patient's corrective exercise program is to avoid stretching the PGM muscle, improve its performance, and decrease the dominance of the TFL muscle.

While in a side-lying position, the patient performs hip abduction with the hip and knee partially flexed (level I) to improve the performance of the PGM muscle.

From a prone position the patient performs hip abduction while maintaining a slightly lateral rotation of her hip. When performing hip extension in this position, an emphasis is placed on contracting the gluteus maximus muscle and rotating the hip laterally. She is instructed to flex her knee, and while maintaining her knee in 90 degrees of flexion, she rotates her hip laterally to stretch the TFL muscle. She also performs isometric hip lateral rotation by pushing one foot against the other with her knees flexed and her hips abducted and laterally rotated.

In a standing position the patient improves the performance of the hip lateral rotators by standing on her right foot and contracting her right gluteal muscles to prevent medial rotation of the hip.

Correcting Postural Habits. Many of this patient's activities are contributing to her problem. They include sitting with her right leg crossed over her left; sleeping on her left side with her right hip flexed, adducted, and rotated medially; standing with her hip adducted; and performing weight training exercises that consisted of knee extension during which she medially rotated her hip and abducted her hip with it in flexion. She is instructed to stop crossing her leg and to use a footstool. It is recommended that she (1) place her right lower extremity on a body pillow while sleeping on her side; (2) stand with her weight equally distributed on both feet; (3) replace the racing style of walking which emphasizes hip adduction and medial rotation by contracting the buttocks of her right hip during the stance phase of walking while keeping her knee pointed straight ahead; (4) keep her knees apart when moving from a sitting to a standing position and during the reverse motion; and (5) omit the resistive hip abduction and knee extension exercises.

Outcome. The patient has complied with her exercise program and has corrected her postural habits within 1 week. Her pain has decreased to a rating of 2 to 3 on a scale of 10 during walking distances of 1 mile, and she does not have pain at rest. Within 4 weeks and 4 visits she is pain free, and the strength of her PGM muscle has improved to 4+/5. She can stand on one leg without hip medial rotation, and she can move from a sitting to a standing position without pain and can keep her knees pointed anteriorly. She can walk for 3 miles without symptoms.

Case Presentation 2

History. A 28-year-old female operating room nurse is referred for physical therapy. Approximately 5 months earlier, she had fallen on her buttocks, primarily on the right side.

Symptoms and Pain. The patient has pain when walking and a pronounced tenderness to palpation in the posterolateral area of her right buttock. One week after her fall, she begins to experience pain down the back of her thigh. The pain makes it increasingly difficult for her to sit. She is now most comfortable when lying on her left side holding her right lower extremity slightly flexed and adducted. The pain that had been in her posterior thigh has now extended to her ankle. CAT and MRI studies are negative for spinal injuries. Because of the increasing severity of the pain, the patient is experiencing great difficulty walking and sitting and is spending most of her time lying on her left side. Codeine has been prescribed. She rates her pain between 8 and 10 with maximum rating being 10.

Alignment Analysis. The patient stands and walks with her right foot plantar flexed and her weight on her toes. Her knee is flexed and her hip is rotated medially and adducted. Because she cannot stand with both feet flat on the ground, assessment of hip height is difficult; however, her right iliac crest seemed notably higher than her left.

Movement Analysis

Standing. At the time of her initial examination the patient is barely able to walk because of the severity of the pain down the posterior aspect of her right thigh and leg. She is not using hand supports and limits her walking to distances of less than 100 feet.

Supine. The patient is most comfortable when her hip and knee are flexed to 45 degrees and passively supported on pillows. She also experiences pain when she rolls onto her side or changes positions. The length of her hip flexor muscles cannot be tested.

Side-lying. The sciatica is increased if her hip is allowed to rotate and adduct medially. When she performs active knee extension in the side-lying position, the greater trochanter is observed to rotate medially and, at this time, she experiences sciatica. When the femur is manually stabilized by holding the greater trochanter to prevent hip medial rotation, she is able to extend her knee without symptoms.

Sitting. When assuming a sitting position the pain is present, particularly with pressure on her right buttock.

Muscle Length and Strength Analysis. The severity of the patient's symptoms and the obvious range-of-motion limitation prohibits standard testing. The following results are based on modified testing in the supine and side-lying positions.

The TFL-ITB, rectus femoris, and iliopsoas muscles are extremely short. The patient has anterior hip pain when these muscles are stretched by hip extension. The hamstring muscles are short (−35 degrees of complete knee extension), and the hip abductor muscles test 3/5. When the femur is held manually in a neutral position

and not permitted to rotate, abduct, or adduct, the patient is able to move from a side-lying to a sitting position and remain in the sitting position without symptoms. When she stands while the hip is stabilized, there are no symptoms. However, she cannot extend her lower extremity because of the short length of the hip flexor muscles.

Summary. The patient's sciatica is clearly elicited by hip adduction/medial rotation, which is consistent with a piriformis syndrome. The symptoms begin below the gluteal fold and follow the path of the sciatic nerve, which is more consistent with sciatic nerve entrapment than with a spinal source of her symptoms that are usually located higher in the buttock. Her hip abductor and lateral rotator muscles are so weak that she cannot avoid this position. Maintaining the hip in the faulty position caused the hip flexors and hamstring muscles to become short. The TFL muscle is especially short because it provides abduction control when walking but is used in a very short position. The anterior hip pain is the result of stretching her short hip flexor muscles.

Diagnosis. The diagnosis is hip adduction with medial rotation. An associated diagnosis is lengthened piriformis syndrome with sciatica.

Intervention. The patient lives 200 miles from the clinic and has been driven to therapy by her husband, who is interested in helping with her program. To help maintain lateral rotation, her hip is taped with the tape running from her buttocks on a diagonal line toward her thigh, following the lines of the gluteus maximus but extending onto the anterior thigh. The tape is applied when she is in the side-lying position, maintaining the femur in slight lateral rotation.

Starting from a hook-lying position the patient holds a sheet under her right thigh with her hands and uses the sheet to perform actively assisted hip and knee flexion. To return to the starting position, she allows her arms to extend while continuing to support the weight of the lower extremity with the sheet and lowering her right leg to the table. She maintains the contraction of the abdominal muscles allowing the lower extremity to extend, and she stops the extension motion when she experiences discomfort. She also performs hip abduction/lateral rotation from flexion while controlling the lower limb, again by holding a sheet under her thigh with her hands.

From a side-lying position and with a pillow between her knees, the patient rotates her right hip laterally. She is instructed to progress to hip abduction as tolerated, with pain and weakness acting as the limiting factors. With her hip flexed to 45 degrees, her husband helps stabilize her femur at the greater trochanter to prevent medial rotation of the hip while she extends her knee.

When the patient is able to sit symmetrically with equal weight-bearing on each hip, she extends her knee by sliding her foot along the floor, making certain that she does not lift or flex her thigh.

The patient performs a sitting-to-standing exercise by minimizing the use of her hands and contracting the gluteal and quadriceps muscles while moving from a sitting position in a chair to a standing posture. The patient uses crutches when walking and is instructed in a three-point gait.

Outcome. The patient returns 2 weeks after her initial visit and reports that the pain has diminished (now fluctuating between 5 and 8). Her alignment and walking are notably improved. She is still using crutches when walking and cannot place her full weight on her right lower limb. Although she can place her foot on the floor and straighten her lower limb, she is still in anterior pelvic tilt. She is able to sit for 15 to 20 minutes at a time. When in a supine position she can lie on her back and extend her right lower extremity to within 20 degrees of complete extension, and she does not need a sheet under her thigh to control her extremity. The patient has her own tape and has been retaping her thigh. She still has some sciatica when her hip adducts and rotates medially.

The patient's program progresses to lying prone, which she can tolerate by placing a pillow under her abdomen. In this position she flexes her knee and rotates her hip laterally with her knee flexed. The purpose of this exercise is to stretch the ITB. She also performs hip abduction by sliding her lower extremity out to the side. In this position the extensor-abductor muscles are more active than the flexor-abductor muscles. Improving the performance of the hip extensor abductors is a primary goal of the program. In the side-lying position, with a pillow supporting her right lower extremity, the patient abducts her hip with her hip flexed 10 degrees and her knee flexed 30 degrees. The motion is performed with slight lateral rotation of the hip.

The patient returns again in 3 weeks and is free of pain except when walking for distances longer than 1/4 mile or when standing or sitting for prolonged periods of time without changing positions. She stopped taping her hip after her last visit and is no longer taking medication. She can perform all activities requiring basic mobility without pain. Her right PGM muscle is still weak (4−/5), but all muscles are normal length. She plans returning to work on a part-time basis in 2 weeks.

Case Presentation 3

History. An 82-year-old woman is referred to physical therapy for evaluation and intervention. The patient lives out of state and is admitted for diagnostic studies of right lateral thigh pain. During the past year the patient had been experiencing increasing pain down her right lower limb. She had been quite active, driving to volunteer activities in a nursing home, but the pain has become increasing intense, and she has not been able to walk any distances. The patient comments that over the past year she has been re-hemming her skirts because they were hanging crooked. Two orthopedic surgeons in her home city have diagnosed her condition as spinal stenosis and have recommended surgery. Her family, who resides in St. Louis, is seeking another opinion from local physicians. Radiologic studies indicate that her spinal stenosis is affecting the left side of the spine, but not the right.

Symptoms. The patient has pain along the lateral side of her right thigh that extends into the lateral aspect of her leg. The pain is severe when she stands and walks, and it diminishes when she sits or lies in a recumbent position. She is most comfortable when her right lower extremity is rotated medially and is flexed at the hip and knee. There is tenderness with palpation along the lateral aspect of her thigh. Radiologic studies indicate she has cervical disk disease with evidence of cord compression.

Alignment Analysis. The patient is very slender with cervical lordosis and thoracic kyphosis. She stands with a slight posterior pelvic tilt and with a posterior sway of her thorax. Her right iliac crest is 1 inch higher than her left. The right hip is rotated medially, as well as adducted, causing her knee to be in valgus alignment. There is poor definition of her gluteal muscles.

Movement Analysis. The following tests are performed with the patient (1) standing, (2) lying supine, (3) in a prone position, (4) sitting, (5) moving from a sitting position to a standing posture, and (6) walking.

Standing. The patient experiences pain along the lateral thigh when she stands with her weight on the right lower extremity. Forward bending with only hip flexion does not change her symptoms. When standing on her right leg, her trunk laterally flexes to the right and her right hip medially rotates and adducts. When standing on her left leg, her left hip slightly adducts.

Supine. When in a supine position the patient experiences pain along her right lateral thigh with slight movement into hip abduction/lateral rotation from flexion. The pain diminishes and her range of motion increases with each repetition; she does not experience pain along her left thigh when performing the same movement of hip abduction/lateral rotation. The range of motion into hip abduction/lateral rotation is three times greater on the left side than on the right. She is able to lie supine without symptoms if she places a pillow under the thoracic spine (for kyphosis) and a pillow under her right knee to keep her right hip flexed and rotated medially.

Prone. Flexion of the right knee causes anterior pelvic tilt, pelvic clockwise rotation, and hip abduction. Flexion of the left knee causes slight anterior pelvic tilt. Pillows are placed under the patient's chest and abdomen to prevent any cervical extension.

Sitting. The patient experiences slight pain along her right lateral thigh when she sits without support. With back support this pain diminishes. Extension of the right knee is accompanied by medial hip rotation, whereas extension of the left knee is not.

Sit-to-stand movement. The patient stands 5 feet 3 inches; therefore her hips are higher than her knees when she sits, which makes it easier to come to a standing position than if her knees were higher than her hips. However, she must use her hands to push up from a chair. Both lower extremities adduct and rotate medially, causing one knee to touch the other. When one knee braces against the other during a sit-to-stand movement, demands on the hip abductor muscles are reduced.

Gait. During the right stance phase of walking, the patient experiences pain along her right lateral thigh. Observable gait impairments are right hip adduction/medial rotation, in addition to lateral trunk flexion. Using a cane in her left hand and walking with a three-point gait reduce her pain and her limp.

Muscle Length and Strength Analysis. When muscle length and strength are examined, the patient's right hamstring muscles are short with knee extension of -25 degrees on her right side to -15 degrees on her left. Right hip lateral rotation is limited to 10 degrees at which point she experiences pain along the lateral thigh. Lateral rotation of her left hip approaches 25 degrees. Her right TFL-ITB is notably short, and her left TFL-ITB is slightly short. The strength of her lower abdominal muscles is less than 1/5; the strength of her right and left TFL-ITB muscles is 3+/5 and 4/5, respectively. The strength of her right and left hip abductor muscle is 3/5 and 4/5, respectively. The patient has limited ability to perform isometric gluteus maximus contraction, bilaterally.

Summary. The pain with palpation along the lateral thigh is characteristic of ITB fascitis. The decrease in her symptoms with repeated motion as demonstrated with the hip abduction/lateral rotation from flexion movement is also symptomatic of fascitis. The weakness of the TFL-ITB is consistent with muscle strain from overuse. The symptoms that occur during right stance phase of walking and when sitting without back support could be exaggerated by the extended alignment of the lumbar spine in these positions. Medial hip rotation and adduction during weight-bearing activities, medial rotation of the hip during knee extension while in the sitting position, and the obvious weakness of the hip abductor and knee extensor muscles are findings consistent with an overuse of the TFL-ITB. The TFL muscle may have

become strained because it provides most of the support for hip abduction and assists in stabilizing the knee when in extension. Driving her car, which requires hip flexion and medial rotation and knee extension, may have contributed to the strain of her TFL-ITB.

Diagnosis. The diagnosis is hip adduction/medial rotation syndrome with ITB fascitis.

Intervention. Because the ITB is believed to be strained, reducing the stress on the band will enable it to heal, an important part of the intervention. Improving the performance of the muscle synergists of the ITB and a careful progressive strengthening program for the TFL-ITB are two important additional components of the treatment program. Limiting her walking has been facilitated because she is hospitalized. When she begins walking she will use a cane in the contralateral hand. Ice packs are applied along the ITB twice a day.

From the hook-lying position, the patient performs unilateral hip and knee extension and flexion by sliding her foot along the bed while contracting her abdominal muscles. She is instructed to keep her hip slightly rotated laterally and to start the repetitions in slight abduction and then adduct the hip during subsequent repetitions. From the supine position with the hip and knee flexed, she performs hip abduction/lateral rotation, using her hands and abdominal muscles to keep her pelvis from rotating. She is instructed to stop this motion at the onset of pain.

While in the side-lying position, the patient is instructed to place a pillow between her knees and perform hip lateral rotation.

While in a prone position, the patient places pillows under her thorax and abdomen to avoid neck and lumbar extension. When performing knee flexion, she is instructed to prevent motion of the pelvis. She is taught to perform hip lateral rotation with the knee flexed to 90 degrees. She also performs hip abduction by sliding the lower extremity along the bed while avoiding pelvic tilt and lumbar extension.

From a sitting position the patient extends her knee while using a back support, avoiding medial hip rotation or flexion. She is instructed to concentrate on maximal recruitment of musculature on the anterior thigh.

When moving from a sitting to a standing posture, the patient slides to the end of the chair by pushing with her hands. She is instructed to (1) minimize the assistance provided by her hands, (2) contract her buttock muscles to keep her knees pointed straight ahead, (3) contract her quadriceps muscles, (4) keep her trunk erect, and (5) avoid leaning forward while coming to a standing position.

Outcome. The patient remains in the hospital for 3 weeks and then stays with her family for an additional week before returning to her home. During the first

3-week period her symptoms improved progressively as her muscle and movement impairments decreased. By the end of 2 weeks she is able to perform the sitting and spine exercises without symptoms or compensatory motions. She can lie in a supine position with both hips and knees extended, as long as she places a pillow under her thoracic spine and head. She still has a slight rotation and tilt of the pelvis during knee flexion while in the prone position. She can walk for 200 feet without symptoms when using a cane. She experiences right lateral thigh pain when climbing stairs or when standing on her right foot without hand support. Right medial rotation and adduction of the hip are still evident when the patient stands without support.

When she is discharged from the hospital, the patient walks without a cane and remains pain free, displaying minimal gait impairments for 150 feet. She can walk for unlimited distances with her cane. She experiences minimal pain when climbing stairs if she uses the hand rail while stepping up with her right foot. All exercises are performed correctly and without symptoms. When the patient stands on one leg and uses hand support for balance, she has difficulty preventing hip adduction/medial rotation.

At the time of her last outpatient visit before her return home, the patient no longer uses a cane. She can climb one flight of stairs and move from a sitting to a standing position without using her hands and without hip adduction or medial rotation. The difference in her iliac crest levels is only 1/4 inch. She characterizes the time with her family as typical as it relates to her routines and activities, except she is not driving her car.

Approximately 3 months after she has returned to her home, the patient reports that she is doing fine and is re-hemming her skirts because her hips are now level.

Hip Extension With Knee Extension Syndrome

Hip extension with knee extension syndrome is characterized by the insufficient participation of the gluteus maximus during hip extension or the quadriceps muscles during knee extension. Typical of this syndrome is contraction of the hamstring muscles, when the foot is fixed, to assist the quadriceps muscles with knee extension. When this pattern of hamstring participation becomes dominant, the result can be strain of the hamstring muscles from overuse because of the demands for exerting tension at the hip and knee. Another possibility for hamstring strain is the insufficient participation of the gluteus maximus muscle to generate the tension necessary for hip extension. A third example of strain, specifically strain of the biceps femoris muscle, occurs when the biceps femoris muscle is insufficiently assisted by the intrinsic hip lateral

rotators—the gemelli, obturators, piriformis, and quadratus femoris muscles—in producing lateral hip rotation (see Chapter 2).

Symptoms and Pain

Complaints can include pain at the insertion of the hamstring muscle on the ischial tuberosity; pain along the hamstring muscular belly; and pain with resistance to contraction with hip extension, knee flexion, or both. Severe strain can be present without muscle tearing as evident in discoloration or marked swelling. If strain is present, pain is a common symptom when the patient walks or sits with pressure on the ischial tuberosity.

Movement Impairments

STANDING POSITION. When stepping up a step or rising out of a chair, the knee appears to be moving back toward the body rather than the body moving toward the knee that stays in a relatively fixed position. When returning from a forward bending position, the primary motions are the hips swaying forward and the ankles moving into dorsiflexion. The return to a standing position is accomplished by using upper body momentum and ankle dorsiflexion more than tension generated by hip extensor muscles. When the patient is standing on the affected leg, the hip medially rotates and often the knee hyperextends.

PRONE POSITION. During active hip extension the motion of the femur is almost complete before there is an obvious change in the contour of the gluteus maximus muscle.

SITTING POSITION. When the patient is in a sitting position and performs active knee extension, there is simultaneous hip extension.

Summary

In the hip extension syndromes, strong contraction of the hamstring muscles increases symptoms, whereas the increased use of the synergists of the hamstring muscles decreases symptoms. The following common impairments are found in the patient with hip extension with knee extension syndrome.

Alignment

No particular structural variations

ACQUIRED IMPAIRMENTS

1. Swayback posture
2. Postural hip extension
3. Medial hip rotation
4. Knee hyperextension
5. Ankle plantarflexion in standing position

Flexibility and Stiffness Impairments

Hip flexion is often stiff because the hamstring muscle is usually hypertrophied, and the medial hamstring muscles are more stiff than the lateral hamstring muscles. The ankle plantar flexor muscles are also stiff.

Muscle and Recruitment Pattern Impairments

Hamstring activity is more dominant than the activity of the gluteus maximus muscle during hip extension. Hamstring activity is more dominant than what is optimal when performing knee extension with the foot fixed. During hip lateral rotation, hamstring activity is more dominant than the activity of the intrinsic hip lateral rotator muscles.

Muscle Length and Strength Impairments

The hamstring muscles are often short, and the gluteus maximus and lateral rotator muscles are weak. There may be possible weakness of the quadriceps muscles.

Confirming Tests

There is tenderness to palpation of the hamstring muscle belly and when pressure is applied to the ischial tuberosity. Resisted contraction to hip extension or knee flexion elicits pain. The result of the Slump test to assess nerve tension sensitivity is negative.

Summary

Hamstring strain occurs as a result of overuse, which is caused by the insufficient participation of the three synergistic groups of the hamstring muscle actions—gluteus maximus, intrinsic hip lateral rotator, and quadriceps muscles. Manual muscle testing of these synergists, as well as observation of movement patterns, is used to support the hypothesis of altered recruitment patterns.

Intervention

PRIMARY OBJECTIVES. The primary objective of an intervention program is to improve the strength and participation of the deficient synergistic muscles, thereby avoiding hamstring muscular strain by chronic overuse. After improving the performance of these deficient synergistic muscles and after restoring the appropriate movement patterns, exercises designed to strengthen the hamstring muscles can be instituted. Immediate emphasis on hamstring strengthening will contribute to the dominant participation of the hamstring muscles.

CORRECTIVE EXERCISE PROGRAM

Quadruped exercises. Rocking backward improves the flexibility of the gluteus maximus and piriformis muscles if either is short or stiff.

Supine exercises. Unilateral hip and knee flexion improves hip flexion flexibility. The straight-leg raise improves hamstring length. During hip flexion the contralateral hamstring muscles should not be contracted,

thus the patient should be instructed to keep the extremity relaxed.

Prone exercises. With a pillow placed under the abdomen to ensure that the hips remain slightly flexed, the knee is flexed and allowed to remain passively flexed as far as possible to minimize hamstring activity. Then the patient performs hip extension. Emphasis should be placed on initiating the motion with the gluteus maximus muscle, which usually requires performing slight lateral rotation along with hip extension. Isometric lateral hip rotation is performed with the knees flexed and the hips abducted and rotated laterally (i.e., one foot pushing against the other).

Side-lying exercises. Hip abduction is performed with slight lateral rotation of the hip, if the PGM is weak.

Sitting exercises. Knee extension is performed without extending or medially rotating the hip, and then ankle dorsiflexion is performed. This exercise stretches the hamstring muscles and dorsiflexes the ankle at the end of the knee extension motion, which stretches the gastrocnemius-soleus muscle. The sit-to-stand motion is practiced with the body leaning forward over the legs. Strengthening the iliopsoas muscle is indicated when, during standing, the swayback posture with the associated alignment of hip joint extension is evident.

Standing exercise. While standing on one leg, emphasis is on gluteal muscle contraction and minimal hamstring contraction. Contracting the gluteal muscles can also prevent medial hip rotation if this motion occurs during single-leg stance. An emphasis is placed on contracting the gluteus maximus muscle to assist hip extension during the return motion from forward bending. Step-up movements are performed with an emphasis on bringing the thigh to the knee rather than allowing the knee to move back toward the body and contracting the quadriceps muscles maximally.

CORRECTING POSTURAL HABITS AND MOVEMENT PATTERNS. Correct posture is neutral position of the hip and knee and avoids hip extension and knee hyperextension. When in the sitting position, "unconscious" contraction of the hamstring muscles must be avoided. When walking, the gluteus maximus muscle should contract at heel strike. When returning from forward bending, the gluteus maximus muscles are used and the forward hip swaying motion is avoided.

Case Presentation

History. A 60-year-old woman has developed pain in the area of her gluteal fold after completing a cross-state bicycle ride. In spite of her pain she continues to run daily and perform weight-training exercises using her lower extremities twice weekly. One month after the bicycle ride, her pain increased and is now present when she is sitting and walking. She is examined by an orthopedic specialist who diagnoses her condition as hamstring strain and who prescribes exercises to stretch and strengthen her hamstring muscles.

Symptoms. The patient has severe pain in the area of the ischial tuberosities bilaterally, but the right side is more painful than the left. She is experiencing severe pain when she walks, and she can barely sit. She has stopped all of her exercise activities. She rates the pain at 7 to 8 on a scale of 10. She is most comfortable when lying down. She has tenderness with palpation at both ischial tuberosities.

Movement Analysis

Standing. When observed in the standing position the patient has a slight posterior pelvic tilt with a flat lumbar spine, poor gluteal definition, and bilateral tibial torsion. Forward bending causes pain in the ischial tuberosities, and the return movement to the upright position is accomplished by swaying at the ankles and hips. When standing on one leg, the patient experiences pain in the area of the ischial tuberosity, and there is a slight medial rotation of the hip but no hip adduction.

Supine. When tested in the supine position the range of hip flexion is within normal limits. The patient experiences pain when she performs resisted hip extension. Her abdominal muscular strength tests 4/5. With her lumbar spine flat, her hip flexes to 90 degrees during the passive straight-leg raise test. The patient does not report pain with active straight-leg raises, except at the end of her range-of-hip flexion.

Prone. When tested in the prone position the patient experiences pain when resistance is applied to knee flexion. When the patient performs hip extension, the hamstring muscles contract and the motion is 50% complete before there is an obvious change in the contour of the gluteus maximus muscle.

Quadruped. When tested in the quadruped position the patient experiences pain in the ischial tuberosities when her hips are allowed to flex to greater than 90 degrees by extending her back and anteriorly tilting her pelvis. While still in the quadruped position, the pain decreases when the hips are flexed to less than 80 degrees by flexing her back and posteriorly tilting her pelvis. The pain increases when the patient rocks backward into hip flexion.

Sitting. The patient is unable to tolerate sitting in an upright position for longer than 5 minutes. Pain decreases when she slides forward in a chair, which places more weight on her sacrum than on her ischial tuberosities. The Slump test for nerve tension sensitivity is negative.

Walking. The patient reports pain during the stance phase of walking. It diminishes when she sways her trunk backward and maintains exaggerated hip extension, which decreases the participation of the hamstring muscles.

Muscle Length and Strength Analysis. Hamstring length is within normal limits. The pain that the patient reports with resisted hip extension and knee flexion makes it difficult to identify weakness. The manual muscle test grade of the gluteus maximus is 4−/5 and of the quadriceps and lateral rotator muscles is normal.

Diagnosis. The pain with active contraction and passive stretch of the hamstring muscles and with palpation of both ischial tuberosities is consistent with hamstring strain. The poor definition of the gluteal muscles, the weakness of the gluteus maximus muscle, and the dominant hamstring activity during hip extension are all consistent with insufficient activity of the gluteus maximus muscle. The diagnosis is hip extension syndrome with knee extension.

Intervention. The primary emphasis at this stage of severity is to provide as much rest as possible for the hamstring muscles by alleviating the tension exerted by these muscles. The patient's muscles are normal in length, but she has been performing resistive exercises that have only contributed to this syndrome.

While in the quadruped position the patient is instructed to allow her hips to flex, just to the point of eliciting symptoms. The excursion during rocking backward is limited to the onset of symptoms.

While in a supine position the patient performs active hip and knee flexion, completing the last phase of hip flexion by using her hands to pull her knee toward her chest.

When in a prone position the patient is instructed to perform isometric contraction of her gluteus maximus muscles. She also abducts her hip by sliding her lower extremity along the floor.

The patient is instructed to sit on a ring-shaped air cushion, avoiding pressure on both ischial tuberosities.

In a standing position the patient is instructed to practice isometric contractions of her gluteal muscles.

While walking, the patient is instructed to assume an exaggerated swayback posture. She is told to use ice packs on the ischial tuberosities twice a day, minimize the amount of walking, and cease all exercise activity except for upper body weight training.

Outcome. Approximately 1 week after the initial visit, the patient notes only slight improvement in her pain level. The improvement is mostly the result of avoiding the use of her hamstring muscles by walking in the swayback posture. Tape is applied across the right ischial tuberosity area as a means of supporting the insertion of the hamstring muscles, which the patient reports helps reduce the pain. The tape is left in place for 3 days. She returns after 1 week, and again tape is applied over the right ischial tuberosity. She is able to walk in a more upright posture than she could previously. She is able to flex her hips to 100 degrees while in the quadruped position and rock backward through 50% of her range, both without pain. The patient is taught to bend forward slightly while only using hip flexion and then return by contracting her gluteus maximus muscles. Hip extension in a prone position with a pillow under her abdomen and with her knee flexed is added to the program.

By the end of 5 weeks she is able to sit for 20 to 30 minutes before experiencing pain. She can walk in the normal upright alignment, but she cannot take long strides. When walking, she is instructed to contract the gluteal muscles of the swinging leg at heel-strike. During her forward bending she is instructed to increase the range to approximately 70 degrees of hip flexion and return by contracting her gluteus maximus muscles. She is also taught an exercise in which she kneels on one knee with the hip extended and knee flexed; the other foot remains on the floor and both the hip and knee are flexed—similar to the lunge exercise. By the end of the seventh weekly treatments, her last visit, the patient is able to walk for 2 miles and sit for up to 2 hours without developing symptoms. Resisted hip extension and knee flexion does not cause pain. In the quadruped position she can rock backward through the full range without symptoms. The strength of her gluteus maximus muscle is normal, and the strength of her hamstring muscles is 4+/5. She is instructed to begin jogging short distances and alternate this jogging with walking for a total distance of 3 miles. She is advised not to resume her resistive exercises to the hamstring muscles, using the "leg curl" motion. Telephone contact 2 months later indicates that she is able to jog for at least 3 miles and has completed a 5-mile run without difficulty. She is encouraged to continue jogging with an emphasis on contracting her gluteal muscles during heel-strike and during the return to the upright position when performing the forward-bending exercise. She is instructed to periodically perform the forward-bending exercise during the day.

Hip Lateral Rotation Syndrome

The hip lateral rotation syndrome is characterized by the insufficient participation of the intrinsic hip lateral rotator muscles, the piriformis, obturators, gemelli, and quadratus femoris muscles. An associated diagnosis of this syndrome is a shortened piriformis with sciatica.

Symptoms and Pain

Typical of the hip lateral rotation syndrome is pain in the posterior buttock, which originates just above the gluteal fold and radiates down the posterior aspect of the thigh to terminate at the knee. This syndrome is frequently misdiagnosed as hamstring strain.

Movement Impairments

The patient with the hip lateral rotation syndrome will usually walk with a laterally rotated hip and a slight antalgic gait.

Alignment: Structural Variations and Acquired Impairments

The structural variation with hip lateral rotation syndrome is hip retrotorsion. An acquired impairment is hip lateral rotation.

Relative Flexibility and Stiffness Impairments

The piriformis muscle and other lateral rotator muscles are stiffer than the medial rotator muscles.

Muscle and Recruitment Pattern Impairments

Activity of the intrinsic hip lateral rotator muscles (e.g., piriformis, gemelli, obturators, quadratus femoris) is more dominant than the activity of the hip medial rotator muscles. Impairments of muscle length and strength include shortness of the piriformis and intrinsic hip lateral rotator muscles and stiffness or shortness of the hamstring and quadriceps muscles.

Confirming Tests

Pain down the posterior thigh increases with hip adduction or adduction with medial rotation and decreases when the hip is abducted and rotated laterally.

Intervention

PRIMARY OBJECTIVES. For the patient with lateral rotational problems, particularly in the presence of sciatica, the intervention is stretching the hip into medial rotation, but the stretching should be performed carefully to avoid irritating the nerve. Thus the patient should only stretch to the point where symptoms are elicited.

CORRECTIVE EXERCISE PROGRAM. In the quadruped position, the patient's hip is abducted and laterally rotated rather than in a neutral position. The patient is instructed to rock back to the point at which the symptoms are just beginning.

CORRECTING POSTURAL HABITS AND MOVEMENT PATTERNS. The patient is instructed to avoid sitting for prolonged periods of time. He or she is also advised to avoid prolonged periods of hip extension and lateral rotation, such as when lying in a supine position.

Summary

When the shortened piriformis syndrome is present, the patient's symptoms are exaggerated by hip flexion and medial rotation/adduction. These symptoms decrease with extension, lateral rotation, and abduction. Movements of the spine do not affect the patient's symptoms as long as there is no motion at the hip joint. This syndrome can also be mistaken for hamstring strain, but the hamstring muscles are not painful to palpation and no pain is elicited by resisted contraction. Typically, the hamstring muscles do not test weak.

Case Presentation

History. A 16-year-old high school student has been referred to physical therapy for right hamstring strain. The patient is a highly competitive golfer who has experienced an onset of posterior thigh pain after competing in a multistate tournament 1 year earlier. Although he did not have any symptoms while playing in the tournament, the next day when riding home, he began experiencing pain along his right posterior thigh from his buttock to his knee. The pain became increasingly intense. An orthopedic surgeon diagnosed his problem as hamstring strain and referred him to physical therapy for stretching and resistive exercises. The patient has been participating in physical therapy three times a week for 2 months without improvement. The patient is instructed to stop all sporting activities, but he is advised to maintain his stretching program.

Symptoms. Although he has followed this instruction, he still experiences pain in his posterior thigh when walking or sitting, which he rates at a 6 to 7 on a scale of 10. When the symptoms become particularly intense he tries to stretch his hamstring muscles, which gives him only temporary relief. The patient is anxious to return to sports, especially golf.

Alignment Analysis. The patient is 6 feet tall, slender, and right handed. He has a flat back and is in posterior pelvic tilt. His left iliac crest is $\frac{1}{2}$ inch higher than his right. He stands with his right hip in lateral rotation, and he keeps most of his weight on his left lower extremity.

Movement Analysis

Standing. When the patient bends forward; his lumbar spine flexes faster than his hips and his pain in his posterior thigh increases slightly. When he returns from forward bending; he initiates the movement by extending his hips. In spite of this hip extension movement, his primary strategy for returning to an erect position is swaying his pelvis forward and his trunk backward. This maneuver makes his ankles the primary fulcrum of the movement rather than the hip joints, which usually indicates weakness of the hip extensor muscles. When the patient stands on his right leg, his hip extends, causing his trunk to lean posterolaterally. When he stands on his left leg, his trunk and pelvis maintains a constant position.

Supine. Hip flexion, medial rotation, and adduction cause pain in his posterior thigh. When he is in a resting position his right lower extremity assumes a position of marked lateral rotation, but his left lower extremity does not. He does not experience pain in the right posterior thigh during a passive straight-leg raise to 80 degrees.

Side-lying. When lying on his side, hip adduction increases symptoms.

Quadruped. Symptoms in his right posterior thigh increase when the patient rocks backward while in a quadruped position. When his right hip is positioned in abduction and lateral rotation before rocking backward, his symptoms decrease.

Muscle Length and Strength Analysis. When testing hip flexor length; the right TFL-ITB is short and the left is within normal limits. The length of the hamstring muscles is within normal limits, and the hip can be flexed to 180 degrees with the lumbar spine flat during a passive straight-leg raise. Resisted hip extension does not cause posterior thigh pain.

The following are the test results for muscle strength:

- Right and left gluteus medius muscles rate 4+/5 and 4/5, respectively.
- Right and left hip lateral rotator muscles rate 4+/5 and 5/5, respectively.
- Right and left hip medial rotator muscles rate 4−/5 and 5/5, respectively.
- Right and left hip medial rotation in the prone position is 20 degrees and 35 degrees, respectively.
- Resistance to knee flexion in the prone position produces no pain.

Diagnosis. The patient's examination clearly indicates that his piriformis muscle is short and that stretching the muscle elicits symptoms. As a right-handed golfer, the hip lateral rotator muscles should control the counterclockwise rotation of the right hip during the end of the swing. Also, because he is tall with long tibias, he habitually sits with his hips abducted and rotated laterally, contributing to the development of muscle shortness. His previous stretching program had only indirectly addressed the primary source of his problem. When he stretched, he did not use the intensity of the symptoms as a guide; rather, he followed the philosophy of "no pain, no gain," which had been irritating the nerve. The diagnosis is hip lateral rotation syndrome with sciatica (shortened piriformis syndrome).

Intervention. From a sitting position the patient is most comfortable if he slides forward in his chair so that his right hip is extended, rotated laterally, and abducted. Slight hip medial rotation and adduction from this position elicit symptoms. He is instructed to perform hip medial rotation/adduction as his exercise while sitting in class, but he is to move his hip only to the point where symptoms are initiated. He is instructed to stand up as frequently as possible and to limit the degree of hip medial rotation to avoid symptoms.

While in a supine position the patient performs hip adduction/medial rotation from flexion, but again he is advised to move his hip only to the point of the onset of symptoms.

From a side-lying position the patient performs hip lateral rotation and abduction with his knee flexed to 45 degrees. He is also instructed to perform hip abduction while the hip is maintained in slight medial rotation and his knee is flexed slightly. Both exercises are performed with a pillow between his knees to prevent hip adduction/medial rotation in the range that elicits symptoms.

When in a prone position the patient performs hip medial rotation with his knee flexed. He is also instructed to avoid movements that elicit symptoms, which he can accomplish by positioning his hip appropriately and limiting the range into medial rotation.

When walking, the patient is instructed to minimize the degree of right hip lateral rotation. He is to rotate his hip as far toward neutral rotation as possible and yet avoid the onset of symptoms. His preferred hip alignment during walking is with his foot pointing almost 25 degrees laterally.

Outcome. The patient returns after 1 week and states that his symptoms are greatly improved; he now rates them at 2 to 3 on a scale of 10. He still cannot sit normally with his hips flexed and in a neutral position in the frontal plane. He is able to perform side-lying and prone exercises without difficulty or symptoms. His hip abduction exercise has progressed to performing it with his knee extended rather than flexed. The exercise is to be performed with his hip in neutral rotation.

The patient does not return to therapy for 4 weeks because of out-of-town summer travel. During this visit he is able to sit with his hip flexed and in neutral abduction/adduction. He can even slightly rotate his hip medially in the sitting position; his right hip medial rotation is 35 degrees in the prone position and he is able to extend his hip with his knee flexed without symptoms. He is able to walk for 1½ miles without symptoms. The patient is planning to resume his sporting activities, but he is instructed to do so slowly and progressively. He never returns for further evaluation.

Femoral Accessory Motion Hypermobility

Femoral accessory motion hypermobility is a syndrome that is found in patients who have early degenerative changes in their hip joint, but without a great loss of range of motion. In fact, careful examination indicates hypermobility of accessory motions. Although the physiologic motions will not be excessive in range and may even be slightly less than normal, particularly in rotation, the joint motions are not associated with the stiff, end-feel characteristic of advanced degenerative hip joint disease. In the patient with accessory motion hypermobility, impairments that occur with both medial and lateral rotation may be subtle and appear to be associated with superior glide of the femur. An associated diagnosis is degenerative hip joint disease in its early stages. These impairments can also be found in patients with hip pain but without radiologic evidence of joint changes. Some of these patients have tears of the labrum. The rotation is believed to be the result of ex-

cessive compression into the hip joint that occurs when the rectus femoris is stretched (hip extended position) and when the hamstrings are stretched (hip flexed position). The rotation is the femoral head following the path of least resistance. Distraction of the femur during the passive knee flexion and knee extension motion alleviate the rotation.

Symptoms and Pain
Symptoms include pain deep in the hip joint and in the anterior groin that may also extend along the medial and anterior thigh. Walking elicits pain, as well as a stiffness in the hip joint after resting and when initially walking.

Movement Impairments
The patient with femoral accessory motion hypermobility will walk with a slight antalgic gait. During single-leg stance the hip will rotate medially. During passive knee flexion in the prone position, monitoring of the greater trochanter indicates that femur will rotate laterally (not the pelvis but the femur) and occasionally superior glide will be detected. During hip lateral rotation in the prone position the greater trochanter will move through a wide arc, suggesting the femur may be flexing slightly. During knee extension in the sitting position the femur will rotate medially and appear to glide superiorly.

Alignment

- Structural variation: limited hip rotational range of motion
- Acquired impairment: slight hip flexion often with anterior pelvic tilt

Flexibility and Stiffness Impairments
Rotation and superior glide of the femur are movements that are more flexible than maintaining a constant position of the femoral head in the acetabulum. The rectus femoris and the hamstring muscles are stiffer than the iliopsoas and intrinsic hip rotator muscles.

Muscle and Recruitment Pattern Impairments
Hip motions are controlled more by muscles located primarily on the thigh than the muscles located primarily on the pelvis. Therefore the hamstring muscles are more dominant as hip extensors than the gluteus maximus. The rectus femoris and the tensor fascia lata muscles are more dominant as hip flexors than the iliopsoas muscles.

Impairments of muscle length and strength include a stiffness or shortness of both the hamstring and quadriceps muscles, which contributes to superior glide of the femur during knee flexion and knee extension. Manual muscle testing indicates weakness of the gluteus medius and iliopsoas muscles.

Confirming Tests

Motion in all directions elicits pain in the hip joint, and hip abduction/lateral rotation in hip flexion (Fabere's test) causes pain in the anterior groin, when there are early hip joint changes.

Intervention

PRIMARY OBJECTIVES. The primary objectives of an intervention program are to reduce the hypermobility of the accessory motions of the hip and to improve the extensibility of the quadriceps and hamstring muscles. The hypermobility of the accessory motions of the hip is most evident during knee flexion and hip lateral rotation when either is performed in the prone position and during knee extension when performed in the sitting position.

CORRECTIVE EXERCISE PROGRAM

Quadruped exercises. With hips abducted and slightly rotated laterally, the patient rocks backward and stops at the point when the femur begins to rotate laterally. Someone may need to monitor this movement of the femur because of its subtleness. The range of rocking backward should be limited to avoid stretching of the intrinsic hip lateral rotator muscles, the piriformis, obturators, and gemelli.

Prone exercises. The patient places the thumb and first finger around the femur at the greater trochanter to monitor its movement. The knee is flexed, but the movement is stopped when the patient perceives rotation of the femur. Distraction of the femur during knee flexion is helpful.

Side-lying exercises. The patient performs hip abduction in neutral flexion/extension and rotation.

Sitting exercises. The patient places the thumb and first finger around the proximal thigh laterally at the inguinal crease to monitor the motion of the femur. The knee is extended with minimal effort, and the motion is stopped when the femur rotates, which is usually medial. The patient uses his hands to lift the thigh to maximal hip flexion and then releases the hold on the thigh and uses his iliopsoas muscle to keep the hip flexed.

CORRECTING POSTURAL HABITS AND MOVEMENT PATTERNS. The major intervention is to teach the patient to monitor femoral movement and correct the performance of motions that elicit pain. All weight-training exercises of the quadriceps and hamstring muscles are eliminated. An emphasis is placed on improving the performance of the muscles that attach closest to the proximal end of the femur rather than to those muscles that attach more distally on the femur. Therefore the exercises emphasize the performance of the iliopsoas, gluteus medius, gluteus minimus, and intrinsic hip lateral rotator muscles as opposed to the rectus femoris, TFL, and hamstring muscles. The patient avoids exaggerated rotational motion of the hips when sitting or standing. This syndrome can also be found in cyclists. Cycling can hypertrophy the quadriceps and hamstring muscles without commensurate hypertrophy of the intrinsic hip girdle muscles and the iliopsoas. The medial rotation of the proximal femur can often be observed during cycling, particularly in the standing position. Taping the proximal femur in neutral rotation can assist in the retraining program.

Summary

In this syndrome, rotation and exaggerated accessory motions of anterior or superior glide occur during hip flexion and extension and during knee flexion and extension. The patient with degenerative hip joint disease, but without restriction to motion other than pain, experiences both medial and lateral rotation accompanied by subtle faults in accessory motions that occur more readily than they should. For example, the rotation can be observed with knee flexion in the prone position and with knee extension in the sitting position. Superior glide accompanies this rotation. Because the rotation and superior glide occurs when stretching either the quadriceps or hamstring muscles during knee extensions, stiffness of these muscles that contributes to joint compression is suggested as the cause of the movement impairments of the femur in the acetabulum. The wide arc of femoral head movement during hip lateral rotation in the prone position is another indicator of impaired accessory movement.

Case Presentation

History. A 43-year-old man is referred to physical therapy for instruction in a home exercise program for bilateral hip pain. His left hip is more painful than his right. Radiologic studies indicate that the patient has degenerative hip joint disease. He has been told that he should not perform any exercises that involve impact loading of his hip joints, such as jogging. The patient is a computer programmer. Approximately 6 years ago he began to jog regularly. He is most distressed that he has been advised to avoid this activity.

Symptoms. The patient experiences pain when he walks. He does not complain of pain when he sits, he experiences pain when he moves from a sitting to a standing position. He also has pain in his hips when he gets in and out of his car and occasionally when he sleeps.

Alignment Analysis. The patient stands 5 feet 10 inches tall. She has a stocky build with well-developed musculature. He does not perform any weight-training exercises, but he explains that his muscular appearance is characteristic of his family. He has a slight anterior pelvic tilt with increased lower lumbar curve. His iliac crest level is symmetrical, and his hip flexion is exaggerated by a slight flexion of the knee. A slight hip lateral rotation is also observed.

Movement Analysis. Tests are performed in the following five positions: (1) standing, (2) supine, (3) prone, (4) quadruped, and (5) sitting.

Standing. When standing, forward bending and the return motion are normal. When in a single-leg stance, a bilateral slight hip drop is observed.

Supine. The patient experiences pain in the anterior groin at 100 degrees of hip flexion with more intense pain on the left side than on the right side. He has pain in his anterior groin with hip abduction/lateral rotation from flexion in the supine position on both the left and right sides.

Prone. Hip lateral rotation and femoral superior glide with knee flexion is greater on his left side than on his right. In the prone position with the knee flexed, during lateral rotation of the hip, a wide arc of proximal femoral motion is evident during palpation at the level of the greater trochanter.

Quadruped. When the patient rocks backward while in the quadruped position, flexion of the lumbar spine is observed rather than hip flexion. There is lateral rotation of the proximal femurs as indicated by monitoring the greater trochanters but no motion of the distal femurs. With correction and repetition he is able to rock backward so that his hips flex to 115 degrees without lateral rotation and without pain.

Sitting. While in a sitting position, when the patient extends his left knee his left hip rotates medially, but during right knee extension his right hip does not rotate.

Muscle Length and Strength Analysis. The TFL and rectus femoris muscles are short bilaterally. The left and right hip abductor muscles test weak with ratings of 4−/5 and 4/5, respectively. The gluteus maximus muscles also test weak with a rating of 4/5 on both sides.

Diagnosis. Pain patterns are consistent with degenerative hip joint disease. The primary impairments of hip rotation and superior glide motion during knee flexion and extension are consistent with a diagnosis of femoral accessory motion hypermobility syndrome. The repeated motions of rotation and superior glide, as well as the excessive range of accessory motion of the femur, contribute to the patient's hip pain.

Intervention. The primary goal of this patient's therapeutic intervention program is to minimize (1) the excessive repetitions of hip rotation and superior glide during knee flexion and extension, and (2) the range of accessory motion of the femur. The patient is instructed in the correct performance of the following exercises:

- In the side-lying position: abduction of the hip with his knee extended

- In the prone position: knee flexion while monitoring the femur, stopping the flexion at the point the femur rotates laterally or moves superiorly
- In the prone position: hip extension to a neutral position with his knee flexed and a pillow under the abdomen
- In the quadruped position: rocking backward with an assistant to monitor the motion of the proximal femur by palpating the greater trochanter and stopping the motion at the point of rotation of the femur
- In the sitting position: knee extension without hip rotation or superior glide of the femur
- While walking: contraction of the gluteal muscles on heel strike

Outcome. The patient returns to therapy 2 weeks after his initial visit and states that he no longer has pain in his hips when walking and is not experiencing pain when moving from a sitting to a standing position. His exercises are reviewed, and his original movement impairments are no longer evident. The patient chose not to return for further intervention, since he is paying for the therapy directly. He is certain that he understands the exercises and knows that they are beneficial. He is encouraged to perform the exercises daily, particularly after riding his bike, which is his fitness exercise.

Femoral Hypomobility with Superior Glide

Femoral hypomobility with superior glide is a syndrome associated with degenerative hip joint disease with capsular signs. The passive and active ranges of hip flexion, extension, rotation, abduction, and adduction are markedly limited.

Symptoms and Pain

Pain with movement is usually felt deep in the joint and can be referred along the inner or anterior thigh. There is joint stiffness after rest. Later in the course of degeneration, there is pain at rest and at night. Because of the lack of hip extension, the patient with this syndrome usually demonstrates an exaggerated pelvic rotation or an anterior pelvic tilt during the stance phase of walking. An antalgic gait is present when the hip abductors are weak.

Movement Impairments

There is limited range of motion in all movement directions when performed both actively and passively. Hip flexion contractures and limited rotation are the most common faults. The patient with this syndrome will develop compensatory movements of lumbar extension and rotation while walking because of the restricted movement of the hip joint.

Alignment

Structural variations: none in particular

ACQUIRED IMPAIRMENTS

1. Anterior pelvic tilt and hip flexion
2. Limited hip joint range in all movement directions
3. Lack of hip extension, which affects alignment by contributing to pelvic tilt and/or rotation
4. Compensatory pelvic rotation caused by limited hip rotation. If the right hip is hypomobile, the pelvis may rotate clockwise so that the hip joint is in medial rotation.
5. Leg-length discrepancy from subchrondral collapse

Flexibility and Stiffness Impairments

The lumbar spine becomes more flexible than the hip joint.

Muscle and Recruitment Pattern Impairments

The primary recruitment problem is the dominant activity of the hip flexor muscles. During the early stages of this syndrome, avoiding hip flexor muscular activity and improving the participation of the hip extensor muscles can decrease symptoms. The restricted range of motion contributes to an acquired weakness of the hip abductor and extensor muscles.

Impairments of muscle length and strength may also be observed. The hypomobility of the joint itself prohibits distinguishing shortness of specific muscles.

Confirming Tests

With femoral hypomobility with superior glide there is a loss of range of motion in all directions, especially rotation, abduction, and adduction.

Summary

There is reduced joint space, particularly along the superior aspect of the joint. Although motion is lost in all directions, the loss of hip extension range causes gait impairments of excessive lumbar extension or pelvic rotation. Weakness of hip abductor muscles contributes to the antalgic gait.

Intervention

PRIMARY OBJECTIVES. The primary objective of an intervention program is maintaining as much range of motion and muscle strength as possible, because the loss of joint space is the major contributing factor that can limit range of motion.

CORRECTIVE EXERCISE PROGRAM

Standing exercises. Caudal long-axis distraction (inferior glide) is a component of intervention. One method of distraction is to stand on a raised level (such as a step) and suspend the involved leg with a 4- to 7-pound weight attached (depending on patient size and whether frail or in good physiologic condition). The patient should prevent the pelvis from dropping and just allow the weight to exert a downward pull on the hip. While the weight is pulling caudally on the lower extremity, the patient can try to rotate the hip medially and laterally within the pain-free range.

Supine exercises. Stretching the hip flexor muscles is important and can be accomplished by asking the patient to hold the opposite knee to his chest and contract his abdominal muscles while sliding the affected hip into extension. Contracting the hip extensor muscles, particularly the gluteus maximus muscle, can assist the range of motion into extension. Placing a weight on the ankle while in the hip flexor length testing position is not recommended because it can create an anterior-directed force on the femoral head. Instead, the patient should hold one knee to his chest while supine and then place a weight on the proximal femur near the inguinal crease. While the weight is on the anterior proximal thigh, the patient can assist the stretch by contracting his gluteus maximus muscle.

Quadruped exercises. If the patient can be placed in the quadruped position, rocking backward toward the heels is a better method to improve the range of hip flexion than pulling the knee to the chest in the supine position. Because of the limited hip flexion range, the patient should stop the backward motion when there is obvious rotation of the pelvis or spine. The patient should push backward with his hands to rock back toward his heels rather than contracting his hip flexors.

Prone exercises. While in a prone position the patient can perform three exercises: (1) knee flexion, (2) hip lateral rotation with knee flexion, and (3) hip abduction by sliding the lower extremity along a supporting surface. The therapist must ensure that the hip flexion contracture does not cause the patient to be in lumbar extension in the prone position. Therefore pillows usually have to be placed under the patient's abdomen.

Standing exercises. Strengthening the lower abdominal muscles can be accomplished by instructing the patient to stand with his or her back against the wall, allowing the hips and knees to flex to flatten the back. The patient should contract the abdominal muscles to keep the back against the wall while straightening the hips and knees.

Walking exercises. The patient is instructed to contract the gluteal muscles at heel strike and try to extend the hip. In the presence of a hip flexion contracture, the preferred compensatory motion is knee flexion rather than lumbar extension or rotation, which will ultimately cause back pain. Although not desirable, knee flexion when walking will not cause knee pain as readily as the compensatory lumbar motions will cause back pain.

Sitting exercises. If the hip flexes only 90 degrees, the patient can sit on a wedge, requiring less hip flexion.

Sitting-to-standing exercises. The patient should move to the front edge of the chair. To perform this movement the patient should push with his or her hand rather than actively flex the hips. The patient should straighten the hips and knees when rising and not rock forward by flexing the hips.

Case Presentation

History. A 58-year-old man is referred to physical therapy for evaluation and intervention of left hip pain. The patient is an executive who maintains an active exercise program that includes tennis, squash, and regular callisthenic exercises at his health club. Radiologic studies demonstrate that the patient has degenerative changes in his left hip, but he is reluctant to have hip joint replacement because, according to his physician, he would be unable to play tennis or to jog. The patient does not believe the pain is severe enough to justify a replacement. He attributes the development of his hip problem to an episode that occurred when he fell while water-skiing and during which he heard a loud "pop" sound. He had "some pain" for several weeks after the accident, but eventually the pain subsided. His only other orthopedic problem occurred 5 years earlier when he tore his heel cord; it was surgically repaired. The patient has not played tennis for 4 months before his physical examination because of hip pain at night and an increased stiffness during the day. Since he stopped playing tennis he has had minimal pain at night. His wife and friends have commented about the limp that is evident when he walks.

Symptoms. The patient has slight pain in his hip when he walks. His most intense pain occurs after sitting for a period of time and then standing and starting to walk. He also has experienced pain in the morning after rising and beginning to walk.

Alignment Analysis. The patient stands 5 feet 11 inches and has good muscle definition. His left hip is flexed but without anterior pelvic tilt, and his knee is flexed. His right hip is not flexed. Both hips are abducted in standing. If he places his feet together there is pain in his left hip. His right and left iliac crests are level, and his left buttock is notably smaller than his right.

Movement Analysis. Tests are performed in the following five positions: (1) standing, (2) supine, (3) prone, (4) quadruped, and (5) walking.

Standing. Forward bending is normally performed with 80 degrees of hip flexion with the knees flexed. During single-leg stance, the trunk sways laterally because of the abducted position of the hip.

Supine. In a supine position the patient's left hip flexion range of motion is limited to 100 degrees. He has pain at the end of the range. In the flexed position his hip is abducted and cannot be adducted. His right hip flexion range is within normal limits. His left hip abduction/lateral rotation in flexion causes pain in the anterior groin at 50% of the range of the same movement of the right hip.

Prone. During left knee flexion while in the prone position his pelvis anteriorly tilts and rotates counterclockwise and his hip abducts.

Quadruped. When rocking backward while in the quadruped position his pelvis shifts to the right because his right hip flexion range of motion is greater than his left hip flexion range of motion. His range of motion is limited to 100 degrees of left hip flexion and to slightly more flexion of the right hip in this position.

Walking. Hip extension is limited during walking; consequently, he has an exaggerated rotation of the pelvis during stance phase. No hip drop is evident.

Muscle Length and Strength Analysis. The left TFL, rectus femoris, and iliopsoas muscles are short. The hip joint is also a source of limitation, with hip extension limited to 30 degrees less than complete extension. The right hip flexor muscles are normal length. Left hip flexion is limited to 100 degrees. The left hip abductor muscles are short (-15 degrees of neutral). When analyzing the left hip, medial and lateral rotation are 10 and 15 degrees, respectively. When analyzing the right hip, medial and lateral rotation are 25 and 30 degrees, respectively. Specific muscle testing cannot be performed because of the limited hip motion.

Diagnosis. The diagnosis is femoral hypomobility syndrome with superior glide.

Intervention. The primary objectives of the intervention program are to increase the hip range of motion, particularly into extension, and improve the function of the gluteal muscles. Specific exercises in the supine, side-lying, prone, and quadruped positions, as well as during a sit-to-stand motion and walking, are prescribed.

While in a supine position the patient is instructed to hold his right knee to his chest and contract his abdominal muscles while sliding his left hip into extension and contracting the gluteal muscles to assist in hip extension. He is also to perform hip abduction/lateral rotation with the hip flexed, stopping the motion when he has pain in the groin.

In the side-lying position the patient slightly abducts his hip and then allows the extremity to adduct, maintaining this position for a count of 10 to 15. When lying prone the patient performs knee flexion while preventing pelvic motion. Another exercise in the prone position is hip rotation with the knee flexed. From a quadruped position the patient rocks backward with the hips abducted. The patient is instructed to stop at the point of uncontrollable weight shift to the right.

When moving from a sitting to a standing position, the patient contracts his buttock muscles and tries to straighten the hips as much as possible.

While walking, the patient is instructed to tighten his left buttock muscles at heel strike and continue to contract the muscles during the entire stance phase. The patient should actively use the calf muscles to push-off at the end of the stance phase.

The patient is advised to stop performing the bilateral hip flexion with knee extension exercise that he performed while hanging from a bar.

Outcome. The patient returns to physical therapy four times over an 8-week period. Only one exercise is added to his program. While in the prone position and with a pillow under his abdomen, the patient is instructed to perform hip extension with his knee flexed. By the end of this 8-week period, he no longer has hip flexion when standing. He can stand with his feet approximately 2 inches apart, and he can walk with minimal pelvic rotation. The contour of his left buttock is similar to his right, and he can flex his left hip to 120 degrees without pain. During a follow-up visit 3 months later, the patient is playing tennis, but he is not as competitive as he had once been. He does not experience pain at night unless he has been particularly active. He can walk for long distances, and his friends have noticed that he no longer limps. The patient returns 2 years later. Although a radiologic examination indicates that there has been additional deterioration, he maintains his sporting activities and experiences minimal pain. He continues to perform his exercise program on a daily basis.

Femoral Lateral Glide Syndrome With Short-Axis Distraction

Femoral lateral glide syndrome with short-axis distraction is similar to the hip adduction syndrome, except the laxity of the abductor muscles can be severe enough to cause the femoral head to glide laterally to the point of subluxation (i.e., short-axis distraction). When a patient is in the side-lying position, the greater trochanter is quite prominent, slightly anterior of midline, and distal of the center of the acetabulum when compared with the other hip in the same position. To position the femur correctly, the therapist has to flex, abduct, and rotate the femur laterally with one hand while guiding the proximal femur at the trochanter into the appropriate alignment in the acetabulum with the other hand. An associated diagnosis of femoral lateral glide syndrome is a "popping" hip, caused from subluxation.

Symptoms and Pain
The primary symptom of femoral lateral glide syndrome with short-axis distraction is hip pain, and most often the patient will readily demonstrate how he or she can make her hip "pop" while standing and performing a mo-

tion of abrupt hip adduction/medial rotation. This syndrome is most common in dancers, individuals with a congenital hypermobility syndrome, or young women who have had a congenital hip condition such as dislocation.

Movement Impairments
STANDING POSITION. In addition to self-initiated subluxation, the femur rotates medially and the hip adducts in a direction consistent with a weakness of the gluteus medius muscle during single-leg stance.

SUPINE POSITION. During hip and knee flexion the femur usually rotates medially. The straight-leg raise (hip flexion with knee extension) is associated with hip medial rotation, and the PICR does not maintain the normal, relatively constant position as indicated by the excessive superior and anterior path of the greater trochanter.

SIDE-LYING POSITION. During hip abduction, the hip flexes and rotates medially. When returning to the starting position, the hip adducts and rotates excessively medially. Monitoring the greater trochanter and comparing its motion with that of the contralateral trochanter during the same movement can detect the excessive caudal and medial excursion of the affected femur during eccentric hip adduction.

PRONE POSITION. During hip lateral rotation there is a wide axis of movement of the greater trochanter. During hip extension the greater trochanter rotates medially.

QUADRUPED POSITION. Monitoring the greater trochanter indicates that the femur may rotate medially as the patient rocks backward.

SITTING POSITION. Knee extension is often accompanied by hip medial rotation.

GAIT. During the stance phase of walking, there is an increased lateral sway of the pelvis or hip adduction of the affected hip. Medial rotation of the femur is also excessive during the stance phase of walking.

Summary
The primary impairment of femoral lateral glide syndrome with short-axis distraction is excessive hip adduction, which is excessive to the point of lateral or short-axis subluxation.

Alignment

STRUCTURAL VARIATIONS

1. Often a history of congenital hip dislocation
2. Wide pelvis
3. Prominent greater trochanters

ACQUIRED IMPAIRMENT

1. Apparent leg-length discrepancy with the iliac crest of the affected hip higher than the contralateral iliac crest

Flexibility and Stiffness Impairments

The range of motion of hip adduction and often of medial rotation is excessive. The hip joint is less stable than normal because the patient is able to actively sublux the hip.

Muscle and Recruitment Pattern Impairments

The hip flexor and medial rotator muscles are more dominant than the hip abductor and lateral rotator muscles. Impairments of muscle length and strength may also be observed. The gluteus medius and hip lateral rotator muscles are long and weak, and the TFL is short.

Confirming Tests

The alignment of the femur in the side-lying position and the patient's demonstration of hip subluxation both confirm the diagnosis of femoral lateral glide syndrome.

Intervention

PRIMARY OBJECTIVES. The primary goal of an intervention program is to eliminate the laxity of the hip abductor muscles and to avoid subluxation of the femur.

CORRECTIVE EXERCISE PROGRAM

Quadruped exercises. Exercises in the quadruped position should NOT be prescribed because they can further stretch the posterior muscles and joint capsule.

Supine exercises. While in a supine position the patient is instructed to flex the hip and knee actively while attempting to maintain the femur in a constant position of neutral with regard to rotation, thus preventing the anterior and medial movement of the greater trochanter.

Prone exercises. From a prone position the patient performs hip abduction with lateral rotation. With the hips and knees flexed and the hips rotated laterally to ensure that the medial side of the feet are touching, the patient performs isometric hip lateral rotation. A second exercise from the prone position is hip extension with the knee flexed.

Side-lying exercises. While in a side-lying position the patient performs hip abduction with a slight lateral rotation. There should be enough pillows between the knees to ensure that the hip does not adduct past the midline of the body on return to the starting position.

Sitting exercises. If the hip rotates medially during knee extension, the patient should practice performing knee extension without allowing hip rotation.

Standing exercises. The patient is instructed to contract the hip abductor/lateral rotator muscles during single-leg standing and to avoid hip adduction/medial rotation.

CORRECTING POSTURAL HABITS AND MOVEMENT PATTERNS. The patient is instructed to avoid crossing his or her legs when sitting and to avoid standing with the hip in adduction. In the side-lying position the patient should place pillows between the knees to prevent the hip from adducting and rotating medially. Lastly, he or she should avoid "popping" the hip.

Case Presentation

History. A 24-year-old female graduate student is experiencing a deep aching pain in her left hip, primarily during and just after running distances of 1 to 2 miles. She also has slight pain when walking, particularly during distances of 3 to 5 miles. She participates in a variety of intramural sports. The patient reports and demonstrates that she can make her hip "pop" by a rapid voluntary motion of adduction and medial rotation while in a standing position. She also reports that when she was an infant, there was something "wrong" with her hip, which caused her to wear a brace at night. There has not been an orthopedic follow-up because her mother believed that her daughter's hip problem was satisfactorily resolved when she was an infant.

Symptoms. The patient has been running distances of 2 miles with a frequency of five to seven times a week until her hip pain started to increase. She has stopped running but still participates in intramural sports. When the pain is at its worst, she rates its intensity as 3 on a scale of 10. As long as she avoids running or walking long distances, she is free of pain.

Alignment Analysis. When the patient stands her left iliac crest is 1/2 inch higher than her right. Pelvic tilt in the sagittal plane is neutral. Her left lateral thigh in the area of the trochanter appears to be larger than the same area of the right hip, and she has slight valgus of both lower extremities and a rigid foot with a high instep.

Movement Analysis. The following tests are performed with the patient (1) standing, (2) in a quadruped position, (3) lying supine, (4) in a side-lying position, (5) prone, (6) sitting, and (7) walking.

Standing. When the patient is instructed to bend forward to return to the upright position and to laterally flex her trunk, she does not report any symptoms and movement impairments are not observed. When the patient stands on the left lower extremity, there is notable hip adduction that is not evident when she stands on the right lower extremity.

Quadruped. When assessing her alignment in the quadruped position, the left side of her pelvis is higher than the right side and her femur is slightly rotated medially. When she is asked to rock backward, monitoring of the greater trochanter indicates that her left femur rotates slightly medially. Her pelvis also moves slightly to the left; consequently, her left hip flexes slightly more than her right.

Supine. Resistance to passive hip flexion is not felt, and her bilateral range of motion is 125 degrees. There is some tendency for the left hip to rotate medially at the end of the hip flexion range. When performing hip abduction/lateral rotation from hip flexion, there is a slight sensation of pinching at the posterolateral aspect of her left femur by the trochanter at the end range of the motion. Compensatory pelvic rotation is not noted. The left hip rotates medially during a straight-leg raise.

Side-lying. In the side-lying position the left hip adducts and medially rotates excessively. When the patient is in the same side-lying position, her left greater trochanter appears to be more distal and anterior in relation to the acetabulum than her right greater trochanter. The right hip does not adduct or rotate medially to the same degree as the left. When the left hip is placed in the proper position for testing abductor strength, the therapist is required to flex and abduct the hip and to manually reposition the left greater trochanter to achieve correct alignment of the femur in relation to the acetabulum.

Prone. When the patient is asked to extend her hip with the knee extended while in a prone position, the left gluteus maximus does not change in contour until the hip extends to almost 10 degrees. The right gluteus maximus and hamstring muscles contract simultaneously, based on the change in contour of the muscles. During hip lateral rotation, there is a wide arc of motion of the left greater trochanter. The left hip lateral rotation range of motion is 35 degrees. The right greater trochanter does not demonstrate this wide arc of movement during hip lateral rotation. The right hip lateral rotation range of motion is also 35 degrees.

Sitting. During left knee extension in a sitting position, the hip rotates medially, which is evident when the therapist places his or her hand on the anterior thigh as the patient extends her knee.

Walking. During the left stance phase of gait, hip medial rotation is exaggerated and hip adduction (hip drop) is evident. None of these gait impairments are evident during the right stance phase of gait.

Muscle Length and Strength Analysis. The left TFL-ITB is short. During the hip flexor length test, her hip must be abducted 25 degrees to achieve complete hip extension; less than 5 degrees of hip abduction is required to achieve complete hip extension on the right. Not one of the other hip flexor muscles is short. The left hip abductor muscles are weak, grading 4−/5. The right hip abductor muscles are normal, grading 5/5. The left PGM is particularly weak and rates 3+/5, and the patient has a difficult time preventing hip medial rotation when placed in the test position. The left and right hip adductor muscles both grade 5/5, but the left and right gluteus maximus muscles grade 4/5 and 5/5, respectively.

Diagnosis. The diagnosis is femoral lateral glide syndrome. The key findings that support this diagnosis

are (1) the patient's ability to "pop" or subluxate her hip; and (2) the fact that the therapist must guide the greater trochanter manually while abducting and rotating the hip laterally to position the hip correctly while the patient is lying on her side. In this side-lying position the hip appears excessively rotated medially and it adducts. Also, the position of the greater trochanter is distal and anterior compared with the other trochanter when the patient lies in this position. The pain in the hip joint develops because of the excessive motion of the femoral head, particularly during activities that require strong control of the femur during the stance phase (e.g., running).

Intervention. The primary goals of the patient's intervention program are to avoid the lateral glide position of the femoral head and to shorten and strengthen the hip abductor lateral rotator muscles.

While in a supine position, the patient is instructed to hold her right knee to her chest to flatten her back. She is also instructed to tilt her pelvis posteriorly and slide her left lower extremity into extension and abduction while maintaining hip lateral rotation. The purpose of this exercise is to stretch her TFL-ITB.

From a side-lying position the patient places pillows between her legs that are high enough to avoid hip adduction and performs hip abduction while maintaining hip lateral rotation. She is instructed to keep her hip as extended as possible while avoiding lumbar extension. She is instructed to position her pelvis in slight anterior rotation so that she is performing hip abduction in slight extension and against gravity.

When in a prone position the patient's hips are abducted and laterally rotated, the knees are flexed, and the medial sides of both feet are touching. The patient isometrically performs hip lateral rotation by pressing her feet together. In the prone position with her knees flexed, the patient is also instructed to perform hip lateral rotation to stretch the TFL-ITB.

While standing on the left leg, the patient is instructed to contract her left gluteal muscles to prevent hip medial rotation and hip drop. When walking, the patient is instructed to contract her left gluteal muscles at heel strike to prevent hip drop and medial rotation.

To correct postural habits, the patient is instructed to place a pillow between her legs when lying on her side, avoiding hip abduction and medial rotation. She is also advised to avoid sitting with her legs crossed. When moving from a sitting to a standing position, as well as when moving in the reverse direction, she is instructed to keep her knees pointed straight ahead and to avoid letting her hips rotate medially. She is also advised to make a conscious effort to contract her gluteal muscles when moving from a sitting position to a standing posture.

Outcome. Because the patient had not been running at the time of her initial visit, she did not report symptoms. After this first visit she returns 1 week later to check the accuracy with which she is performing her exercises. She has been performing all of them correctly, and the strength of her left PGM muscle improved to a rating of 4−/5. Approximately 3 weeks after her first visit she is allowed to start jogging for only 1 minute and then to walk for 1 minute, alternating for a total of 20 minutes. She is to limit her jogging to every other day for only 3 days a week. She can walk for 30 minutes on the other 4 days. During the jogging and walking routine she is instructed to contract her gluteal muscles at heel strike. After 2 weeks on this schedule the patient has increased her jogging to 2 minutes with 1 minute of walking, and the overall time has been increased to 30 minutes. Observing the patient while jogging indicates that she is able to control the hip drop and medial rotation. After another 2 weeks she is allowed to jog for 5 minutes and walk for 1 minute and increase the overall frequency to four times a week on an every-other-day schedule. Approximately 3 months after her initial visit, the patient no longer demonstrates a shortness of her TFL-ITB and her hip abductor muscles test 5/5. She is told that she can jog for 20 minutes at a time and that she can increase the duration of her running as long as the activity does not elicit symptoms and as long as she can continue to prevent hip medial rotation and abduction. Approximately 1 month after her last visit the patient reports that she is running for 30 minutes four times a week and is not experiencing any symptoms.

Conclusion

Based on the author's experience in treating patients referred to physical therapy for hip pain, this chapter offers movement impairment syndromes of the hip in the order of the frequency in which they have been observed. However, the actual distribution of these syndromes needs verification by a larger database.

References

1. Bogduk N, Pearcy M, Hadfield G: Anatomy and biomechanics of psoas major, *Clin Biomech* 7:109, 1992.

2. Deusinger R: Validity of pelvic tilt measurements in anatomical neutral position, *J Biomech* 25:764, 1992.

3. Ebrall PS: Some antropometric dimensions of male adolescents with idiopathic low back pain, J Manipulative Physiol Ther 17:296, 1994.

4. Fagerson TL: *The hip handbook*, Boston 1998, Butterworth-Heinemann.

5. Freiberg AH, Vinke TH: Sciatica and sacro-iliac joint, *J Bone Joint Surg Am* 16:126, 1934.

6. Gelberman RH, Cohen MS, Hekhar S et al: Femoral anteversion, *J Bone Joint Surg Br* 69-B:75, 1987.

7. Goldman JM et al: An electromyographic study of the abdominal muscles during postural and respiratory maneuvers, *J Neurol Neurosurg Psychiatry* 50:866, 1987.

8. Inman VT, Ralston HJ, Todd F: *Human walking*, Baltimore, 1981, Williams & Wilkins.

9. Jukar D et al: Quantitative intramuscular myoelectric activity of lumbar portions of psoas and the abdominal wall during a wide variety of tasks, *Med Sci Sports Exerc* 30:301, 1998.

10. Kaplan EB: The iliotibial tract, *J Bone Joint Surg Am* 40A(4):817, 1958.

11. Kendall FP, McCreary EK, Provance PG: *Muscles, testing and function*, ed 4, Baltimore, 1993, Williams & Wilkins.

12. Lieb FJ, Perry J: Quadriceps function: an EMG study under isometric conditions, *J Bone Joint Surg Am* 53:749, 1971.

13. Merriam WF et al: A study revealing a tall pelvis in subjects with low back pain, *J Bone Joint Surg Br* 65B:153, 1983.

14. Mueller MJ et al: Relationship of plantar-flexor peak torque and dorsiflexion range of motion to kinetic variables during walking, *Phys Ther* 75:684, 1995.

15. Norkin CC, Levangie PK: *Joint structure and function: a comprehensive analysis*, ed 2, Philadelphia, 1992, FA Davis.

16. Pare EB, Stern JT, Schwartz JM: Functional differentiation within the tensor fascia latae: a telemetered electromyographic analysis of its locomotor roles, *J Bone Joint Surg Am* 63(9):1457, 1981.

17. Pritchard B: Get hip, *Golf Magazine* August:78, 1993.

18. Reid DC: *Sports injury assessment and rehabilitation*, Edinburgh, UK, 1992, Churchill Livingstone.

19. Richardson C et al: *Therapeutic exercise for spinal segmental stabilization in low back pain*, Sydney, 1999, Churchill-Livingstone.

20. Ruwe PA, Gage JR, Ozonoff MB, Deluca PA: Clinical determination of femoral anteversion: a comparison with established techniques, J *Bone Joint Surg Am* 74:820, 1992.

21. Shields RK, Heiss DG: An electromyographic comparison of abdominal muscle synergies during curl and double straight leg lowering exercises with control of the pelvic position, *Spine* 22(16):1873, 1997.

22. *Stedman's Dictionary*, Baltimore, 1997, Williams & Wilkins.

Chapter 4
Appendix

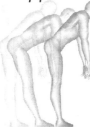

FEMORAL ANTERIOR GLIDE SYNDROME

Without Medial Rotation

The primary movement dysfunction in this syndrome is insufficient posterior glide of the femur during hip flexion. The stiffness of the hip extensors and posterior hip joint structures and the excessive flexibility of the anterior hip joint structures as the result of maintained hip extension create a path of least resistance of anterior glide.

SYMPTOMS AND HISTORY

- Groin pain with hip flexion or standing
- May experience generalized hip pain
- Often occurs in younger people, distance runners, dancers, martial arts (stance leg)

KEY TESTS AND SIGNS

Standing alignment

- Posterior tilt, hip extension, knee hyperextension, decreased gluteal definition

Supine position

HIP AND KNEE FLEXION

- *Active:* Increased pain after 90 degrees
- *Passive:* If posteroinferior glide is applied at the inguinal crease, stiffness is evident and range of pain-free flexion increases

STRAIGHT-LEG RAISE

- *Active:* Slight deviation of PICR indicated by greater trochanter
- *Passive:* If posteroinferior glide is applied at the inguinal crease, stiffness increases and range decreases
- At maximum hip flexion, patient actively contracts hip flexors; results in deviation of greater trochanter

Prone hip and knee extension

- Anterior displacement of the greater trochanter
- Onset of gluteal maximus contraction after hip extension is 50% of complete range of motion

Manual muscle test

- Weak iliopsoas (may be weak and painful), weak gluteal maximus

Quadruped position

- Pelvis on the involved side appears higher (less than 90 degrees of hip flexion); hip on the affected side does not flex as easily as the hip on the other side; as a result, pelvis tilts during rocking backward

ASSOCIATED SIGNS
(contributing factors)

Long iliopsoas muscles

Short hamstring muscles

Short TFL-ITB

Gait: knee hyperextended

Habit of sitting with legs crossed

DIFFERENTIAL MOVEMENT AND ASSOCIATED DIAGNOSES

Movement diagnoses

- Femoral anterior glide with medial rotation

- Femoral anterior glide with lateral rotation

- Femoral accessory hypermobility

Associated diagnosis

- Iliopsoas tendinopathy iliopsoas bursitis

SCREENING FOR POTENTIAL MEDICAL DIAGNOSES REQUIRING REFERRAL

- Avascular necrosis

- Osteoarthritis

- *Stress fractures:*
  Lesser trochanter
  Proximal medial femur
  Pubic symphysis

- Iliopsoas abscess

- Spinal cord tumor

- Ascites

- Hemophilia (GI bleeding)

- Aortic aneurysm

- Ureteral pain

- Interior oblique avulsion

- Pubalgia

- Osteitis pubis

- Inguinal hernia

- Pelvic organ prolapse

GI, Gastrointestinal; *PICR,* path of the instant center of rotation.

Chapter 4
Appendix

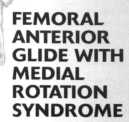

FEMORAL ANTERIOR GLIDE WITH MEDIAL ROTATION SYNDROME

The primary movement dysfunction in this syndrome is insufficient posterior glide and excessive medial rotation of the femur during hip flexion. An impaired PICR of the hip joint occurs as indicated by upward and medial movement of the greater trochanter during hip flexion. There is failure of the hip flexor lateral rotators to counteract the hip flexor medial rotators. The stiffness of the hip extensors and posterior hip joint structures and the excessive flexibility of the anterior hip joint structures as the result of maintained hip extension create a path of least resistance of anterior glide.

SYMPTOMS AND HISTORY

- Groin pain during active hip flexion
- Groin pain may progress to aching pain of whole hip
- Often seen in runners, dancers, martial arts (kicking leg) participants, soccer players

KEY TESTS AND SIGNS

Standing alignment

- Posterior tilt, hip extension, and medial rotation; knee hyperextension, decreased gluteal definition

Standing on one leg

- Observed medial rotation

Active and passive straight-leg raises

- *Active:* See anteromedial deviation of PICR of greater trochanter (may be painful)
- *Passive:* If posteroinferior glide is applied at the inguinal crease, stiffness is evident and range of pain-free flexion increases
- Place at end range, ask patient to hold; observe anterior glide

Hip and knee flexion

- *Active:* Increased pain after 90 degrees
- *Passive:* If posteroinferior glide is applied at the inguinal crease, stiffness is evident and range of pain-free flexion increases; range may also increase with lateral rotation

Prone hip and knee extension (severe cases)

- Anterior displacement of the greater trochanter
- Onset of gluteus maximus after initiation of hip extension

Quadruped position

- Pelvis on the involved side appears higher at less than 90 degrees of hip flexion; femur does not glide posteriorly or flex easily during backward rocking

MMT

- Weak or weak and painful iliopsoas, posterior gluteus medius, or intrinsic hip lateral rotators; weak gluteus maximus

Sitting position

- *Knee extension:* Observe hip medial rotation with lateral rotation; range decreases or movement into extension is slower

ASSOCIATED SIGNS
(contributing factors)

- Apparent leg-length discrepancy
- Asymmetric hamstring muscles (medial shorter than lateral)
- Medial hamstring muscles recruited over lateral hamstring muscles
- Shortened length of TFL-ITB
- *Acquired faults:* Ankle pronation
- *Structural variations:*
  Femoral antetorsion
  Retroversion
  Genu valgus
- *Gait:*
  Hip medial rotation
  Knee hyperextension

DIFFERENTIAL MOVEMENT AND ASSOCIATED DIAGNOSES

Movement diagnoses

- Femoral accessory hypermobility
- Femoral anterior glide
- Femoral anterior glide with lateral rotation
- Hip adduction with medial rotation

Associated diagnoses

- Iliopsoas tendinopathy
- Iliopsoas bursitis
- Obturator internus trigger point
- Snapping hip syndrome

SCREENING FOR POTENTIAL MEDICAL DIAGNOSES REQUIRING REFERRAL

- Avascular necrosis
- Osteoarthritis
- *Stress fractures:*
  Lesser trochanter
  Proximal medial femur
  Pubic symphysis
- Iliopsoas abscess
- Spinal cord tumor
- Ascites
- Hemophilia (GI bleeding)
- Aortic aneurysm
- Ureteral pain
- Interior oblique avulsion
- Pubalgia
- Osteitis pubis
- Inguinal hernia
- Pelvic organ prolapse

GI, Gastrointestinal; *MMT,* manual muscle test; *PICR,* path of the instant center of rotation; *TFL-ITB,* tensor fascia lata–iliotibial band.

Chapter 4
Appendix

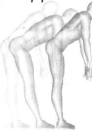

FEMORAL ANTERIOR GLIDE WITH LATERAL ROTATION SYNDROME

Faulty standing alignment (hip extension and lateral rotation) causes the head of the femur to push into anterior structures. The stiffness of the hip extensors, the stretched anterior joint structures, and the dominance of the hamstring muscles over the gluteal maximus contributes to excessive anterior glide of the femoral head during extension.

SYMPTOMS AND HISTORY

- Groin pain with hip extension and lateral rotation; worse in weight bearing (e.g., running, jumping)
- Pain may be located more medially than in anterior glide with medial rotation syndrome
- Participation in activities (e.g., ice skating, soccer, ice hockey) with emphasis on lateral rotation and abduction
- *Incidence:* Moderate to frequent

KEY TESTS AND SIGNS

Standing alignment

- Posterior pelvic tilt, hip extension and lateral rotation, knee hyperextension (pain may decrease with medial rotation)

Supine position

- *Hip and knee flexion:* Observe lateral rotation and short gluteus maximus
- Stiffness noted during hip flexion

Manual muscle test

- Weak iliopsoas muscle (may be weak and painful)

Prone position

- *Hip and knee extension:* Anterior displacement of greater trochanter (in severe cases)
- Onset of gluteus maximus after initiation of hip extension
- *Hip rotation:* Limited medial rotation (short lateral rotator muscles)

Quadruped position

- Pelvis on the involved side appears higher than the other side because that hip is not as flexed and does not flex as easily during backward rocking (femur does not easily glide posteriorly)
- *Hip lateral rotation:* Alignment and movement improve

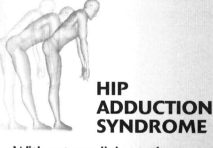

HIP ADDUCTION SYNDROME

Without medial rotation

Excessive hip adduction and overstretch of the superior and posterolateral capsule of the hip is the result of impaired alignment in standing activities. There is an impaired recruitment pattern of hip adductor muscles over abductor muscles for control of the pelvis.

SYMPTOMS AND HISTORY

- Buttock pain or lateral thigh pain during standing, walking, stair climbing, sitting-to-standing movement, or occasionally sitting with legs crossed
- May report pain along inner thigh or medial groin area
- History of sleeping in the side-lying position (hip in adduction)

KEY TESTS AND SIGNS

Manual muscle test

- Weak primary hip abductor muscles (gluteus medius, gluteus minimus)

Standing on one leg

- Hip adduction (drop) or lateral trunk flexion

Gait

- Hip adduction (drop)

Resisted test

PATIENTS WITH BUTTOCK OR LATERAL THIGH PAIN

- Weak and painful hip abduction
- Strong hip adductors muscles

PATIENTS WITH INNER THIGH PAIN

- Both hip abductor and adductor muscles may be weak and painful

ASSOCIATED SIGNS
(contributing factors)

- *Standing on one leg:* Observe lateral rotation
- *Supine hip abduction and lateral rotation in flexion:* May produce groin pain
- Short hamstring muscles
- Weakness of gluteus maximus, anterior gluteus medius and minimus
- *Structural variations:* Femoral retroversion, tibial torsion, rigid foot (history of exercises to include lateral rotation with antetorsion of the hips)
- Habit of sitting with legs crossed (foot on thigh)

DIFFERENTIAL MOVEMENT AND ASSOCIATED DIAGNOSES

Movement diagnoses
- Femoral accessory hypomobility with superior glide
- Femoral accessory hypermobility
- Femoral anterior glide
- Hip adduction syndrome

Associated diagnoses
- Iliopsoas tendinopathy or bursitis
- Adductor muscle strain or tendinopathy

SCREENING FOR POTENTIAL MEDICAL DIAGNOSES REQUIRING REFERRAL

- Avascular necrosis
- Osteoarthritis
- *Stress fractures:*
    Lesser trochanter
    Proximal medial femur
    Pubic symphysis
- Iliopsoas abscess
- Spinal cord tumor
- Ascites
- Hemophilia (gastrointestinal bleeding)
- Aortic aneurysm
- Ureteral pain
- Interior oblique avulsion
- Pubalgia
- Osteitis pubis
- Inguinal hernia
- Pelvic organ prolapse

ASSOCIATED SIGNS
(contributing factors)

- *Standing alignment:* Increased hip adduction
- Habit of standing in hip add with increased weight bearing on involved lower extremity
- Apparent leg-length discrepancy (pain on side of high iliac crest)
- Short adductor muscles (less than 35 degrees of hip abduction)
- *Structural variations:* Broad pelvis, prominence of greater trochanter, genu valgus, pronated feet

DIFFERENTIAL MOVEMENT AND ASSOCIATED DIAGNOSES

Movement diagnoses
- Low back syndrome
- Hip adduction with medial rotation
- Femoral lateral glide

Associated diagnoses
- Gluteal medius strain or tendinopathy
- Adductor strain or tendinopathy
- Trochanteric bursitis
- Iliotibial band fasciitis
- Ischiogluteal bursitis

SCREENING FOR POTENTIAL MEDICAL DIAGNOSES REQUIRING REFERRAL

- *Patients with buttock or lateral thigh pain:*
    Peripheral neuropathy
    Neurogenic claudication
    Neoplasm
    Disk protrusion
- *Stenosis:*
    Osteophyte formation
    Thickening ligament
- *Patients with inner thigh or medial groin pain:*
    Hip joint pathologic condition (e.g., early stage osteoarthritis) or avascular necrosis
    Stress fracture (pubic symphysis or lesser trochanter)
    Iliopsoas abscess

Chapter 4
Appendix

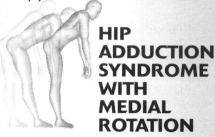

HIP ADDUCTION SYNDROME WITH MEDIAL ROTATION

Lack of posterolateral stabilization of the proximal femur is caused by impaired positioning and overstretch of the posterolateral capsule and muscles of the hip. The impaired movement is exaggerated hip adduction and medial rotation with recruitment of the hip adductor muscles over the abductor muscles for control of the pelvis and hip medial rotators over lateral rotators. In some cases, the lengthened piriformis muscle may compress the sciatic nerve (lengthened piriformis syndrome). The syndrome may also be associated with inflammation of the ITB from overuse of the TFL-ITB (recruitment of TFL-ITB for hip abduction and flexion).

SYMPTOMS AND HISTORY

- Posterior lateral hip pain; *or*
- Sciatica (no low back pain, lengthened piriformis syndrome); *or*
- Aching or burning pain along lateral thigh (ITB); *or*
- Pain along inner thigh or medial groin area
- Pain occurs with weight on the lower extremity (e.g., standing, walking, stair climbing, sitting-to-standing movement, prolonged sitting, occasionally sitting with legs crossed)
- History of a fall or surgery (soft tissue damage to gluteal muscles present)
- *Incidence:* Infrequent to moderate

KEY TESTS AND SIGNS

Standing alignment

- Hip adduction and medial rotation
- Habit of standing in hip adduction with increased weight bearing on involved lower extremity; apparent leg length discrepancy (pain on side of high iliac crest)
- Pain decreases with increased hip lateral rotation or gluteal contraction

Gait

- Trendelenburg's or antalgic test

Standing on one leg

- Hip adduction (drop)

Ober's test

- *Short TFL-ITB:* Observe prominence of the greater trochanter if hip is in adduction and medial rotation; may be painful in patients with lateral thigh pain

Manual muscle test

- Weak or weak and painful; lateral rotation, gluteus medius, gluteus maximus

Prone hip rotation

- Increased medial rotation

Functional mobility

- Medial rotation associated with gait, sitting-to-standing movement, stair climbing

Patients with sciatica

Supine position

- *Hip flexion, adduction, medial rotation:* May reproduce pain

Slump test

- May be positive
- Resisted knee flexion (hamstring muscles): Negative strong and painless

Patients with lateral thigh pain

Supine position

- *Hip flexion, abduction, lateral rotation:* Reproduces pain with limited range; range increases and pain decreases if repeated
- *Resisted TFL:* Weak and painful
- *Palpation of ITB:* Tenderness

ASSOCIATED SIGNS
(contributing factors)

- *Muscle length:* Short adductor muscle
- *Structural variations:*
  Broad pelvis, prominent greater trochanter
  Femoral antetorsion, genu valgus, ankle pronation, hallux valgus
  Sleeping position is often side-lying with hip in medial rotation and adduction
- *Patients with lateral thigh pain:*
  May experience numbness along lateral lower leg
  Numbness may be reproduced with inversion of the ankle during the modified Ober's test
  May experience weakness in quadriceps and iliopsoas muscles

DIFFERENTIAL MOVEMENT AND ASSOCIATED DIAGNOSES

Movement diagnoses
- Low back syndrome with radiating symptoms
- Hip adduction syndrome
- Hip extension with medial rotation
- Hip extension with knee extension
- Femoral lateral glide
- Hip lateral rotation syndrome

Associated diagnoses
- Lengthened piriformis
- Sciatica
- Hamstring strain
- Ischiogluteal bursitis
- ITB fasciitis
- Gluteal medius strain or tendinopathy
- Trochanteric bursitis
- Snapping hip syndrome
- Superior iliac region dysfunction
- Obturator internus strain
- Adductor strain
- Posterior facet syndrome
- Fibromyalgia

SCREENING FOR POTENTIAL MEDICAL DIAGNOSES REQUIRING REFERRAL

- *Patients with sciatica:*
  Disk herniation
  Stenosis
  Neoplasm
  Diabetic neuropathy
  Megacolon
  Pregnancy
  Staph infection
  Intrapelvic aneurysm
  Abscess
- *Patients with lateral thigh pain:*
  Stenosis
- *Patients with medial thigh pain:*
  Hip joint pathologic condition (early stages osteoarthritis) or avascular necrosis
  Stress fracture (pubic symphysis or lesser trochanter)
  Iliopsoas abscess

ITB, Iliotibial band; *TFL,* tensor fascia lata;
TFL-ITB, tensor fascia lata–iliotibial band.

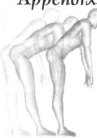

FEMORAL LATERAL GLIDE SYNDROME

The movement dysfunction in this syndrome is associated with a lateral glide or short axis distraction of the femoral head. It is usually a progression in severity from the hip adduction or hip adduction with medial rotation syndrome or associated with femoral hypermobility syndrome.

SYMPTOMS AND HISTORY

- Deep hip pain
- Popping hip
- Active subluxation by sudden hip adduction and medial rotation (may have habit of "popping" hip in standing)
- May report general hyperflexibility
- *Incidence:* Moderate to frequent
- Occurs in dancers or activity with excessive stretching (e.g., yoga)

KEY TESTS AND SIGNS

Standing alignment
- Hip adduction

Standing on one leg
- Observe hip adduction and may see exaggerated lateral glide

Side-lying position
- Greater trochanter appears prominent, anterior and distal, compared with the greater trochanter of the other hip; correct by placing hip in flexion, abduction, lateral rotation position and guiding proximal femur into the joint

Manual muscle test
- Primary hip abductors and lateral rotators are weak

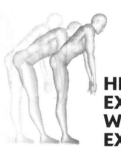

HIP EXTENSION WITH KNEE EXTENSION

Hamstring strain

Hip extension is the primary movement dysfunction in this syndrome associated with a dominance of the hamstring muscles over the gluteus maximus. The syndrome may also be associated with a dominance of the hamstring muscles over the quadriceps during a combination of hip extension with knee extension.

SYMPTOMS AND HISTORY

- Pain along ischial tuberosity, in the hamstring muscle belly or at the insertion
- May be sudden (i.e., trauma) or insidious onset
- Pain with gait, stairs, running
- Often occurs with athletes

KEY TESTS AND SIGNS

Standing alignment
- Hip extension and knee hyperextension

Gait
- Observe knee hyperextension heelstrike to flat foot

Resisted test for hamstring in prone or end range of straight-leg raise
- Increased pain (strong and painful or weak and painful)

Passive stretch
- *Hip flexion with knee extension (straight-leg raise):* Increased pain

Palpation
- Point tender on hamstring muscle belly—origin or insertion

Steps up or down
- Poor knee control (decreased muscle performance of quadriceps muscles)

Prone hip extension and knee extended
- Onset of gluteus maximus after initiation of hip extension
- Weak gluteus maximus with manual muscle test

Functional mobility
- *Stair climbing and sitting-to-standing movement:* Observe knee back to body as the knee is extended with foot fixed (hamstring over quadriceps muscles)

ASSOCIATED SIGNS
(contributing factors)

- *Muscle length:*
  Lengthened hip abductors
  Lengthened hip lateral rotators
  Short tensor fascia lata–iliotibial band
- Sleeping position with hip in adduction and medial rotation
- Habit of sitting with legs crossed
- *Structural variations:*
  Broad pelvis, prominent greater trochanter
  Femoral antetorsion, genu valgus, ankle pronation
  Hallux valgus

DIFFERENTIAL MOVEMENT AND ASSOCIATED DIAGNOSES

Movement diagnoses

- Hip adduction syndrome
- Hip adduction with medial rotation syndrome

Associated diagnoses

- Trochanteric bursitis
- Snapping hip syndrome
- Hypermobility syndrome

SCREENING FOR POTENTIAL MEDICAL DIAGNOSES REQUIRING REFERRAL

- Hip joint pathologic conditions (early stage of osteoarthritis) or avascular necrosis
- Stress fractures (pubic symphysis, lesser trochanter)
- Iliopsoas abscess

ASSOCIATED SIGNS
(contributing factors)

- Shortened length of hamstrings and gastrocnemius muscles
- May observe bruising in hamstring muscles
- *Standing alignment:* Swayback posture
- *Return from forward bending:* Hips sway forward; ankles dorsiflex; upper body momentum and ankle dorsiflexion are used more than gluteus maximus and rotation around the hip axis; greater rotation around the hip and less about the ankles are the ideal

DIFFERENTIAL MOVEMENT AND ASSOCIATED DIAGNOSES

Movement diagnoses

- Hip extension with medial rotation
- Proximal tibiofibular glide syndrome
- Hip adduction with medial rotation
- Low back syndrome

Associated diagnoses

- Sciatica
- Hamstrings strain
- Piriformis syndrome
- Ischiogluteal bursitis

SCREENING FOR POTENTIAL MEDICAL DIAGNOSES REQUIRING REFERRAL

- *Patients with sciatica or posterior thigh pain:*
  Disk herniation
  Stenosis
  Neoplasm
  Diabetic neuropathy
  Megacolon
  Pregnancy
  Staph infection
  Intrapelvic aneurysm
  Abscess

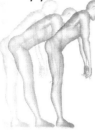

HIP EXTENSION WITH MEDIAL ROTATION

Hamstring strain

Hip extension with medial rotation is the primary movement dysfunction in this syndrome. The syndrome is also associated with recruitment of the biceps femoris for hip lateral rotation rather than recruitment of the intrinsic hip lateral rotator muscles.

SYMPTOMS AND HISTORY

- Pain along ischial tuberosity in the hamstring muscle belly or at the insertion
- Insidious onset is often sudden (i.e., trauma)
- Pain with gait, stair climbing, running
- Occurs most often in athletes, especially runners

KEY TESTS AND SIGNS

Standing alignment
- Hip medial rotation

Standing on one leg
- Observe increased hip medial rotation

Tests for soft tissue differential diagnosis
- Resisted contraction of the hamstring muscle is positive for pain when tested in prone or supine position (SLR) positions
- Hamstring muscles may be strong or weak

Passive stretching
- Hip flexion with knee extended (SLR) is positive for pain

Palpation
- Point tender on hamstring muscle belly, origin, or insertion
- Bruising may appear

Manual muscle test
- Weak lateral rotator muscles, posterior gluteus medius and maximus

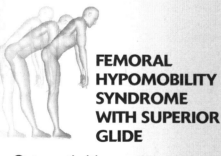

FEMORAL HYPOMOBILITY SYNDROME WITH SUPERIOR GLIDE

Osteoarthritis

The movement dysfunction in this syndrome is associated with a decreased hip joint space and degenerative changes in the joint and surrounding soft tissue. As a result, the physiologic motion of the hip is limited in a variety of directions, particularly flexion.

SYMPTOMS AND HISTORY

- Deep hip and groin pain or referred pain along inner thigh or medial knee
- Pain may be constant but varies in intensity; associated with weight-bearing activities and sitting-to-standing movement
- Pain described as discomfort or ache
- Stiffness noted after rest or in morning
- X-ray findings include narrowing of joint space
- Typically occurs in ages 55 and older

KEY TESTS AND SIGNS

Gait
- Trendelenburg or antalgic gait; limited hip extension during midstance (push off); compensatory lateral extension or lumbopelvic rotation

Passive ROM
- Limited in capsular pattern (medial rotation and flexion greater than extension)
- *Supine position:* Hip abduction/lateral rotation from flexion is positive for pain in groin

Hip flexor length test
- Short iliopsoas, rectus femoris, TFL-ITB

Quadruped position
- Limited hip flexion, observe shift toward uninvolved side or pelvic rotation at end of hip flexion ROM

Sitting-to-standing movement
- Painful if initiated with hip flexion; decreased pain if initiated with gluteus maximus

ASSOCIATED SIGNS
(contributing factors)

- *Muscle length:*
  Short hamstring muscles—observe hip medial rotation with sitting knee extension (asymmetrical hamstring length)
  Short gastrocnemius
- *Standing alignment:*
  Knee hyperextension
  Ankle pronation
- *Structural variation:*
  Femoral antetorsion
  Genu valgus

DIFFERENTIAL MOVEMENT AND ASSOCIATED DIAGNOSES

Movement diagnoses

- Hip extension with knee extension
- Hip adduction with medial rotation
- Tibiofemoral rotation
- Proximal tibiofibular glide syndrome
- Low back syndrome

Associated diagnoses

- Sciatica
- Hamstrings strain
- Lengthened piriformis syndrome
- Ischiogluteal bursitis

SCREENING FOR POTENTIAL MEDICAL DIAGNOSES REQUIRING REFERRAL

- *Patients with sciatica or posterior thigh pain:*
  Disk herniation
  Stenosis
  Neoplasm
  Diabetic neuropathy
  Megacolon
  Pregnancy
  Staph infection
  Intrapelvic aneurysm
  Abscess

ASSOCIATED SIGNS
(contributing factors)

- Decreased gluteal definition
- Weakness of lower abdominal and posterior gluteus medius and maximus muscles
- Stand with lordosis, anterior pelvic tilt, hip joint flexion (may also see pelvic rotation)
- Relative flexibility in back and hip

DIFFERENTIAL MOVEMENT AND ASSOCIATED DIAGNOSES

Movement diagnoses

- Femoral anterior glide
- Femoral anterior glide with lateral rotation
- Femoral anterior glide with medial rotation
- Hip adduction syndrome
- Hip adduction with medial rotation
- Low back syndrome

Associated diagnoses

- Osteoarthritis
- Degenerative joint disease
- Adductor strain

SCREENING FOR POTENTIAL MEDICAL DIAGNOSES REQUIRING REFERRAL

- Avascular necrosis
- Osteoarthritis
- *Stress fractures:*
  Greater trochanter
  Proximal medial femur
  Pubic symphysis
- Spinal cord tumor
- Ascites
- Hemophilia (GI bleeding)
- Aortic aneurysm
- Ureteral pain
- Interior oblique avulsion
- Pubalgia
- Osteitis pubis
- Inguinal hernia

GI, Gastrointestinal; *ROM*, range of motion; *SLR*, straight-leg raise; *TFL-ITB*, tensor fascia lata–iliotibial band.

Chapter 4
Appendix

FEMORAL ACCESSORY HYPERMOBILITY SYNDROME

The movement dysfunction in this syndrome is associated with degenerative hip joint disease and hypermobility of the hip joint associated with movements of the knee. The physiologic motion of the hip is NOT limited in a capsular pattern but may be associated with early osteoarthritis. There is dominance of the thigh musculature over the pelvic girdle muscles.

SYMPTOMS AND HISTORY

- Deep hip and groin pain associated with weight-bearing activities (e.g., standing, walking, running)
- Increased pain when sitting on a soft couch
- Childhood history of lower extremity structural problems
- Often occurs in: High level athletes or fitness training
- X-ray: may show early degenerative joint disease of hip joint

KEY TESTS AND SIGNS

Appearance
- Hypertrophied quadriceps and hamstring muscles

Standing on one leg
- Observe medial rotation
- *Passive and active SLR:* See antero-medial deviation of PICR (greater trochanter); may be painful
- *Passive:* If posteroinferior glide is applied at the inguinal crease, stiffness is evident and the range of pain-free flexion increases.
- Place at end range, ask patient to hold; observe anterior glide

Prone knee flexion
- Lateral rotation of femur associated with passive knee flexion (monitored at the trochanter)
- Distraction of the femur decreases lateral rotation during knee flexion

Prone hip lateral rotation
- Observe impaired axis of rotation (greater trochanter moves through wide arc); correction of wide arc, ROM decreases

Manual muscle test
- Weak posterior gluteus medius and maximus, lateral rotator, and iliopsoas muscles
- *Sitting knee extension:* Observe medial rotation (monitored at proximal thigh)

ASSOCIATED SIGNS
(contributing factors)

- *Standing alignment:* Knee hyperextended
- May appear to have increased length of hip flexors in length test
- *Quadruped position:* Increased hip flexion
- *Gait:* Trendelenburg's or antalgic test
- Knee hyperextension noted from initial contact to midstance

DIFFERENTIAL MOVEMENT AND ASSOCIATED DIAGNOSES

Movement diagnoses

- Femoral anterior glide
- Femoral anterior glide with lateral rotation
- Femoral anterior glide with medial rotation
- Femoral hypomobility
- Hip adduction syndrome
- Hip adduction with medial rotation
- Femoral lateral glide syndrome
- Low back syndrome

Associated diagnoses

- Osteoarthritis
- Degenerative joint disease (early)
- Labral tear

SCREENING FOR POTENTIAL MEDICAL DIAGNOSES REQUIRING REFERRAL

- Avascular necrosis
- Osteoarthritis (early stages)
- *Stress fractures:*
  Greater trochanter
  Proximal medial femur
  Pubic symphysis
- Spinal cord tumor
- Ascites
- Hemophilia (GI bleeding)
- Aortic aneurysm
- Ureteral pain
- Interior oblique avulsion
- Pubalgia
- Osteitis pubis
- Inguinal hernia

PICR, Path of the instant center of rotation; *ROM,* range of motion; *SLR,* straight-leg raise.

Chapter 4
Appendix

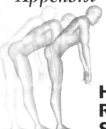

HIP LATERAL ROTATION SYNDROME

Shortened piriformis

Shortened muscle compresses the sciatic nerve (entrapment syndrome of sciatic nerve).

SYMPTOMS AND HISTORY

- Pain along sciatic nerve distribution that begins at gluteal fold (no back pain)
- Pain is worse with standing and walking than it is with sitting
- *Incidence:* Moderate to frequent
- Male golfers

KEY TESTS AND SIGNS

Standing alignment

- *Hip lateral rotation:* May have reduced lumbar curve, posterior pelvic tilt, or hip joint extension
- If apparent leg-length discrepancy, pain is experienced on side of lower iliac crest (may also be true for lower back pain with radiculopathy)
- Pain may be relieved by increased lateral rotation in standing or walking
- *Hip flexion, adduction, medial rotation:* Reproduces pain

Prone position

- *Hip rotation:* Limited medial rotation
- *Palpation:* Tenderness in buttocks
- *Resisted testing:* Hamstring muscles (strong and painless)

Quadruped position

- *Alignment:* Involved hip angle is less than 90 degrees or in lateral rotation or abduction
- *Functional mobility:* Lateral rotation associated with sitting-to-standing movement, gait, stair climbing

ASSOCIATED SIGNS
(contributing factors)

Decreased range of hip flexion

May have a positive slump test

Weak or long iliopsoas muscles

Short hamstrings muscles

Resisted lateral rotation may reproduce symptoms

Habit of sitting with legs crossed (foot on thigh)

Structural variation: Femoral retroversion

DIFFERENTIAL MOVEMENT AND ASSOCIATED DIAGNOSES

Movement diagnoses
- Low back syndrome
- Hip adduction with medial rotation
- Hip extension with knee extension

Associated diagnoses
- Sciatica
- Hamstring muscle strain
- Piriformis syndrome (shortened)

SCREENING FOR POTENTIAL MEDICAL DIAGNOSES REQUIRING REFERRAL

- Disk herniation
- Stenosis
- Neoplasm
- Diabetic neuropathy
- Megacolon
- Pregnancy
- Staph infection
- Intrapelvic aneurysm
- Abscess

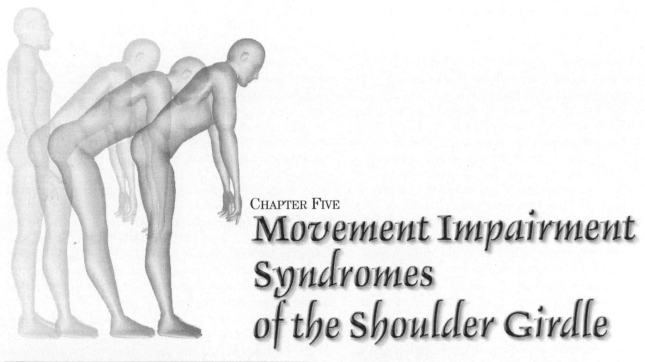

Movement Impairment Syndromes of the Shoulder Girdle

Chapter Highlights

Normal Alignment of the Shoulder Girdle
Motions of the Shoulder Girdle
Muscular Actions of the Shoulder Girdle
Movement Impairment Syndromes of the Scapula
 Relationship Between Alignment and Movement
 Criteria for the Diagnosis of a Scapular Syndrome
 Scapular Syndromes in Observed Frequency
Movement Impairment Syndromes of the Humerus
 Relationships Between Alignment and Movement
 Criteria for a Diagnosis of a Humeral Syndrome
 Order of Observed Frequency of Humeral Syndromes

Chapter Objectives

After considering the information presented in this chapter, the reader will be able to:

1. Describe kinesiology of the musculature of the shoulder girdle with emphasis on the counterbalancing actions of muscles and their roles in the force-couples that control shoulder motion.
2. Identify the characteristics of each movement impairment syndrome of the scapulothoracic and glenohumeral joints.

In treating the patient with shoulder pain, the reader will be able to:

1. Perform an examination, consider the contributing factors, and establish the diagnoses, both primary and secondary, if indicated.
2. Develop and instruct the patient in a diagnosis-specific treatment program and modification of life's activities, which contribute to the formation of the movement impairment syndrome.

Introduction

The premise of this approach, which diagnoses and manages musculoskeletal pain problems, is that minor alterations in the precision of movement cause micro-trauma and, if allowed to continue, will cause macro-trauma and pain. These alterations in the precision of movement result in the development of compensatory movements that occur in specific directions and can be categorized as movement impairments. The contributing factors to these movement impairments are changes in muscle length, strength, stiffness, and patterns of participation that arise from repeated movements and sustained postures.

The purpose of the examination is to identify the movement impairments and the contributing factors. This information leads to a diagnosis that directs treatment.

The therapeutic exercises and the correction of the movement patterns used to perform daily activities become the means to remedy the identified movement impairments. The observation of the movement characteristics and their effect on symptoms are the primary guides to the diagnosis and treatment of the movement impairments. If symptoms are associated with the impairment, the correction of the movement will alleviate the symptoms. For example, increasing the amount of lateral humeral rotation during shoulder flexion/elevation often eliminates the shoulder pain caused by one form of impingement. Because the scapula plays a critical role in controlling the position of the glenoid, relatively small changes in the action of thoracoscapular muscles can affect the alignment and forces involved in movement around the glenohumeral joint.[31,32] Clinically based observations suggest that most syndromes involving the shoulder arise from impairments in the timing and control of scapular motion.

Specific pain problems of the muscles and tendons arise from repeated movements that have altered their normal patterns rather than from a single episode of isolated stress placed on the specific painful tissue. For example, supraspinatus tendinitis or tendinopathy is a common pain problem that is attributed to overuse or to impingement from altered biomechanics of the shoulder, rather than from using the arm excessively on a particular occasion. Supraspinatus tendinopathy can begin as vascular insufficiency in the "critical zone" of the tendon.[26] *Tendinopathy* refers to the whole range of painful conditions caused by overuse of the tendon. Tendinopathy is the preferred term to designate a condition such as tendinitis because most painful tendon conditions result from tendinosis, which has a different pathology than tendinitis and a longer healing time than the 1 to 2 weeks of tendinitis.[13] Tendinopathy can be the result of mechanical impingement, compression of the rotator cuff by its surrounding local anatomic structures,[18] damage of the undersurface of the cuff muscles,[17] or the overuse of the muscle during movement. Neer was the first to categorize impingement syndromes into either outlet or non-outlet. Outlet impingement resulted from damage to the cuff from contact with the structures of the coracoacromial arch, whereas non-outlet impingement occurs when there is a normal supraspinatus outlet.[22] Jobe and colleagues suggest that outlet syndromes occur in individuals who are over 35 years of age and nonoutlet syndromes in those younger than 35 years of age and who participate in sports requiring overhead activities. In non-outlet syndrome, hyperangulation of the humerus that causes stretching of the anterior shoulder structures is a precipitating factor.[17]

Inadequate upward rotation of the scapula during shoulder flexion causes impingement if the patient performs 180 degrees of flexion, with the scapula only accounting for 45 degrees rather than the desired 60 degrees of upward rotation. If the participation of the other humeral depressors is insufficient, the result could be overuse of the supraspinatus muscle. If the teres minor, infraspinatus, or subscapularis muscles do not generate sufficient tension during shoulder flexion and abduction, the demand on the supraspinatus muscle to exert an inferior pull on the humeral head to counterbalance the compressive force by the deltoid muscle is increased.

Neer was the first to describe a continuum of shoulder problems that begins with impingement and progresses to rotator cuff tears.[20] The limited subacromial space combined with the development of relatively small imbalances in muscle control of the scapula and humerus can lead to a wide range of soft tissue and even osseous changes. Other investigators have described the self-perpetuating cycle that can develop when the humeral depressor mechanism is dysfunctional.[19] The premise that underlies movement impairment concepts is that this continuum arises from alterations in the control of scapular and humeral motions because of the changes in neuromuscular components that result from repeated use. This chapter emphasizes the need to identify the movement impairments and the component impairments that, when analyzed, form the basis of the diagnosis. Identifying these factors requires careful examination and testing. Remediation requires the appropriate selection of and instruction in the therapeutic exercises that will result in correction of the movement impairments.

The key elements of the examination are assessment of alignment, movement patterns, and specific tests of muscle length and strength. Normal and impaired alignment, movement patterns, and muscle length tests are presented as guidelines for the performance of the examination that is required to establish a diagnosis.

Normal Alignment of the Shoulder Girdle

Alignment is an indicator of possible muscle length changes and of the joint alignments that need to be corrected to allow for optimal motion. For example, if the patient has medially rotated shoulders, when shoulder abduction is being performed, a greater amount of lateral rotation must occur during the motion than if the starting alignment was more neutral. If the humerus does not rotate enough to correct for the impaired initial alignment, the greater tuberosity of the humerus can impinge against the coracoacromial ligament. Similarly, if the scapula is downwardly rotated at rest, then the amount of upward rotation must be more than the optimal 60 degrees to correct for the faulty starting position. Most often, the impairments that allow or create the alignment faults are the ones that interfere with achieving optimal movement. For example, if the rhomboid muscles are short contributing to postural downward rotation of the scapula, then during shoulder flexion the shortness of the rhomboid muscles will interfere with optimal upward rotation. Deviations in alignment are those that differ from the ideal postural standard.

Shoulders

Normal Alignment
The shoulders should be positioned slightly below the horizontal axis through T1 in the front or back view. In the side view, the plumb line should bisect the acromion.

Impaired Alignment

The impairments of shoulder alignment are discussed in greater detail in the scapula section because scapular alignment determines shoulder position.

- *Elevated.* The neck appears to be short and the shoulders appear to be closer to the ears than ideal (Figure 5-1). Clarification of the anatomic reference point used to assess shoulder position is important because of the variation in muscle impairments associated with different scapular positions. The reference points for observation of shoulder height are discussed in the scapula section.
- *Depressed.* The clavicles appear to be horizontal or the acromioclavicular joint is lower than the sternoclavicular joint (Figure 5-2). The superior angle of the scapula is lower than T2.
- *Forward.* When viewing the entire shoulder girdle, the tip of the shoulder at the acromion can appear to be forward because of several possible impaired scapular positions. In the forward shoulder position, the scapula can be abducted, tilted, or moved in a combination of these positions. Because each of these impaired scapular positions is associated with different muscle imbalances and requires different management, they are discussed in relation to the alignment of the scapula.

Scapula

Normal Alignment

The vertebral border of the scapula is parallel to the spine and is positioned approximately 3 inches from the midline of the thorax.[28] It is situated on the thorax between the second and seventh thoracic vertebrae. The scapula is flat against the thorax and is rotated 30 degrees anterior to the frontal plane.

Impaired Alignment

- *Downwardly rotated.* The inferior angle of the scapula is medial to the root of the spine of the scapula rather than the vertebral border being parallel to the spine (Figure 5-3). Most often, the levator scapula muscle and rhomboid muscles are short and the upper trapezius muscle is long. The serratus anterior muscle may also be long. This is

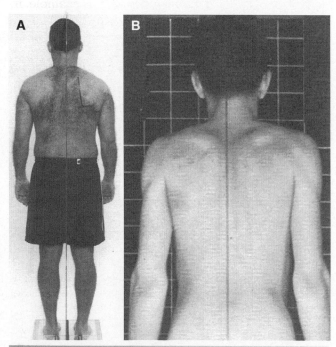

Figure 5-1

Elevated shoulders. *A,* The shoulders may appear elevated if the superior angle of the scapula is elevated with depression of the acromion. *B,* The entire scapula is elevated including the acromion, which causes the appearance of a short neck. (From Kendall et al: *Muscles: testing and function,* ed 4, Baltimore, 1993, Williams & Wilkins.)

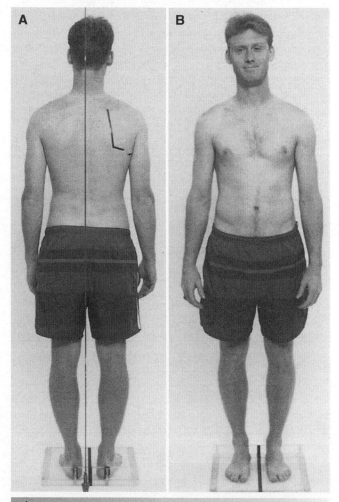

Figure 5-2

Depressed shoulders. *A,* The superior angle of the scapula is positioned below T2, which causes the patient to appear to have a long neck. *B,* In the front view, the clavicle appears horizontal or the acromioclavicular joint is lower than the sternoclavicular joint.

one of the most common alignment impairments in individuals with shoulder pain.

- *Depressed.* The superior border of the scapula is positioned lower than the second and seventh thoracic vertebral landmarks (see Figure 5-2). This postural position infers that the upper trapezius muscle is long. Muscles that may contribute to this depressed position are the pectoralis major and the latissimus dorsi muscles. This alignment is also common in patients with shoulder pain. A postural alignment of depression that is not corrected during shoulder flexion and abduction contributes to stress at the glenohumeral and acromioclavicular joints.

- *Elevated.* The elevation of the superior angle of the scapula, but not the acromion, suggests that the levator scapula muscle is short (see Figure 5-1). The elevation of the entire scapula, including the acromion, infers that the upper trapezius muscle is short. In this condition the lateral portion of the clavicle appears notably higher than the medial portion. If the levator scapula, rhomboid, and upper trapezius muscles are all short, then the entire spine of the scapula will appear higher and will be positioned closer to the seventh cervical

vertebra than to the second thoracic vertebra and the scapula may also appear adducted.

- *Adducted.* The vertebral border of the scapula is less than 3 inches from the midline of the thorax (Figure 5-4). The rhomboid and the trapezius mus-

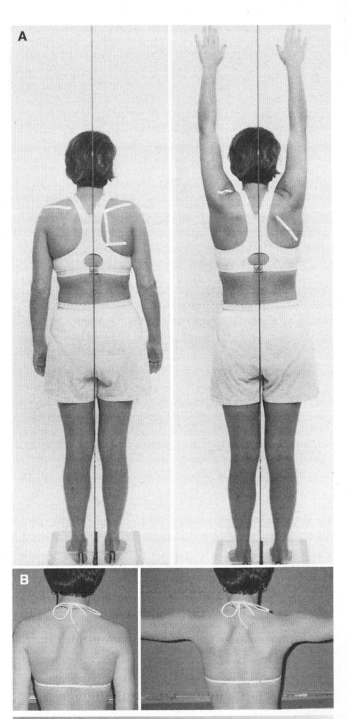

Figure 5-4

Adducted scapula. *A,* The vertebral border of the scapula is less than 3 inches from the vertebral spine. At the completion of shoulder flexion, the scapulae are more adducted than the optimum. *B,* The scapulae are adducted at rest and remain adducted even when the shoulders are abducted to 90 degrees.

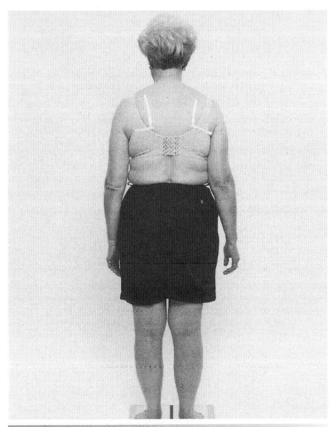

Figure 5-3

Downwardly rotated scapula. The thoracic kyphosis contributes to this alignment of the scapula.

cles may be short while the serratus anterior muscle is long.

- *Abducted.* The vertebral border of the scapula is more than 3 inches from the midline of the thorax (Figure 5-5). When the scapula is abducted, it is also rotated more than 30 degrees anterior to the frontal plane. When the scapula is abducted and rotated anteriorly, the glenoid will face anteriorly and the humerus will appear medially rotated. The medial rotation of the humerus in this condition should not be corrected because the orientation of the humerus in the glenoid is correct. When the patient adducts his or her scapula, the humeral position will be correct and appears normal. In the abducted-rotated scapular alignment, if the humeral position appears correct with the cubital fossa facing anteriorly, the actual alignment is one of lateral rotation. Often specific examination of the length of the lateral rotators indicates that they are short. The most common cause of the abducted-rotated scapular position is shortness of the serratus anterior and/or the pectoralis major muscles.

- *Tilted or tipped.* The inferior angle protrudes away from the rib cage (Figure 5-6). Most often, this alignment is associated with shortness of the pectoralis minor muscle. Another cause of the tilted alignment is shortness of the biceps brachii muscle, the short head attaches to the coracoid process or to the anterior deltoid muscles or to both. If the biceps brachii muscle is short, then the elbow will flex when the scapular alignment is corrected. If the elbow is passively flexed while the scapula is held in the corrected position, then the shoulder will extend if the biceps brachii muscle is the source of the tilted scapula. If the shoulder remains flexed, then the most likely source of the tipped shoulder is the anterior deltoid muscle and/or the coracobrachialis muscle.

- *Depressed and tilted.* The scapula is depressed as described previously, but the scapula is also anteriorly tilted.

- *Abducted and tilted.* This alignment is the combination of the conditions of abduction and tilted, each of which has been described previously.

- *Winged.* The vertebral border protrudes posteriorly from the thorax (Figure 5-7). This alignment is often associated with weakness of the serratus anterior muscle. Other alignment impairments that can contribute to the appearance of winged scapula include a flat thoracic spine, a rounded

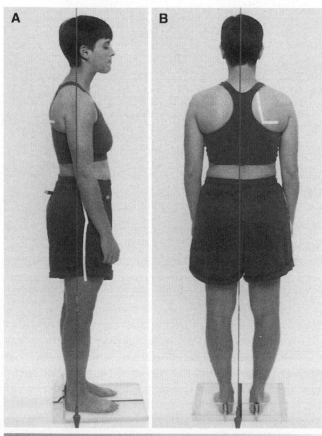

Figure 5-5

Abducted forward shoulders. *A,* In the side view the shoulder joint appears forward of the midline of the body. *B,* In the back view the shoulders also appear forward and the hands are forward of the hips.

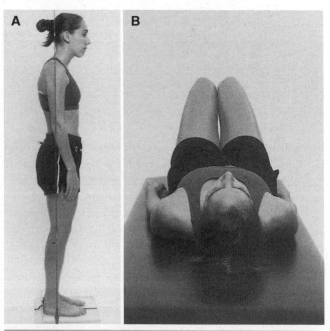

Figure 5-6

Tilted scapula. *A,* The inferior angle of the scapula protrudes from the thorax and the coracoid process tilts anteriorly The increased curvature of the thoracic spine contributes to the anterior tilt of the scapula. *B,* In the supine position, the forward position of the scapula is associated with shortness of the pectoralis minor muscle.

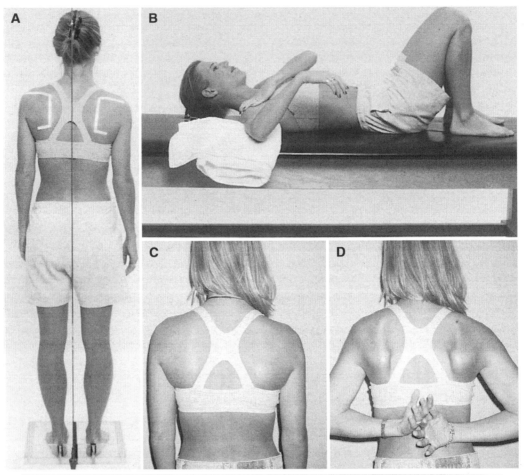

Figure 5-7

Winged scapula. *A,* The vertebral border protrudes from the thorax rather than lying flat. *B,* In the supine position during shoulder medial rotation when the scapula motion is prevented, the shortness of the lateral rotator muscles does not permit shoulder medial rotation. *C,* Scapulae appear to be in the winging position at rest. *D,* During shoulder medial rotation, shortness of the scapulohumeral muscles is contributing to winging of the scapulae.

back, or scoliosis. In scoliosis, the scapulae appear notably asymmetrical in their alignment. When the subscapularis is hypertrophied, the scapulae will appear to be winged because the vertebral borders of the scapulae are prominent. However, they are not actually rotated in the frontal plane but are no longer flat on the thorax. Careful examination of the scapula indicates that the entire scapula is protruding from the thorax and not just from the vertebral border. This condition is seen most often in patients who regularly perform chin-up exercises or wall-climbing activities.

- *Upwardly rotated.* The root of the spine of the scapula is medial to the inferior angle. The muscle most likely to be short is the trapezius muscle.

Humerus

Normal Alignment

There should be less than one third of the humeral head protruding in front of the acromion. Neutral rotation should be present so that the antecubital crease faces anteriorly and the olecranon faces posteriorly, with the palm of the hand facing the body. In some cases, the palm of the hand may face posteriorly without the olecranon facing posteriorly. Most often this condition is the result of short finger flexor muscles (Figure 5-8). The proximal and distal ends of the humerus should be in the same vertical plane when viewed from the side, the front, or the back. As discussed previously, the scapula must be in ideal alignment when properly assessing the glenohumeral joint position.

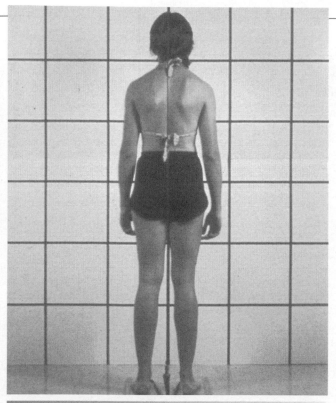

Figure 5-8

Humerus neutral rotation with forearm pronated. The position of the olecranon is neutral, thus the shoulder is not medially rotated, although the palm of the hand is facing posteriorly. This alignment is frequently associated with short finger flexor muscles.

Impaired Alignment

- *Anterior.* More than one third of the humeral head is positioned anterior to the acromion (Figure 5-9).
- *Superior.* The humeral head appears superior in relation to the acromion.
- *Abducted.* The distal part of the humerus is away from the side of the body, or the scapula is downwardly rotated or depressed (Figure 5-10).
- *Rotated medially.* The cubital fossa faces medially, the olecranon faces laterally, and often the palm of the hand faces posteriorly. As discussed previously the position of the scapula must be assessed for accurate assessment of humeral rotation.
- *Rotated laterally.* Lateral rotation of the humerus is not common except when the scapula is abducted and the humerus appears to be in the correct alignment (Figure 5-11).
- *Flexion/extension.* With flexion of the humerus, the distal aspect of the humerus is anterior to the proximal aspect of the humerus. With extension of the humerus, the distal end of the humerus is posterior to the proximal end of the humerus, which may also be associated with anterior position of the humeral head. The position of the humerus

must be assessed in relation to the position of the scapula. What appears to be the correct alignment can be impaired depending on the position of the scapula, and vice versa.

Thoracic Spine

Normal Alignment

There should be a slight posterior curve of the thoracic vertebrae.

Impaired Alignment

- *Kyphosis.* There is increased outward (posteriorly orientated) curve or flexion of the thoracic spine (Figure 5-12).
- *Scoliosis.* Kyphosis and rotation of the spine with a rib hump that often results in malalignment of the scapula. When the alignment of the scapulae are markedly different, scoliosis is the most common cause. If a rib hump causes the scapula to wing, the patient should not be encouraged to correct the alignment by sustained contraction of the scapular adductors. The resulting shortness of the adductors restricts the abduction and upward rotation of the scapula and can lead to impingement, rotator cuff tears, and neck pain. The neck pain occurs because of the additional stress exerted on the cervical spine by contraction of the upper trapezius muscle in its role as an upward rotator of the scapula.
- *Flat.* The loss of the normal outward curve resulting in a straight or flat thoracic spine. A flat thoracic spine makes the scapula appear to be winged.

Motions of the Shoulder Girdle
Glossary of Scapular Motions[14]

The following definitions are described to ensure commonality in understanding the segmental movements upon which the syndromes are based (Figure 5-13).

- Rotation, lateral or upward, is movement about a sagittal axis in which the inferior angle moves laterally and the glenoid cavity moves cranially.
- Rotation, medial or downward, is movement about a sagittal axis in which the inferior angle moves medially and the glenoid cavity moves caudally.
- Elevation is a gliding movement in which the scapula moves cranially, as in shrugging the shoulder.
- Depression is a gliding movement in which the scapula moves caudally and is the reverse of elevation and anterior tilt.

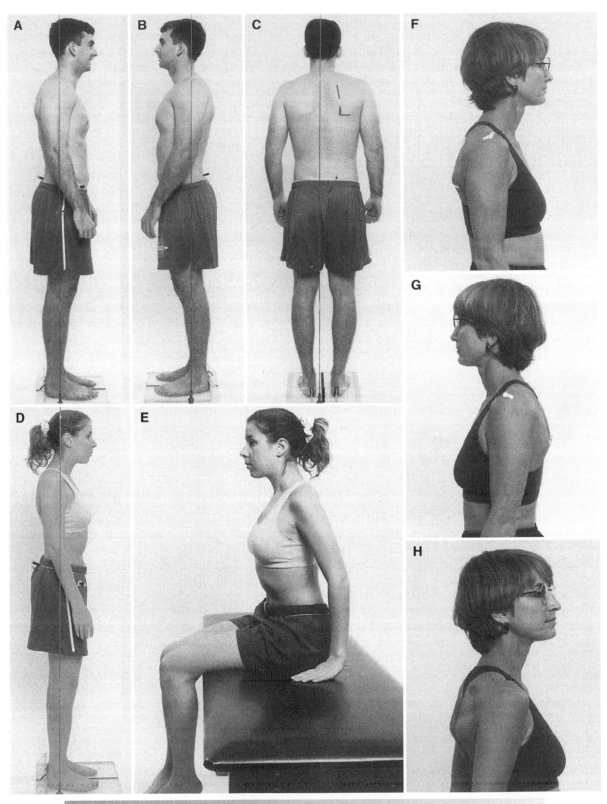

Figure 5-9

Humerus anterior of acromion. *A,* More than one third of the humeral head is anterior of the acromion. On the right, the distal humerus is posterior to the proximal humerus. *B,* The left humeral head is not as anterior, and the distal humerus is more in line with the proximal humerus. *C,* The posterior view indicates that the left shoulder is abducted and medially rotated, which contributes to the proximal end of the humerus being aligned with the distal end. *D,* The anterior position of the humerus is shown. *E,* The anterior position of the humerus is exaggerated and demonstrated by the way the patient is stabilizing her body. *F,* The right humeral head appears anterior and superior. *G,* The left humeral head is less anterior and superior than the right. *H,* Shoulder extension, as occurs during walking, can contribute to further anterior glide of the humeral head.

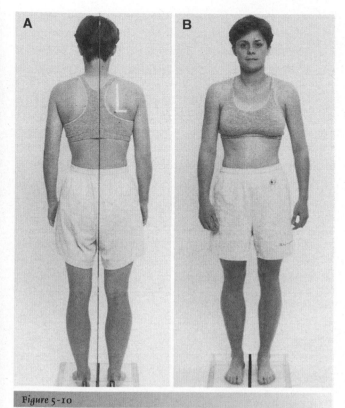

Figure 5-10

Humerus abducted and medially rotated. The humerus is away from the side of the body rather than lying parallel to the thorax. The olecranon faces laterally *(A)* and the cubital fossa faces medially *(B)*. The left shoulder is more abducted and medially rotated than the right. If the shoulder is depressed, the glenohumeral joint alignment is abducted.

- Adduction is a gliding movement in which the scapula moves toward the vertebral column.
- Abduction is a gliding movement in which the scapula moves away from the vertebral column and into full abduction, following the contour of the thorax until it assumes a posterolateral position.
- Anterior tilt is a movement about the coronal axis in which the coracoid process moves in an anterior and caudal direction. The coracoid process may be said to be depressed anteriorly.
- Winging occurs around the vertical axis at the acromioclavicular joint. The vertebral border of the scapula moves away from the thorax, and the glenoid fossa moves anteriorly. This motion occurs to maintain the contact of the scapula with the curve of the thorax as the scapula slides (glides) around the thorax into abduction or adduction. The movement becomes abnormal when the motion of the vertebral border of the scapula away from the thorax becomes obvious.[24]

Shoulder Girdle Movement Patterns

The key observations for assessing the optimal performance of shoulder girdle movement are as follows:

- *Starting alignment.* As discussed previously, if the scapula and humerus are not in the correct starting position, then during movement these faults must be corrected. For example, if the

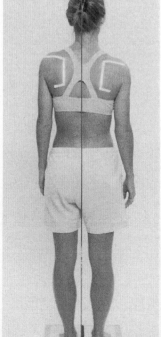

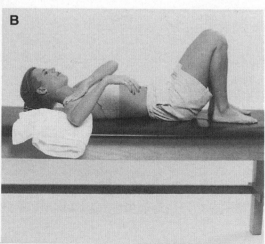

Figure 5-11

Laterally rotated humerus. *A,* It is uncommon to have the olecranon face medially in the resting position, but if the scapula is markedly abducted and the olecranon faces posteriorly, the humerus is actually laterally rotated. *B,* The lateral rotator muscles are short, which is consistent with a slight laterally rotated position of the humerus.

scapula is downwardly rotated, then during shoulder flexion the amount of upward rotation must be greater than the normal 60 degrees to compensate for the faulty starting position.

- *Scapulohumeral rhythm.* During the first 60 degrees of shoulder flexion and 30 degrees of abduction the movement of the scapula is highly variable. Inman and Saunders termed this the *setting phase.*[10] After the setting phase the humerus and scapula move in a constant ratio. A ratio of 2 degrees of glenohumeral motion for 1 degree of scapulothoracic motion results in 120 degrees of glenohumeral joint motion and 60 degrees of scapular motion at the completion of shoulder flexion (Figure 5-14). More recent studies have reported some variability in the exact timing of that motion.[2,6,7] In analyzing patients who have pain, comparing one shoulder with the other provides a reference point to guide the examiner in making a decision as to whether the movement is impaired or just a normal variation. Observations of deviations in timing and range of scapular motion combined with the timing of the onset of pain and identification of impairments of muscle performance further guide decisions regarding the importance of the deviations.

- *Timing and range of scapular motion.* During flexion the scapula will often stop its movement when the shoulder is flexed to about 140 degrees; the rest of the motion occurs almost entirely at the glenohumeral joint. Placing the thumb and first finger on the inferior angle of the scapula and

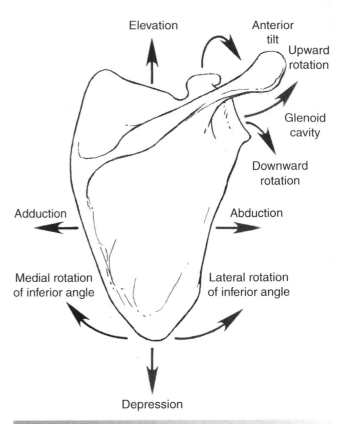

Figure 5-13

Motions of the scapula. (From Kendall et al: *Muscles: testing and function,* ed 4, Baltimore, 1993, Williams & Wilkins.)

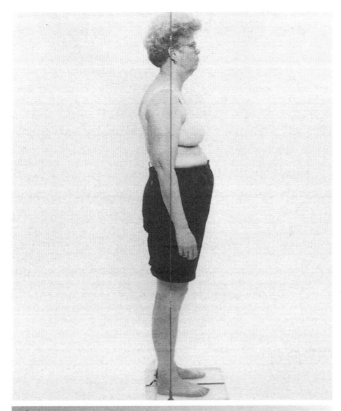

Figure 5-12

Thoracic kyphosis. Increased outward curve of the thoracic spine.

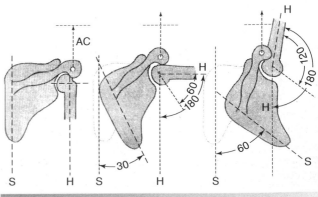

Figure 5-14

Scapulohumeral rhythm. The scapula moves 1 degree for 2 degrees of humeral motion. On completion of shoulder flexion, the glenohumeral joint motion is 120 degrees and the scapulothoracic motion is 60 degrees. (From Calliet R: *Shoulder pain,* ed 2, Philadelphia, 1981, FA Davis.)

following the motion of the scapula while observing the humerus is a good way to assess the movement pattern. Comparing one side with the other during unilateral and bilateral motion is also helpful.

Upon the completion of flexion, the inferior angle of the scapula should be close to the midline of the thorax and the vertebral border of the scapula should be rotated 60 degrees (Figure 5-15). The inferior angle should not be forward of this line, nor should it protrude laterally more than ½ inch in full glenohumeral joint flexion or abduction. The movement of the inferior angle beyond the midline or the protrusion of the scapula laterally beyond the thorax indicates excessive scapular abduction (Figure 5-16).

- *Scapular winging.* The scapula should not wing during arm movement, either during the flexion/ abduction phase or during the return from flexion/abduction phase (Figures 5-17 and 5-18).

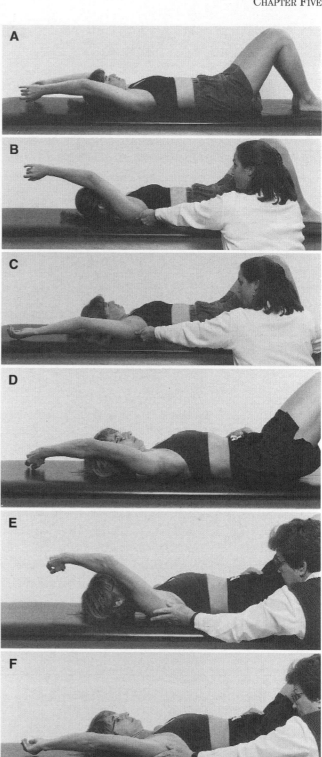

Figure 5-16

Excessive scapular abduction on completion of shoulder flexion. *A, D,* The inferior angle protrudes more than ½ inch lateral of the side of the thorax. *B, E,* Correcting the scapular position decreases the range of shoulder flexion, indicating the scapulohumeral muscles are short. *C, F,* Medial rotation of the humerus increases the range of shoulder flexion, which indicates the teres major muscle is short.

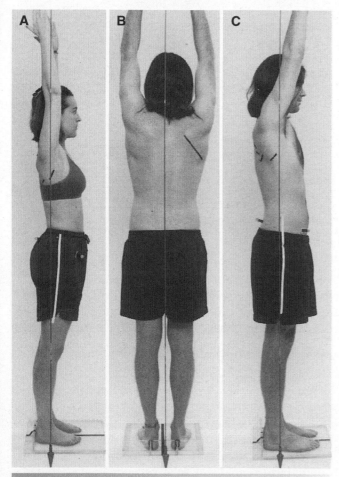

Figure 5-15

Scapular position at completion of shoulder flexion. *A,* Inferior angle of scapula is posterior to the midaxillary line. *B,* Scapula is not upwardly rotated 60 degrees. *C,* The inferior angle of the scapula is not positioned correctly on the lateral thorax.

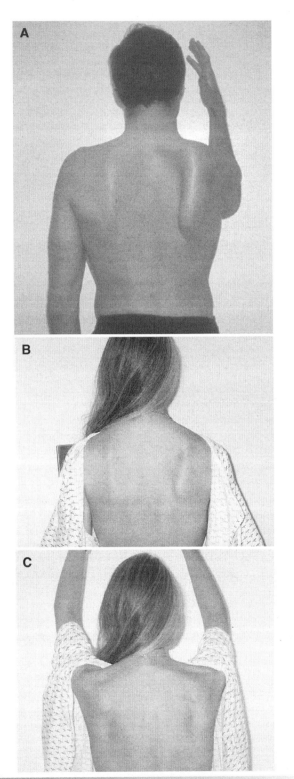

Figure 5-17

Winging of the scapula during shoulder flexion. *A,* During shoulder flexion the vertebral border of the scapula protrudes from the posterior aspect of the thorax because the scapulohumeral muscles are short. The axioscapular muscles are not providing adequate control to prevent the winging. B, Scapular winging, depression, and downward rotation is demonstrated. C, During shoulder flexion, the scapula wings and abducts excessively.

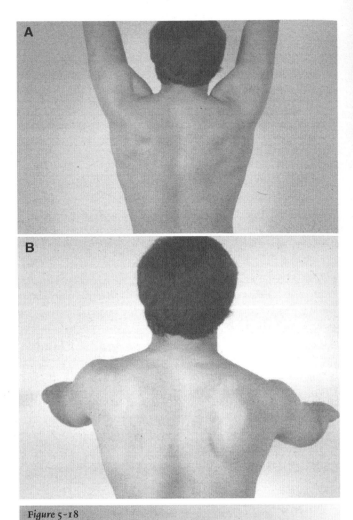

Figure 5-18

Scapular winging during return from shoulder flexion. *A,* Scapula does not wing during shoulder flexion. *B,* Scapula wings during the return from shoulder flexion, suggesting that timing of muscle relaxation, not of muscle strength, is the problem.

- *Scapular elevation.* There should be some elevation of the shoulder (as in the shrugging motion), but it should not be excessive during the flexion/abduction phase. If the shoulder is depressed at rest, then elevation of the scapula is particularly important.
- *End of the range.* The scapula should slightly depress, posteriorly tilt, and adduct to complete the motion of 180 degrees. The presence of a kyphosis or shortness of the pectoralis minor muscle can impede this depression (Figure 5-19).
- *Humeral head.* The axis of rotation of the humeral head should stay relatively constant so that it is centered in the glenoid throughout the motion (Figure 5-20). Therefore the scapulohumeral muscles that depress the head of the humerus must offset the strong upward pull of the deltoid muscle

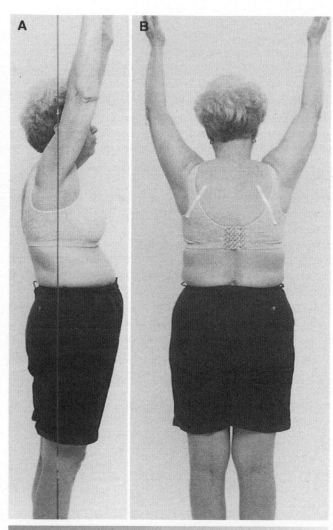

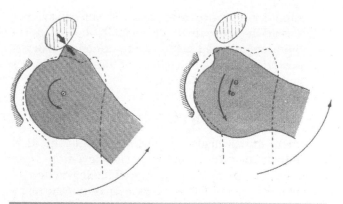

Figure 5-20

Depression and lateral rotation of the humeral head during shoulder flexion. (From Calliet R: *Shoulder pain*, ed 2, Philadelphia, 1981, FA Davis.)

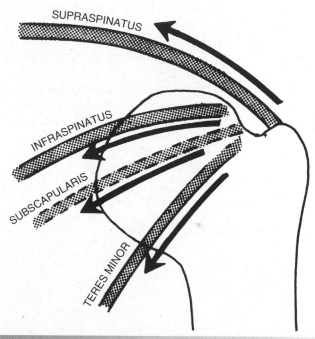

Figure 5-21

The rotator cuff muscles exert a downward pull on the humeral head during shoulder flexion. The infraspinatus and teres minor muscles also laterally rotate the humerus during shoulder flexion. (From Calliet R: *Shoulder pain*, ed 2, Philadelphia, 1981, FA Davis.)

Figure 5-19

Thoracic kyphosis interfering with scapular motion during shoulder flexion. *A,* The thoracic kyphosis is evident in the side view. *B,* Inadequate upward rotation and adduction of scapula at the completion of shoulder flexion is demonstrated. The scapula cannot adduct because it must follow the contour of the rib cage.

and must laterally rotate the humerus to prevent the greater tuberosity from impinging on the coracoacromial ligament or the acromion (Figure 5-21). If the pectoralis major and latissimus dorsi muscles depress the head of the humerus, they will also medially rotate it and can alter the timing of humeral motion with the scapula and the position of the humerus relative to the glenoid.

- *Spine.* Minimal movement of the spine should occur during full abduction or flexion of the shoulder. If the thoracic spine is kyphotic, the scapula will be tilted anteriorly by the convexity of the ribs, thus limiting the apparent range of shoulder flexion. Decreasing the degree of the thoracic kyphosis will improve the range of shoulder flexion.

- *Test for rhomboid dominance.* When the patient has his arms at his sides with the elbows flexed and is instructed to perform shoulder lateral rotation, the scapula should not adduct, particularly during the first 35 degrees of the motion (Figure 5-22). Adduction of the scapula is interpreted as a sign of rhomboid dominance and poor control of glenohumeral lateral rotation. The desired motion is one in which the humerus is rotating in the glenoid about a vertical axis. The humeral head should not move anteriorly or superiorly; nor should the arm extend. These faulty movements of the humeral head demonstrate dominance of the posterior deltoid muscle over the infraspinatus and teres minor muscles.

Muscular Actions of the Shoulder Girdle

Movement impairments are deviations from the ideal kinesiologic pattern of motion. The deviation is an alteration of the normal counterbalancing action of muscular synergists. Often the assessment of the alignment of the shoulder girdle at rest indicates the presence of muscle impairments, which can be associated with movement impairments. This section reviews the important shoulder girdle muscles and their actions with an emphasis on their counterbalancing effects. This review is not intended to be a detailed anatomic description but to focus on the counterbalancing actions of muscles. Alterations in the counterbalancing actions are a major factor in the development of movement impairment syndromes.

The muscle is described under a group designation determined by the muscle attachments. The groups discussed are the thoracoscapular, thoracohumeral, and scapulohumeral muscles. Based on the kinesiology of shoulder motion, the thoracoscapular muscles must move the scapula correctly for the scapulohumeral muscles to provide optimal control of the humerus and to maintain an optimal relationship of the glenoid and the humeral head. Alteration in the actions of the thoracohumeral muscles can be a major source of movement impairment because of the large size of these muscles and their direct attachment to the humerus.

Thoracoscapular Muscles

The correct length, strength, and pattern of participation of the muscles attaching to the thorax and to the scapula are important. The thoracoscapular muscles are responsible for the movement of the scapula, which must maintain an optimal relationship with the humerus to minimize abnormal stresses at the glenohumeral joint. *A key to optimal glenohumeral joint motion is that the head of the humerus remains centered in relationship to the glenoid as motion occurs at the shoulder joint.* The path of the instantaneous center of rotation (PICR) of the humerus in the glenoid defines motion in the glenoid (see Figure 5-20). This requires relatively precise timing of the muscles that produce scapular motion. The force couple action of

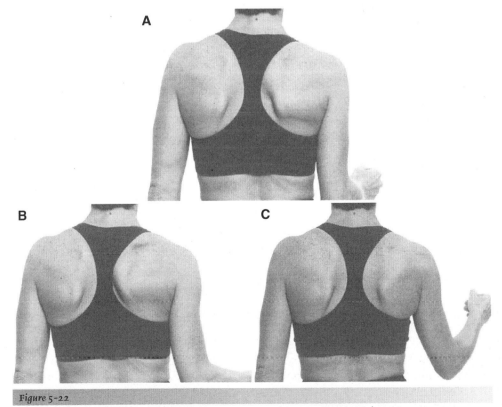

Figure 5-22

Rhomboid muscle dominance. *A,* In the starting position for shoulder lateral rotation, rhomboid muscle definition is evident. *B,* Instead of shoulder lateral rotation, the patient adducts the scapula. *C,* Without scapular adduction, the lateral rotation range of motion appears to be decreased.

the trapezius and serratus anterior muscles must be carefully assessed because this action is a key to motion of the scapula (Figure 5-23). Alterations in the relative participation of these muscles or restriction of motion by their antagonists disrupt the pattern of movement. Because shoulder motion does not involve true reciprocal muscular activity, most of the thoracoscapular muscles are active during shoulder motion although they have antagonistic actions.

Alteration in the dominance or the length of any one muscle can compromise the muscle balance. Understanding the synergistic and antagonistic actions of these muscles is essential for the analysis of shoulder girdle motion. Impairments in alignment observed in the resting position are manifested as muscle impairments during movement. Knowledge of the anatomy of the thoracoscapular muscles provides the examiner with the basic information necessary to analyze muscle length and movement faults. Based on clinical experience, the author believes that most patients with shoulder pain *develop their condition as a result of movement impairments of the scapula*, which has disrupted the relationship between the humerus and the glenoid. This disruption causes alterations in the accessory motions of the humerus, particularly anterior and superior glide.

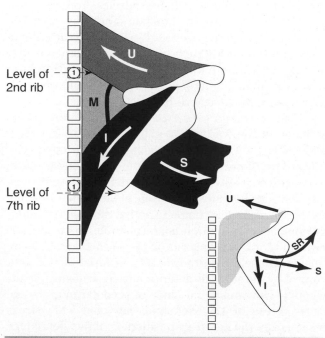

Figure 5-23

Scapular force couple. The upper and lower trapezius muscles are one component of the force couple acting to rotate the scapula upwardly. The serratus anterior muscle is the other component. The adduction action of the trapezius is counterbalanced by the abduction action of the serratus anterior muscle. (Adapted from Calliet R: *Shoulder pain,* ed 2, Philadelphia, 1981, FA Davis.)

The *trapezius muscle* (Figure 5-24) adducts and upwardly (laterally) rotates the scapula. The upper trapezius muscle elevates the scapula, whereas the lower trapezius muscle depresses the scapula. The trapezius muscle attaches to the acromion and clavicle. When the upper trapezius muscle is short and the shoulder girdle is posturally elevated, the entire shoulder, including the distal end of the acromion, should be elevated. When the upper trapezius muscle is long, the shoulder is depressed (see Figure 5-2). If the scapula fails to elevate during shoulder flexion or abduction, the action of the upper trapezius muscle is considered to be insufficient.

The *upper trapezius muscle,* through its attachment to the ligamentum nuchae, can affect the cervical spine. An impairment is present if monitoring the spinous processes of the cervical vertebrae while the patient with neck pain flexes the shoulder indicates that the spinous processes rotate to the same side as the shoulder being flexed. The most likely explanation for the rotation of the cervical vertebrae is that the cervical vertebrae are excessively flexible; thus when the upper trapezius muscle contracts, the spine rotates instead of remaining stable. This motion is often eliminated by bilateral shoulder flexion as the simultaneous bilateral contraction of the trapezius muscle stabilizes the spine. Most often, the cervical rotation occurring with shoulder flexion is seen only when one shoulder is moving.

The *levator scapula muscle* (see Figure 5-24) adducts and downwardly (medially) rotates the scapula. This muscle is a synergist of the trapezius for adduction but an antagonist for rotation. The levator scapula muscle attaches to the transverse processes of the first four cervical vertebrae. This muscle can restrict cervical rotation and in the presence of excessive cervical joint flexibility may rotate the cervical spine during shoulder motions. For example, during shoulder flexion, the levator scapula muscle is stretched as the scapula upwardly rotates. If the cervical vertebrae are more flexible than the levator scapulae muscle is extensible, the stretch of the muscle will rotate the cervical vertebrae and, in some instances, actually rotate the head to the same side as the muscle being stretched.

Because the levator scapula muscle attaches to the medial aspect of the superior angle of the scapula, shortness of this muscle can give the impression of an elevated shoulder if the examiner observes the shoulder height near the base of the neck (Figure 5-25). The attachment of the levator scapula muscle to the superior angle of the scapula can elevate the most medial portion of the scapula but does not elevate the acromial region (see Figure 5-25). Differentiating between shortness of the levator scapula and

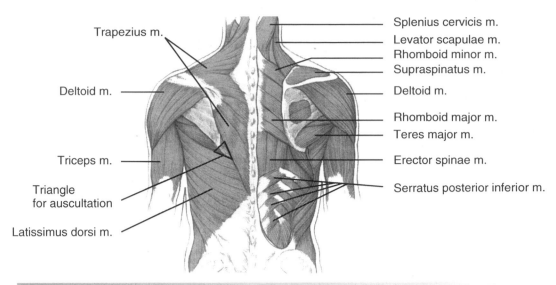

Trapezius m.

Deltoid m.

Triceps m.

Triangle
for auscultation

Latissimus dorsi m.

Splenius cervicis m.
Levator scapulae m.
Rhomboid minor m.
Supraspinatus m.
Deltoid m.
Rhomboid major m.
Teres major m.
Erector spinae m.
Serratus posterior inferior m.

Figure 5-24

Posterior axioscapular and scapulohumeral muscles. (From Mathers et al: *Clinical anatomy principles,* St Louis, 1996, Mosby.)

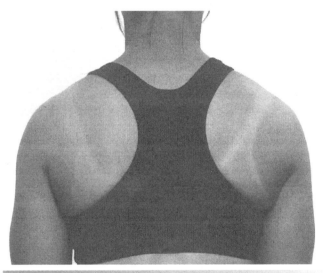

Figure 5-25

Elevation of the superior angle of the scapula with depression of the acromion. This shoulder alignment is association with shortness of the levator scapulae and excessive length of the upper trapezius muscles.

rhomboid muscles versus the upper trapezius muscle is extremely important in designing the correct therapeutic exercises.

The *rhomboid muscles* (see Figure 5-24) adduct and downwardly (medially) rotate the scapula. Similar to the levator scapula muscle, the rhomboid muscles are both synergists and antagonists of the trapezius muscles. These muscles usually become more dominant than the trapezius muscles and can restrict

upward rotation of the scapula. The exercise of shoulder shrugging with the arms at the sides (the glenohumeral joint is in downward rotation) is usually not a desirable exercise because it reinforces the activity of the rhomboid and levator scapulae muscles, contributing to the dominance of these muscles. To emphasize upper trapezius activity, shoulder shrugging should be performed with arms overhead so that the scapula is in upward rotation (Figure 5-26). Based on many postural assessments, the author has found that depressed shoulders are a common postural impairment; thus the upper trapezius muscle is frequently elongated.

The *serratus anterior muscle* (Figure 5-27) abducts and upwardly (laterally) rotates the scapula and holds the scapula flat against the rib cage. The upward rotation is produced by the force couple action of the serratus anterior muscle with the trapezius muscle. The serratus anterior muscle is the primary abductor of the scapula. Complete active range of shoulder flexion/elevation motion is not possible when the serratus anterior is paralyzed or becomes severely weak (manual muscle test grade of 2/5). In addition, deficient control by the serratus anterior muscle, causing impairments in the timing and range of scapular motion, can cause stress at the glenohumeral joint. This stress results from the incorrect positioning of the glenoid for glenohumeral joint motion when there is insufficient abduction and upward rotation of the scapula. If the scapula is not correctly positioned during shoulder flexion or abduction, the scapulohumeral muscles will not be able to maintain their optimal length and tension relationships.

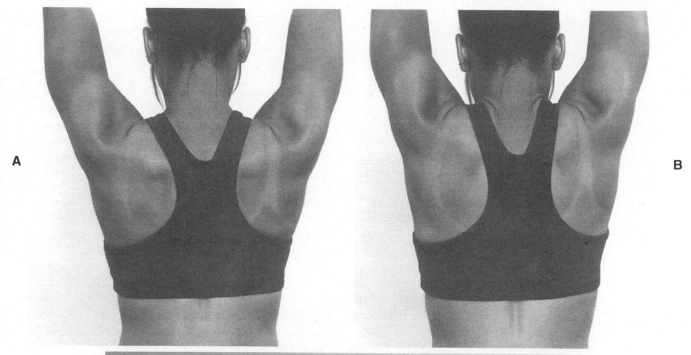

A   B

Figure 5-26

Shoulder flexion with emphasis on upper trapezius muscle activity. *A,* The shoulders remain depressed during shoulder flexion. *B,* To emphasize participation of the upper trapezius, the patient shrugs her shoulders at 90 degrees of flexion. The continued motion should be a smooth combination of shrugging and flexion.

The author has found that impaired control of the scapula by the serratus anterior muscle is common. The impaired control results from the serratus anterior muscle being weak, long, short, or altered in the timing of its movement of the scapula in relation to the movement of the humerus. Careful observation of the degree of abduction or adduction of the scapula is necessary to distinguish between insufficient performance of the trapezius or of the serratus anterior muscle. Although both muscles are upward rotators, because the trapezius is an adductor and the serratus an abductor, the medial/lateral position of the scapula can be a guide as to which muscle should be emphasized during the corrective exercise program. The primary indicators of impaired performance are inadequate abduction and inadequate upward rotation of the scapula during shoulder flexion and abduction. The inferior angle of the scapula reaching the midline of the lateral side of the thorax when the shoulder is in full flexion, as well as the scapula being upwardly rotated 60 degrees at the completion of shoulder flexion, is a guide to the correct action of the serratus anterior muscle (Figure 5-28).

Patients with adducted scapulae and large acromioclavicular joints should be carefully examined and tested for impaired performance of the serratus anterior muscle. If the serratus anterior muscle does

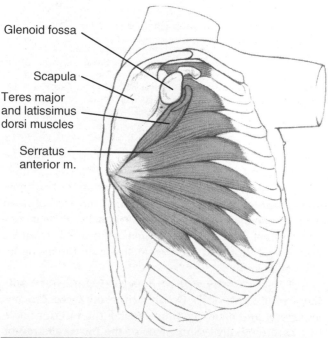

Glenoid fossa

Scapula

Teres major and latissimus dorsi muscles

Serratus anterior m.

Figure 5-27

Axioscapular muscle: serratus anterior. The serratus anterior muscle is the only effective abductor of the scapula. The serratus has an important role in upward rotation of the scapula and in keeping the scapula adhered to the thorax. (From Mathers et al: *Clinical anatomy principles,* St Louis, 1996, Mosby.)

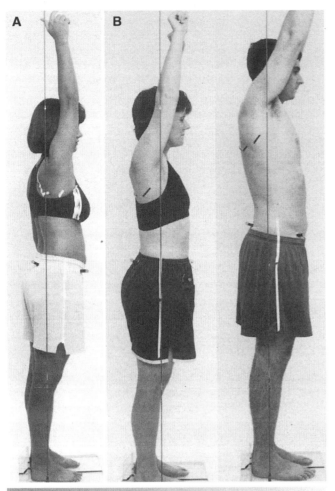

Figure 5-28

Scapular position on completion of shoulder flexion. *A,* With optimal abduction and upward rotation of the scapula during shoulder flexion, the inferior angle reaches the midline of the lateral side of the thorax. *B,* If the serratus anterior muscle does not exert optimal control of the scapula, the inferior angle will be posterior to the midline of the thorax.

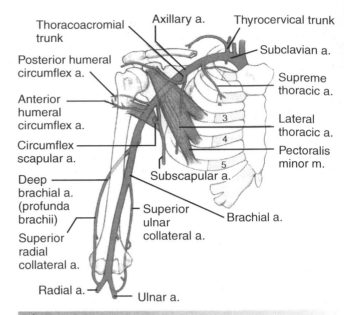

Figure 5-29

Attachments of the pectoralis minor muscle. The brachial plexus and the axillary artery run beneath the pectoralis minor muscle and above the rib cage. Anterior tilt of the scapula produced by the pectoralis minor, which attaches to the coracoid process of the scapula, can compress the nerves and vessels. (From Mathers et al: *Clinical anatomy principles,* St Louis, 1996, Mosby.)

not sufficiently upwardly rotate the scapula, then the participation of the upper trapezius muscle, another upward rotator, may be increased. The upper trapezius muscle attaches to the clavicle. According to Johnson et al, this segment of the trapezius muscle exerts its primary effect during the terminal portion of scapular upward rotation and can create stress on the acromioclavicular joint.[13]

The *pectoralis minor muscle* (Figure 5-29) tilts the scapula anteriorly by tilting the coracoid process anteriorly and caudally, thus causing the inferior angle to rotate medially.[14] Shortness of the pectoralis minor muscle interferes with the upward rotation of the scapula. If the patient has short or stiff abdominal muscles, this restriction by the pectoralis minor muscle can be even more exaggerated. Short or stiff abdominal muscles restrict the elevation of the rib cage, thus adding greater resistance to movement of the scapula

than if the rib cage elevates as a compensation for the lack of extensibility of the pectoralis minor muscle. Shortness of the pectoralis minor muscle can also contribute to thoracic outlet syndrome (see Figure 5-29). This muscle is difficult to stretch because the pressure must be applied to the coracoid process, not to the humerus, while the chest is stabilized (see Figure 5-30). Therefore the most effective stretching requires an assistant. These techniques are described in the therapeutic exercise section.

Correcting the scapular position (see Figure 5-30) with the glenohumeral joint in neutral position must be performed carefully. Because the emphasis should be on posterior tilt and not on adduction of the scapula, the exercise of scapular posterior tilt performed in the standing position must be taught carefully so that adduction is not exaggerated. This exercise may not stretch the pectoralis minor muscle, and the contraction of the rhomboid muscles can reinforce the downward rotation of the scapula, which is a common problem. The author prefers that the patient try to acquire the correct scapular alignment by abducting and depressing (posteriorly tilting) the scapula when the shoulders are flexed or abducted to at least 90 degrees and the elbows are flexed. The patient should then carefully return the arms to his or her sides by moving in the shoulder joint and not allowing the scapula to anteriorly tilt during the return to neutral position of

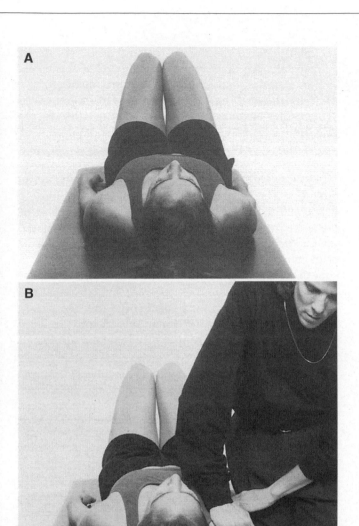

Figure 5-30

A, Shoulders tilted forward because of shortness of the pectoralis minor muscle. The lateral border of the spine of the scapula is more than an 1 inch off the table. *B,* Passive stretch of the pectoralis minor corrects the scapular position. The therapist applies pressure to the coracoid process of the scapula in a diagonal direction that is the line of the muscle fibers. The rib cage must be stabilized if the chest elevates or rotates during the application of stretch.

the glenohumeral joint. Management of shoulder pain syndromes requires a careful examination of the length and stiffness of the pectoralis minor muscle and the implementation of a precise stretching program when an impairment is identified.

Thoracohumeral Muscles

Impairments of the *pectoralis major* (Figure 5-31) and the *latissimus dorsi* (see Figure 5-24) muscles can contribute to glenohumeral joint dysfunction. These

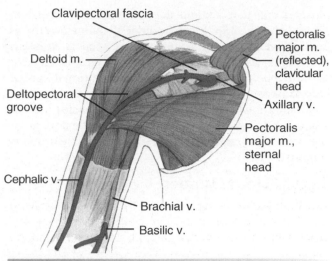

Figure 5-31

Axiohumeral muscle: pectoralis major. The pectoralis major flexes, medially rotates, and horizontally adducts the humerus. (From Mathers et al: *Clinical anatomy principles,* St Louis, 1996, Mosby.)

muscles essentially bypass the scapula and attach directly to the humerus and can contribute to disruption of scapulohumeral rhythm. Because both of these muscles are medial rotators of the humerus and are powerful muscles with strong and extensive attachments to the axial skeleton, the range of shoulder lateral rotation can be limited during the last one third of the range of shoulder flexion if they become short or stiff. In addition, both muscles attach farther away from the axis of rotation of the glenohumeral joint than the scapulohumeral medial rotators. When they become the dominant muscles, they can be a source of faulty control of the humerus in the glenoid.

The pectoralis major muscle, if not appropriately counterbalanced by muscles such as the subscapularis muscle, can contribute to excessive anterior glide of the humeral head. Because both the latissimus dorsi and pectoralis major muscles depress the shoulder girdle, if one or both are short or dominant, they can become sources of restriction of shoulder girdle elevation, which is a motion that should accompany shoulder flexion.

The pectoralis major muscle adducts and medially rotates the humerus. The upper fibers flex and horizontally adduct the shoulder. The lower fibers depress the shoulder girdle through their attachments on the humerus. A common clinical finding is that the fibers forming the sternal portion of the pectoralis major muscle test short, whereas the fibers forming the clavicular portion test long (Figure 5-32).

The latissimus dorsi muscle medially rotates, adducts, and extends the shoulder and depresses the shoulder girdle. Acting bilaterally, the latissimus dorsi muscles can help extend the spine and anteriorly tilt the pelvis. The range of shoulder flexion/elevation is limited when the latissimus dorsi muscle is short (Figure 5-33). If the abdominal muscles are short or stiff, the back will maintain a relatively normal lumbar curvature even without an active effort to contract the abdominal muscles. If the abdominal muscles are not taut when the patient performs shoulder flexion, he or she will compensate with lumbar spine extension (Figure 5-34).

Scapulohumeral Muscles

The counterbalancing effects of the scapulohumeral muscles are critical to optimal control of the humerus in its relationship to the glenoid. The most common impairments are as follows:

1. Shortness or stiffness of the lateral rotators.
2. Insufficient activity of the lateral rotators and therefore inadequate lateral rotation of the humerus to prevent the greater tuberosity from contacting the acromion.
3. Insufficient activity of the subscapularis muscle, which in turn allows the humeral head to glide anteriorly and superiorly.
4. Dominance of the deltoid muscle, causing the humeral head to glide superiorly.

5. Shortness of the lateral rotators and teres major muscle also impeding the maintenance of the correct axis of rotation for the humeral head.
6. Shortness of the capsule, particularly the posterior or inferior part. Because the rotator cuff muscles are an intrinsic part of the capsule, shortness or stiffness of these muscles should also imply similar effects on the capsule.

The *deltoid muscle* (see Figure 5-24) abducts the humerus. The anterior portion of the deltoid muscle flexes and medially rotates the humerus, the posterior portion extends and laterally rotates the humerus, and the middle portion abducts the humerus. This is a powerful muscle and from the rest position generates a superiorly directed vector that pulls the humeral head toward the acromion. Therefore it is essential that the depressors of the humeral head, primarily the supraspinatus, infraspinatus, teres minor, and subscapularis muscles, adequately offset the proximal pull of the deltoid muscle.

Often when the deltoid muscle becomes dominant as the patient performs shoulder abduction, the humeral head glides superiorly because the downward pull of the rotator cuff muscles is insufficient and cannot counterbalance the upward pull of the deltoid. As the humerus continues to abduct, the compression forces

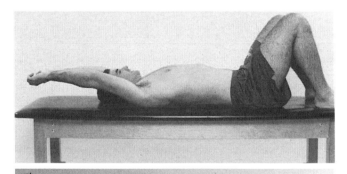

Figure 5-33

Length assessment of the latissimus dorsi muscle. The flat lumbar spine and limited range of shoulder flexion are indicative of shortness of the latissimus dorsi muscle.

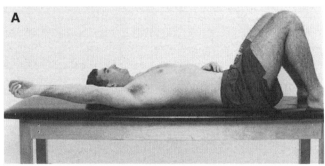

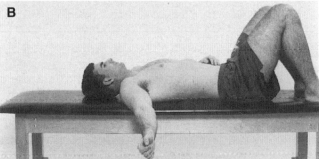

Figure 5-32

Length assessments of the pectoralis major muscle. *A,* Shortness of the sternal portion of the pectoralis major muscle, limits the range of shoulder motion in 155 degrees of abduction. *B,* The clavicular portion of the pectoralis major muscle is often excessively long, as indicated by the excessive horizontal abduction of the shoulder, even in individuals with shortness of the sternal portion.

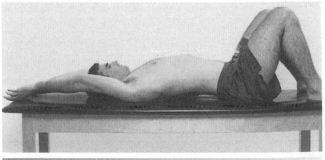

Figure 5-34

Shoulder flexion increased by extension of the lumbar spine. When this patient allows his lumbar spine to extend (taking some of the stretch off of the latissimus dorsi), the range of shoulder flexion is increased.

generated by the deltoid muscle maintain the humerus in this position. If the same patient flexes rather than abducts the humerus, the movement impairment is not evident. This can be explained by the reduced participation of the deltoid muscle. During flexion, the primary activity is in the anterior portion, which is just one third of the muscle, as compared with activity of the entire deltoid muscle during abduction.

Another dominance pattern involves the posterior deltoid. When the posterior deltoid has become the dominant lateral rotator, the result is anterior glide of the humeral head during the motion. One of the most challenging aspects of developing exercises for the rotator cuff muscles is ensuring that the infraspinatus and teres minor muscles are participating optimally and that the posterior deltoid muscle is not the primary rotator. One method of assessing the degree of participation of the different lateral rotators is to monitor the head of the humerus during the motion and not just the distal motion of the humerus. In the prone position with the shoulder in 90 degrees of abduction, the elbow flexed to 90 degrees, and the forearm over the edge of the table, the patient is instructed to laterally rotate the shoulder. The therapist places his or her fingers under the humeral head to monitor the motion. The humeral head should not anteriorly glide and exert pressure against the therapist's fingers. When the deltoid is dominant, in addition to the humeral anterior glide, the shoulder often extends, and the posterior deltoid muscle belly becomes prominent with dimpling evident just inferior to the posterior deltoid muscle belly. When the teres minor and infraspinatus are the dominant lateral rotator muscles, the motion is pure rotation and the head of the humerus is pulled toward the glenoid and does not glide anteriorly. Careful performance of this exercise is critical to correction of rotator cuff dysfunction.

Depressed shoulder joint alignment is actually abduction of the glenohumeral joint despite the patient being at rest with his arms by his sides (Figure 5-35). When the glenohumeral joint is abducted, the deltoid and supraspinatus muscles are in shortened positions. If the resting glenohumeral joint position is one of medial rotation, the combination of abduction and medial rotation of the humerus predisposes the subject to an impingement syndrome (Figure 5-36). In some cases the deltoid muscle is short; to compensate, the shoulders become depressed or downwardly rotated or both so the arms will be close to the thorax while in a standing posture. The therapist can assess this by correcting the scapular position. If the humerus then assumes an abducted position, the deltoid muscle and possibly the supraspinatus muscle are short.

Another cause of depressed shoulders, besides short deltoid and supraspinatus muscles, is when the upper trapezius muscle has become lengthened. In this condition the deltoid and supraspinatus muscles are not necessarily short as described. Normally, the scapula must upwardly rotate during abduction or the deltoid muscle will become too short to work effectively (Figure 5-37). In patients with depressed shoulders, the amount of shoulder girdle elevation must exceed that of the normal situation to compensate for

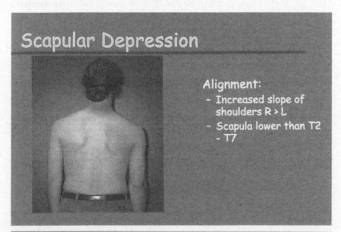

Figure 5-35

Shoulder alignment of abduction associated with depressed shoulders.

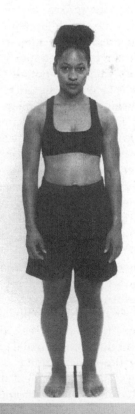

Figure 5-36

Depressed shoulders. When the shoulders are depressed, the glenohumeral joint is in an abducted position.

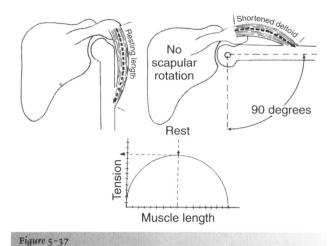

Figure 5-37

Deltoid contractile inefficiency. When the scapula is not upwardly rotated, the deltoid becomes too short to develop effective contractile tension. (From Calliet R: *Shoulder pain,* ed 2, Philadelphia, 1981, FA Davis.)

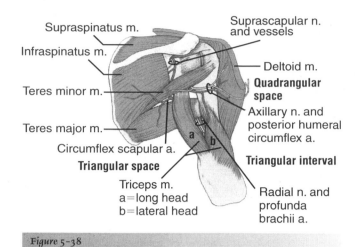

Figure 5-38

Scapulohumeral muscle. The supraspinatus muscle abducts, slightly laterally rotates, and depresses the humerus. (From Mathers et al: *Clinical anatomy principles,* St Louis, 1996, Mosby.)

the impaired starting alignment. Typically the optimal degree of elevation does not occur. Precise function of the thoracoscapular muscles is critical in providing the required control of the scapula to position the glenoid and to optimize the action of the scapulohumeral muscles.

The *supraspinatus muscle* (Figure 5-38) abducts and laterally rotates the shoulder, depresses, and stabilizes the humeral head in the glenoid. Because this muscle passes under the acromion, it is particularly vulnerable to injury when the shoulder is depressed. If the humeral head (1) glides superiorly, (2) does not glide inferiorly during shoulder flexion and abduction, or (3) does not laterally rotate enough to prevent impingement of the greater tuberosity against the coracoacromial ligament, then the supraspinatus muscle and tendon are exposed to compression forces (Figure 5-39). A commonly used exercise that increases the risk of impingement of the greater tuberosity of the humerus against the coracoacromial ligament is shoulder abduction to 90 degrees or more with the humerus medially rotated. Because of the increased risk of impingement, this exercise should be avoided particularly in the range of 70 to 90 degrees of abduction. Many patients performing this exercise have depressed shoulders; when they abduct to shoulder height, they are abducting more than 90 degrees. In addition, performing shoulder abduction in medial rotation can contribute to anterior tilt of the scapula.

If the resting postural alignment of the scapula is one of exaggerated abduction, the apparent shoulder medial rotation is actually the correct alignment of the humeral head in its relationship to the glenoid (Figure

5-40). Because the scapula follows the contour of the rib cage during abduction, the degree of rotation in the frontal plane increases. The result is that the glenoid faces more anteriorly than if the scapula is positioned correctly on the thorax. Therefore when the scapula is abducted and the glenoid faces more anteriorly than laterally, the humerus will appear to be medially rotated because the cubital fossa is facing medially. However, this alignment helps to maintain the correct relationship between the humeral head and the glenoid.

Correct performance of glenohumeral joint abduction requires that the humerus is in the plane of the scapula. Therefore if the scapula is abducted and rotated in the frontal plane, the humerus during abduction should be in the same plane as the scapula and will appear slightly forward of the side of the body. If the arm is maintained in line with the frontal plane of the body and not the scapula, the humerus is actually in an extended position and the humeral head will be in an anterior position in relation to the acromion. Careful assessment of the position of the scapula and of the humerus in relationship to the glenoid is essential when developing exercise programs for shoulder pain problems and when correcting alignment and movement impairments during functional activities.

The following example illustrates the importance of careful assessment. A patient is referred to physical therapy for biceps tendonitis of the right shoulder. The magnetic resonance imaging (MRI) indicates a tendon pathologic condition and superior position of the humeral head. The patient also has subluxation of the sternoclavicular joint, scoliosis,

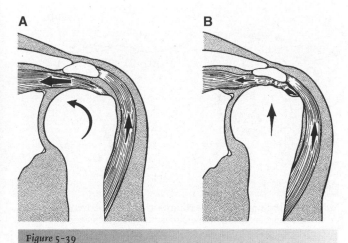

Figure 5-39

Compression of the supraspinatus tendon. If downward pull of the humerus by the rotator cuff muscles is insufficient to counteract, the upward pull from the deltoid, the supraspinatus tendon can be impinged. (From Rockwood CA, Matsen FA: *The shoulder,* vol 1, Philadelphia, 1990, WB Saunders.)

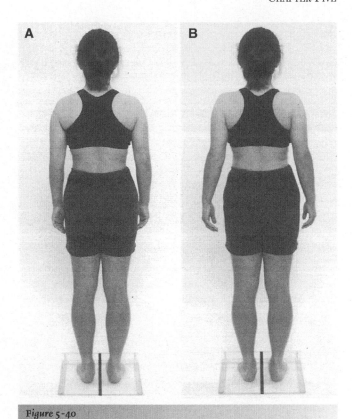

Figure 5-40

Abducted scapula and humeral rotation. *A,* When the scapula is abducted the humerus appears to be medially rotated because the olecranon faces laterally. *B,* When the scapular position is corrected, the humerus no longer appears to be medially rotated.

and a right rib hump contributing to abduction of the scapula. In the resting position, her cubital fossa is directed anteriorly. She does not have any range of motion limitations. Her shoulder becomes painful with use of her right dominant hand, even when she is not doing overhead or lifting activities. Based on the belief that what appears to be the correct degree of humeral rotation with her arm at her side is actually lateral rotation, she is instructed to change the manner of using her arm. She is instructed to turn the cubital fossa medially, which also means that she has to be in slight abduction to use her arm for activities such as cutting and chopping food and working on her computer. This change in alignment coincides with a major improvement in her condition. No improvement had occurred in her condition during the month before changing the degree of rotation of her shoulder during daily activities.

The *infraspinatus muscle* (see Figure 5-38) laterally rotates and depresses the head of the humerus. The infraspinatus and teres minor muscles are the primary lateral rotator muscles that depress the head of the humerus, with some assistance from the supraspinatus. The posterior deltoid, a powerful lateral rotator, causes superior glide of the humeral head. Based on comparison of the number of muscles and their size, the medial rotators should be able to generate greater tension than the lateral rotators. The lateral rotator muscles and the posterior capsule often become short or stiff and can interfere with the posterior glide of the humeral head; thus it is extremely important that they be monitored for both their length and strength properties.[19]

The *teres minor muscle* (see Figure 5-38) laterally rotates and depresses the head of the humerus. This muscle has the same important role in depressing and laterally rotating the humeral head as the infraspinatus muscle. Deficiencies in performance of these two muscles are very common. Shortness or greater stiffness of the teres minor and infraspinatus muscles relative to the stiffness of the axioscapular muscle is common (Figure 5-41). Shortness of the lateral rotators can contribute to excessive anterior and superior glide of the humeral head. Restricted posterior glide and excessive anterior glide of the humeral head are factors in shoulder impingement syndromes.[12] Neer has described how the lack of posterior capsular length contributes to impingement during flexion[21] (Figure 5-42).

The *subscapularis muscle* (see Figure 5-38) medially rotates the humerus and depresses the head of the humerus. This muscle has a particularly important role because of its angle of pull, acting not only to depress the head of the humerus but also to pull it posteriorly, thus offsetting the muscles acting to cause an anterior-superior glide of the humerus. Because large powerful muscles such as the pectoralis major and latissimus

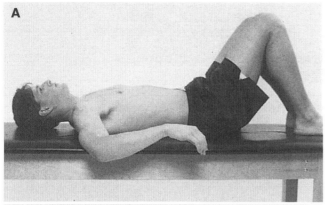

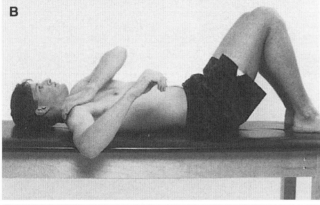

Figure 5-41

Test of the length of the lateral rotator muscles. *A,* In the supine position with the shoulder abducted to 90 degrees and the elbow flexed, the shoulder is allowed to rotate medially and the scapula anteriorly tilts, rather than the range of shoulder medial rotation increasing. *B,* When the scapular tilt is prevented, the shortness of the lateral rotators is evident.

dorsi muscles are also medial rotators, the subscapularis muscle often becomes less dominant. The subscapularis and the joint capsule provide anterior glenohumeral stability.[29,30] If the subscapularis becomes long or weak, the result can be excessive anterior glide of the humeral head, which has been cited as a precursor to impingement syndrome.[11] If the lateral rotators are short or stiff, this can contribute further to the anterior and superior glide of the humeral head and can limit the medial rotation range, resulting in lengthening or weakening of the subscapularis muscle. In addition, if the pectoralis major is the dominant medial rotator, its attachment on a more distal portion of the humerus and its anterior pull on the humerus will further exaggerate the anterior glide of the humeral head and place pressure on the anterior joint capsule during shoulder flexion or horizontal adduction.

The *teres major muscle* (see Figure 5-38) medially rotates, adducts, and extends the shoulder joint. Shortness of this muscle limits shoulder flexion and can impede depression and lateral rotation of the humeral head. Accurate assessment of the length of the

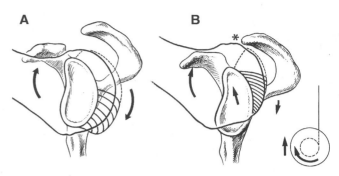

Figure 5-42

Stiffness of the posterior glenohumeral capsule. *A,* Normally lax posterior capsule allows the humeral head to remain centered in the glenoid during shoulder flexion. *B,* Stiffness of the posterior joint capsule forces the humeral head upward against the anteroinferior acromion as the shoulder is flexed. (From Rockwood CA, Matsen FA: *The shoulder,* vol 1, Philadelphia, 1990, WB Saunders.)

teres major muscle is particularly important when the range of shoulder flexion is limited and when the PICR of the humeral head does not remain centered but drops inferiorly during humeral flexion or abduction.

Movement Impairment Syndromes of the Scapula

Relationship Between Alignment and Movement

As discussed in Chapter 1, optimal movement performance is more easily achieved if the alignment of body segments is closer to ideal than if marked deviations in segmental alignment are present. However, several combinations of movement patterns and alignments are possible with each combination having a different implication for the examination process and the subsequent management. The following examples illustrate how alignment and movement faults are used to define the various syndromes:

- *The scapular alignment is correct, but the movement of the scapula is impaired.* Impaired scapular movement refers to insufficient or excessive range, alteration in orientation, or inappropriate timing of scapular movement in relation to humeral motion. For example, although the subject has ideal shoulder girdle alignment, the scapula only upwardly rotates 40 degrees at the completion of shoulder flexion.

- *The scapular alignment is impaired, and the movement is impaired.* For example, the scapula is downwardly rotated in the starting position and upwardly rotates only 40 degrees by the time the range of shoulder flexion is completed. The result could be only 35 of the 60 degrees of upward rotation that are standard for scapular rotation during shoulder flexion.

- *The scapular alignment is impaired, and the movement is of normal range but does not correct or compensate for the initial impaired position.* For example, the scapula is downwardly rotated 10 degrees and the range of scapular upward rotation is 60 degrees, but the final position of upward rotation is still 10 degrees less than that required for optimal scapular motion during shoulder flexion.

- *The scapular alignment is impaired, but the movement is of sufficient range (greater than ideal) to compensate for the initial position.* For example, the scapula is downwardly rotated 10 degrees, and during shoulder flexion the scapula upwardly rotates 70 degrees. Because the scapular motion is correct, the glenohumeral joint motion is not particularly impaired, but the impaired alignment of the scapula is usually associated with neck pain. Correcting scapular alignment often alleviates the neck pain or the associated referred pain arising from myofascial stress or from radiculopathy.

The syndromes are identified by naming the bony segment, scapula or humerus, followed by the name of the primary movement impairment. Although both the scapula and humerus may be involved, usually one is the source of the primary movement problem and is designated as the primary diagnosis. Correction of this segment's pattern of movement is the most important part of the treatment program. A major fault of the other segment, when present, is designated as the secondary diagnosis.

Criteria for the Diagnosis of a Scapular Syndrome

- The primary problem is impaired scapular movement.
- The impaired scapular movement often causes or is associated with impaired humeral motion.
- Symptoms are reduced when the patient performs the scapular motion correctly or the therapist corrects the scapular impairment during active movement performed by the patient. For example, the therapist assists the upward rotation of the scapula when this is identified as being insufficient during shoulder flexion/elevation. Because this correction decreases or eliminates the pain, the therapeutic program is designed to correct the movement impairment and the contributing impairments.
- The syndrome is named for the observed impairment that may present as abnormal, an exaggeration of normal, or an insufficient range of motion.

For example, scapular downward rotation syndrome is the name assigned to the condition when either the scapular downward rotation is exaggerated during the early phases of shoulder flexion/abduction or its upward rotation movement is less than the kinesiologic standard at the completion of the motion.

Scapular Syndromes in Observed Frequency of Occurrence

Establishing a specific diagnosis of a syndrome does not require the presence of all of the impairments described for a syndrome. The relationship between the behavior of the symptoms and the impaired movement pattern should be present. The greater the number of impairments, the greater the severity of the syndrome, although it is also possible to have only one impairment that is particularly severe.

As with all musculoskeletal pain syndromes, various stages of severity can be present. For example, shoulder pain at rest suggests an acute inflammatory state. If positioning the shoulder girdle in the correct alignment and alleviating compression forces on the humeral head (such as the force on the superior aspect of the humerus associated with leaning on the elbow) does not alleviate the pain, then the exercise program should be limited to relatively pain-free exercises. This is consistent with established treatment during the acute stages of the inflammatory process.[3,8]

Pain-free motion through at least 60% of the normal glenohumeral joint range into flexion and rotation should be available before a major emphasis is placed on using scapular motions in the treatment program. Thus the treatment with patients with marked glenohumeral hypomobility is directed primarily at improving mobility at the glenohumeral joint with less attention directed toward scapular motion. Correction of scapular resting alignment is always indicated. Once these criteria are met and the pain occurs primarily at the end of the range of glenohumeral joint motion rather than during movement, the management of impaired scapular movement becomes particularly important. In those conditions in which the passive range of shoulder motion is not restricted by more than 20 degrees, the impairments in scapular control are most likely the key to alleviating the pain. However, very often there is also a humeral component as discussed in the next section.

Scapular Downward Rotation Syndrome

SYMPTOMS, PAIN PROBLEMS, AND ASSOCIATED DIAGNOSES. Many of the pathoanatomic or associated diagnoses described for this syndrome are also found in the other movement impairment syndromes. Because the same pain problem is present with different movement impairments, using a diagnosis based on the name of the painful anatomic structure, such as supraspinatus tendinopathy, or an associated diagnosis, such as impingement, is not adequate for directing treatment. A diagnosis that provides information about the cause and direction for remediation of the problem is more useful for directing physical therapy than for just identifying the potential anatomic source of the pain. Describing the movement impairment syndrome and its contributing factors provides guidelines for directing the treatment for alleviating the pain problem.

Supraspinatus or rotator cuff tendinopathy and impingement. The pinching of any structure between the head of the humerus and the acromion is referred to as impingement of the shoulder. This may include the bursa, the rotator cuff tendons, or the tendon of the long head of the biceps brachii muscle. Other associated diagnoses include tendinopathy, bursitis, and minor rotator cuff tears or strains. Sharp or pinching pain is usually present around the anterior, lateral, or posterior aspect of the acromial process of the scapula during shoulder abduction or flexion. Often the pain will be referred to the area of the insertion of the deltoid muscle. The insufficient upward rotation of the scapula causes the humerus to impinge against the coracoacromial ligament. This situation becomes particularly exaggerated if the humeral depressor muscles do not counteract the upward pull of the deltoid muscle or if the humerus does not adequately laterally rotate. Possible sources of this pain are the various soft tissues beneath the acromial process. Four stages leading to the development of rotator cuff disorders have been described.[9] In stage 1, the edema and hemorrhage are attributed to repeated microtrauma. Unless the cause of the microtrauma is addressed, the process can lead to more severe pathology.

Rotator cuff tear. Deep pain can be present at the insertions of any of the rotator cuff muscles. The downward rotation of the scapula and the compensatory glenohumeral joint motion can cause microtrauma leading to rotator cuff tear. The most obvious clinical sign of a large rotator cuff tear is when a patient has full range of passive shoulder motion but is unable to perform complete range of active shoulder flexion even without pain. Manual muscle testing indicates that the lateral rotator muscles are weak and significant atrophy of the rotator cuff musculature is evident. If the tear is severe, even if the shoulder is passively placed in shoulder flexion or abduction, the patient is unable to hold the arm in that position (positive drop arm test).

Thoracic outlet and neural entrapment. Symptoms of this condition include numbness and tingling in the forearm and hand, particularly on the ulnar side of the forearm. This condition is most frequently seen when the scapula is depressed and downwardly rotated or tilted forward.

Humeral subluxation. Humeral subluxation can occur during shoulder flexion when the inferior joint capsule and other supporting structures such as the glenohumeral ligaments are stretched. Restriction of the upward rotation of the scapula with extreme flexibility of the glenohumeral joint predisposes the humerus to inferior subluxation (the humerus moves without maintaining the proper relationship with the glenoid).

Humeral instabilities. During shoulder motion, there is a discontinuity in the coordinated movement of the scapula and humerus, such that the humerus seems to suddenly alter its movement and "pop" into a new position.

Neck pain (with or without radiating pain into the arm). This occurs because of the downward or asymmetric rotational pull on the cervical vertebrae or the cervical plexus by the levator scapulae muscle, the upper trapezius muscle, and the weight of the upper extremity.

Pain in the levator scapula and the upper trapezius muscles. This occurs from strain as the result of the muscles being in a stretched or lengthened position.

Acromioclavicular joint pain. If the serratus anterior muscle is not functioning adequately, extra stress is placed on the acromion and clavicle by the trapezius muscle as it attempts to upwardly rotate the scapula. When the serratus anterior muscle is participating optimally, this stress is reduced by the action of the serratus anterior muscle on the vertebral border of the scapula. If the rhomboid muscles are short or stiff, the resistance they create also adds to the stress at the acromioclavicular joint as the trapezius muscle attempts to upwardly rotate the scapula.

Sternoclavicular joint pain. The sternoclavicular joint acts as a fulcrum for shoulder motion and can be subject to stress if (1) the pectoralis minor muscle is short restricting scapular motion, (2) the upper trapezius muscle attaching to the lateral part of the clavicle is exerting a strong pull, and (3) the performance of the serratus anterior muscle is not optimal. The joint is often swollen, painful to touch, and painful with shoulder motion.

MOVEMENT IMPAIRMENTS. After approximately the first 30 degrees of shoulder motion into abduction and 60 degrees into flexion, the scapula downwardly rotates during glenohumeral flexion/abduction instead of rotating upwardly as is the normal pattern. Scapular upward rotation or glenohumeral elevation or both are insufficient (scapula does not rotate 60 degrees), particularly during the final phase of humeral elevation.

The inferior angle of the scapula does not reach the midaxillary line of the thorax upon completion of shoulder flexion because of insufficient abduction and upward rotation.

Alignment

STRUCTURAL VARIATIONS

- **Thoracic kyphosis.** The accompanying rib deformity contributes to impaired scapular starting position. In addition, the curvature of the ribs interferes with the scapular upward rotation and depression at the completion of shoulder flexion.

- **Scoliosis.** Depending on the degree of curvature, the rib deformity contributes to the impaired scapular posture.

- **Obesity with a large thorax.** The shoulder girdle is usually downwardly rotated with the humerus in abduction at the glenohumeral joint because of the width of the thorax and the weight of the arms.

- **Large breasts.** The weight of the breasts that is exerted on the lateral aspect of the scapula via bra straps adds to downwardly rotated scapula.

- **Heavy arms.** The weight of the arms can contribute to downward pull on the shoulder girdle and cause an excessive load on the muscles during arm movements.

- **Long trunk with relatively short arms.** The standard height of the armrests on most chairs is too low for individuals with this type of structure. They are unable to rest their forearms on the armrests unless they downwardly rotate or depress their shoulder.

ACQUIRED IMPAIRMENTS

- A downwardly rotated scapula, with the inferior border more medial than the superior border, can result from shortness of the deltoid and the supraspinatus muscles, from excessive length of the upper trapezius muscle, or from shortness or stiffness of the levator scapulae and the rhomboid muscles (Figure 5-43).

- The shoulders are lower and downwardly sloped at the acromial end but may appear higher at the base of the neck because of shortness of the levator scapulae muscle, which attaches to the superior border of the scapula.

- Forward shoulders are frequently seen secondary to tilting of the scapula and a forward head posture.

- Abduction of the humerus can be secondary to the downwardly rotated position of the scapula.

- The scapula may be adducted, the vertebral border is less than 3 inches from the vertebral spine.

RELATIVE FLEXIBILITY AND STIFFNESS IMPAIRMENTS. The glenohumeral joint moves through its range more readily than does the thoracoscapular joint. Because the scapula does not fully upwardly rotate, the glenohumeral joint becomes the site of compensatory movement. To achieve 180 degrees of shoulder flexion/elevation, the humerus must rotate on the glenoid fossa for more than 120 degrees to compensate for the lack of the ideal 60 degrees of scapular upward rotation. Increased stiffness of the rhomboids and/or the levator

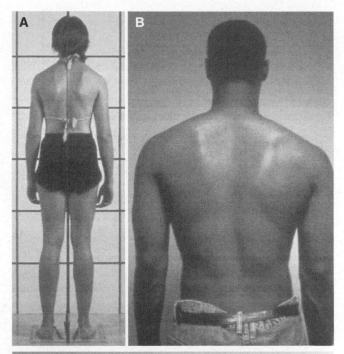

Figure 5-43

Downwardly rotated scapula. *A,* The obvious definition of the left rhomboid muscle suggests that the dominance of this muscle contributed to the downward rotation. The position of the right scapula can be attributed to shortness of the deltoid and supraspinatus. *B,* Excessive length of the upper trapezius and serratus anterior are contributing factors to the position of the scapula.

scapulae muscles creates an impediment to scapular upward rotation. If the glenohumeral joint does not compensate for the deficient scapular motion, shoulder flexion range will be limited.

MUSCLE IMPAIRMENTS

Recruitment pattern impairments. During the initiation of flexion, the action of downward rotation by the rhomboids and the levator scapulae muscles is dominant over the action of upward rotation by the trapezius and the serratus anterior muscles.

During the initiation of abduction, the action of the deltoid muscle can cause the scapula to downwardly rotate if the upward rotating activity of the trapezius and serratus anterior muscles is insufficient to counteract the effect of the deltoid muscle during glenohumeral abduction.

During shoulder flexion, the activity of the trapezius and serratus anterior muscles, which are the primary upward rotators of the scapula, is insufficient and does not upwardly rotate the scapula the desired 60 degrees (Figure 5-44).

Muscle length and strength impairments. Passive upward rotation and, if necessary, assisted upward rotation of the scapula by the therapist as the patient

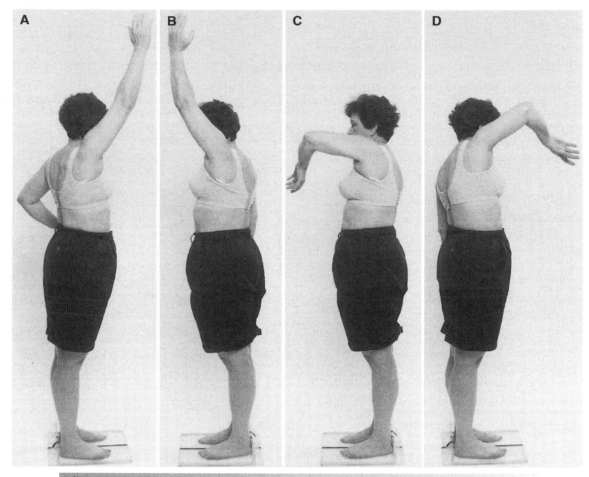

Figure 5-44

Insufficient scapular upward rotation and excessive glenohumeral flexion. *A,* The inferior angle of the right scapula does not reach the midline of the lateral thorax during maximum shoulder flexion. *B,* The left scapula reaches the midline during maximum shoulder flexion. *C,* With the humerus maximally medially rotated, shoulder flexion should be only slightly greater than 90 degrees if scapular movement is limited. *D,* Because of the limited scapula upward rotation, flexion of the right shoulder is excessive.

performs shoulder flexion indicates the degree of resistance to this motion and/or the limitation of scapular abduction and upward rotation.

Shortness of the rhomboids and levator scapulae muscles can restrict the range of abduction or upward rotation of the scapula or both.

Shortness of the pectoralis minor muscle can interfere with scapular upward rotation because of the resultant anterior tilting of the scapula. Maintaining the scapula in an anteriorly tilted position does not allow the scapula to upwardly rotate during shoulder flexion and to depress, adduct, and posteriorly tilt at the end of the range.

The latissimus dorsi muscle can exert a downward pull on the humerus and on the inferior angle of the scapula. Although the attachment of the latissimus dorsi to the inferior angle is inconsistent, if the attachments are present and the latissimus dorsi is short, the effect could be depression of the shoulder girdle. If the latissimus dorsi is short, depression of the shoulder girdle allows a greater range of shoulder flexion or abduction than if the shoulder girdle is not depressed.

Shortness of the deltoid and supraspinatus muscles can cause the resting position of the humerus to be in abduction. Instead of the arm remaining in the undesirable and awkward position of abduction with the elbow positioned away from the body, the scapula downwardly rotates to allow the entire humerus to be closer to the body.

If the upper and lower trapezius muscles are long or weak or both, they cannot generate sufficient tension to assist in upward rotation of the scapula. Optimal performance of the upper trapezius is necessary to elevate the acromial end of the scapula during the first part of the glenohumeral motion. Optimal performance of the lower trapezius is necessary to upwardly rotate the scapula, particularly at the end of the range. Scapular motion must be optimal to prevent undue stress on the glenohumeral joint.

CONFIRMING TESTS

- Insufficient upward rotation of the scapula can be observed during active glenohumeral joint flexion/abduction with the presence of any of the symptoms listed previously.
- Passive support of the scapula in the correct alignment results in reduction or elimination of the patient's symptoms in the neck region and often results in improved range of motion of the cervical spine into rotation. Scapular downward rotation syndrome is a secondary diagnosis for the cervical problem.
- The therapist can passively upwardly rotate the scapula during glenohumeral flexion and decrease the patient's symptoms.
- The therapist feels resistance while attempting to passively correct the scapular alignment or while assisting in upwardly rotating the scapula.

TREATMENT. The downwardly rotated position of the scapula must be corrected throughout the day and during sleep whenever possible. The patient should sit with his or her arm supported so that the scapula is maintained in the correct alignment and the glenohumeral joint is not abducted. Chairs must have armrests adjusted high enough to correctly support the arm and maintain the shoulder in the correct alignment. Sitting on a sofa with low armrests or no armrests should be discouraged. The patient must find support for his or her arm if not provided by the furniture.

If possible, the patient's shoulder girdle should be passively supported while working or driving a car. The patient can use his or her contralateral hand, placed under the elbow like a sling, to support the affected shoulder when standing for a prolonged time. Any activities that exaggerate the downward rotation of the scapula should be eliminated. An example of this is resistive exercises requiring scapular adduction with the shoulder at less than 120 degrees of flexion.

If pressure from bra straps is contributing to the impaired alignment, a sports bra with straps that cross closer to the neck is recommended. Carrying a backpack or a waist pack instead of a purse supported on the painful shoulder is recommended. Carrying a briefcase or suitcase with the affected arm should be avoided. All activities of daily living should be reviewed and modified accordingly.

Important exercises emphasize the serratus anterior muscle and the trapezius muscle performance. The patient must be taught how to abduct and to upwardly rotate his or her scapulae. Exercises to emphasize these motions of the scapula can be performed in the prone position or standing and facing a wall. The range of glenohumeral motion should not be emphasized because of the possibility of increasing or causing compensatory glenohumeral joint hypermobility.

Shoulder shrugs with the arms in the anatomic position should be avoided because this movement pattern encourages levator scapulae and rhomboid muscle activity rather than the desired activity of the upper trapezius muscle. However, with the arms held in elevation, the shoulder shrug exercise emphasizes upper trapezius activity.

The patient may need assistance with scapular upward rotation and abduction if the rhomboid and levator scapulae muscles are short or are particularly stiff. In the supine position with the shoulder flexed, the patient can use the opposite hand to pull the inferior angle of the scapula to assist in its upward rotation.

Prescribing stretching exercises for the muscles found to be short during the examination is important. Of equal importance is ensuring that the patient does and continues to do the exercises correctly. The passive support of the shoulders and exercises performed facing the wall should be repeated frequently during the day and evening. Often the patient needs assistance in effectively carrying out the therapist's advice during daily routines.

Exercises in the quadruped position, such as rocking backward and exaggerating the correct scapular motion, are particularly helpful to increase the participation of the serratus anterior muscles. When the patient is sitting back on his or her heels and the shoulder is flexed to almost 160 degrees, the scapula should be almost maximally upwardly rotated and there will be minimal demands on the serratus anterior muscles. If the patient performs the exercise on a table or bed, he or she can grasp the sides of the table or the top of the bed while rocking backward to assist in upward rotation of the scapula and in the stretching of the rhomboid and the levator scapulae muscles.

The patient must be careful not to allow compensatory activity at the glenohumeral joint. Often when the levator scapulae muscle is short, the head and neck will extend as the patient rocks backward. This occurs because as the scapula is being upwardly rotated and abducted, the levator scapulae muscle is lengthening. However, when the muscle is stiff, compensatory motion can occur at its cranial attachments instead of restricting the scapular motion. If the patient holds the chin toward the chest as he or she rocks backward in the quadruped position, the levator scapulae muscles will be stretched, the compensatory motion will be stopped, and the intrinsic neck flexor muscles will be strengthened. All of these corrective measures should help correct the forward head posture.

As the patient rocks forward in the quadruped position, a greater percentage of the body weight is placed on the serratus anterior muscle. If the demand exceeds the strength of the serratus anterior muscle, the scapula will wing. At this point the forward rocking motion should be stopped. Shortness of the scapulohumeral muscles also contributes to the winging of the scapula as the weight is transferred from the hips to the shoulders while rocking forward. The patient should be instructed to lift the acromion, as in shrugging, and bring the scapula around into abduction whenever he or she brings an arm overhead during functional activities.

Case Presentation 1

History. The patient is a 45-year-old male professional violinist with right shoulder pain and mild neck pain. He is right handed. In addition to the pain, he is particularly concerned about his ability to control his bow when playing on the low strings on the left side of the violin. This lack of control is most evident when playing very lightly on the strings for prolonged periods of times.

Alignment Analysis. The patient stands very erect without a kyphosis, but he has a very large chest. His right shoulder is markedly depressed. The entire spine of the right scapula is $3/4$ inch lower than the left. The scapula is downwardly rotated at rest with the inferior angle of the scapula less than 2 inches from the vertebral column. The spine of the scapula is $2^{1}/_{2}$ inches from the vertebral column. The humerus is slightly medially rotated.

Movement Analysis. During shoulder flexion the scapula wings slightly. The downward rotation of the scapula during 0 to 100 degrees of shoulder flexion is readily apparent. Upon completion of shoulder flexion, the inferior angle of the scapula reaches the lateral border of the thorax but does not move anteriorly to the midaxillary line. There is slight pain around the acromion at the end of shoulder flexion range. When performing shoulder abduction, the winging of the scapula is even more evident than during flexion. The shoulder also remains partially depressed at the end range of flexion and elevation.

When the scapular rotation/abduction is assisted during shoulder flexion, the patient no longer experiences pain in his shoulder and does not feel strain on his neck. When the patient holds his arm in 90 degrees of abduction, similar to the position used while playing the violin, and the therapist supports the scapula to prevent downward rotation, the patient indicates that he does not feel the weakness and lack of control that

was usually present in this position. When his scapula is held in neutral rotation by the therapist, the glenohumeral joint is in slight abduction. Horizontal adduction is limited to 40 degrees as compared with 60 degrees on the left side.

Muscle Length and Strength Analysis. The pectoralis minor, pectoralis major, latissimus dorsi, shoulder lateral rotators (medial rotation range is 50 degrees), deltoid, supraspinatus, and rhomboid muscles all test short. The serratus anterior and lower trapezius muscles test 3/5. The upper trapezius muscle tests 4/5.

Muscle Stiffness Analysis. The rhomboid muscles are stiff by assessment of resistance to passive movement.

Assessment. The effect of the downwardly rotated position of the scapula is as follows:

• Placing excessive strain on his neck because of the pull from the upper trapezius muscle and the lack of suitable assistance from the lower trapezius and serratus anterior muscles

• Creating a condition of "active insufficiency" for the deltoid muscle and thus compromising the patient's control of his or her arm in the abducted position. (Active insufficiency occurs when the muscle is in such a shortened position that the contractile elements overlap enough to reduce the tension generated during active contraction [see Figure 2-16].)

• Contributing to impingement of the glenohumeral joint because of the inadequate upward rotation of the glenoid

Diagnosis. The patient is diagnosed with scapular downward rotation syndrome.

Treatment

Supine exercises

• The patient performs shoulder flexion to stretch the latissimus dorsi and pectoralis major muscles.

• The therapist assists with stretching of the pectoralis minor muscle.

• Shoulder medial rotation is performed with the arm in 90 degrees of abduction.

Prone exercises. Scapular upward rotation and abduction initially required assistance from the therapist to facilitate the scapular motion.

Quadruped exercises. The patient does quadruped rocking backward with emphasis on the upward rotation of scapula. He then rocks forward to the neutral position.

Standing exercises

• The patient faces the wall, slides his arms up the wall, and shrugs his shoulders after the shoulders are flexed to 90 degrees. He continues the shrugging motion as he completes the full range of shoulder flexion.

• The patient faces the wall with the arms at maximum shoulder flexion. He adducts his scapulae to lift his arms off the wall. He is instructed not to depress his shoulders.

• The patient stands with his back to the wall, fixes his right scapula against the wall, and pulls the shoulder into horizontal adduction.

Education. The patient is instructed to have his right arm supported while sitting to keep his shoulder at the correct height. While playing the violin, he is to hold the acromial end of his right shoulder up and to move primarily at the glenohumeral joint when playing on the higher strings. When playing on the low strings, he is to pull his scapula forward into abduction and upward rotation to help correctly position the arm.

Outcome. The patient is extremely conscientious about his exercise program. Over a period of 6 weeks, with review of his program every 2 weeks, he has corrected his scapular position and can sustain a constant position of shoulder horizontal adduction and control his bow enough to play lightly on the strings. Although the initial objective of the program is accomplished, the patient returns for follow-up visits because his playing has improved markedly and he is anxious to optimize his exercise program to achieve as high a level of performance as possible.

Scapular Depression Syndrome

This syndrome is similar to the scapular downward rotation syndrome except that the rhomboids and levator scapulae muscles are not usually short. The upper trapezius muscle is particularly long and/or weak. Shortness of the latissimus dorsi and pectoralis major and minor muscles is common.

SYMPTOMS, PAIN PROBLEMS, AND ASSOCIATED DIAGNOSES
• Glenohumeral joint impingement
• Rotator cuff tear
• Humeral subluxation
• Acromioclavicular joint pain
• Neck pain with or without radiating pain into the arm
• Pain in the regions of the trapezius and levator scapulae muscles
• Thoracic outlet syndrome

MOVEMENT IMPAIRMENTS. The scapula is depressed in the starting position and fails to elevate sufficiently during glenohumeral joint flexion/abduction. If the scapula is not depressed at rest, there are two phases of movement during which the faulty movement can occur: the last phase of glenohumeral joint elevation (90 to 180 degrees) or during the initial phase of glenohumeral flexion/abduction (0 to 90 degrees).

ALIGNMENT IMPAIRMENTS
Structural variations
• Long neck, often associated with narrow shoulders and long arms
• Long trunk, typically tall and lanky

• Short arms
• Heavy arms
• Large breasts

In all of these conditions the arms exert a downward pull on the entire scapula. When sitting, the arms do not reach the armrest unless the entire shoulder girdle is depressed.

Acquired impairments
• The shoulders are depressed with the clavicles lying horizontally or slightly lower laterally than medially.
• The position of the superior angle of the scapula is lower than the second thoracic vertebra (Figure 5-45).

RELATIVE FLEXIBILITY AND STIFFNESS IMPAIRMENT. The glenohumeral joint is more flexible than the scapulothoracic joint and therefore becomes the site of compensatory motion.

MUSCLE IMPAIRMENTS
Recruitment pattern impairments
• The upper trapezius muscle does not elevate the shoulder girdle during shoulder flexion/abduction.
• The lower trapezius muscle (depressor of the scapula) is more dominant than the upper trapezius muscle (elevator of the scapula) during shoulder motions.

Muscle length and strength impairments
• Shortness of the latissimus dorsi muscle can depress the shoulder girdle and interfere with elevation of the scapula.

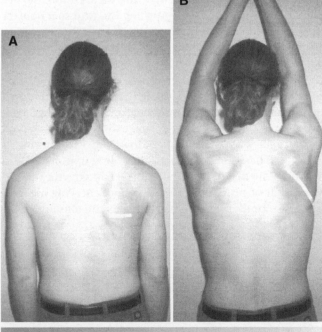

Figure 5-45

Depressed shoulders. *A,* The acromial ends of both shoulders are low. *B,* During shoulder flexion the shoulders remain depressed.

- Shortness of the pectoralis major muscle can depress the shoulder girdle and interfere with elevation of the scapula.
- Shortness of the pectoralis minor muscle can tilt the scapula anteriorly and interfere with elevation of the scapula.
- A long or weak upper trapezius muscle is unable to generate enough tension at the correct length to elevate the scapula.

CONFIRMING TESTS. Active-assisted elevation of the scapula during shoulder flexion results in reduction or elimination of the shoulder pain. Passive elevation of the shoulders while the patient completely relaxes the shoulder girdle muscles should decrease symptoms around the neck, along the upper trapezius, or along the levator scapula muscles.

TREATMENT. The most important treatment is to passively support the shoulders so that they are not constantly in the depressed position. The carrying and holding of objects that contribute to the downward pull must be avoided as much as possible. Shoulder shrugs with the glenohumeral joint in the anatomic position and with the shoulder flexed to more than 120 degrees should be repeated frequently.

When the latissimus dorsi, pectoralis major, and pectoralis minor muscles are short, they must be stretched to eliminate downward pull on the shoulder girdle. Emphasis must be on performing upper trapezius exercises and avoiding lower trapezius exercises that result in scapular depression.

The patient must also practice shoulder flexion with emphasis on correcting the depression of the shoulder girdle and then returning the arm to a neutral position without allowing depression of the shoulder. Because impaired movement patterns become very automatic, the patient should use a mirror to observe the impaired pattern and should be instructed in how to restore a normal pattern if the movement pattern becomes less than optimal. Patients with this syndrome must follow the same suggestions as those given to patients with the scapular downward rotation syndrome. These suggestions include supporting the shoulder in the correct position, reducing the downward pull of bra straps, and avoiding carrying a heavy briefcase or an object that depresses the shoulder.

Case Presentation 2

History. A 35-year-old mother of three children presents with pain at the insertion of her left deltoid muscle. The patient states that her neck feels stiff, particularly in the morning. She has some tenderness bilaterally around the upper trapezius muscle by the base of her neck. She works 10 to 15 hours per week as a secretary for her church but is otherwise a "stay-at-home" mother. Her children are all under 6 years of age. She breast fed all of her children until they were 1 to 2 years of age. She has never been physically active and prefers reading and gardening to aerobic or sporting activities. She is right handed.

Alignment Analysis. The patient is 5 feet, 10 inches tall, slightly overweight, and stands in a swayback posture with the associated kyphosis and posterior pelvic tilt. Both shoulders are depressed and slightly forward. The vertebral borders of her scapulae are parallel and positioned approximately 3 inches from the midline of her thorax.

Movement Analysis. During left shoulder flexion and shoulder abduction, the patient's scapula abducts and upwardly rotates but remains depressed. The scapula and humerus maintain a one- to two-movement ratio until the last 15 degrees of motion when the scapula stops moving and the humerus alone completes the motion. During this phase of motion, the patient experiences pain in her left shoulder. Her range of cervical rotation is limited to 50 degrees bilaterally. When asked to rotate her head and neck, she partially extends her neck, performing a twisting motion rather than a pure rotation of the cervical spine about the vertical axis.

Confirming Tests. Passive elevation of her shoulder girdles with complete relaxation of her trapezius muscles eliminated the aching type pain she had in the region of the base of the neck. Her cervical rotation range increased by 15 degrees in both directions. Passively supporting her left shoulder to eliminate the depressed position while she performed shoulder flexion and abduction eliminated the pain that she had been experiencing at the end of left shoulder flexion. She demonstrated excessive shoulder flexion, exceeding 180 degrees of flexion when her scapula was supported.

Muscle Length and Strength Analysis. Muscle shortness is not found. The upper trapezius muscle tests 3+/5. The lower trapezius and serratus anterior muscles test 4/5.

Diagnosis. The patient is diagnosed with scapular depression syndrome.

Treatment. The primary contributing factors are the previous lack of physical activity, which suggests that the shoulder girdle muscles are chronically underused and underdeveloped. Because the patient is tall, most armrests on chairs are too low to support her shoulders at the correct level for her structure. She does not have armrests on the chair she uses at work.

Her bra straps add to the depressed shoulder posturing. The downward pull from the bra straps was exaggerated because her breast size increased as the result of having breast-fed three children. Lifting and holding her three children also contributed to the downward pull on her shoulders.

The patient should identify ways that she can support her arms with the shoulders horizontal rather than depressed. Even when lifting and holding her children, she should shrug her shoulders before lifting and should maintain this position while lifting. After lifting or holding her children, she should perform shoulder flexion with the shrugging exercise. When holding her children while sitting, she should have a pillow under her forearms so that her shoulders are at the correct level.

Outcome. The patient's symptoms are immediately decreased when passive support is applied to her shoulders. She returned three times over 5 weeks for monitoring and modification of her program. Although her shoulders remain somewhat depressed, she is pain free during all activities and has corrected her movement patterns for most activities. Her muscle strength grades improve by one grade over the treatment period.

Scapular Abduction Syndrome

SYMPTOMS, PAIN PROBLEMS, AND ASSOCIATED DIAGNOSES
- Glenohumeral joint impingement
- Humeral subluxation (anterior)
- Tendinopathy—biceps, infraspinatus, and supraspinatus
- Bursitis—infra deltoid
- Interscapular pain in the rhomboids and middle trapezius
- Sternoclavicular joint pain

MOVEMENT PATTERN IMPAIRMENTS. There is excessive scapular abduction during glenohumeral joint flexion/abduction. At the end of shoulder flexion/elevation, the axillary border of the scapula protrudes laterally more than ½ inch beyond the thorax or the inferior angle of the scapula reaches beyond the midaxillary line of the thorax (Figure 5-46).

The scapula remains relatively stationary during the first half of shoulder flexion with movement of the humerus being the source of most of the motion, which is markedly different than the 1 degree of scapular motion to 2 degrees of glenohumeral motion. During the phase from about 90 to 180 degrees of flexion, the scapula and humerus move in a one-to-one ratio. One reason for this movement pattern impairment is postural abduction of the scapula. The abducted scapular position is associated with excessive length of the

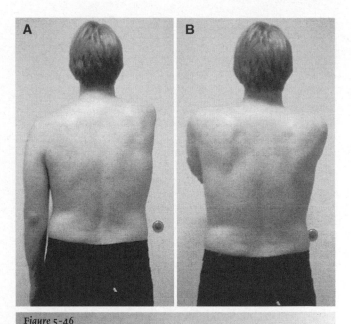

Figure 5-46

Excessive scapular abduction. *A,* The scapula is excessively abducted during shoulder flexion. *B,* The patient can actively limit the degrees of scapular abduction.

trapezius, possibly the rhomboid muscles, and shortness of the serratus anterior muscle. Alterations in the length-tension relationships of these muscles interfere with their ability to properly control the scapula, particularly for the final phase of scapular upward rotation and depression.

When the patient is prone with his or her arm abducted to 90 degrees, the scapula will abduct during glenohumeral lateral rotation instead of remaining in a constant position on the chest wall during arm motion. This is a direct result of the excessive length of the thoracoscapular muscles and accompanied by shortness of the scapulohumeral muscles. The contraction of the lateral rotators moves the lighter segment, namely the scapula, because it is not well controlled by the trapezius and rhomboid muscles.

The impaired scapular abduction can occur during active glenohumeral joint flexion/abduction but may not be observed when the same motions are performed passively by the examiner. This movement pattern impairment occurs not because of a lack of length of the thoracoscapular muscles but because the thoracohumeral muscles do not work effectively at the length that would hold the scapula correctly on the thorax. The contraction of the scapulohumeral muscles moves the scapula toward the humerus until the adapted longer length of the rhomboids and trapezius muscles is reached.

Alignment

STRUCTURAL VARIATIONS

- With kyphosis, the curvature of the ribs contributes to an abducted position of the scapula because the curvature moves the scapula laterally, lengthening the thoracoscapular muscles.

- With long arms, the weight of the arms contributes to abduction of scapulae.

- Often a large thorax contributes to shoulder abduction and shortness of the deltoid muscle. Shortness of the deltoid muscle can contribute to the abducted scapula position. Individuals with a large thorax often need a greater excursion of the scapulae to reach in the front of the body. This excursion contributes to the shortness of the serratus anterior muscle.

- Large breasts contribute to abducted scapulae because the increased dimension of the chest forces the patient to abduct the scapula to increase the excursion of the arms in front of the body.

- With scoliosis, the thoracic rib hump causes the ipsilateral scapula to be abducted because of the structural barrier.

ACQUIRED IMPAIRMENTS

- A posturally abducted scapula (more than 3 inches from the vertebral spine) can result from performing activities in the front of the body, such as playing the cello or the double bass or doing weight-training exercises that include many repetitions of bench presses that require contraction of the pectoralis major and minor muscles. Push-up exercises that are performed with excessive scapular abduction result in a posturally abducted scapula.

- Medial rotation of the humerus, particularly when the pectoralis major muscle is short, can contribute to scapular abduction. Medial rotation of the humerus is often incorrectly interpreted as being an abnormal posture. When the scapula is abducted and the glenoid is facing anteriorly, what appears to be humeral medial rotation is actually the correct alignment of the humerus. This alignment can be verified by correcting the scapular position and reassessing the humeral position.

- Lateral rotation of the humerus associated with scapular abduction may be misinterpreted as the correct degree of rotation when the antecubital fossa is aligned forward. If the abducted scapular position is corrected, the humerus will be in lateral rotation. Assessment of the length of the lateral rotators, which should be short, is necessary to confirm the impression of humeral lateral rotation.

- An abducted scapula in the quadruped position must be carefully assessed. When the scapula is allowed to adduct to the correct position on the thorax, the scapula will wing. The winging of the scapula is attributed to the adaptive shortening of the serratus anterior muscle that alters its length-tension properties. When subjected to a load at a longer length, the muscle cannot develop sufficient tension to prevent winging. Stiffness or shortness of the scapulohumeral muscles can also contribute to the winging of the scapula because of their effect on limiting horizontal adduction of the glenohumeral joint and contribute to excessive scapular abduction.

RELATIVE FLEXIBILITY AND STIFFNESS IMPAIRMENT. Thoracoscapular joint motion occurs more readily than glenohumeral joint motion, thus the scapular movement into abduction may exceed the normal range. The patient is unable to dissociate glenohumeral joint motion from thoracoscapular joint motion. The stiffness or shortness of the scapulohumeral muscles contributes to compensatory motion of the scapula.

MUSCLE IMPAIRMENTS

Muscle recruitment patterns. The scapulohumeral muscles, along with the pectoralis minor, pectoralis major, and serratus anterior muscles, exert a more dominant effect than the rhomboid and trapezius muscles. This is evident in the excessive abduction and limited upward rotation of the scapula.

The posterior deltoid may also be more dominant than the infraspinatus and teres minor. Dominance of the posterior deltoid muscle contributes to the development of shortness of this muscle, which can pull the scapula into abduction because contraction of the deltoid causes the scapula to move toward the humerus.

Muscle length and strength impairments

- Shortness of the deltoid or supraspinatus muscles that holds the humerus in an abducted position at rest can pull the scapula into the abducted position when the counterbalancing rhomboid and trapezius muscles are not performing effectively.

- Hypertrophied and short scapulohumeral muscles, along with hypertrophy of the pectoralis major muscle can lead to scapular abduction.

- Long and/or weak trapezius and rhomboid muscles are unable to hold the scapula in normal alignment, which is approximately 3 inches from the vertebral spine. The result is a position of scapular abduction.

- Short pectoralis major muscles hold the humeri in medial rotation and horizontal adduction. Combined with the shortness of the scapulohumeral muscles, the pectoralis major muscles acting on the humeri passively pull the scapulae into abduction during shoulder flexion and horizontal adduction.

CONFIRMING TESTS. The therapist passively corrects the scapular position at rest and then passively controls the degree of scapular abduction. The therapist assists with upward rotation at the end of the motion during shoulder flexion and assesses whether the postural correction results in reduction in symptoms.

TREATMENT. The focus of treatment is to stretch the short glenohumeral and thoracohumeral muscles. Treatment should also be directed toward improving the performance of the adductor components of the lower and middle trapezius muscles in particular. Therefore the key exercises are the progressions for the lower trapezius muscles with the emphasis placed on scapular adduction and not on scapular depression. A good initial exercise for the patient is to face a wall, slide the arms up the wall, and at the end of the range adduct the scapulae, avoiding movement into depression. The progression is to perform the exercise with the back to the wall so that the patient is lifting the full weight of the arms. The next stage of the progression is to perform the exercise in the prone position.

Stretching the pectoralis major and minor muscles may be necessary. It may be helpful to stretch the humeral rotators in the supine position, using light hand weights to achieve greater ranges of medial and lateral rotation if these motions are limited.

The quadruped position can be used to stretch and strengthen the serratus anterior muscles and to stretch the scapulohumeral muscles. The patient can stretch his or her scapulohumeral muscles by standing with his or her back to the wall and fixing the scapula against the wall while passively adducting the humerus in a horizontal plane. If rhomboid-strengthening exercises are indicated, then scapular adduction motions while sitting can be performed periodically during the day. However, it is unusual to find the true weakness of the rhomboid muscles.

Case Presentation 3

History. A 33-year-old male professional cellist develops right anterior shoulder pain that is diagnosed as subdeltoid bursitis. The pain occurs only after playing and subsides after resting for 3 to 4 hours. The onset of his problem was 1 month before his visit to physical therapy, but the frequency and intensity of the pain has been increasing over the past week.

Alignment Analysis. The patient is slightly overweight with poor definition of the muscles of his shoulder girdle and trunk. He has a large abdomen. His right scapula is abducted when examined in the standing position, measuring 3½ inches from the vertebral spine. The vertebral border of the scapula is vertical, and his shoulder is only slightly depressed. The left scapula is 3 inches from the vertebral spine.

Movement Analysis. The scapula abducts so that the entire axillary border almost reaches the midaxillary line during right shoulder flexion. Scapular upward rotation is slightly limited. The patient experiences some pain in the anterior area of his shoulder during shoulder flexion. During shoulder abduction, the amount of scapular abduction is not as marked as during shoulder flexion, but he still experiences pain in the shoulder at 120 degrees of elevation. Slight winging of the scapula is evident during the return from abduction. The patient has a reduction in shoulder pain when the therapist manually restrains the scapula from abducting excessively during shoulder flexion and when she assists with the upward rotation of the scapula.

Muscle Length and Strength Analysis. There is a compensatory anterior tilt of the scapula during right shoulder medial rotation. With his scapula stabilized, the medial rotation range is limited to 55 degrees. Testing indicates that the pectoralis minor muscle is stiff but not short. His shoulder is forward in the supine position but can be manually stretched so that the spine of the scapula contacts the supporting surface. His latissimus dorsi muscle is short, and shoulder flexion is limited to 160 degrees. His humerus rotates medially during shoulder flexion. The lower trapezius tests 4−/5 and is unable to withstand resistance applied throughout the range. The middle trapezius tests 4/5.

Diagnosis. The patient is diagnosed with a primary scapular abduction syndrome and a secondary shoulder medial rotation syndrome.

Treatment. The patient is instructed to stretch the pectoralis minor and latissimus dorsi muscles in the supine position. He is also instructed to stretch his shoulder lateral rotators. Emphasis is placed on the shortening and strengthening of the lower trapezius muscles. Rhomboid muscle exercises are not indicated because of the limitation of scapular upward rotation. Lower and middle trapezius exercises are prescribed using the face-to-the-wall, back-to-the-wall, and prone positions.

He is also prescribed quadruped rocking with an emphasis on allowing the scapula to adduct. Quadruped rocking is performed by sitting back on the heels and rocking forward through a limited range so that a low load will be placed on the serratus anterior muscle. He also practices humeral horizontal adduction with the scapula fixed against the wall. After this exercise, he practices with his cello bow trying to confine the bowing action to the glenohumeral joint and restricting his movement of the scapula into abduction.

Outcome. The patient is seen only once a month for 4 months because of his performance schedule. He has painful episodes during the first month directly related to the amount of playing he does. He does the standing exercises during the concert intermissions, after each concert, and several other times during the day. As he becomes more consistent in doing his corrective exercises, he has fewer episodes of pain and has resolution of pain by the end of the second month of treatment.

He returns for two additional visits at which time he commences a light weight-training program. Resistive exercise is recommended for shoulder flexion, shoulder rotation, and prone scapular adduction with the shoulder in 135 degrees of abduction. Resistive exercises for elbow flexion and extension are also recommended. The emphasis of the program is on building endurance, with the recommendation to increase the repetitions to three sets of ten and to progress the weights to 10 pounds in each hand. The patient is discharged pain free after 4 months.

Scapular Winging Syndrome

SYMPTOMS, PAIN PROBLEMS, AND ASSOCIATED DIAGNOSES
- Glenohumeral impingement, often anteriorly
- Tendinopathy
- Bursitis
- Rotator cuff tear
- Thoracic outlet syndrome and neural entrapment

The inability to flex the shoulder actively above 120 degrees with severe winging of the scapula occurring during the motion is characteristic of the denervation of the serratus anterior muscle because of neuropathy of the long thoracic nerve.

MOVEMENT PATTERN IMPAIRMENTS. There can be observable tilting of the inferior angle or winging of the vertebral border of the scapula during glenohumeral joint flexion or abduction/elevation or both. This can also occur during the return from glenohumeral joint elevation that is particularly evident during the first half of the movement from 180 to 90 degrees of extension. The winging is usually more exaggerated during the return from flexion than from abduction.

Alignment

STRUCTURAL VARIATIONS
- As the thoracic flexion deformity increases with progression of a kyphosis, the scapulae are forced into a position of increased winging and abduction, placing the serratus anterior in a shortened position.
- With scoliosis, the increased rib prominence can cause winging of the vertebral border of the scapula.
- A flat thoracic spine can make the scapula appear winged, although no muscle impairments are present.
- Heavy arms, as in weight lifters, can cause the scapula to be pulled forward.

ACQUIRED IMPAIRMENTS
- Forward shoulders can be accompanied by the scapulae being tipped forward with prominence of the inferior angles of the scapulae.
- Winging of the vertebral border of the scapula can be a result of muscle imbalances of the serratus anterior and scapulohumeral muscles (Figure 5-47).
- The scapula can be abducted with winging of the vertebral border so that the scapula is rotated more than 30 degrees in the horizontal plane, thus having a greater anterior-posterior orientation than a medial-lateral orientation. Most often this alignment change is present in patients who have done a great deal of upper extremity weight training and who have an increased slope of their shoulders at rest.

RELATIVE FLEXIBILITY AND STIFFNESS IMPAIRMENT. Scapular motion seems to exceed the normal amount because thoracoscapular joint motion occurs more readily than glenohumeral joint motion. At various points in the range, the scapula and humerus can move in a one-to-one ratio for a prolonged period of the motion. In this situation, the motion is almost exclusively at the thoracoscapular joint during the initial return to neutral after completion of shoulder flexion.

MUSCLE IMPAIRMENTS

Muscle recruitment impairments. During the initiation of shoulder flexion, the pectoralis minor muscle action is dominant as evident by the anterior tilt of the scapula (winging of the inferior angle). If the pectoralis minor muscle is short, the scapula will already be in the anteriorly tilted position, which becomes more exaggerated upon the contraction of the muscle.

There is insufficient activity of the serratus anterior muscle to maintain the scapula against the thorax.

During the return from shoulder flexion/elevation, the thoracoscapular joint is the primary site of movement with limited change in the glenohumeral joint angle. The scapula can often be observed to downwardly rotate and wing, which can be associated with pain. The deltoid and supraspinatus muscles do not appear to be elongating (their action appears to be more of an isometric than an eccentric contraction), whereas the serratus anterior and the trapezius muscles are elongating more rapidly.

MUSCLE LENGTH AND STRENGTH IMPAIRMENTS
- Short or weak serratus anterior muscle that does not maintain the scapula against the thorax can cause winging.
- Short pectoralis minor muscles can tilt the scapula anteriorly.
- Often, short scapulohumeral muscles can contribute to the winging of the scapula (see Figure 5-7).

CONFIRMING TESTS. During shoulder flexion, the scapula is passively restrained by the therapist to prevent tilting or winging. This correction of the scapular alignment during motion decreases or eliminates the patient's pain. When the scapula wings during the return from flexion or abduction, the patient flexes his or her elbow to reduce the length of the lever that is being lowered. The patient is instructed to relax his or her glenohumeral joint as completely as possible and to control the scapula. The initial motion should then be primarily at the glenohumeral joint and not at the thoracoscapular joint.

TREATMENT. The emphasis is on correcting the scapular tilting or winging. The tilting is most readily corrected by stretching the pectoralis minor muscle, which usually requires another person's assistance.

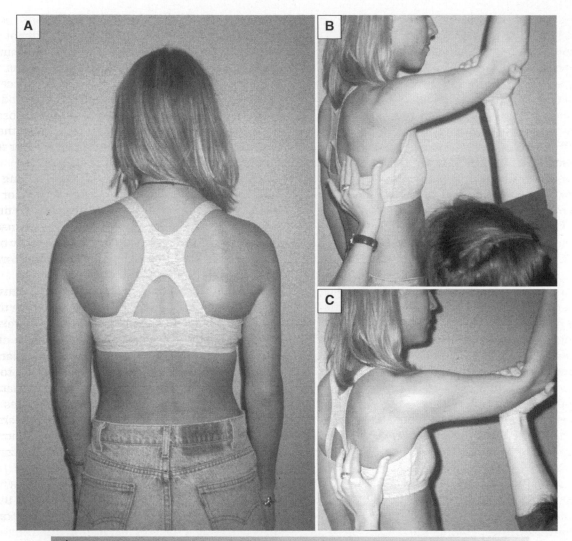

Figure 5-47

Winging of scapula. Impairment of serratus anterior and scapulohumeral muscles. *A,* The vertebral borders of the scapula are prominent in the rest position. *B,* The serratus anterior muscle tests weak. *C,* Weakness is indicated by scapular downward rotation with pressure on the humerus.

Serratus anterior muscle retraining and strengthening is also necessary. Quadruped rocking from the position of sitting on the heels where the weight on the shoulder girdle is minimal and rocking forward to the neutral position is a good exercise for controlling the force demands on the serratus anterior muscle.

If the scapula wings in the resting position and during shoulder flexion, then the serratus anterior muscle is weak and strengthening is indicated. If the scapula only wings during the first phase of the motion, the quadruped rocking is a good exercise, but the therapist should monitor to ensure that the scapula does not wing because of excessive load. The exercise with the

patient positioned against the wall keeping the scapula fixed against the wall, with the elbow flexed to 120 degrees and then flexing the shoulder to no more than about 60 degrees, is a good way to control the winging occurring on initiation of motion. If the patient can complete shoulder flexion with the elbow flexed and without scapular winging, then he or she should move away from the wall so that the scapula is not restricted while doing upward rotation.

If the scapula wings markedly throughout the entire active motion, then the serratus anterior muscle is very weak. If the weakness of the serratus anterior muscle is secondary to a lesion of the long thoracic nerve, then a slowly progressive strengthening program must be prescribed and carefully monitored. The patient should not be expected or encouraged to perform complete shoulder flexion in the presence of a very weak serratus anterior muscle because his or her inability to upwardly rotate the scapula will contribute to the development of an impingement syndrome.

Case Presentation 4

History. The patient is a 34-year-old man whose primary fitness activity is swimming. He has been experiencing pain in the anterior area of his left shoulder in the region of the humeral head near the acromioclavicular joint. The pain has been present for 2 weeks. The patient swims competitively once per week but trains at least 2 other days per week. He has a routine program of strengthening and stretching exercises that he performs before swimming. The pain is most pronounced after swimming but usually subsides within 24 hours. He applies ice to the area and takes an antiinflammatory medication. His occupation is relatively sedentary and does not require unusual lifting or physical activity.

Alignment Analysis. The patient is slender with a depressed chest, slight kyphosis, and a tendency to shift his upper back posteriorly. His abdominal muscles are taut suggesting shortness. His shoulders are tipped forward with the left positioned farther forward than the right. From the posterior view, the inferior angle of his left scapula is protruding. The scapula is slightly abducted, with the vertebral border positioned 3½ inches from the vertebral spine. The vertebral borders of the scapulae are parallel to the spine.

Movement Analysis. During the initial phase of shoulder flexion, anterior tilting of the left scapula is observed until shoulder flexion reaches 90 degrees. At 150 degrees the patient notes pain in the anterior shoulder region. The scapula is observed to be appropriately abducting but was limited in the amount of upward rotation and does not depress on the thorax at the end of the shoulder flexion range.

Confirming Test. The therapist controls the inferior angle of the scapula to prevent anterior tilting during shoulder flexion. During the last phase of shoulder flexion the therapist assists with depression of the scapula. Considerable resistance is felt by the therapist while attempting to assist the scapular motion. The patient attempts to extend his back to compensate for the lack of scapular motion.

Muscle Length and Strength Analysis. The pectoralis minor muscle is short. The patient's shoulder is 2 inches away from the support surface and cannot be manually stretched to the table without rotation of his thorax. His rectus abdominis muscle and the sternal portion of the pectoralis major muscle are both short. Shoulder medial rotation is associated with compensatory scapular tilt. The left lower trapezius tests 4/5. The right lower trapezius tests 5/5. The shoulder rotator muscles test normal in strength.

Diagnosis. The patient is diagnosed with scapular winging syndrome.

Treatment. The emphasis of the program is on stretching the pectoralis minor muscle, improving the performance of the lower trapezius muscle, which can be considered an antagonist of the pectoralis minor, and correcting abdominal muscle imbalances. The patient is instructed in assisted pectoralis minor and pectoralis major muscle stretching. Other exercise recommendations include shoulder medial rotation while in the supine position. An emphasis is placed on keeping the scapula still and allowing the shoulder lateral rotators to lengthen by having them relax rather than using active contraction of the medial rotators to produce the motion. He is instructed in the lower trapezius exercise performed facing the wall. With his back to the wall, he performs shoulder flexion with his elbows flexed and shoulder abduction with his elbows flexed. In the abduction exercise, he cannot get his arms against the wall because of the shortness of the pectoral muscles. Thus he is instructed to abduct to 90 degrees and then to try to adduct his scapula and not to attempt to get the posterior aspect of his elbows against the wall. When he reaches the end range of shoulder flexion and abduction, he is instructed to take a deep breath to stretch his abdominal muscles. He performs lateral flexion of his thorax while standing with his back against the wall and his forearms on top of his head. The purpose of this exercise is to stretch his abdominal and rib cage musculature. He does quadruped rocking, with an emphasis on allowing his thoracic spine to flatten, particularly when he rocks all the way back to sit on his heels.

Outcome. The patient is told to stop swimming and avoid overhead activities for the first 2 weeks of his rehabilitation program. He is seen weekly for 6 weeks. The patient is able to have a friend help him with stretching his pectoralis minor muscle, which has regained normal length after 2 weeks. At the end of 2 weeks he has shoulder pain only at the end of shoulder flexion range. By the end of 4 weeks he is pain free during all active motions performed in the clinic but develops some pain after swimming for more than 20 minutes. At the end of 6 weeks, he can swim for 40 minutes without experiencing pain in his shoulder. He is discharged after 6 weeks, at which time all muscles are of normal length and he no longer has winging of his scapula at rest or during motion.

Movement Impairment Syndromes of the Humerus

Relationships Between Alignment and Movement

As discussed in the introductory chapter, ideal alignment of body segments with one another is important because ideal alignment facilitates ideal movement. However, several combinations of movement patterns and alignments are possible. The following examples illustrate how alignment and movement can be related to the various humeral syndromes:

- Humeral alignment is correct, but the movement of the humerus is impaired. For example, the humerus is correctly positioned at rest, but during shoulder flexion the humerus medially rotates excessively.
- Humeral alignment is impaired, and the movement is of normal range but does not correct or compensate for the initial impaired position. For example, the humerus is medially rotated in the standing position and laterally rotates during abduction but not enough to correct for the impaired starting position.
- Humeral alignment is impaired, and the movement pattern is impaired. For example, the humerus is medially rotated in the standing position and does not rotate during abduction.

Criteria for a Diagnosis of a Humeral Syndrome

- The primary source of pain is movement impairment of the humeral head on the glenoid, although often scapular motion is impaired as well.
- The symptoms are decreased or eliminated when the patient corrects the movement impairment of the humerus or when the therapist manually corrects the impairment during active movement performed by the patient. For example, the therapist assists in lateral rotation of the humerus during the appropriate range of shoulder flexion, resulting in decreased pain. Because this correction alleviates or eliminates the pain, the focus of the therapeutic program is correction of this impairment.
- The syndrome is named for the observed humeral movement impairment, which may be an insufficient or exaggerated accessory or physiologic normal motion. An example of humeral accessory movement impairment is observing notable humeral anterior glide during shoulder hyperextension as occurs during arm swing when walking. An example of humeral physiologic movement impairment is to observe the humerus positioned

in medial rotation and failing to rotate laterally during shoulder abduction (Figure 5-48).

Order of Observed Frequency of Humeral Syndromes

- Humeral anterior glide
- Humeral superior glide (abduction)
- Shoulder medial rotation
- Glenohumeral hypomobility

Establishing a specific diagnosis of a syndrome does not require the presence of all of the impairments described for a syndrome. The symptom pattern and impaired movement must be present. Generally the more impairments that are present, the greater the severity of the syndrome, although it is also possible to have just one fault that is particularly severe.

As with all musculoskeletal pain syndromes, various stages of severity can be present. Pain in the shoulder at rest suggests an acute inflammatory state. Exercise should be avoided when it is found to

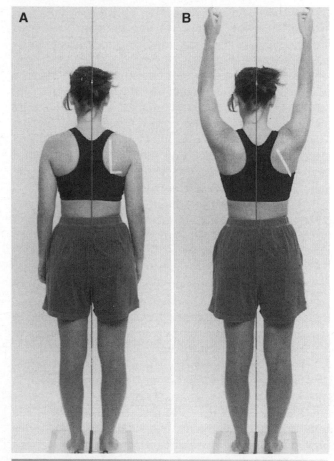

Figure 5-48

Deficient left humeral lateral rotation during shoulder flexion and abduction. *A,* The left humerus is medially rotated in the rest position. *B,* The left humerus remains medially rotated during shoulder flexion.

increase the pain in the shoulder joint after the exercise has ceased or if exercise increases the pain with the shoulder at rest.

Humeral Anterior Glide Syndrome

SYMPTOMS, PAIN PROBLEMS, AND ASSOCIATED DIAGNOSES. Pain is present in the anterior or anteromedial aspect of the shoulder joint. The pain is increased by glenohumeral medial rotation, by shoulder hyperextension, and by horizontal abduction. Pain can also be increased by shoulder flexion, particularly in the range from 80 to 180 degrees of flexion.

There can also be pain along the proximal one third of the biceps brachii tendon. The pain can increase in this area with manual resistance to elbow flexion or with shoulder abduction performed with the elbow flexed and the glenohumeral joint laterally rotated. The symptoms can be similar to those that are characteristic of the early stages of impingement syndrome or bicipital tendinopathy.

Anterior dislocation can occur if the anterior joint capsule has been weakened by previous episodes of dislocation. Other symptoms can be associated with impingement syndrome, including supraspinatus tendinopathy and bursitis.

MOVEMENT PATTERN IMPAIRMENTS. Excessive anterior motion of the humeral head into the anterior joint capsule is present during glenohumeral abduction, during the initiation of glenohumeral flexion, and on the return from the end range of flexion (elevation). During glenohumeral joint rotation with the shoulder in 90 degrees of abduction, the anterior movement of the head of the humerus can be readily palpated.

ALIGNMENT IMPAIRMENTS. In the anatomic position, there are three alignment impairments:

- More than one third of the humeral head is anterior to the acromial process of the scapula.
- The humeral head is more anterior than the distal humerus. The proximal and distal aspects of the humerus do not lie in the same vertical plane.
- The shoulder appears forward, but usually the humerus is forward of the acromion in addition to the anterior tilt of the scapula.

On the posterior surface, there is a slight indentation below the acromion because the humeral head is anterior with respect to the glenoid.

RELATIVE FLEXIBILITY AND STIFFNESS IMPAIRMENTS. The anterior joint capsule is more flexible than the posterior capsule and/or the glenohumeral lateral rotators.

MUSCLE IMPAIRMENTS

Recruitment patterns. The action of the pectoralis major muscle as a medial rotator of the glenohumeral joint is more dominant than the action of the subscapularis muscle. Because of the attachment of the pectoralis major muscle onto the crest of the

greater tubercle of the humerus, contraction of this muscle pulls the head of the humerus into the anterior joint capsule. This anterior pull should be counteracted by the downward, posteriorly directed pull of the subscapularis muscle. If the subscapularis muscle is too long or weak to counteract the pull of the pectoralis major muscle and the anterior joint capsule is stretched, contraction of the pectoralis major muscle would contribute to anterior glide of the humeral head.

The infraspinatus and teres minor muscles are recruited more strongly than the subscapularis muscle when acting as depressors of the humerus. In this situation, the dominant activity of the lateral rotator-depressors would add to the stiffness of the posterior joint capsule, restricting the posterior glide of the humeral head.

Muscle length and strength impairments. The lengthened or weak subscapularis muscle permits the anterior glide of the humeral head as discussed previously. Shortness of the scapulohumeral lateral rotators (infraspinatus and teres minor muscles) contributes to the stiffness of the posterior capsule, thus preventing the posterior glide of the humeral head as discussed previously[19,27] (see Figure 5-42). Shortness of the pectoralis major muscle can contribute to medial rotation of the humerus and the anterior position of the humeral head. In addition, shortness of the pectoralis major can contribute to the abducted position of the scapula and to increased anterior glide of the humerus during shoulder lateral rotation and horizontal abduction.

CONFIRMING TEST. The therapist prevents the anterior glide of the humeral head during shoulder rotation and flexion, which decreases the patient's symptoms.

TREATMENT. The emphasis of the treatment program is to correct the anterior position of the humeral head at rest and to prevent the anterior glide during motion. Therefore it is necessary to shorten and strengthen the subscapularis muscle. Frequently, stiffness or shortness of the humeral lateral rotators is present and must be corrected to enable the humeral head to glide posteriorly. A key exercise improves the passive range into medial rotation. The exercise used most frequently is performed in the supine position with the glenohumeral joint abducted to approximately 90 degrees and with the elbow flexed. The patient uses the contralateral hand to prevent anterior glide of the humeral head while allowing the shoulder to medially rotate. If the humeral lateral rotators are short, a light weight may be held in the hand to assist the medial rotational force. The weight should be heavy enough to pull the arm into medial rotation but not so heavy that the patient cannot allow the lateral rotators to relax.

Another exercise is horizontal adduction, performed passively with the scapula stabilized against a wall when the patient is standing or against the floor when the patient is in the supine position. The shoulder and elbow are flexed to 90 degrees, and the patient uses the contralateral hand to grasp the arm at the elbow and passively pull the arm into horizontal adduction. In the standing position facing a wall, the patient can perform shoulder flexion while maintaining lateral rotation. He or she can also lean onto the arm while performing this exercise, after the shoulder is flexed to more than 90 degrees to assist in the inferior and posterior glide motions. If shortness of the pectoralis major muscle is present, it should be stretched. Once the optimal medial rotation range has been achieved, strengthening the subscapularis muscle becomes particularly important.

The best exercise to strengthen the subscapularis muscle is performed lying on a table or bed in the prone position with the shoulder abducted to 90 degrees and the elbow flexed to 90 degrees. The forearm is positioned so that it is hanging over the edge of the bed. Often the patient must initially learn to maintain the glenohumeral joint at the end range of medial rotation before performing the strengthening exercise. If an assistant is available, the arm is positioned at the end range, and the patient must maintain this position with an isometric contraction. The patient then gradually allows the glenohumeral joint to laterally rotate (eccentric contraction) about 40 to 50 degrees before concentrically contracting the medial rotators. The primary challenge is to elicit the participation of the subscapularis muscle and not the pectoralis major and teres major muscles. The position just described with the emphasis on the end of the range appears to be the most optimal for this purpose.

In the quadruped position, rocking from the neutral position backward toward the heels also helps by creating forces that favor posterior glide of the humeral head. The patient should push back with his arms rather than flexing his hips to rock backward. The exercise previously described with the patient facing the wall and gliding the hand up the wall from an elbow flexed position to full shoulder flexion with the elbow extended also promotes humeral head depression and posterior glide.

Another treatment to assist in reducing the stress on the anterior joint capsule is taping the anterior shoulder joint directing the force to pull the humeral head posteriorly. Correcting scapular alignment, which is often the forward or depressed position, is also necessary.

Case Presentation 5

History. A 34-year-old woman has pain in the anterior superior area of her left shoulder. The pain occurs primarily during shoulder abduction, particularly against resistance, and during shoulder flexion at the end of the range. The pain has been present for 3 weeks and is rated at a severity of 3 to 4 out of 10 during these motions. She does not have pain at rest, nor is she awakened by pain at night. Her primary recreational activity is ballroom dancing. She has been performing a program of upper extremity weight training.

Alignment Analysis. The patient has a slight thoracic kyphosis, and her scapulae are abducted and slightly depressed. Both scapulae are positioned more than 3 inches from her vertebral spine. More than one third of the head of the left humerus extends beyond the acromion. The proximal end of the humerus is anterior to its distal end. The humeral alignment of the right upper extremity is normal.

Her thoracic kyphosis is decreased when the therapist provides support at the apex of the outward curve of the thoracic spine and the patient lifts her chest. Shortness of her rectus abdominis muscles is the primary cause of the thoracic kyphosis. Passive posterior tilting and adduction of her scapula is met with resistance, suggesting shortness of the pectoralis minor muscle.

Movement Analysis. During shoulder flexion, the scapula remains depressed and does not adduct at the end range of shoulder flexion. Medial rotation of the humerus is observed during shoulder flexion, initiated with the elbow flexed; however, the elbow then extends as the shoulder flexion motion is completed. At the end of the range, she notes some pain in the shoulder. If she slides her hand up a wall, creating a slight posteroinferior force on the humerus while maintaining lateral rotation, the motion is performed without symptoms. A similar test is performed in the prone position with the same findings. In the standing position, with the shoulder in the anatomic position and the elbow flexed, the humeral head can be observed to glide anteriorly when she performs lateral rotation.

Muscle Length and Strength Analysis. Shortness of the pectoralis minor muscles is found, indicated by forward shoulders in the supine position and by marked resistance noted on attempting to stretch the pectoralis minor muscles. The left lateral rotators are short, indicated by medial rotation limited to 50 degrees. Anterior glide of the humeral head is observed during glenohumeral medial rotation. Medial rotation of the right humerus is 70 degrees. Lateral rotation range of humeral motion is 90 degrees bilaterally. The left shoulder flexion range of motion is 180 degrees, but the lateral border of scapula extends 1 inch beyond the lateral border of thorax, indicating shortness of the teres major. The range of right shoulder flexion is 180 degrees with normal scapular position. The left shoulder medial rotators test 3+/5, and the right medial rotators test 5/5. The left lower trapezius muscle tests 4/5, and the right trapezius muscle tests 5/5.

Diagnoses. The patient is diagnosed with humeral anterior glide and scapular abduction syndromes.

Treatment

Supine Exercises

• The patient is instructed in the correct technique to stretch the pectoralis minor muscle using an assistant.

• The patient performs shoulder flexion while maintaining a flat back and takes a deep breath at the end of the range of shoulder flexion to stretch her abdominal muscles.

• She performs shoulder medial rotation, being careful to avoid anterior glide of the humeral head.

Prone Exercises. The patient is lying in the prone position on a plinth with her left shoulder and elbow flexed to 90 degrees and her forearm hanging off the edge of the table. The left arm is placed in maximal medial rotation with her hand supported on a small table placed along side the plinth and a towel roll placed under the humeral head to ensure avoidance of anterior glide. The patient extends her elbow just enough to clear her hand from the table, thus eliminating the passive support of her shoulder in medial rotation. She then allows the shoulder to laterally rotate (eccentric medial rotation) through a range of 20 degrees and then returns the arm to the starting position. Care is taken to avoid substitution by shoulder extension.

Quadruped Exercises. The patient starts in a neutral position and then rocks backward toward the heels.

Standing Exercises

Facing the wall. The patient is positioned with the ulnar side of her hand against the wall, the elbows flexed, and the shoulders laterally rotated. The patient slides her hands up the wall from the starting position to complete shoulder flexion with elbow extension. During this motion, when the shoulder has become flexed to 90 degrees, the patient shrugs her shoulders to exaggerate the activity of the upper trapezius as she continues to reach into full flexion. At the end of the range, she lifts her arms off the wall by adducting the scapula.

Back to the wall. With elbows flexed, the patient performs shoulder flexion, being sure to maintain lateral rotation as the shoulder flexes. At the end of shoulder flexion, the patient takes a deep breath to stretch the rectus abdominis muscles. From the same starting position, the patient performs shoulder abduction. If pain is present, she tries to adduct her left scapula before abducting her shoulder from 90 degrees to full elevation, which relieves the pain.

Outcome. The patient is seen weekly for 4 weeks and then once every 2 weeks for two additional visits. Within 2 weeks the patient achieves 70 degrees of medi-

al rotation but has to apply strong pressure to the proximal humerus to prevent anterior glide of the head. In the prone position she can medially rotate her arm from a neutral position to 70 degrees. She does not have pain with abduction or flexion as long as she adducts her scapula before reaching the end of the range of shoulder flexion. After 4 weeks the shoulder rotation exercises in the supine and prone positions are performed using 2-pound weights. She also performs the lower trapezius exercise (level 3) in prone. The muscle shortness is corrected quickly.

She returns for two more sessions, at which time she is told to increase her weights to 3 and then to 4 pounds in each hand. She also begins using 2-pound weights during the motion of elbow and shoulder flexion to elbow extension. At the end of 6 weeks she is pain free with all motions and no longer demonstrates anterior glide of the humeral head during prone or supine shoulder rotational movements.

Humeral Superior Glide Syndrome

SYMPTOMS, PAIN PROBLEMS, AND ASSOCIATED DIAGNOSES. Typically sharp pain is present around the anterior and lateral aspects of the acromial process during shoulder abduction, medial rotation, and lateral rotation. Sometimes the pain is referred to the area around the insertion of the deltoid muscle.

• Impingement syndrome
• Supraspinatus tendinopathy
• Subacromial or subdeltoid bursitis
• Bicipital tendinopathy
• Calcific tendinitis
• Rotator cuff tear
• Early stages of adhesive capsulitis

MOVEMENT PATTERN IMPAIRMENT. During glenohumeral flexion, abduction, or elevation, there is excessive proximal movement of the head of the humerus against the acromion (the humeral head fails to depress or to inferior-glide). This impairment is most evident during glenohumeral joint abduction. Often this syndrome is accompanied by the scapular downward rotation syndrome.

Alignment

STRUCTURAL VARIATIONS

None have been identified that specifically contribute to this syndrome.

ACQUIRED IMPAIRMENTS

• The shoulders are elevated, and the head of the humerus appears to be superior, positioned very close to the acromion (Figure 5-49). Normally there are about 9 to 10 mm between the humeral head and the acromion in the anatomic position.[25] The shoulders are abducted.

ASSOCIATED SIGNS
(contributing factors)

Alignment and appearance

- May have normal resting alignment
- Large breasts
- Heavy arms

Structural variations

- Long arms
- Long neck
- Long trunk
- Short arms

Common activities

- Habitual depression of shoulder girdle
- Computer keyboard too low
- Arm rests on chair too low

Movement impairments

SHOULDER FLEXION

- *Associated with impingement:* May have slight end range limitation and may have painful arc
- *Associated with TOS:* May have numbness and tingling or other symptoms associated with TOS during arm elevation
- *Associated with instability:* May observe increased crease distal to acromion; may also observe increased prominence of humeral head in axilla

Palpation

- *Associated with impingement:* May be tender over coracoacromial ligament, bicipital groove, or rotator cuff tendons—especially supraspinatus
- *Associated with TOS:* May be tender over scalenes and pectoralis minor muscles

Special tests

- *Associated with impingement:* Tests reproduce pain; resisted tests of rotator cuff and biceps for soft tissue differential diagnosis may be strong and painful or weak and painful
- *Associated with TOS:* May reproduce symptoms
- *Associated with instability:* May have increased accessory glide at GH joint in any direction
- *Associated length impairments:* Short lower trapezius and latissimus

DIFFERENTIAL MOVEMENT AND ASSOCIATED DIAGNOSES

Differential scapular diagnoses

- *Rule:* If scapular depression is associated with another movement impairment (e.g., scapular downward rotation, abduction), scapular depression is the diagnosis if passive correction of the depression alleviates the symptoms
- Scapular downward rotation
- Scapular abduction
- Scapular winging and tilting

Differential primary diagnoses

- Humeral anterior glide
- Humeral inferior glide
- Humeral superior glide
- Cervical rotation
- Cervical extension
- Cervical rotation and extension

Associated diagnoses

- Rotator cuff tendinopathy
- Shoulder impingement
- Partial rotator cuff tear
- Bicipital tendinopathy
- Supraspinatus tendinopathy
- Humeral subluxation
- TOS and neural entrapments
- Neck pain with or without radiating pain
- Pain or trigger points in levator scapulae, rhomboids, upper trapezius
- Bursitis
- AC joint pain
- Calcific tendinopathy
- Subscapular bursitis
- Snapping scapulae
- Drooping shoulder
- Long thoracic nerve injury
- Cervical or cervical thoracic junction pain

SCREENING FOR POTENTIAL MEDICAL DIAGNOSES REQUIRING REFERRAL

Musculoskeletal origin

- Cervical radiculopathy
- Peripheral nerve entrapment
- Brachial plexus injury
- Rotator cuff tear
- Fracture
- OA or RA
- Glenoid labrum tear
- Spinal accessory nerve palsy
- Long thoracic nerve palsy

Visceral origin

- Neoplasms
- Cardiovascular disease
- Pulmonary disease
- Breast disease
- Abdominal organ abnormality

Systemic origin

- Collagen vascular disease
- Gout
- Syphilis and gonorrhea
- Sickle cell anemia
- Hemophilia
- Rheumatic disease

AC, Acromioclavicular; *GH,* glenohumeral; *OA,* osteoarthritis; *RA,* rheumatoid arthritis; *TOS,* thoracic outlet syndrome.

Chapter 5
Appendix

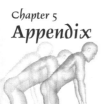

SCAPULAR ABDUCTION SYNDROME

The primary movement impairment in this syndrome is excessive scapular abduction. Muscle impairments are a dominance of scapular abductor muscles (pectoralis major, serratus anterior) and insufficient activity of the scapular adductor (primarily trapezius) muscles, primarily their alignment and appearance.

SYMPTOMS AND HISTORY

Associated with impingement

- Pain in anterior or posterior shoulder or deltoid area
- May experience pain with overhead activities and reaching forward
- Unable to sleep on affected side
- *May be associated with thoracic or cervical pain*

Associated with adductor strain

- Pain between scapula and spine or along vertebral border of scapula

Associated with TOS

- May experience numbness and tingling in hand
- May experience decreased circulation or feeling of coldness or whole arm falling asleep with arms overhead
- Pain in interscapular area, medial arm, forearm, and hand

Associated with instability

- "Clunking" with arm movements or the sensation of the shoulder slipping out of socket

Activities

- Weight lifters or heavy laborers
- Cellist
- Hairdressers
- Swimmers

KEY TESTS AND SIGNS

Alignment and appearance

- Vertebral border of scapula is greater than 3 inches from spine
- Plane of scapula is greater than 30 degrees anterior to frontal plane
- *Correction of alignment impairment decreases symptoms; if associated with TOS, distal symptoms may increase with correction of scapular impairment*

Movement impairments

SHOULDER FLEXION

- Excessive scapular abduction; *correction of abduction decreases symptoms*
- Axillary border of scapula protrudes laterally $^1/_2$ inch or more beyond posterior lateral border of thorax with arm over head
- Scapula and humerus moves in 1:1 ratio
- Insufficient scapular adduction during GH horizontal abduction

Lifting or holding

- Unable to maintain proper scapular alignment (scapula abducts) during lifting or when loads are added to arm

Impairments in muscle length

BASED ON LENGTH

- Short pectoralis major and minor, SH muscles

BASED ON ALIGNMENT

- Short serratus anterior muscles
- Long trapezius, rhomboid muscles

Impairments in muscle strength

- Weak or long trapezius (middle to upper and lower) and rhomboid muscles
- Associated with muscle strain, resisted tests of scapular adductors will be weak and painful

ASSOCIATED SIGNS
(contributing factors)

Alignment and appearance

- May have normal resting alignment
- Obesity
- Large abdomen
- Large breasts
- Heavy arms
- Thoracic kyphosis
- Hypertrophied scapulohumeral

Structural variations

- Long arms
- Thoracic kyphosis
- Scoliosis
- Large or wide thorax

Common activities

- Habitual abduction of shoulder girdle
- Sit with slouched posture
- Activities requiring reaching forward

Movement impairments

SHOULDER FLEXION

- *Associated with impingement:* May have slight end range limitation and may have painful arc
- *Associated with TOS:* May have numbness and tingling or other symptoms during arm elevation
- *Associated with instability:* May observe increased crease distal to acromion; may also observe increased prominence of humeral head in axilla

Palpation

- May be tender over adductor muscle bellies if strained
- *Associated with impingement:* May be tender over coracoacromial ligament, bicipital groove, or rotator cuff tendons (e.g., supraspinatus)

Special tests

- *Associated with TOS:* May be tender over scalenes and pectoralis minor; may reproduce symptoms
- *Associated with impingement:* Tests reproduce pain; resisted tests of rotator cuff and biceps for soft tissue differential diagnosis may be strong and painful or weak and painful
- *Associated with instability:* May have increased accessory glide at GH joint in any direction

DIFFERENTIAL MOVEMENT AND ASSOCIATED DIAGNOSES

Differential scapular diagnoses

- Scapular downward rotation
- Scapular depression
- Scapular winging and tilting

Differential primary diagnoses

- Humeral anterior glide
- Humeral superior glide
- Humeral medial rotation
- GH hypomobility
- Cervical extension

Associated diagnoses

- Rotator cuff tendinopathy
- Shoulder impingement
- Partial rotator cuff tear
- Bicipital tendinopathy
- Supraspinatus tendinopathy
- Humeral subluxation
- TOS and neural entrapments
- Neck pain with or without radiating pain
- Pain or trigger points in rhomboids
- Bursitis
- AC joint pain
- Calcific tendinopathy
- Subscapular bursitis
- Snapping scapulae
- Thoracic pain
- Costochondritis
- Teres syndrome
- Sternal pain
- Cervical or cervical thoracic junction pain

SCREENING FOR POTENTIAL MEDICAL DIAGNOSES REQUIRING REFERRAL

Musculoskeletal origin

- Cervical radiculopathy
- Brachial plexus injury
- Rotator cuff tear
- Fracture
- OA or RA
- Glenoid labrum tear
- Spinal accessory nerve palsy
- Peripheral nerve entrapment

Visceral origin

- Neoplasms
- Cardiovascular disease
- Pulmonary disease
- Breast disease
- Abdominal organ pathologic condition

Systemic origin

- Collagen vascular disease
- Gout
- Syphilis and gonorrhea
- Sickle cell anemia
- Hemophilia
- Rheumatic disease

AC, Acromioclavicular; *GH,* glenohumeral;
OA, osteoarthritis; *RA,* rheumatoid arthritis;
SH, scapulohumeral; *TOS,* thoracic outlet syndrome.

Chapter 5
Appendix

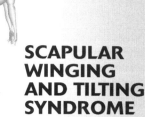

SCAPULAR WINGING AND TILTING SYNDROME

The primary movement impairment in this syndrome is scapular winging and tilting during shoulder flexion and extension. This impairment may also be evident during shoulder rotation. In some cases, the winging is caused by weakness of the serratus anterior. In other cases, the impairment is the result of a timing problem between the axioscapular muscles and the scapulohumeral muscles. The scapulohumeral muscles do not elongate as rapidly as the axioscapular muscles or there is poor eccentric control (neural drive) of the serratus anterior during the return from flexion.

SYMPTOMS AND HISTORY

Associated with impingement
- Pain in anterior or posterior shoulder or deltoid area
- Pain with overhead activities
- Unable to sleep on affected side

Associated with TOS
- May experience numbness and tingling in hand
- May experience decreased circulation or feeling of coldness or whole arm falling asleep with arms overhead
- Pain in interscapular area, medial arm, forearm, and hand

Associated with instability
- "Clunking" with arm movements or sensation of the shoulder slipping out of socket

Activities
- Jobs requiring sustained arm positions at 90 degrees shoulder flexion (e.g., pipe fitters)
- Swimmers
- Weight lifters
- Laborers
- Kayakers
- Cross-country skiers

KEY TESTS AND SIGNS

Alignment and appearance
- Inferior angle of scapula protrudes from thorax
- Vertebral border of scapula protrudes from thorax
- *Correction of alignment impairment decreases symptoms; if associated with TOS, distal symptoms may increase with correction of scapular impairment*

Movement impairments
ASSOCIATED WITH WEAKNESS OF SERRATUS ANTERIOR
- Pronounced scapular winging noted during arm elevation and during the return; *correction decreases symptoms*
- May note scapular adduction during arm elevation
- Scapula will not achieve 60 degrees upward rotation at end-range shoulder flexion or abduction

Movement impairment without profound weakness
- Winging and tilting of scapula noted only on return from arm elevation; *correction decreases symptoms*
- Scapula and humerus move in 1:1 ratio during arm elevation
- Insufficient scapular posterior tilt at end-range arm elevation; *correction decreases symptoms*

Lifting and holding
- Unable to maintain proper scapular alignment (scapula wings and tilts) during lifting or when loads are added to arm
- Associated with weakness of serratus anterior

Impairments in strength
- Weak and paralyzed serratus anterior

Impairments in muscle length
BASED ON LENGTH TESTS
- Short pectoralis minor and major, SH, biceps muscles
BASED ON ALIGNMENT
- Long lower and middle trapezius

Impairments in muscle strength
- Long trapezius (primarily lower)
- Weak or long serratus anterior

ASSOCIATED SIGNS
(contributing factors)

Alignment and appearance

- May have normal resting alignment
- May have downwardly rotated scapula
- Heavy arms
- Large breasts
- Hypertrophy of rhomboid muscles

Structural variations

- Long arms
- Flat thoracic spine (winging)
- Scoliosis
- Thoracic kyphosis (tilting)

Common activities

- Sit with slouched posture
- Activities requiring reaching forward
- *Associated with profound weakness of serratus anterior*

Impairments in length

BASED ON ALIGNMENT OR PASSIVE MOVEMENT

- May develop shortened trapezius, rhomboids, and lengthened serratus anterior

Movement impairments

SHOULDER FLEXION

- *Associated with impingement:* May have slight end-range limitation; may have painful arc
- *Associated with TOS:* May have numbness and tingling or other symptoms during arm elevation
- *Associated with instability:* May observe increased crease distal to acromion; may also observe increased prominence of humeral head in axilla

Palpation

- *Associated with impingement:* May be tender over coracoacromial ligament, bicipital groove, or rotator cuff tendons (especially supraspinatus)
- *Associated with TOS:* May be tender over scalenes and pectoralis minor

Special tests

- *Associated with impingement:* Tests reproduce pain; resisted tests of rotator cuff and biceps for soft tissue differential diagnosis may be strong and painful or weak and painful
- *Associated with TOS:* May reproduce symptoms
- *Associated with instability:* May have increased accessory glide at GH joint in any direction

DIFFERENTIAL MOVEMENT AND ASSOCIATED DIAGNOSES

Differential scapular diagnoses

- Scapular downward rotation
- Scapular abduction

Differential primary diagnoses

- Humeral anterior glide
- Humeral superior glide
- Humeral medial rotation

Associated diagnoses

- Rotator cuff tendinopathy
- Shoulder impingement
- Partial rotator cuff tear
- Bicipital tendinopathy
- Supraspinatus tendinopathy
- Humeral subluxation
- TOS and neural entrapments
- Neck pain with or without radiating pain
- Pain or trigger points in rhomboids
- Bursitis
- AC joint pain
- Calcific tendinopathy
- Subscapular bursitis
- Snapping scapulae
- Cervical or cervical thoracic junction pain
- Long thoracic nerve injury

SCREENING FOR POTENTIAL MEDICAL DIAGNOSES REQUIRING REFERRAL

Musculoskeletal origin

- Long thoracic nerve palsy
- Cervical radiculopathy
- Brachial plexus injury
- Rotator cuff tear
- Fracture
- OA or RA
- Glenoid labrum tear
- Peripheral nerve entrapment
- Spinal accessory nerve palsy

Visceral origin

- Neoplasms
- Cardiovascular disease
- Pulmonary disease
- Breast disease
- Abdominal organ abnormality

Systemic origin

- Collagen vascular disease
- Gout
- Syphilis and gonorrhea
- Sickle cell anemia
- Hemophilia
- Rheumatic disease

AC, Acromioclavicular; *GH,* glenohumeral; *OA,* osteoarthritis; *RA,* rheumatoid arthritis; *SH,* scapulohumeral; *TOS,* thoracic outlet syndrome.

Chapter 5
Appendix

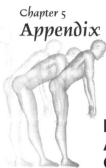

HUMERAL ANTERIOR GLIDE SYNDROME

Excessive anterior or insufficient posterior glide of the humeral head is noted during shoulder motions. This syndrome may be associated with laxity of the anterior structures and stiffness or shortness of the posterior structures of the GH joint. The subscapularis is frequently lengthened or weak and the posterior deltoid dominates over the infraspinatus and teres minor muscles. The muscles that attach farther from the axis of rotation (e.g., pectoralis major, latissimus, teres major) dominate over the subscapularis.

SYMPTOMS AND HISTORY

Associated with impingement

- Pain in anterior or posterior shoulder or deltoid area
- Pain with overhead activities, reaching out to the side or backward (e.g., reaching into passenger seat or back seat of car)
- Unable to sleep on affected side

Associated with instability

- "Clunking" with arm movements or sensation of the shoulder slipping out of socket
- *Might be associated with distal neurological symptoms in more severe cases*
- History of trauma
- More common in younger population versus older

Activities

- Racquet sports (especially forehand and overhead)
- Volleyball
- Swimmers
- Throwing athletes

KEY TESTS AND SIGNS

Alignment and appearance

- Greater than on third of humeral head protrudes anterior to anterolateral corner of acromion
- Distal humerus posterior to proximal humerus (shoulder extension) in side view
- Correction of humeral alignment decreases symptoms

Movement impairments

- May note excessive humeral anterior glide during shoulder abduction, horizontal abduction, return from flexion, medial or lateral rotation, and elbow extension
- Passive correction of anterior glide of humerus decreases symptoms
- Humeral anterior glide may be more evident during prone active lateral rotation versus passive
- Humeral anterior glide and pain may be more evident during shoulder rotation in the frontal plane versus the scapular plane
- Horizontal adduction may reproduce pain at the anterior shoulder caused by insufficient posterior glide
- Accessory joint motion increased anteriorly and decreased posteriorly

Impairments in muscle length

- *Based on length tests:* Short lateral rotators and pectoralis major

Impairments in muscle strength

- Long or weak medial rotators

ASSOCIATED SIGNS
(contributing factors)

Alignment and appearance
- May have normal resting alignment
- May be associated with forward shoulders
- Poor upper body muscle definition

Structural variations
- Thoracic kyphosis
- Elbow flexion contracture

Common activities
- Posturing with arms in extension (hands on hips or clasped behind back)
- May note decreased distance between humeral head and base of neck at end-range shoulder flexion
- Commonly associated with a scapular syndrome
- Ineffective passive restraint by the long head of biceps

Movement impairments
SHOULDER FLEXION
- *Associated with impingement:* May have slight end-range limitation and may have painful arc
- *Associated with instability:* May also observe increased prominence of humeral head in axilla with arm over head

Palpation
- May be tender over coracoacromial ligament, bicipital groove, or rotator cuff tendons (especially subscapularis)

Special tests
- *Associated with impingement:* Tests reproduce pain; resisted tests of rotator cuff and biceps for soft tissue differential diagnosis may be strong and painful or weak and painful
- *Associated with TOS:* May reproduce symptoms
- *Associated with instability:* May have increased accessory glide at GH joint in any direction

DIFFERENTIAL MOVEMENT AND ASSOCIATED DIAGNOSES

Differential humeral diagnoses
- *Rule:* If superior and anterior glide co-exist, assign anterior glide
- Humeral superior glide

Differential primary diagnoses
- Scapular downward rotation
- Scapular depression
- Scapular abduction
- Scapular winging and tilting

Associated diagnoses
- Rotator cuff tendinopathy
- Shoulder impingement
- Partial rotator cuff tear
- Bicipital tendinopathy
- Supraspinatus tendinopathy
- Humeral subluxation
- Bursitis
- AC joint pain
- Calcific tendinopathy
- Inlet syndrome

SCREENING FOR POTENTIAL MEDICAL DIAGNOSES REQUIRING REFERRAL

Musculoskeletal origin
- Cervical radiculopathy
- Brachial plexus injury
- Rotator cuff tear
- Fracture
- OA or RA
- Glenoid labrum tear

Visceral origin
- Neoplasms
- Cardiovascular disease
- Pulmonary disease
- Breast disease
- Abdominal organ pathologic condition

Systemic origin
- Collagen vascular disease
- Gout
- Syphilis and gonorrhea
- Sickle cell anemia
- Hemophilia
- Rheumatic disease

AC, Acromioclavicular; *GH,* glenohumeral;
OA, osteoarthritis; *RA,* rheumatoid arthritis;
SH, scapulohumeral; *TOS,* thoracic outlet syndrome.

Chapter 5
Appendix

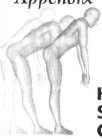

HUMERAL SUPERIOR GLIDE SYNDROME

Excessive superior or insufficient inferior glide of the humeral head is noted during shoulder motions. This may be associated with stiffness or shortness of the superior or inferior structures of the GH joint. Insufficiency of the rotator cuff because of weakness, recruitment impairments, or tear is a major causative factor. This disrupts the normal force couple between the rotator cuff and the deltoid.

SYMPTOMS AND HISTORY

Associated with impingement

- Pain in superior, anterior or posterior shoulder or deltoid area
- Pain with overhead activities or reaching out to the side
- Unable to sleep on affected side
- More common in middle aged to older people

Activities

- Weight lifters and body builders
- Swimmers

KEY TESTS AND SIGNS

Alignment and appearance

- Flattened deltoids (greater tuberosity not prominent just distal to acromion)
  - Arms in abduction relative to scapulae
  - Associated with scapula aligned in downward rotation
  - Correction of scapular alignment causes humerus to abduction
- Hypertrophied deltoid (arm rests in abduction)

Movement impairments

- Excessive humeral superior glide noted during shoulder abduction, flexion, and medial or lateral rotation
- Humeral superior glide more evident during active abduction versus passive
- Manual correction decreases symptoms. Active correction by increasing rotator cuff and decreasing deltoid activity decreases symptoms
- Decreased GH crease noted just distal to acromion with arm overhead
- Decreased distance between humeral head and base of neck noted at end range arm elevation

Special tests

- Accessory joint motion decreased inferior glide (more evident with 90 degrees arm abduction) and lateral distraction

Impairments in muscle length

BASED ON LENGTH TESTS

- Short subscapularis and lateral rotators
- Shortness of supraspinatus, deltoid (limitation of humeral adduction)

BASED ON ALIGNMENT

- Short deltoid and supraspinatus

Impairments in muscle strength

- Weak rotator cuff muscles

ASSOCIATED SIGNS
(contributing factors)

Alignment and appearance

Obesity

May have normal resting alignment

May see atrophy of rotator cuff muscles

Structural variations

May have generalized increased muscle bulk

Common activities

Repetitive arm activities

Leaning on elbows or arms

Commonly associated with a scapular syndrome

Movement impairments

Shoulder flexion

Associated with impingement: May have slight end range limitation and may have painful arc

Impairments in muscle length

BASED ON LENGTH TESTS

Shortness of latissimus, teres major muscles

Palpation

May be tender over coracoacromial ligament, bicipital groove, or rotator cuff tendons

Special tests

Associated with impingement: Tests reproduce pain; resisted tests of rotator cuff and biceps for soft tissue differential diagnosis may be strong and painful or weak and painful

Drop arm: Test may be positive

Empty can test positive for reproduction of pain

DIFFERENTIAL MOVEMENT AND ASSOCIATED DIAGNOSES

Differential humeral diagnoses

- *Rule:* If superior and anterior glide co-exist, assign anterior glide
- *Rule:* If shoulder medial rotation and superior glide co-exist, superior glide is the diagnosis
- Humeral anterior glide
- Shoulder medial rotation
- GH hypomobility

Differential primary diagnoses

- Scapular downward rotation
- Scapular depression
- Scapular abduction
- Scapular winging and tilting

Associated diagnoses

- Rotator cuff tendinopathy
- Shoulder impingement
- Partial or complete rotator cuff tear
- Bicipital tendinopathy
- Supraspinatus tendinopathy or tear
- Humeral subluxation
- Bursitis
- AC joint pain
- Calcific tendinopathy
- Frozen shoulder and adhesive capsulitis
- Outlet syndrome (Jobe)

SCREENING FOR POTENTIAL MEDICAL DIAGNOSES REQUIRING REFERRAL

Musculoskeletal origin

- Cervical radiculopathy
- Brachial plexus injury
- Rotator cuff tear
- Fracture
- OA or RA
- Glenoid labrum tear

Visceral origin

- Neoplasms
- Cardiovascular disease
- Pulmonary disease
- Breast disease
- Abdominal organ pathologic condition

Systemic origin

- Collagen vascular disease
- Gout
- Syphilis and gonorrhea
- Sickle cell anemia
- Hemophilia
- Rheumatic disease

AC, Acromioclavicular; *GH,* glenohumeral; *OA,* osteoarthritis; *RA,* rheumatoid arthritis.

Chapter 5
Appendix

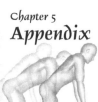

SHOULDER MEDIAL ROTATION SYNDROME

Excessive humeral medial rotation or insufficient lateral rotation is noted during shoulder flexion and abduction. The shoulder medial rotators dominate over the lateral rotators.

SYMPTOMS AND HISTORY

Associated with impingement

- Pain most often in anterior shoulder but may also be posterior shoulder or deltoid area
- Pain with overhead activities or with activities involving shoulder rotation arm elevated
- Unable to sleep on affected side

Activities

- Weight lifters
- Heavy laborers
- Swimmers (water polo)

KEY TESTS AND SIGNS

Alignment and appearance

- Humerus is medially rotated with or without corrected scapular alignment

Movement impairments

- Excessive humeral medial rotation noted during shoulder flexion and abduction
- *Correction of the excessive medial rotation may lessen the pain*
- *May increase the pain if capsular structures are shortened leading to increased compressive forces (e.g., superior glide)*

Special test

- Accessory joint motion can be decreased posteriorly

Impairments in muscle length

- *Based on length tests:* Short medial rotators (e.g., teres major, latissimus dorsi, pectoralis major)

Impairments in muscle strength

- Weak lateral rotators

ASSOCIATED SIGNS
(contributing factors)

Alignment and appearance

- May have normal resting alignment
- Humerus may be abducted
- Forward shoulders (abducted or tilted scapulae)
- Obesity

Structural variations

- Generalized increased muscle bulk
- Wide thorax
- Barrel chest
- Also commonly associated with a scapular syndrome.

Movement impairments

SHOULDER FLEXION

- *Associated with impingement:* May have slight end range limitation and may have painful arc
- *Associated with instability:* During shoulder flexion see a sudden shift of humerus into medial rotation

Impairments in muscle length

- Short or stiff deltoid
- Short lateral rotators

Impairments in muscle strength

- Weak subscapularis associated with impingement

Palpation

- May be tender over coracoacromial ligament, bicipital groove, or rotator cuff tendons (especially supraspinatus)

Special tests

- *Impingement tests:* Reproduce pain; resisted tests of rotator cuff and biceps for soft tissue differential diagnosis may be strong and painful or weak and painful.

DIFFERENTIAL MOVEMENT AND ASSOCIATED DIAGNOSES

Differential humeral diagnoses

- Humeral superior glide (if shoulder medial rotators and superior glide co-exist, superior glide is the diagnosis)

Differential primary diagnoses

- Scapular downward rotation
- Scapular depression
- Scapular abduction
- Scapular winging and tilting

Associated diagnoses

- Rotator cuff tendinopathy
- Shoulder impingement
- Partial rotator cuff tear
- Bicipital tendinopathy
- Supraspinatus tendinopathy
- Bursitis
- AC joint pain
- Calcific tendinopathy

SCREENING FOR POTENTIAL MEDICAL DIAGNOSES REQUIRING REFERRAL

Musculoskeletal origin

- Cervical radiculopathy
- Brachial plexus injury
- Rotator cuff tear
- Fracture
- OA or RA
- Glenoid labrum tear

Visceral origin

- Neoplasms
- Cardiovascular disease
- Pulmonary disease
- Breast disease
- Abdominal organ pathologic condition

Systemic origin

- Collagen vascular disease
- Gout
- Syphilis and gonorrhea
- Sickle cell anemia
- Hemophilia
- Rheumatic disease

AC, Acromioclavicular; *OA,* osteoarthritis; *RA,* rheumatoid arthritis; *SH,* scapulohumeral.

Chapter 5
Appendix

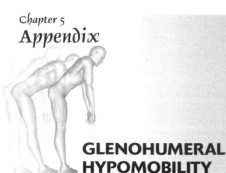

GLENOHUMERAL HYPOMOBILITY SYNDROME

This syndrome is characterized by a loss of motion at the GH joint in all directions. In most cases a capsular pattern of restriction is noted and associated with the medical diagnosis of adhesive capsulitis. This syndrome progresses through three stages. The patient presentation and treatment may vary, depending on the stage. GH hypomobility refers to the second two stages.

SYMPTOMS AND HISTORY

- Pain in superior, anterior, or posterior shoulder or deltoid area
- Pain may radiate down lateral arm to elbow
- Stiffness and loss of ROM
- Unable to sleep on affected side; pain at night; may awaken frequently
- Common functional limitations (e.g., unable to fasten bra, remove coat, remove shirt overhead, reach behind back)
- Most common from ages 40 to 60 years
- Diabetes
- More women than men
- History of trauma

KEY TESTS AND SIGNS

Movement impairments

- Loss of both passive and active ROM in all directions, most commonly in a capsular pattern
- Typically, pain increases toward the limits of the ROM
- Excessive humeral superior glide noted during shoulder abduction and flexion
- Decreased GH just distal to acromion with arm overhead
- Compensatory movements
  - During shoulder flexion and abduction scapula elevates excessively
  - During shoulder lateral rotation, scapula adducts or depresses
  - During shoulder medial rotation, scapula anteriorly tilts or abducts

Special tests

- Accessory joint motion decreased GH glide in all directions

ASSOCIATED SIGNS
(contributing factors)

Alignment and appearance

May have normal resting alignment

May develop scapular elevation secondary to compensatory motion

Decreased distance between humeral head and base of neck at end range arm elevation

Impairments in muscle recruitment

Deltoid dominates over rotator cuff muscles

Upper trap dominates over lower trapezius as a result of compensation

Impairments in muscle length

Muscles are probably short but difficult to test initially because of restriction of ROM pectoralis, latissimus dorsi, medial and lateral rotators

Long middle and lower trapezium muscles

Impairments in muscle strength

Weak rotator cuff muscles

DIFFERENTIAL MOVEMENT AND ASSOCIATED DIAGNOSES

Differential humeral diagnoses

- *Rule:* If GH hypomobility exists, it supercedes other diagnoses
- Humeral superior glide

Differential primary diagnoses

- Scapular downward rotation
- Scapular abduction

Associated diagnoses

- Frozen shoulder
- Adhesive capsulitis
- Rotator cuff tendinopathy
- Shoulder impingement
- Partial or complete rotator cuff tear
- Bicipital tendinopathy
- Supraspinatus tendinopathy or tear
- Bursitis
- AC joint pain
- Calcific tendinopathy
- Postsurgical or postfracture

SCREENING FOR POTENTIAL MEDICAL DIAGNOSES REQUIRING REFERRAL

Musculoskeletal origin

- Cervical radiculopathy
- Brachial plexus injury
- Rotator cuff tear
- Fracture
- OA or RA
- Glenoid labrum tear

Visceral origin

- Neoplasms
- Cardiovascular disease
- Pulmonary disease
- Breast disease
- Abdominal organ pathologic condition

Systemic origin

- Collagen vascular disease
- Gout
- Syphilis and gonorrhea
- Sickle cell anemia
- Hemophilia
- Rheumatic disease

GH, Glenohumeral; *OA,* osteoarthritis; *RA,* rheumatoid arthritis; *ROM,* range of motion.

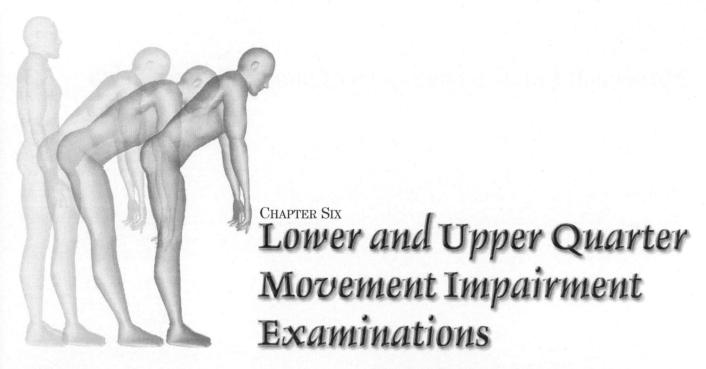

CHAPTER SIX

Lower and Upper Quarter Movement Impairment Examinations

Introduction

Formulating a diagnosis requires the performance of an examination and the accurate interpretation of the tests included in the examination. An examination has been designed that can be used to determine movement impairments of the lower quarter (e.g., thoracic spine, lumbar spine, hip, knee, ankle). The examination for movement impairment syndromes of the low back and hip includes the same test items, but the focus of the examination is concentrated on the painful area. A few special tests are used when assessing hip pain, and some tests can be eliminated when the focus is the lumbar spine. The advantages of this system are that it allows the therapist to determine whether (1) the low back is referring pain to the hip, (2) the pain arises from the hip joint, (3) hip dysfunction is contributing to back pain, or (4) both the hip and back are sources of pain. The test results also provide direction for the treatment. In fact, for most patients a positive finding for a test usually means that the test will become one of the patient's exercises. On completion of the examination the therapist should be able to establish a diagnosis, which is the directional susceptibility to movement (DSM) that is causing the pain and the factors that are contributing to make this movement direction the path of least resistance.

The examination is performed with the patient standing, supine, side-lying, prone, quadruped, sitting, and standing against a wall. The charts in this chapter describe the test items in these seven positions. For each test, the segment to be examined, the normal stan-dard for performance, the faults and criteria for the faults, the resulting impairments, and the possible DSM of the joint are identified. The listed impairments are considered as possible conditions and are not to be considered as always present with a given fault. The examination is provided in detail; however, this does not imply that all patients with low back pain will need to be examined for all the lower extremity alignment faults. A patient with hip or knee pain will need a more thorough examination of lower extremity alignment than the patient with low back pain. The details of these relationships are provided as a guide to the anatomic structures that the examiner is assessing and may need to be addressed by the treatment. Separate charts are provided for the lower and upper quarter parts of the body.

Additional check-off charts are provided that allow the therapist to check the test result and the most likely DSM. On completion of this chart, the DSM with the most positive findings should be the diagnosis. This check-off chart will also guide the therapist as to the contributing factors that are to be addressed by the treatment program and the instructions to the patient about how to modify his or her daily and sports activities. When several movement directions elicit symptoms, the therapist will also have to weigh the intensity of symptoms to select which movement direction is the most important. Only through the performance of a thorough examination and the identification of all contributing factors will the therapist be able to develop a comprehensive program that will be effective for both immediate restitution of the problem and for reducing the chance of reoccurrence.

Movement Impairments: Lower Quarter Examination

Test items, test criteria, and associated impairments

TEST	SEGMENT	FAULT
Standing tests		
Position	**Lumbar spine**	**Normal**
		Dysfunction
Alignment	**Thoracic spine**	**Normal**
		Kyphotic
		Flat
		Swayed back
	Infrasternal angle	**Normal**
		Narrow
		Wide
	Lumbar spine	**Normal**
		Lordotic
		Flat
	Paraspinal symmetry	**Normal**
		Asymmetry

ASIS, Anterior superior iliac spine; *DSM*, directional susceptibility to movement; *ITB*, iliotibial band; *MMT*, manual muscle test; *PIP*, proximal interphalangeal; *PICR*, path of the instantaneous center of rotation; *PSIS*, posterior superior iliac spine; *SLR*, straight-leg raise; *TFL*, tensor fascia lata; *TFL-ITB*, tensor fascia lata–iliotibial band.

CRITERIA	IMPAIRMENT	DSM
No pain		
Extension stress or compression	Pain Confirming test: flatten lumbar spine decreases pain	Lumbar extension
Outward curve		
Outward curve—increased	Rectus abdominis muscles—short, thoracic Paraspinal muscles—long	
Outward curve—absent	Thoracic paraspinal muscles—short	
Shoulders more than 2" posterior to greater trochanters	External oblique muscles—long Rectus abdominis muscles—short Internal oblique muscles—short	
90 degrees		
75 degrees	External oblique muscles—short	
More than 100 degrees	Internal oblique muscles—short External oblique—long	
Inward curve—20 to 30 degrees		

Inward curve greater than
    30 degrees
	External oblique muscles—long
	Iliopsoas muscle short; lumbar
	Paraspinal muscles—short
	Pain
	Confirming test: flatten lumbar spine to
	    decrease pain
		Extension

Inward curve—absent (may be normal for men)	Paraspinal muscles—long Iliopsoas muscle—long	

Left and right regions from lumbar
    spinous processes to 2" lateral
    are less than ½" different in
    prominence		

One side is more than ½" larger than other side	Paraspinal muscles—hypertrophied Spine rotated toward most prominent side	Lumbar rotation

Movement Impairments: Lower Quarter Examination — cont'd

TEST	SEGMENT	FAULT
Standing tests — cont'd		
Alignment—cont'd	Scoliosis	Rib hump
	Pelvis	Normal
		Anterior tilt
		Posterior tilt
		Lateral tilt
		Rotation
	Hip joint	Normal
		Flexed
		Extended
	Knees	Normal
		Hyperextended
		Flexed

ASIS, Anterior superior iliac spine; DSM, directional susceptibility to movement; ITB, iliotibial band; MMT, manual muscle test; PIP, proximal interphalangeal; PICR, path of the instantaneous center of rotation; PSIS, posterior superior iliac spine; SLR, straight-leg raise; TFL, tensor fascia lata; TFL-ITB, tensor fascia lata–iliotibial band.

CRITERIA	IMPAIRMENT	DSM
Ribs more prominent on one side Lumbar paraspinal asymmetry		Rotation
Line between ASIS and PSIS within 15 degrees of horizontal line (may vary in women)		
ASIS is 20 degrees lower than PSIS	External oblique muscles—long Hip flexor muscles—short Pain Confirming test: posterior tilt decreases pain	Extension
ASIS is 20 degrees higher than PSIS	Abdominal muscles—short Iliopsoas muscles—long	Flexion
One iliac crest is more than ½" higher than other iliac crest Lateral lumbar flexion toward high side	High side hip abductor muscles—long Low side hip abductor muscles—short	Rotation
ASIS on one side is anterior to ASIS on other side Hip on side to which pelvis is rotated—medially rotated, other hip-laterally rotated	TFL—short on side toward which pelvis is rotated	Rotation
Neutral position No angle at hip Peak of iliac crest to greater trochanter (axis) to line along thigh		
Hip angle of flexion is more than 10 degrees	Hip flexor muscles—short	
Hip angle of extension is more than 10 degrees	Iliopsoas muscle—long Hamstring muscles—short	Anterior glide
Neutral position		
Bowing of knee joint—backward Tibia may be posterior to femur	Quadriceps muscles—weakness Gastrocnemius muscles—short	
Forward angulation of knees		

Movement Impairments: Lower Quarter Examination — cont'd

TEST	SEGMENT	FAULT
Standing tests — cont'd		
Alignment—cont'd		Varum
		Valgum
	Tibia	Normal
		Bowed
		Varum
		Torsion
	Ankles	Normal
		Pronated
		Rigid
	Toes	Normal
		Hammer
		Hallux valgus
Standing movement tests		
Bilateral hip/knee flexion (partial squat)		Normal
		Hip dysfunction

ASIS, Anterior superior iliac spine; *DSM*, directional susceptibility to movement; *ITB*, iliotibial band; *MMT*, manual muscle test; *PIP*, proximal interphalangeal; *PICR*, path of the instantaneous center of rotation; *PSIS*, posterior superior iliac spine; *SLR*, straight-leg raise; *TFL*, tensor fascia lata; *TFL-ITB*, tensor fascia lata–iliotibial band.

CRITERIA	IMPAIRMENT	DSM
Bowing outward of knee joint **Nonstructural—hyperextended** knees with hip medial rotation	Hip lateral rotator muscles—long and weak	
Knees directed inward **Knock-knees** **Nonstructural—hip medial rotation**		
Shaft is perpendicular		
Posterior curve in sagittal plane		
Lateral curve in frontal plane		
Rotation of shaft of bone in horizontal plane		
Longitudinal arch—neutral		
Longitudinal arch—flattened	Posterior tibialis muscle—long	
Increased height of longitudinal arch **Does not flatten during hip and knee flexion**	Dorsiflexion range—limited	
Neutral alignment of joints		
PIP joint flexion	Toe flexor and extensor muscles—short Tendency to keep weight line posterior during sit to stand	
Lateral deviation of big toe		
Knee flexes 45 degrees with heel staying in contact with floor **Knee stays in line with 2nd toe** **Longitudinal arch decreases (pronates)**		
Medial rotation **Knee moves in line medial to big toe**	Hip medial rotation, hallux valgus	Medial rotation

Movement Impairments: Lower Quarter Examination — cont'd

TEST	SEGMENT	FAULT
Standing movement tests — cont'd		
Bilateral hip/knee flexion—cont'd		**Lateral rotation**
	Ankle	**Longitudinal arch**
Single leg stance **Other hip flexed to 70 degrees**	Normal	
		Lateral trunk flexion
		Hip adduction
		Pelvic rotation
		Hip rotation
Forward bending		**Normal**
	Lumbar	**Dysfunction**

ASIS, Anterior superior iliac spine; *DSM*, directional susceptibility to movement; *ITB*, iliotibial band; *MMT*, manual muscle test; *PIP*, proximal interphalangeal; *PICR*, path of the instantaneous center of rotation; *PSIS*, posterior superior iliac spine; *SLR*, straight-leg raise; *TFL*, tensor fascia lata; *TFL-ITB*, tensor fascia lata–iliotibial band.

CRITERIA	IMPAIRMENT	DSM
Knee moves in line lateral to fourth toe Hip lateral rotation		
Pronation—excessive flattening Supination—no change in arch Knee flexion less than 45 degrees		
No change in pelvic tilt or rotation No change in hip joint rotation		
Side bending of trunk toward stance leg	Stance side hip abductor weakness	Lumbar rotation
Downward tilting of opposite side of pelvis	Stance side hip abductor muscles—weak and long	Lumbar rotation Hip adduction
Toward stance leg	Hip lateral rotator muscles—long Medial rotator muscles—short	Lumbar rotation Hip medial rotation
Femur rotates medially	Hip lateral rotator muscles—long and weak	Hip medial rotation
Associated knee rotation only		Tibial femoral rotation
Associated ankle pronation only (femur and tibia maintain constant relationship)		Ankle pronation
Lumbar spine curve—0 to 20 degrees Hips flex to 80 degrees and move faster than spine		
Final alignment—more than 25 degrees of flexion	Lumbar back extensor muscles—long Hip extensor muscles—stiff	Lumbar flexion
	Pain Confirming test: forward bend with only hip flexion decreases pain	Flexion
Final alignment—inward lumbar curve	Lumbar back extensor muscles—short	Extension

Movement Impairments: Lower Quarter Examination — cont'd

TEST	SEGMENT	FAULT
Standing movement tests — cont'd		
Forward bending—cont'd		
		Hip dysfunction
		Ankle dysfunction
Return from forward bending		Normal
		Lumbar dysfunction
		Hip sway
Side bending		Normal
		Lumbar dysfunction
		Lumbar dysfunction

ASIS, Anterior superior iliac spine; *DSM*, directional susceptibility to movement; *ITB*, iliotibial band; *MMT*, manual muscle test; *PIP*, proximal interphalangeal; *PICR*, path of the instantaneous center of rotation; *PSIS*, posterior superior iliac spine; *SLR*, straight-leg raise; *TFL*, tensor fascia lata; *TFL-ITB*, tensor fascia lata–iliotibial band.

CRITERIA	IMPAIRMENT	DSM
Lumbar spine flexes faster than hips during first 50% of motion		Lumbar flexion
Men—flexes less than 75 degrees Women—less than 85 degrees	Hip extensor muscles—short and stiff Trunk—long, high center of gravity	
Flexes more than 100 degrees	Hamstring muscles—long	
Hips shift posteriorly more than 5"	Plantar flexor muscles—short	
Movement initiated with hip extension Hips continue to extend as lumbar spine moves toward extension		
Movement initiated with spine Hips extend after first third of range	Back extensor muscles more dominant than hip extensors Short hip flexors	Extension
	Pain Confirming test: return with hip extension only to decrease pain	
Marked dorsiflexion and forward sway of hips with lumbar extension	Hip extensor muscles—weak	
Symmetrical curve throughout lumbar spine		
Pain Limited range of motion toward *prominent* side Single site of motion rather than curve throughout spine Lateral glide of spine	Spine rotated toward prominent side	Lumbar rotation
Limited range of motion toward *nonprominent* side Single site of motion at lumbo-pelvic junction corrected by blocking movement site	Paraspinal muscles on side opposite limited range—stiff	Lumbar rotation

Movement Impairments: Lower Quarter Examination—cont'd

TEST	SEGMENT	FAULT
Standing movement tests—cont'd		
Spinal rotation	**Thoracic spine**	**Normal**
		Dysfunction
	Lumbar spine	**Normal**
		Dysfunction
Supine tests		
Double knee to chest (both knees are pushed toward chest)		**Normal**
		Lumbar dysfunction
		Thoracic dysfunction

ASIS, Anterior superior iliac spine; *DSM,* directional susceptibility to movement; *ITB,* iliotibial band; *MMT,* manual muscle test; *PIP,* proximal interphalangeal; *PICR,* path of the instantaneous center of rotation; *PSIS,* posterior superior iliac spine; *SLR,* straight-leg raise; *TFL,* tensor fascia lata; *TFL-ITB,* tensor fascia lata–iliotibial band.

CRITERIA	IMPAIRMENT	DSM
Symmetrical rotation of about 30 degrees to each side mostly between T8 and T11		
Pain **Increased rotation to one side**	**Abdominal and back extensor muscles—long**	**Thoracic rotation**
Rotation is less than 6 degrees to each side		
Rotation is more than 10 degrees to one side	**Abdominal and back extensor muscles—long** **Pain** **Confirming test: hand at side at waist level during side bending to same side to decrease pain**	**Lumbar rotation**

CRITERIA	IMPAIRMENT	DSM
Hips flex to 120 degrees without flexion of lumbar spine (spine should be flat)		
Lumbar spine flexes when hips are flexed less than 120 degrees **Sacrum lifts off table**	**Lumbar paraspinal muscles—long** **Hips—stiff**	**Lumbar flexion**
Thoracic spine flexes **Lumbar spine does not flatten when hips are flexed less than 120 degrees**		**Thoracic flexion**

Movement Impairments: Lower Quarter Examination—cont'd

TEST	SEGMENT	FAULT

Supine tests—cont'd

Hip flexor length test 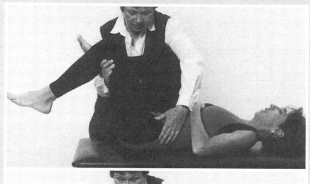	Back flat; monitor ASIS while lowering the relaxed limb; keep hip in neutral abduction/adduction	**Normal**
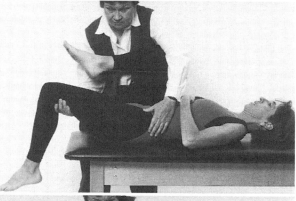	Thigh does not reach table, indicating hip flexor muscle shortness	
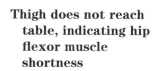 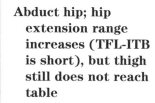	Abduct hip; hip extension range increases (TFL-ITB is short), but thigh still does not reach table	
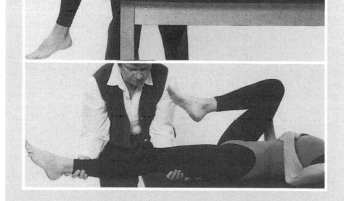	Passively extend knee; hip extension range increases (rectus femoris is short)	

ASIS, Anterior superior iliac spine; *DSM*, directional susceptibility to movement; *ITB*, iliotibial band; *MMT*, manual muscle test; *PIP*, proximal interphalangeal; *PICR*, path of the instantaneous center of rotation; *PSIS*, posterior superior iliac spine; *SLR*, straight-leg raise; *TFL*, tensor fascia lata; *TFL-ITB*, tensor fascia lata–iliotibial band.

CRITERIA	IMPAIRMENT	DSM
Extended thigh lies on table with lumbar spine flat Femur in midline without hip rotation or abduction Knee flexed to 80 degrees without abduction of tibia or lateral tibial rotation Hip extended 10 degrees		

Movement Impairments: Lower Quarter Examination — cont'd

TEST	SEGMENT	FAULT
Supine tests — cont'd		
Hip flexor length test—cont'd		**Lumbopelvic dysfunction**
	Hip muscle	**Dysfunction**
	Hip joint	**Dysfunction**
	Knee joint	**Dysfunction**
Supine position		**Normal**
	Lumbar	**Dysfunction**

ASIS, Anterior superior iliac spine; *DSM*, directional susceptibility to movement; *ITB*, iliotibial band; *MMT*, manual muscle test; *PIP*, proximal interphalangeal; *PICR*, path of the instantaneous center of rotation; *PSIS*, posterior superior iliac spine; *SLR*, straight-leg raise; *TFL*, tensor fascia lata; *TFL-ITB*, tensor fascia lata–iliotibial band.

CRITERIA	IMPAIRMENT	DSM
Pelvis tilts anteriorly	Abdominal control—deficient Spine too flexible	Lumbar extension
Pelvis rotates or laterally tilts	Abdominal control—deficient Spine too flexible	Lumbar rotation
Hip extension: greater when the hip is allowed to abduct and/or medially rotate	Tensor fascia lata muscle—short	
Hip extension: greater when the knee is passively extended while the femur is abducted	Rectus femoris—short	
Hip extension: limited when hip is abducted and knee is extended	Iliopsoas muscle—short	
Femoral head—glides anteriorly	Iliopsoas—long Anterior joint capsule—stretched	Femoral anterior glide
Anterior knee pain with hip extension/adduction	TFL-ITB—short and stiff	Patellar glide lateral
Lateral tibial rotation	TFL-ITB—short and stiff	Tibiofemoral rotation
Tibia glides laterally	ITB—short and stiff	Tibiofemoral lateral glide
Able to lie with hips and knees extended		
Lumbar spine extended	Abdominal muscles performance—insufficient Hip flexor muscles—short and stiff Pain Confirming test: hips and knees flexed; decreases pain	
Lumbar spine flexed	Back extensor muscles—long Abdominal muscles—short Pain Confirming test: hips and knees extended; decreases pain	

Movement Impairments: Lower Quarter Examination — cont'd

TEST	SEGMENT	FAULT
Supine tests — cont'd		
Lower abdominal, external oblique and rectus abdominis performance		Normal
	Level 3: hip flexed 90 degrees, extending other hip and knee; unsupported	
	Level 2: hip flexed 90 degrees, other hip/knee extended; supported	
	Hip flexed to greater than 90 degrees; other hip/knee extended; supported	
	On hip held passively in flexion, lift other limb off table	
	Keep one foot on table; slide other hip/knee into extension	
		Normal
	Lumbar spine	Dysfunction
	External oblique	Dysfunction

ASIS, Anterior superior iliac spine; *DSM*, directional susceptibility to movement; *ITB*, iliotibial band; *MMT*, manual muscle test; *PIP*, proximal interphalangeal; *PICR*, path of the instantaneous center of rotation; *PSIS*, posterior superior iliac spine; *SLR*, straight-leg raise; *TFL*, tensor fascia lata; *TFL-ITB*, tensor fascia lata–iliotibial band.

CRITERIA	IMPAIRMENT	DSM
Maximal performance: double-leg lowering, while maintaining flat lumbar spine and posterior pelvic tilt	MMT grade 5/5	
Minimal performance: maintain one hip at 90 degrees of flexion, back flat, while other lower extremity is extended and lowered to supporting surface while maintaining lumbar spine flat and pelvis in posterior pelvic tilt	MMT grade 3/5	
Anterior shear on lumbar spine	Pain with hip flexion	
One hip flexed to 90 degrees while other lower extremity is extended while lightly touching heel to supporting surface and able to maintain lumbar spine flat and pelvis in posterior tilt	MMT grade 2/5	

Movement Impairments: Lower Quarter Examination—cont'd

TEST	SEGMENT	FAULT
Supine tests—cont'd		
Lower abdominal, external oblique and rectus abdominis performance—cont'd	**External oblique**	**Dysfunction**
Trunk curl–sit up: internal oblique and rectus abdominis performance **Position: supine with hands on head, hips and knees extended with small support under knees**		**Normal**
	MMT grade 5/5	
	MMT grade 4/5	
	MMT grade 3/5	
	Spine	**Dysfunction**

ASIS, Anterior superior iliac spine; *DSM,* directional susceptibility to movement; *ITB,* iliotibial band; *MMT,* manual muscle test; *PIP,* proximal interphalangeal; *PICR,* path of the instantaneous center of rotation; *PSIS,* posterior superior iliac spine; *SLR,* straight-leg raise; *TFL,* tensor fascia lata; *TFL-ITB,* tensor fascia lata–iliotibial band.

CRITERIA	IMPAIRMENT	DSM
One hip flexed to 90 degrees while the other, lower extremity is lifted from supporting surface, back stays flat	MMT grade 1/5	
Flexion of cervical and upper thoracic spines Posterior pelvic tilt with reversal of lumbar curve, flexion of thoracic spine Thoracic and lumbar flexion reaches the limit of spinal flexibility, at the point the hip flexors contract and the hip flexes until the hip flexes to 80 degrees	MMT grade 5/5	
Unable to segmentally flex spine throughout trunk curl	Stiff spine	

Movement Impairments: Lower Quarter Examination — cont'd

TEST	SEGMENT	FAULT
Supine tests — cont'd		
Trunk curl–sit up: internal oblique and rectus abdominis performance—cont'd	Hip muscle	Dysfunction
	Internal oblique	Dysfunction
	Internal oblique	Dysfunction
	Internal oblique	Dysfunction
Straight-leg raise (SLR)	Monitoring greater trochanter Hip remains in neutral position; correct greater trochanter position Hip medially rotated; greater trochanter moves anteriorly	Normal

ASIS, Anterior superior iliac spine; *DSM*, directional susceptibility to movement; *ITB*, iliotibial band; *MMT*, manual muscle test; *PIP*, proximal interphalangeal; *PICR*, path of the instantaneous center of rotation; *PSIS*, posterior superior iliac spine; *SLR*, straight-leg raise; *TFL*, tensor fascia lata; *TFL-ITB*, tensor fascia lata–iliotibial band.

CRITERIA	IMPAIRMENT	DSM
Initiation: limited posterior tilt Lumbar spine does not reverse its curve	Iliopsoas muscle—short	
Able to flex the vertebral column through the same range and hold it flexed while coming to a sitting position with forearms folded across chest	Muscle weakness MMT 4/5	
Able to flex the vertebral column through the same range and hold it flexed while coming to a sitting position with forearms extended forward	Muscle weakness MMT 3/5	
Able to flex the vertebral column to the same range with forearms extended forward but loses curl when hip flexors contract	Muscle weakness MMT 3−/5	
Greater trochanter maintains a constant position (PICR) during passive and active SLR Hip flexes to 80 degrees		

Movement Impairments: Lower Quarter Examination — cont'd

TEST	SEGMENT	FAULT
Supine tests — cont'd		
SLR—cont'd	Hip	Dysfunction
	Lumbar	Neural dysfunction
Iliopsoas	Muscle performance	Normal
	Hip muscle	Dysfunction

ASIS, Anterior superior iliac spine; *DSM*, directional susceptibility to movement; *ITB*, iliotibial band; *MMT*, manual muscle test; *PIP*, proximal interphalangeal; *PICR*, path of the instantaneous center of rotation; *PSIS*, posterior superior iliac spine; *SLR*, straight-leg raise; *TFL*, tensor fascia lata; *TFL-ITB*, tensor fascia lata–iliotibial band.

CRITERIA	IMPAIRMENT	DSM
Greater trochanter moves anterior and superior (medial rotation and insufficient posterior glide) during active SLR During passive SLR, greater trochanter maintains a relatively constant position, but the examiner may need to control the axis of rotation by placing their thumb along the inguinal crease Active SLR may produce anterior hip pain while passive SLR is pain free	Stiff posterior hip joint structures Hamstring muscles—short	Femoral anterior glide
Femoral medial rotation	Iliopsoas muscles—long Hip lateral rotator muscles—long and stiff	Femoral medial rotation
Hip flexion less than 80 degrees Lumbar flexion	Hamstring muscles—short and stiff	Lumbar flexion
Pain down lower extremity with hip flexion of less than 45 degrees	Neural entrapment Confirming test: same pain, patient is completely relaxed Hip flexor effect on spine if pain is less when patient is completely relaxed	
Able to maintain constant position of hip flexion/abduction/lateral rotation with knee extended Pelvis stabilized by examiner, when resistance is applied in direction of hip extension/adduction		
Hip flexed/abducted/laterally rotated with knee extended Pelvis stabilized by examiner with pressure on contralateral iliac crest—unable to maintain position with application of resistance, but able to after change of 10 to 15 degrees	Iliopsoas muscle—long Usually TFL will be strong or dominant	

Movement Impairments: Lower Quarter Examination — cont'd

TEST	SEGMENT	FAULT
Supine tests — cont'd		
Iliopsoas—cont'd		
Iliopsoas performance		Normal
	Hip muscle	Dysfunction
Hip abduction/lateral rotation with hip flexed		Normal
	Right hip abduction/ lateral rotation; monitoring anterior superior iliac crest	
	Left hip abduction/ lateral rotation; no pelvic rotation	

ASIS, Anterior superior iliac spine; *DSM*, directional susceptibility to movement; *ITB*, iliotibial band; *MMT*, manual muscle test; *PIP*, proximal interphalangeal; *PICR*, path of the instantaneous center of rotation; *PSIS*, posterior superior iliac spine; *SLR*, straight-leg raise; *TFL*, tensor fascia lata; *TFL-ITB*, tensor fascia lata–iliotibial band.

CRITERIA	IMPAIRMENT	DSM
Hip flexed/abducted/laterally rotated with knee extended Pelvis stabilized by examiner with pressure on contralateral iliac crest—unable to maintain position with application of maximum resistance, at any point in range of motion	Iliopsoas muscle—strained and weak	
Able to maintain constant position with hip flexed/abducted/medially rotated with knee extended Pelvis stabilized by examiner when maximum pressure is applied in direction of hip extension/adduction		
Hip flexed/abducted/medially rotated with knee extended Pelvis stabilized by examiner with pressure on contralateral iliac crest—unable to maintain position with application of resistance (most often the hip will medially rotate)	TFL muscle—strained and weak	
Lower extremity moves through full range of motion (hip flexion, abduction, and lateral rotation) and in opposite direction (hip flexion, adduction, and medial rotation) without associated pelvic rotation		

Movement Impairments: Lower Quarter Examination—cont'd

TEST	SEGMENT	FAULT
Supine tests—cont'd		
Hip abduction/lateral rotation with hip flexed—cont'd	**Lumbopelvic**	**Dysfunction**
	Hip joint	**Dysfunction**
Unilateral hip and knee flexion (single knee to chest); passive and active		**Normal**
	Passive hip flexion	
	Pressure at inguinal crease during passive hip flexion	
	Active hip flexion to 90 degrees; patient then uses hands to pull knee toward chest	
	Lowering leg with incorrect lumbar extension	

ASIS, Anterior superior iliac spine; *DSM*, directional susceptibility to movement; *ITB*, iliotibial band; *MMT*, manual muscle test; *PIP*, proximal interphalangeal; *PICR*, path of the instantaneous center of rotation; *PSIS*, posterior superior iliac spine; *SLR*, straight-leg raise; *TFL*, tensor fascia lata; *TFL-ITB*, tensor fascia lata–iliotibial band.

CRITERIA	IMPAIRMENT	DSM
Pelvis rotates more than ½" during first 50% of lower extremity motion	Abdominal muscle control deficiency (internal & contralateral external obliques)	Lumbar rotation
Limited range of hip motion	Pain in groin	
Hip flexes 120 degrees in neutral rotation without lumbar flexion Additional hip flexion causes posterior pelvic tilt, flattening of lumbar spine while opposite lower extremity remains in contact with supporting surface (comparable to 10 degrees of hip extension)		

Movement Impairments: Lower Quarter Examination—cont'd

TEST	SEGMENT	FAULT
Supine tests—cont'd		
Unilateral hip and knee flexion (single knee to chest); passive and active—cont'd	Ipsilateral hip	Dysfunction
	Lumbopelvic	Dysfunction
	Contralateral hip	Dysfunction
Side-lying tests		
Position		Normal
	Lumbar	Dysfunction
Hip abduction/lateral rotation		Normal
	Patient could rest foot of top leg on bottom leg and upwardly rotate knee of top leg to produce hip abduction/lateral rotation motion	

ASIS, Anterior superior iliac spine; *DSM,* directional susceptibility to movement; *ITB,* iliotibial band; *MMT,* manual muscle test; *PIP,* proximal interphalangeal; *PICR,* path of the instantaneous center of rotation; *PSIS,* posterior superior iliac spine; *SLR,* straight-leg raise; *TFL,* tensor fascia lata; *TFL-ITB,* tensor fascia lata–iliotibial band.

CRITERIA	IMPAIRMENT	DSM
Hip flexes less than 115 degrees	Gluteus maximus, piriformis—short Lumbar paraspinal muscles—long Pain in groin Greater trochanter moves anterior/superior Restricting trochanter movement by pressure at inguinal crease, increases the resistance to hip flexion Stiffness of posterior hip joint structures	Femoral anterior glide
Pelvis tilts posteriorly and lumbar spine flexes (sacrum lifts off supporting surface)		Lumbar flexion
Opposite hip flexes (hip does not extend 10 degrees)	Iliopsoas muscles—short	
No discomfort		
Pain	Spinal lateral flexion Confirming test: support placed at waist to eliminate lateral flexion to decrease pain	Lumbar rotation
Able to abduction/laterally rotate hip without movement of the pelvis		

Movement Impairments: Lower Quarter Examination—cont'd

TEST	SEGMENT	FAULT
Side-lying tests—cont'd		
Hip abduction/lateral rotation—cont'd	**Lumbopelvic**	**Dysfunction**
Hip abduction (other hip joint positions neutral) (gluteus medius, minimus, TFL strength)		**Normal**
	Hip abductor test position; pressure applied above ankle	
	Hip	**Dysfunction**
	Lumbopelvic	**Dysfunction**
Hip abduction in lateral rotation and extension (posterior gluteus, medius strength)		**Normal**
	Posterior gluteus medius test position	
	Iliotibial band length assessment	

ASIS, Anterior superior iliac spine; *DSM,* directional susceptibility to movement; *ITB,* iliotibial band; *MMT,* manual muscle test; *PIP,* proximal interphalangeal; *PICR,* path of the instantaneous center of rotation; *PSIS,* posterior superior iliac spine; *SLR,* straight-leg raise; *TFL,* tensor fascia lata; *TFL-ITB,* tensor fascia lata–iliotibial band.

CRITERIA	IMPAIRMENT	DSM
Pelvis rotates during hip abduction/lateral rotation	Abdominal muscle—deficient control	Lumbar rotation
Able to tolerate maximum resistance at end of range	MMT 5/5	
Unable to tolerate maximum resistance at any point in the range of motion	Hip abductor muscles—weak	
Unable to tolerate maximum resistance at the end of the range but can after 10 to 15 degrees of adduction	Hip abductor muscles—long	
Lateral pelvic tilt during active hip abduction	Lateral abdominal muscles—dominant	Lumbar rotation
Able to tolerate maximum resistance applied at the end of range	MMT grade 5/5	

Movement Impairments: Lower Quarter Examination — cont'd

TEST	SEGMENT	FAULT
Side-lying tests — cont'd		
Hip abduction in lateral rotation and extension—cont'd	Hip	Dysfunction
Hip adduction (uppermost lower extremity) **Starting position: hip abduction, lateral rotation, and slight extension with knee extended**		Normal
	Hip	Dysfunction
	Lumbopelvic	Dysfunction
Hip adduction (lowermost lower extremity) **Position: hip adducted, neutral rotation, neutral flexion/extension, knee extended**		Normal
	Hip	Dysfunction
Prone tests		
Position		Normal
	Lumbopelvic	Dysfunction

ASIS, Anterior superior iliac spine; *DSM*, directional susceptibility to movement; *ITB*, iliotibial band; *MMT*, manual muscle test; *PIP*, proximal interphalangeal; *PICR*, path of the instantaneous center of rotation; *PSIS*, posterior superior iliac spine; *SLR*, straight-leg raise; *TFL*, tensor fascia lata; *TFL-ITB*, tensor fascia lata–iliotibial band.

CRITERIA	IMPAIRMENT	DSM
Unable to tolerate maximum resistance at any point in range	Posterior gluteus medius muscle—weak	
Unable to tolerate resistance at end of range but can after hip adducts 10 to 15 degrees	Posterior gluteus medius muscle—long	
Hip flexes when maximum resistance is applied	TFL—dominant	
Hip adducts 10 degrees		
Hip adducts less than 5 degrees	Hip abductor muscles—short	
Hip flexes and/or medially rotates	TFL and/or anterior gluteus medius and minimus—short	Hip medial Rotation and/or adduction
Excessive hip adduction with anterior distal position of greater trochanter	Hip abductor muscles—long	Femoral lateral glide
Lateral pelvic tilt	Lateral abdominal muscle control—deficient	Lumbar rotation
Able to tolerate maximum resistance applied to lower thigh	MMT grade 5/5	
Unable to tolerate maximum resistance	Adductor muscle—weak	
No pain		
Pain	Lumbar extension—increased Compression or anterior shear from psoas muscle—increased Confirming test: pillow under abdomen; decreases pain	

Movement Impairments: Lower Quarter Examination — cont'd

TEST	SEGMENT	FAULT
Prone tests — cont'd		
Knee flexion		Normal
	Muscle performance	
	Muscle	Dysfunction
	Lumbopelvic	Dysfunction
	Tibiofemoral	Dysfunction
Hip medial rotation		Normal

ASIS, Anterior superior iliac spine; *DSM*, directional susceptibility to movement; *ITB*, iliotibial band; *MMT*, manual muscle test; *PIP*, proximal interphalangeal; *PICR*, path of the instantaneous center of rotation; *PSIS*, posterior superior iliac spine; *SLR*, straight-leg raise; *TFL*, tensor fascia lata; *TFL-ITB*, tensor fascia lata–iliotibial band.

CRITERIA	IMPAIRMENT	DSM
Knee flexes to 120 degrees without pelvic tilt, rotation, or lumbar extension		
Able to maintain knee flexion of 80 degrees when maximum resistance is applied	MMT grade 5/5	
Unable to maintain knee flexion when resistance is applied	Hamstring muscles—weak	
Knee flexion less than 110 degrees	Quadriceps muscles—short	
Anterior pelvic tilt	Rectus femoris muscle—stiff Abdominal muscle control—deficient	Lumbar extension
Pelvic rotation	TFL muscle—stiff Abdominal muscle control—deficient	Lumbar rotation
Tibia lateral rotation	TFL muscle—stiff	Tibiofemoral rotation
35 degrees of medial rotation without pelvic rotation Hip rotation range of motion is highly variable and does not necessarily imply muscle shortness		

Movement Impairments: Lower Quarter Examination—cont'd

TEST	SEGMENT	FAULT
Prone tests—cont'd		
Hip medial rotation—cont'd	Hip	Dysfunction
	Lumbopelvic	Dysfunction
	Tibiofemoral	Dysfunction
Hip lateral rotation		Normal
	Hip	Dysfunction
	Lumbopelvic	Dysfunction
	Tibiofemoral	Dysfunction

ASIS, Anterior superior iliac spine; *DSM*, directional susceptibility to movement; *ITB*, iliotibial band; *MMT*, manual muscle test; *PIP*, proximal interphalangeal; *PICR*, path of the instantaneous center of rotation; *PSIS*, posterior superior iliac spine; *SLR*, straight-leg raise; *TFL*, tensor fascia lata; *TFL-ITB*, tensor fascia lata–iliotibial band.

CRITERIA	IMPAIRMENT	DSM
Less than 30 degrees of hip medial rotation	Lateral rotators: obturators, quadratus femoris, gemelli, piriformis, posterior gluteus medius—short	
Less than 10 degrees	Structural variation: retroversion of femur	
More than 50 degrees	Structural variation: antetorsion of femur	
Pelvic rotation during first 50% of range	Lumbar spine excessive flexibility	Lumbar rotation
Tibia glides laterally on femur	Knee joint laxity	Tibiofemoral rotation
35 degrees of lateral rotation without pelvic motion, with limited arc of movement Hip rotation range of motion is highly variable and does not necessarily imply muscle shortness		
Less than 30 degrees of lateral rotation	Medial rotators: TFL-ITB, anterior gluteus medius, gluteus minimus—short	
Less than 10 degrees of lateral rotation	Structural variation: possible antetorsion of femur	
More than 50 degrees of lateral rotation	Structural variation: possible retrotorsion of femur	
Greater trochanter moves antero-lateral, making a wide arc of movement	TFL-ITB muscle—short	Anterior femoral glide
Pelvic rotation during first 50% of motion	Lumbar excessive flexibility	Lumbar rotation
Tibia glides on femur	Knee joint laxity	Tibiofemoral rotation

Movement Impairments: Lower Quarter Examination — cont'd

TEST	SEGMENT	FAULT
Prone tests — cont'd		
Hip extension with knee extended		Normal
	Muscle	Dysfunction
	Lumbopelvic	Dysfunction
Hip	Dysfunction	
Hip extension with knee flexed		Normal

ASIS, Anterior superior iliac spine; *DSM*, directional susceptibility to movement; *ITB*, iliotibial band; *MMT*, manual muscle test; *PIP*, proximal interphalangeal; *PICR*, path of the instantaneous center of rotation; *PSIS*, posterior superior iliac spine; *SLR*, straight-leg raise; *TFL*, tensor fascia lata; *TFL-ITB*, tensor fascia lata–iliotibial band.

CRITERIA	IMPAIRMENT	DSM
Hip extends 10 degrees with slight lumbar extension, and simultaneous contraction of gluteus maximus and hamstring muscles		
Hip extends 5 degrees	Iliopsoas muscle—short	
Lumbar extension/anterior pelvic tilt	Abdominal muscle control—deficient Iliopsoas muscle—short	Lumbar extension
Gluteal muscle contraction, as indicated by change in muscle contour, delayed until hip is extended	Hamstring recruitment—dominant	
Greater trochanter moves anteriorly	Hamstring recruitment—dominant, short and stiff TFL—stretched anterior joint capsule	Femoral anterior glide
10 degree hip extension with slight lumbar extension		

Movement Impairments: Lower Quarter Examination—cont'd

TEST	SEGMENT	FAULT
Prone tests — cont'd		
Alignment	**Muscle performance**	
	Muscle	**Dysfunction**
	Hip	**Dysfunction**
	Lumbopelvic	**Dysfunction**
Quadruped tests		
Alignment	**Head and neck**	**Normal**
		Dysfunction
	Thoracic	**Normal**
		Dysfunction
	Scapula	**Normal**

ASIS, Anterior superior iliac spine; *DSM*, directional susceptibility to movement; *ITB*, iliotibial band; *MMT*, manual muscle test; *PIP*, proximal interphalangeal; *PICR*, path of the instantaneous center of rotation; *PSIS*, posterior superior iliac spine; *SLR*, straight-leg raise; *TFL*, tensor fascia lata; *TFL-ITB*, tensor fascia lata–iliotibial band.

CRITERIA	IMPAIRMENT	DSM
Able to maintain hip extension when maximum resistance is applied	MMT grade 5/5	
Hip extension less than 5 degrees	Rectus femoris, TFL-ITB muscles—short	
Unable to take maximum resistance to hip extension	Gluteus maximus muscle—weak MMT grade 3 to 4/5	
Anterior displacement of greater trochanter during hip extension	Stretched anterior joint capsule Hamstring muscle—dominance	Femoral anterior glide
Anterior pelvic tilt–hip flexion/lumbar extension	Hip flexor muscles—stiff Abdominal muscle control—deficient	Lumbar extension
Head neutral, cervical spine slight inward curve, levator scapulae not prominent		
Cervical extension, prominence of levator scapula	Neck extensor muscles—short Levator scapulae muscles—short	
Slight outward curve		
Increased outward curve	Thoracic paraspinal muscles—long Rectus abdominis muscles—short	Rotation
Asymmetry; scoliosis	Abdominal muscle imbalance	Rotation
Flat on thorax, positioned between T2-7, approximately 3 inches from spine		

Movement Impairments: Lower Quarter Examination — cont'd

TEST	SEGMENT	FAULT
Quadruped tests — cont'd		
Alignment—cont'd		Dysfunction
	Lumbar spine	Normal
		Dysfunction
	Hip joint	Normal
		Dysfunction
	Ankle	Normal

ASIS, Anterior superior iliac spine; *DSM,* directional susceptibility to movement; *ITB,* iliotibial band; *MMT,* manual muscle test; *PIP,* proximal interphalangeal; *PICR,* path of the instantaneous center of rotation; *PSIS,* posterior superior iliac spine; *SLR,* straight-leg raise; *TFL,* tensor fascia lata; *TFL-ITB,* tensor fascia lata–iliotibial band.

CRITERIA	IMPAIRMENT	DSM
Winging	Serratus anterior muscles—weak and long	
Abducted, more than 3¼" from spine	Serratus anterior muscles—short Rhomboid and trapezius muscles— may be short	
Adducted, less than 2½" from spine	Serratus anterior muscle—long Rhomboid muscles—may be short	
Flat or level; no pain		
Flexed, kyphotic	Lumbar back extensor muscles—long Abdominal muscles—short Psoas muscle—imbalanced Pain Confirming test: flatten lumbar spine to decrease pain	Lumbar flexion
Confirming test: flatten lumbar spine to increase pain		Extension or rotation
Extended, lordotic	Lumbar back extensor muscles—short Abdominal muscles—long and weak Pain Confirming test: flatten lumbar spine; decreases pain	Lumbar extension
Asymmetry, one paraspinal area more than ½" more prominent than opposite side	Abdominal and back extensor imbalance	Rotation
90-degree angle between femur and pelvis Neutral rotation Abduction/adduction		

Less than 90 degrees	Posterior hip joint capsule, gluteus
	   maximus, piriformis muscles—short and
	   stiff	

Hip lateral rotation	Gluteus maximus, piriformis muscles— short and stiff	
Plantarflexed with dorsum of foot almost on supporting surface		

Movement Impairments: Lower Quarter Examination — cont'd

TEST	SEGMENT	FAULT
Quadruped tests — cont'd		
Alignment—cont'd		Dysfunction
Rocking backward toward heels		Normal
	Lumbar	Dysfunction
	Hip	Dysfunction
Rocking forward		Normal
	Lumbar	Dysfunction

ASIS, Anterior superior iliac spine; *DSM*, directional susceptibility to movement; *ITB*, iliotibial band; *MMT*, manual muscle test; *PIP*, proximal interphalangeal; *PICR*, path of the instantaneous center of rotation; *PSIS*, posterior superior iliac spine; *SLR*, straight-leg raise; *TFL*, tensor fascia lata; *TFL-ITB*, tensor fascia lata–iliotibial band.

CRITERIA	IMPAIRMENT	DSM
Dorsiflexion	Dorsiflexor and toe extensor muscles—short	
Hips flex, lumbar spine remains flat No pain		
Flexion of spine during first 50% of motion	Lumbar back extensor muscles—long Rectus abdominis muscles—short Hip extensor muscles—short and stiff Pain with lumbar flexion Confirming test: prevent lumbar flexion and increase hip flexion: decreases pain	Lumbar flexion
	Pain with flat or lordotic lumbar spine Confirming test: push back with hands and avoid use of hip flexors; decreases pain	Lumbar extension
Rotation of lumbar spine	Paraspinal muscle—imbalance	Rotation
Decreased hip flexion	Gluteus maximus, piriformis muscles—short and stiff Confirming test: abduct and/or laterally rotate hips; increases hip flexion	
Pelvic rotation	Gluteus maximus, piriformis muscles—asymmetric short and stiff Confirming test: abduct/laterally rotate hip with less hip flexion, high side of pelvis	
Even distribution of extension throughout the lumbar spine No pain		
Marked extension at lower segments	Excessive extension flexibility of spine Hip flexor muscles—short Pain	Extension

Movement Impairments: Lower Quarter Examination — cont'd

TEST	SEGMENT	FAULT
Quadruped tests — cont'd		
Shoulder flexion		**Normal**
	Thoracic	**Dysfunction**
	Lumbar	**Dysfunction**
Sitting tests		
Alignment		**Normal**
	Lumbar	**Dysfunction**
Sitting knee extension and ankle dorsiflexion		**Normal**

ASIS, Anterior superior iliac spine; *DSM*, directional susceptibility to movement; *ITB*, iliotibial band; *MMT*, manual muscle test; *PIP*, proximal interphalangeal; *PICR*, path of the instantaneous center of rotation; *PSIS*, posterior superior iliac spine; *SLR*, straight-leg raise; *TFL*, tensor fascia lata; *TFL-ITB*, tensor fascia lata–iliotibial band.

CRITERIA	IMPAIRMENT	DSM
Thoracic and lumbar spines remain motionless		
Rotation of thoracic spine more than ½ inch with shoulder flexion	Abdominal muscle—poor control	Rotation
Rotation of lumbar spine more than ½ inch with shoulder flexion	Abdominal muscle—poor control	Rotation
Lumbar spine is flat; hip flexed to 90 degrees without pain		
Lumbar spine is flexed	Lumbar back extensor muscles—long Pain	Lumbar extension
Lumbar spine is extended	Lumbar back extensor muscles—short Hip flexor activity—excessive Pain	Extension
Lumbar spine remains flat, knee extends to within 10 degrees of complete extension with hip flexed to 90 degrees, ankle dorsiflexes to 10 degrees		

Movement Impairments: Lower Quarter Examination — cont'd

TEST	SEGMENT	FAULT
Sitting tests — cont'd		
Sitting knee extension and ankle dorsiflexion—cont'd	Lumbar	**Dysfunction**
	Hip	**Dysfunction**
	Ankle	**Dysfunction**

ASIS, Anterior superior iliac spine; *DSM*, directional susceptibility to movement; *ITB*, iliotibial band; *MMT*, manual muscle test; *PIP*, proximal interphalangeal; *PICR*, path of the instantaneous center of rotation; *PSIS*, posterior superior iliac spine; *SLR*, straight-leg raise; *TFL*, tensor fascia lata; *TFL-ITB*, tensor fascia lata–iliotibial band.

CRITERIA	IMPAIRMENT	DSM
Lumbar spine flexes during knee extension	Lumbar paraspinal muscles—long Hamstring muscles—stiffer than lumbar spine Pain Confirming test: lumbar spine remains flat; decreases pain	Flexion
Lumbar spine rotates during knee extension	Lumbar paraspinal muscles—unilaterally long Hamstrings—stiffer than lumbar spine Pain Confirming test: prevent rotation; decreases pain	Rotation
Knee extends less than 75 degrees with hip flexed to 90 degrees	Hamstring muscles—short	
Hip medially rotates	Medial hamstring muscles—short TFL muscle—inappropriately recruited	
Dorsiflexion less than 10 degrees with knee extended	Gastrocnemius muscle—short Soleus muscles—short	
Dorsiflexion less than 10 degrees with knee flexed	Soleus muscles—short	
Toe extension during dorsiflexion	Extensor digitorum longus muscle—dominant	
Eversion of ankle during dorsiflexion	Peroneal muscle—dominant	Pronated foot

Movement Impairments: Lower Quarter Examination—cont'd

TEST	SEGMENT	FAULT
Sitting tests—cont'd		
Sitting hip flexion		Normal
	Muscle	Dysfunction
Hip rotation		Normal
	Hip	Dysfunction
	Leg	

CRITERIA	IMPAIRMENT	DSM
Hip is flexed to 120 degrees Maximum resistance to iliopsoas is tolerated		
Unable to tolerate resistance with hip in 120 degrees of flexion but can at 105 to 110 degrees of hip flexion	Iliopsoas muscle—long	
Unable to tolerate resistance to hip flexion at any point in range	Iliopsoas muscle—weak	
Hip medial and lateral rotation is symmetrical and approximately 30 degrees Hip medial and lateral rotators can tolerate maximum resistance		
In maximum medial or lateral rotation, maximum resistance cannot be tolerated at the end of the range of motion	Tested hip rotator muscle—long	
Maximum resistance cannot be tolerated at any point in the range of motion	Tested hip rotator muscle—weak	
Medial rotation range of motion much greater than lateral rotation range	Structural variation: hip antetorsion	
Lateral rotation range of motion much greater than medial rotation range	Structural variation: hip retrotorsion	
Tibial structural variation	Line between medial and lateral malleoli is more than 25 degrees off horizontal	

Movement Impairments: Lower Quarter Examination—cont'd

TEST	SEGMENT	FAULT
Standing: back to wall tests		
Flatten back with arms at sides		Normal
	Lumbopelvic	Dysfunction

ASIS, Anterior superior iliac spine; DSM, directional susceptibility to movement; ITB, iliotibial band; MMT, manual muscle test; PIP, proximal interphalangeal; PICR, path of the instantaneous center of rotation; PSIS, posterior superior iliac spine; SLR, straight-leg raise; TFL, tensor fascia lata; TFL-ITB, tensor fascia lata–iliotibial band.

CRITERIA	IMPAIRMENT	DSM
With arms at side, feet 3 inches forward of the wall, lumbar spine can be flattened against the wall without pain		
Unable to flatten lumbar spine	Abdominal muscles—weak Iliopsoas muscle—short Back extensor muscles—short Pain with lumbar flexion	Extension Extension Extension Flexion

Gait

COMPONENT	DYSFUNCTION	CRITERIA
Pelvic rotation	Normal	Pelvis rotates 4 degrees on either side of a central axis (total 8 degrees) during swing phase with right and left sides
	Lumbopelvic dysfunction	Increased rotation of pelvis at end of stance phase when hip is extending
		Increased anterior pelvic tilt at end of stance phase when hip is extending
Lateral pelvic shift	Normal	Trunk shifts laterally over weightbearing leg 1 inch
	Lumbopelvic dysfunction	Lateral pelvic shift less than 1 inch
Pelvic drop (hip rotation)	Normal	5 degrees of hip adduction of stance leg
	Lumbopelvic dysfunction	More than 5 degrees of hip adduction of stance leg
		Lateral trunk flexion toward stance leg
Hip medial rotation of stance leg from heel strike to midstance	Normal	5 to 7 degrees of hip medial rotation from heel strike to midstance
	Hip dysfunction	More than 5 to 7 degrees of hip medial rotation
		Less than 5 to 7 degrees of hip lateral rotation
Hip lateral to rotation on stance leg from midstance to push-off	Normal	5 to 7 degrees of hip lateral rotation from foot flat toe off associated with supination
	Lumbopelvic dysfunction	Less than 5 to 7 degrees of hip lateral rotation
Knee angle from heel strike to midstance	Normal	At heel strike the knee flexes 15 degrees then extends to neutral until push-off
	Knee dysfunction	At heel strike or shortly afterwards, the knee hyperextends
Ankle motion from midstance to push-off	Normal	From midstance to push-off the ankle plantar flexors increase their activity to create heel rise and contribute to knee flexion
	Ankle dysfunction	Push-off decreased, appears to walk "flat-footed

Inman VT, Ralston HJ, Todd F: *Human walking*, Baltimore, 1981, Waverly Press.
Kendall FP, McCreary EK, Provance PK: *Muscles: testing and function*, ed 4, Baltimore, 1993, Williams and Wilkins.

IMPAIRMENT	DSM
Hip flexor muscles of stance leg—short and stiff	Lumbar rotation
Hip flexor muscles of stance leg—short and stiff	Lumbar extension
Hip abductor muscles of stance leg—short	
Hip abductor muscle—weak	
Hip abductor—markedly weak	
Hip lateral rotator muscles—long and weak Hip abductor medial rotator muscles—dominant	
Hip lateral rotator muscles—short	
Lateral rotator muscle—inefficient performance	
Gastrocnemius and soleus muscles—short Quadriceps muscles—decreased performance	
Gastrocnemius and soleus muscles—decreased performance	

Movement Impairments: Lower Quarter Examination

POSITION	TEST	IMPAIRMENT STRUCTURAL VARIATION		DSM EXT	DSM ROT	DSM FLEX	NT	ACC
Standing	**Alignment** Thoracic	❑ Kyphosis ❑ Flat ❑ Asymmetry: prominent	R L	❑	❑	❑		
	Lumbar	❑ Lordotic ❑ Flat ❑ Asymmetric ❑ Pain ❑ Decreased pain when flatten spine		❑	❑	❑		
	Pelvis	❑ Anterior tilt ❑ Posterior tilt ❑ Lateral tilt ❑ Rotation to	R < > L R L	❑	❑	❑		
	Hip	❑ Flexed ❑ Extended ❑ Medially rotated ❑ Laterally rotated	R L R L	❑	❑	❑		
	Knees	❑ Bowed ❑ Varum ❑ Torsion	R L R L R L					
	Foot	❑ Pronated ❑ Supinated	R L R L					
Standing movement tests	Forward bending	❑ Pain ❑ Lumbar spine flexion > 25 degrees ❑ Lumbar spine extended ❑ Spine faster > hips ❑ Hip flexion < 70 degrees		❑	❑	❑		
	Corrected forward bending	❑ Pain increase ❑ Pain same ❑ Pain decrease		❑	❑	❑		
	Return forward bending	❑ Pain ❑ Mostly leads with back ❑ Hip sway		❑	❑	❑		
	Corrected return	❑ Pain increase ❑ Pain same ❑ Pain decrease		❑	❑	❑		
	Side bending	❑ Pain ❑ Limited to ❑ Asymmetry ❑ Sharp angle of bend ❑ Lateral glide to	R L R L R > < L R L R L		❑			

Abd, Abduction; *acc*, accessory; *DSM*, directional susceptibility to movement; *ext*, extension; *flex*, flexion; *lat*, lateral; *LE*, lower extremity; *NT*, nerve tension; *PICR*, path of the instantaneous center of rotation; *PGM*, posterior gluteus medius; *Rot*, rotation.

POSITION	TEST	IMPAIRMENT STRUCTURAL VARIATION		DSM EXT	DSM ROT	DSM FLEX	NT	ACC
Standing movement tests— cont'd	Corrected side bending	❑ Pain increase ❑ Pain same ❑ Pain decrease			☐			
	Rotation Thoracic	❑ Pain ❑ Asymmetric	R L R > < L					
	Lumbar	❑ Pain ❑ Asymmetric	R L R > < L		☐			
	Backward sway	❑ Pain		☐		☐		
	True lumbar extension	❑ Pain						
	Single-leg stance	❑ Lateral trunk flexion ❑ Hip adduction ❑ Pelvic rotation ❑ Hip rotation	R L R L R L R L		☐			
	Hip/knee flex partial squat	❑ Hip medial rotation ❑ Hip lateral rotation ❑ Ankle pronation ❑ Ankle supination	R L R L R L R L					
Supine (edge of table)	Double knee to chest	❑ Pain ❑ Lumbar flexion, sacrum off table				☐		
	Hip flexor length Pelvis	❑ Anterior tilt ❑ Lateral tilt ❑ Rotation	R L R L R L	☐	☐	☐		
	Muscle length short	❑ TFL ❑ Rectus femoris ❑ Iliopsoas	R L R L R L	☐	☐			
	Hip joint	❑ Iliopsoas—long ❑ Femoral head prominent (anterior glide)	R L R L					☐
	Knee joint	❑ Lateral tibial rotation	R L		☐			
On table	**Position** Hips/knees flexion	**(Compared to standing)** ❑ Pain increase ❑ Pain same ❑ Pain decrease	R L R L R L	☐		☐		

Movement Impairments: Lower Quarter Examination — cont'd

POSITION	TEST	IMPAIRMENT STRUCTURAL VARIATION			DSM EXT	DSM ROT	DSM FLEX	NT	ACC
On table—cont'd	Hips/knees extension	☐ Pain	R L	both only					
		☐ Pain onset < 50% of ext	R	L	☐		☐		
		☐ Pain onset > 75% of ext	R	L					
	Support under lumbar spine	☐ Pain increase			☐		☐		
		☐ Pain same							
		☐ Pain decrease							
	Unilateral hip/knee flexion Passive Active	☐ < 110 degrees hip flexion	R	L			☐		
		☐ Associated lumbar flexion	R	L			☐		
		☐ Pain in groin	R	L					☐
		☐ PICR deviation	R	L					☐
		☐ Pain with LE motion	R	L	☐				
		☐ Lumbopelvic rotation with	R	L		☐			
	Hip abd/lat rot from flexion	☐ Lumbopelvic rotation	R	L	☐	☐			☐
		☐ Limitation hip motion	R	L					
		☐ Pain in groin	R	L					
		☐ Lateral hip pain	R	L					
Supine	Lower abdominal muscle performance	☐ Pain with hip flexion	R	L	☐	☐			
		☐ Hold knee to chest	R	L					
		☐ Hip flex > 110 degrees	R	L					
		☐ 1/5	R	L					
		☐ 2/5							
		☐ 3/5, 4/5, 5/5							
	Upper abdominal muscle performance	☐ Trunk curl < 1/5							
		☐ Trunk curl–sit up, arms out		3/5					
		☐ Trunk curl–sit up, arms folded		4/5					
		☐ Trunk curl–sit up, hands on head 5/5							
	Hip flexion/knee extended	☐ < 80 degrees with back flat	R	L	☐	☐	☐		
		☐ Pain into thigh < 45 degrees	R	L				☐	
	Straight-leg raise	☐ No pain; totally passive	R	L	☐				
		☐ PICR deviation	R	L					☐
	From SLR: hip extension—resisted	☐ Pain	R	L					
	Iliopsoas performance	☐ Long	R	L					
		☐ Weak/strained, 3/5, 4/5	R	L					
	TFL performance	☐ Weak/strained, 2/5, 3/5, 4/5	R	L					
		2/5, 3/5, 4/5	R	L					

Abd, Abduction; *acc*, accessory; *DSM*, directional susceptibility to movement; *ext*, extension; *flex*, flexion; *lat*, lateral; *LE*, lower extremity; *NT*, nerve tension; *PICR*, path of the instantaneous center of rotation; *PGM*, posterior gluteus medius; *Rot*, rotation.

POSITION	TEST	IMPAIRMENT STRUCTURAL VARIATION			DSM EXT	DSM ROT	DSM FLEX	NT	ACC
Side-lying	**Position**	☐ Pain				☐			
	Support under side	☐ Pain increase	R	L		☐			
		☐ Pain same	R	L					
		☐ Pain decrease	R	L					
	Hip lateral rotation/ abduct	☐ Pain	R	L		☐			
		☐ Lumbopelvic rotation	R	L					
	Hip abduction (top LE)	☐ Pain	R	L		☐			
		☐ Lateral pelvic tilt	R	L		☐			
	Muscle performance (top LE)	☐ Long	R	L					
		☐ Weak/strained	R	L					
		3, 4, 5	R						
		3, 4, 5		L					
	Hip adduction (top LE)	☐ Lateral pelvic tilt	R	L		☐			
		☐ Medial rotation	R	L					☐
		☐ Excessive ROM	R	L					
		☐ Limited ROM (Ober test < 10 degrees)	R	L					
	Muscle performance (bottom LE)	Weak; 2, 3, 4, 5	R						
	Hip abduction/lat rotation/ extension (PGM)	Long	R	L					
		Weak/strained	R	L					
		Hip flexion/medial rotation	R	L					
		3, 4, 5	R						
		3, 4, 5		L					
Prone	**Position**	☐ Pain increase			☐		☐		
		☐ Pain same							
		☐ Pain decrease							
	Support under abdomen	☐ Pain increase			☐		☐		
		☐ Pain same							
		☐ Pain decrease							
	Knee flexion Passive	☐ Pain	R	L	☐	☐			
		☐ Anterior pelvic tilt	R	L					
		☐ Lumbopelvic rotation	R	L					
	Active	☐ Pain	R	L	☐	☐			
		☐ Anterior pelvic tilt	R	L					
		☐ Lumbopelvic rotation	R	L					
	Stabilize pelvis	☐ Pain increase	R	L	☐	☐			
		☐ Pain same	R	L					
		☐ Pain decrease	R	L					

Movement Impairments: Lower Quarter Examination—cont'd

POSITION	TEST	IMPAIRMENT STRUCTURAL VARIATION			DSM EXT	DSM ROT	DSM FLEX	NT	ACC
Prone— cont'd	Passive flexion femur	❏ Lateral rotation	R	L					❏
	Muscle performance	❏ Weak, 3/5, 4/5	R						
		3/5, 4/5		L					
	Resisted knee flexion	❏ Strained	R	L					
	Hip medial rotation	Pain	R	L		❏			
		Lumbopelvic rotation	R	L					
		Pain increase	R	L		❏			
	Stabilize pelvis	Pain same	R	L					
		Pain decrease	R	L					
		Range of motion	R	L					
		Antetorsion	R	L					
		Retrotorsion	R	L					
	Hip lateral rotation	Pain	R	L		❏			
		Lumbopelvic rotation	R	L		❏			
		Pain increase	R	L		❏			
		Pain same	R	L					
		Pain decrease	R	L					
		Range of motion	R	L					
		Antetorsion	R	L					
		Retrotorsion	R	L					
	Hip extension with knee extended	❏ Pain	R	L	❏	❏			
		❏ > Lumbar extension	R	L	❏				
		❏ Lumbopelvic rotation	R	L		❏			
		❏ Onset gluteus maximus after hip extension	R	L					❏
		❏ PICR anterior deviation	R	L					❏
	Hip extension with knee flexed	❏ Pain	R	L	❏				
		❏ > Lumbar extension	R	L	❏				
		❏ < 5 degrees hip extension	R	L					
		❏ PICR anterior deviation	R	L					❏
		❏ Weak/long							
	Gluteus maximus performance	3, 3+, 4−, 4, 4+/5	R						
		3, 3+, 4−, 4, 4+/5		L					
Quadruped	**Alignment** Thoracic spine	❏ Kyphosis							
		❏ Scoliosis							

Abd, Abduction; *acc*, accessory; *DSM*, directional susceptibility to movement; *ext*, extension; *flex*, flexion; *lat*, lateral; *LE*, lower extremity; *NT*, nerve tension; *PICR*, path of the instantaneous center of rotation; *PGM*, posterior gluteus medius; *Rot*, rotation.

POSITION	TEST	IMPAIRMENT STRUCTURAL VARIATION		DSM EXT	DSM ROT	DSM FLEX	NT	ACC
Quadruped —cont'd	Lumbar spine	❑ Flexed		☐	☐			
		❑ Flat						
		❑ Lordotic						
		❑ Asymmetric, prominent	R　L					
	Pelvis	❑ Asymmetric, prominent	R　L	☐	☐			
		❑ Pain		☐	☐			
	Correct alignment	❑ Pain increase		☐	☐			
		❑ Pain same						
		❑ Pain decrease						
	Rocking backward	❑ Pain						
	Lumbar spine	❑ Flexes		☐	☐	☐		
		❑ Rotates						
		❑ Extends						
	Pelvis	❑ Rotates	R　L		☐			
		❑ Lateral tilt	R　L					
	Corrected lumbar alignment	❑ Pain increase		☐	☐	☐		
		❑ Pain same						
		❑ Pain decrease						
	Push with arms	❑ Pain increase		☐	☐			
		❑ Pain same						
		❑ Pain decrease						
	Hip laterally rotated/ abducted	❑ < Pelvic rotation/tilt			☐			
		❑ < Lumbar rotation						
	Rocking forward	❑ Pain		☐				
	Shoulder flexion	❑ Pain			☐			
		❑ Lumbar rotation with shoulder motion	R　L					
Sitting	**Alignment** Flexion Flat Extended	❑ Pain ❑ Pain ❑ Pain		☐	☐	☐		
	Knee extension	❑ Pain	R　L	☐	☐	☐		
		❑ Lumbar flexion	R　L					
		❑ Lumbar rotation/flexion	R　L					
		❑ < 80 deg of knee extension	R　L					
		❑ Hip medial rotation	R　L					
	Dorsiflexion	❑ < 10 deg of dorsiflexion	R　L					

Movement Impairments: Lower Quarter Examination—cont'd

POSITION	TEST	IMPAIRMENT STRUCTURAL VARIATION			DSM EXT	DSM ROT	DSM FLEX	NT	ACC
Sitting— cont'd	Hip flexion— iliopsoas performance	❏ Long	R	L					
		❏ Weak/strained	R	L					
		3, 4, 5	R							
		3, 4, 5		L						
	Hip medial rotation	Range of motion	R	L					
		❏ Antetorsion	R	L					
		❏ Retrotorsion	R	L					
	Muscle performance	❏ Weak/long							
		3, 3+, 4−, 4, 4+/5	R							
		3, 3+, 4−, 4, 4+/5		L						
	Hip lateral rotation	Range of motion	R	L					
		❏ Antetorsion	R	L					
		❏ Retrotorsion	R	L					
		❏ Weak/long							
		3, 3+, 4−, 4, 4+/5	R							
		3, 3+, 4−, 4, 4+/5		L						
Standing: back to wall	Flatten back	❏ Pain increase			☐		☐		
		❏ Pain same							

Abd, Abduction; *acc*, accessory; *DSM*, directional susceptibility to movement; *ext*, extension; *flex*, flexion; *lat*, lateral; *LE*, lower extremity; *NT*, nerve tension; *PICR*, path of the instantaneous center of rotation; *PGM*, posterior gluteus medius; *Rot*, rotation.

❑ Pain decrease

POSITION	TEST	IMPAIRMENT STRUCTURAL VARIATION	DSM EXT	DSM ROT	DSM FLEX	NT	ACC
	Shoulder flexion	❑ Pain increase ❑ Pain same ❑ Pain decrease	☐				
Gait	Lumbar extension	❑ Increased during stance of R L ❑ Pain increase	☐				
	Pelvic rotation	❑ Increased during stance of R L ❑ Pain increase		☐			
	Lateral trunk flexion	❑ Increased during stance of R L ❑ Pain increase		☐			
	Hip adduction (pelvic drop)	❑ Increased during stance of R L ❑ Pain increase		☐			
	Hip medial rotation during stance	❑ Increased during stance of R L					
	Knee angle at midstance	❑ Hyperextension R L					
	Heel rise	❑ Flexion ❑ Decreased R L					

Au: We cannot have a blank right-hand page, thus the reason we need to balance the table on the last two pages of this table.

Movement Impairments: Upper Quarter Examination

Test items, test criteria, and associated impairments

TEST	SEGMENT	FAULT
Standing tests		
Alignment	**Head and neck**	**Normal**
		Dysfunction
		Extended
		Forward
		Flat
	Thoracic spine	**Normal**
		Kyphotic
		Flat
		Swayed back
		Scoliotic
	Infrasternal angle	**Normal**
		Narrow
		Wide
	Lumbar spine	**Normal**
		Lordotic **Confirming test:** **flatten lumbar** **spine decreases pain**

ASIS, Anterior superior iliac spine; *DSM*, directional susceptibility to movement; *ITB*, iliotibial band; *MMT*, manual muscle test; *PIP*, proximal interphalangeal; *PICR*, path of the instantaneous center of rotation; *PSIS*, posterior superior iliac spine; *SLR*, straight-leg raise; *TFL*, tensor fascia lata; *TFL-ITB*, tensor fascia lata–iliotibial band.

CRITERIA	IMPAIRMENT	DSM
Head erect in neutral position with inward cervical curve		
Pain in neck, between neck and acromion Confirming test: passive elevation of shoulder girdle to decrease pain		
Head forward with increased cervical curve (lordotic)	Intrinsic neck flexor muscles—long Extensor muscles—short	
Head forward with straight cervical spine	Degenerative disk disease	
Decrease in cervical curve	Neck extensor muscles—long	
Outward curve		
Outward curve—increased	Rectus abdominis muscle—short Thoracic paraspinal muscles—long	
Outward curve—absent	Thoracic paraspinal muscles—short	
Shoulders more than 2" posterior to greater trochanter muscles	External oblique muscles—long Rectus abdominis muscle—short Internal oblique muscles—short	
Rotation with rib hump	Asymmetric abdominal and back musculature performance	
90 degrees		
75 degrees	External oblique muscle—short	
More than 100 degrees	External oblique muscles—short and/or long	
Inward curve—20 to 30 degrees		
Inward curve more than 30 degrees	External oblique muscles—long Iliopsoas muscles—short Lumbar paraspinal muscles—short Pain	Extension

Movement Impairments: Upper Quarter Examination — cont'd

TEST	SEGMENT	FAULT
Standing tests — cont'd		
Alignment—cont'd		Flat
	Scapula	Normal
		Downwardly rotated
		Depressed
		Abducted
		Adducted
		Winging/tilt
		Elevated
	Humerus	Normal
		Anterior

ASIS, Anterior superior iliac spine; *DSM*, directional susceptibility to movement; *ITB*, iliotibial band; *MMT*, manual muscle test; *PIP*, proximal interphalangeal; *PICR*, path of the instantaneous center of rotation; *PSIS*, posterior superior iliac spine; *SLR*, straight-leg raise; *TFL*, tensor fascia lata; *TFL-ITB*, tensor fascia lata–iliotibial band.

CRITERIA	IMPAIRMENT	DSM
Inward curve—absent (may be normal for men)	Paraspinal muscles—long Iliopsoas muscle—long	
Horizontal, situated between T2-6, flat on thorax, vertebral border parallel to and approximately 3" from spine Rotated 30 degrees in frontal plane		
Superior angle farther from spine than inferior angle	Upper trapezius—long Levator scapula and rhomboid muscles—short and stiff Serratus anterior lower fibers—long Deltoid and supraspinatus muscles—short	
Lower than T2, acromioclavicular joint lower than sternoclavicular joint	Upper trapezius muscles—long	
Vertebral border is more than 3" from spine Rotated in frontal plane is more than 30 degrees	Serratus anterior muscles—short Rhomboid and trapezius muscles—long Scapulohumeral muscles—short and stiff	
Vertebral border less than 3" from spine	Serratus anterior muscles—long Rhomboid and trapezius muscles—short	
Vertebral border or inferior angle protrudes from thorax	Flat thorax Serratus anterior muscles—weak Pectoralis minor muscles—short Scapulohumeral muscles—short and stiff Rib hump	
Higher than T2 and acromion high	Upper trapezius muscles—short Levator scapula and rhomboid muscles—short	
Superior aspect extends slightly lateral of acromion, less than one third of head is forward of the acromion, neutral rotation, parallel to thorax, proximal and distal ends in same vertical plan		
More than one third of head forward of acromion	Anterior joint capsule—stretched Subscapularis muscle—long	

Movement Impairments: Upper Quarter Examination—cont'd

TEST	SEGMENT	FAULT
Standing tests—cont'd		
Alignment—cont'd	**Humerus—cont'd**	**Superior**
		Medially rotated
		Laterally rotated
		Abducted
Shoulder flexion—elevation		**Normal**
	Shoulder	**Dysfunction**
	Scapular	**Dysfunction**

ASIS, Anterior superior iliac spine; *DSM*, directional susceptibility to movement; *ITB*, iliotibial band; *MMT*, manual muscle test; *PIP*, proximal interphalangeal; *PICR*, path of the instantaneous center of rotation; *PSIS*, posterior superior iliac spine; *SLR*, straight-leg raise; *TFL*, tensor fascia lata; *TFL-ITB*, tensor fascia lata–iliotibial band.

CRITERIA	IMPAIRMENT	DSM
Up against acromion	Deltoid muscles—short Rotator cuff—inefficient	Superior glide
Cubital fossa faces medially Olecranon faces laterally: if scapula abducted may not be medially rotated	Lateral rotator muscles—ineffective control Medial rotator muscles—short and stiff	Medial rotation
Not common, except when scapula is adducted and humerus appears neutral	Lateral rotator muscles—short	
Distal aspect of humerus away from side of body, humerus does not extend beyond acromion	Deltoid muscles—short Supraspinatus muscles—short Scapula downwardly rotated	Superior glide
180 degrees without abduction of scapula more than $\frac{1}{2}$" beyond posterolateral border of thorax, inferior angle of scapula reaches midaxillary line by abducting and upwardly rotating to 60 degrees, without excessive elevation or depression of shoulder girdle, or movement of spine		
Less than 180 degrees of motion	Latissimus dorsi muscles—short Pectoralis minor muscles—short Pectoralis major muscles—short Pain, extension of trunk Shoulder flexor muscles—weak	Anterior glide
Inferior angle does not reach midaxillary line Insufficient abduction/upward rotation	Serratus anterior muscles—long and weak Rhomboid muscles—short and stiff	
Upward rotate less than 60 degrees	Serratus anterior muscles—long and weak Trapezius muscles—long and weak Rhomboid muscles—short and stiff	
Does not depress at end of range	Lower trapezius muscles—long and weak Pectoralis minor muscles—short	
Elevation—excessive	Upper trapezius muscle—dominant	Humerus—excessive superior glide

Movement Impairments: Upper Quarter Examination — cont'd

TEST	SEGMENT	FAULT
Standing tests — cont'd		
Shoulder flexion—elevation—cont'd	Scapula	Dysfunction
	Humerus	
		Dysfunction
Shoulder extension (return from elevation)		Normal
	Scapula	Dysfunction

ASIS, Anterior superior iliac spine; *DSM,* directional susceptibility to movement; *ITB,* iliotibial band; *MMT,* manual muscle test; *PIP,* proximal interphalangeal; *PICR,* path of the instantaneous center of rotation; *PSIS,* posterior superior iliac spine; *SLR,* straight-leg raise; *TFL,* tensor fascia lata; *TFL-ITB,* tensor fascia lata–iliotibial band.

CRITERIA	IMPAIRMENT	DSM
Abduction—excessive	Serratus anterior muscles—short and dominant Trapezius muscles—long and weak Rhomboid muscles—long	
Winging of scapula	Serratus anterior—long and weak Scapulohumeral muscles—short and weak	
Anterior glide more than one third of head—excessive	Subscapularis muscle—long and weak Anterior joint capsule—stretched Pectoralis major muscle—dominant	
Superior glide—excessive	Deltoid muscle—dominant Rotator cuff—decreased performance	
Medial rotation—excessive (scapula not abducted)	Lateral rotator muscles—insufficient performance Medial rotator muscles—short and stiff	
Scapula downwardly rotates and adducts while remaining close to thorax Humerus moves in a 2:1 relationship to scapula Humerus remains centered in the glenoid as extends		
Winging of scapula	Scapulohumeral muscles not elongating as rapidly as the thoracoscapular muscles Often associated with shortness of scapulohumeral muscles Pectoralis minor muscle—dominant	
Scapular depression—excessive	Upper trapezius muscle—decreased performance Lower trapezius muscle—dominant	
Downward rotation—excessive	Serratus anterior and lower trapezius muscles—decreased performance Scapulohumeral muscles—short and stiff	
Adduction—excessive	Serratus anterior muscle—decreased performance	

Movement Impairments: Upper Quarter Examination — cont'd

TEST	SEGMENT	FAULT
Standing tests — cont'd		
Shoulder extension—cont'd	Humerus	Dysfunction
Shoulder abduction—elevation		Normal
	Scapula	Dysfunction
	Humerus	Dysfunction

ASIS, Anterior superior iliac spine; *DSM,* directional susceptibility to movement; *ITB,* iliotibial band; *MMT,* manual muscle test; *PIP,* proximal interphalangeal; *PICR,* path of the instantaneous center of rotation; *PSIS,* posterior superior iliac spine; *SLR,* straight-leg raise; *TFL,* tensor fascia lata; *TFL-ITB,* tensor fascia lata–iliotibial band.

CRITERIA	IMPAIRMENT	DSM
Anterior displacement of humeral head (often associated with insufficient scapular adduction)	Subscapularis muscles—long and weak Anterior joint capsule—stretched Posterior deltoid muscle—dominant	Anterior glide
After first 30 degrees of abduction, the scapula upwardly rotates and abducts, moving in a 1:2 ratio with the humerus, which is laterally rotating while remaining centered in the glenoid On completion of 180 degrees of motion, the inferior angle of the scapula reaches the midaxillary line of the thorax Scapula is upwardly rotated 60 degrees		
Inferior angle does not reach midaxillary line, insufficient abduction/upward rotation—insufficient	Serratus anterior—long and weak Rhomboid muscles—short and stiff	
Upward rotate less than 60 degrees	Serratus anterior muscles—long and weak Trapezius muscles—long and weak Rhomboid muscles—short and stiff	
Does not depress at end of range	Lower trapezius muscles—long and weak Pectoralis minor muscle—short	
Elevation excessive	Upper trapezius muscle—dominant Humerus—excessive superior glide	
Abduction excessive	Serratus anterior muscle—short and dominant Trapezius muscle—long and weak Rhomboid muscles—long	
Winging of scapula	Serratus anterior muscle—long and weak Scapulohumeral muscles—short and weak	Superior glide
Superior glide excessive (most likely to occur during abduction)	Deltoid muscle—dominant Rotator cuff—decreased performance	

Movement Impairments: Upper Quarter Examination — cont'd

TEST	SEGMENT	FAULT
Standing tests — cont'd		
Shoulder abduction—elevation—cont'd	Humerus	Dysfunction
Shoulder adduction—return from shoulder abduction		Normal
	Scapula	Dysfunction
		Humeral dysfunction
Supine tests		
Pectoralis minor length		Normal

ASIS, Anterior superior iliac spine; *DSM*, directional susceptibility to movement; *ITB*, iliotibial band; *MMT*, manual muscle test; *PIP*, proximal interphalangeal; *PICR*, path of the instantaneous center of rotation; *PSIS*, posterior superior iliac spine; *SLR*, straight-leg raise; *TFL*, tensor fascia lata; *TFL-ITB*, tensor fascia lata–iliotibial band.

CRITERIA	IMPAIRMENT	DSM
Excessive anterior glide more than one third of head (most often when scapula is abducted) Humerus is not in plane of scapula but in plane of lateral trunk	Subscapularis muscle—long and weak Anterior joint capsule—stretched Pectoralis major—dominant	Anterior glide
Lateral rotation—decreased	Lateral rotator muscles—insufficient performance Medial rotator muscles—short and stiff	Medial rotation
Scapula downwardly rotates and adducts while remaining close to thorax Humerus moves in a 2:1 relationship to scapula and remains centered in the glenoid as the humerus extends to the neutral position		
Winging of scapula	Scapulohumeral muscles not elongating as rapidly as the thoracoscapular muscles Often associated with shortness of scapulohumeral muscles Pectoralis minor—dominant	
Scapular depression—excessive	Upper trapezius—decreased performance Lower trapezius muscle—dominant	
Downward rotation—excessive	Serratus anterior and lower trapezius muscles—decreased performance Scapulohumeral muscles—short and stiff	
Adduction—excessive	Serratus anterior muscle—decreased performance	
Superior glide of humeral head	Deltoid muscle—dominant Rotator cuff—decreased performance	Humeral superior glide
Posterior border of acromion no greater than 1 inch from table with arms at side and elbows flexed		

Movement Impairments: Upper Quarter Examination — cont'd

TEST	SEGMENT	FAULT
Supine tests — cont'd		
Pectoralis minor length—cont'd		
		Muscle dysfunction
Shoulder flexion—maximum (latissimus dorsi length)		Normal
		Shoulder dysfunction
		Muscle dysfunction

ASIS, Anterior superior iliac spine; *DSM*, directional susceptibility to movement; *ITB*, iliotibial band; *MMT*, manual muscle test; *PIP*, proximal interphalangeal; *PICR*, path of the instantaneous center of rotation; *PSIS*, posterior superior iliac spine; *SLR*, straight-leg raise; *TFL*, tensor fascia lata; *TFL-ITB*, tensor fascia lata–iliotibial band.

CRITERIA	IMPAIRMENT	DSM
Stretch applied in superior-lateral direction can place the posterior border of acromion against the table without rotation or elevation of rib cage, when the thoracic spine has a normal curve		
Posterior border of the acromion is more than 1 inch from table and cannot be passively stretched to the table when elbow is flexed or shoulder is slightly flexed (absence of kyphosis or scoliosis)	Pectoralis minor muscle—short	
Posterior border of the acromion is more than 1 inch from table and cannot be passively stretched to the table when arm is at patient's side and the elbow is extended	Short head of biceps brachii muscles—short	
Shoulders flex to 180 degrees (arms in contact with table) with lumbar spine flat and scapula does not protrude more than $1/2$ inch beyond posterolateral border of thorax		
Humeral anterior or superior glide, medial rotation, insufficient scapular upward rotation	Pain	
Shoulder flexion less than 180 with back flat	Latissimus dorsi muscle—short	
Lumbar spine extends during shoulder flexion	Latissimus dorsi muscle—short and stiff Abdominal muscles—less stiff Lumbar spine flexible into extension	
Inferior angle of scapula extends more than $1/2$ inch beyond posterolateral border of thorax	Teres major muscle—short Confirming test: medially rotate humerus—increased range of motion into flexion No change in flexion range of motion All scapulohumeral muscles—short	

Movement Impairments: Upper Quarter Examination — cont'd

TEST	SEGMENT	FAULT
Supine tests — cont'd		
Shoulder positioned in 135 degrees of abduction (pectoralis major length—sternal)		Normal
		Shoulder dysfunction
		Muscle dysfunction
		Glenohumeral dysfunction
Shoulder positioned in 90 degrees of abduction (pectoralis major length—clavicular)		Normal
		Shoulder dysfunction
		Muscle dysfunction
		Glenohumeral dysfunction
Lateral rotation of shoulder (medial rotator muscle length) Shoulder positioned in 90 degrees of abduction Elbow flexed to 90 degrees		Normal
		Shoulder dysfunction
		Muscle dysfunction
Medial rotation of shoulder (lateral rotator muscle length) Shoulder positioned in 90 degrees of abduction Elbow flexed to 90 degrees		Normal
		Shoulder dysfunction
		Shoulder dysfunction
		Muscle dysfunction

ASIS, Anterior superior iliac spine; *DSM,* directional susceptibility to movement; *ITB,* iliotibial band; *MMT,* manual muscle test; *PIP,* proximal interphalangeal; *PICR,* path of the instantaneous center of rotation; *PSIS,* posterior superior iliac spine; *SLR,* straight-leg raise; *TFL,* tensor fascia lata; *TFL-ITB,* tensor fascia lata–iliotibial band.

CRITERIA	IMPAIRMENT	DSM
Arm rests on table without anterior displacement of humeral head		
Humeral anterior or superior glide	Pain in glenohumeral joint	Anterior to superior glide
Arm does not contact table	Pectoralis major, sternal portion—short	
Head of humerus is displaced anteriorly	Laxity of anterior joint capsule	Anterior glide
Arm contacts table without anterior displacement of the humeral head		
Humeral anterior or superior glide	Pain glenohumeral joint	
Arm does not contact table	Pectoralis major, clavicular portion—short	
Anterior displacement of humeral head	Laxity of anterior joint capsule	Anterior glide
90 degrees of humeral abduction and lateral rotation with minimal movement of scapula		
Anterior or superior glide of humeral head	Pain Lateral rotator muscles—stiff Laxity of anterior joint capsule	Anterior or superior glide
Less than 90 degrees of lateral rotation	Teres major, subscapularis, pectoralis major (clavicular portion) muscles—short	
90 degrees of abduction, shoulder should rotate 70 degrees medially (fingers touch table with wrist flexed), without scapular tilt or humeral anterior glide		
Scapular anterior tilt	Lateral rotators stiffer than lower trapezius	Anterior glide
Humeral anterior glide	Laxity of anterior joint capsule	
Less than 70 degrees of medial rotation	Infraspinatus, teres minor muscles— short and stiff with 6 to 8 repetitions; range improves—stiff very frequent finding	

Movement Impairments: Upper Quarter Examination — cont'd

TEST	SEGMENT	FAULT
Prone tests		
Shoulder medial rotation		**Normal**
		Shoulder dysfunction
		Muscle dysfunction

ASIS, Anterior superior iliac spine; *DSM*, directional susceptibility to movement; *ITB*, iliotibial band; *MMT*, manual muscle test; *PIP*, proximal interphalangeal; *PICR*, path of the instantaneous center of rotation; *PSIS*, posterior superior iliac spine; *SLR*, straight-leg raise; *TFL*, tensor fascia lata; *TFL-ITB*, tensor fascia lata–iliotibial band.

CRITERIA	IMPAIRMENT	DSM
90 degrees of abduction, with humerus in scapular plane, the patient is able to medially rotate the humerus 70 degrees without scapular movement or anterior glide of humeral head Able to maintain medially rotated position with application of maximum resistance		
Humeral anterior glide	Pain Teres minor, infraspinatus, posterior deltoid muscles—stiff and short Laxity of anterior joint capsule	Anterior glide
Scapular anterior tilt	Lower trapezius muscle—long and weak	
Scapular elevation	Upper trapezius muscle—dominant	
Less than 70 degrees of medial rotation	Teres minor, infraspinatus, posterior deltoid muscles—short	
Unable to maintain medial rotation with application of maximum resistance	Subscapularis muscle—weak and long	

Movement Impairments: Upper Quarter Examination — cont'd

TEST	SEGMENT	FAULT
Prone tests — cont'd		
Shoulder lateral rotation		**Normal**
		Shoulder dysfunction

ASIS, Anterior superior iliac spine; *DSM*, directional susceptibility to movement; *ITB*, iliotibial band; *MMT*, manual muscle test; *PIP*, proximal interphalangeal; *PICR*, path of the instantaneous center of rotation; *PSIS*, posterior superior iliac spine; *SLR*, straight-leg raise; *TFL*, tensor fascia lata; *TFL-ITB*, tensor fascia lata–iliotibial band.

CRITERIA	IMPAIRMENT	DSM
90 degrees of abduction with humerus in scapular plane Scapula not abducted Able to rotate humerus laterally 90 degrees without scapular depression Able to maintain laterally rotated position with application of maximum resistance		
Anterior or superior glide of humeral head	Pain Anterior joint capsule—lax Posterior deltoid muscle—dominant (note extension of arm)	Anterior or superior glide
Abduction of scapula (only able to be detected if scapula correctly positioned and not resting in abduction for test)	Trapezius and rhomboid muscles—long and weak	

Movement Impairments: Upper Quarter Examination — cont'd

TEST	SEGMENT	FAULT
Prone tests — cont'd		
Shoulder lateral rotation—cont'd		
		Muscle dysfunction
Lower trapezius performance		Normal
		Muscle dysfunction
Middle trapezius performance		Normal

ASIS, Anterior superior iliac spine; *DSM*, directional susceptibility to movement; *ITB*, iliotibial band; *MMT*, manual muscle test; *PIP*, proximal interphalangeal; *PICR*, path of the instantaneous center of rotation; *PSIS*, posterior superior iliac spine; *SLR*, straight-leg raise; *TFL*, tensor fascia lata; *TFL-ITB*, tensor fascia lata–iliotibial band.

CRITERIA	IMPAIRMENT	DSM
Scapular depression	Lower trapezius or latissimus dorsi muscles—dominant Timing problem with glenohumeral lateral rotators	
Less than 90 degrees of lateral rotation	Teres major, subscapularis muscles—short	
Unable to tolerate maximum resistance when laterally rotated	Infraspinatus, teres minor, posterior deltoid muscle—weak	
Able to maintain scapular upward rotation/adduction/depression and lateral rotation of humerus (thumb upward) with shoulder abducted to 135 degrees with application of maximum resistance		
Difficulty passively placing the arm in test position	Pectoralis minor muscles—short	
Unable to maintain test position with maximum resistance, but can after 10 to 15 degrees of position change	Lower trapezius muscle—long	
Unable to tolerate maximum resistance at any point in range of motion	Lower trapezius muscle—weak	
Shoulder girdle elevates with application of maximum resistance	Upper trapezius muscle—dominant	
Scapula downwardly rotates or humerus medially rotates	Rhomboid muscles—dominant	
Able to maintain scapular upward rotation/adduction/depression and lateral rotation of humerus (thumb upward) with shoulder abducted to 90 degrees with application of maximum resistance		

Movement Impairments: Upper Quarter Examination — cont'd

TEST	SEGMENT	FAULT
Prone tests — cont'd		
Middle trapezius performance—cont'd		**Muscle dysfunction**
Rhomboid muscles		
Quadruped tests		
Alignment (see Figure 6-16)	**Head and neck**	**Normal**
		Dysfunction
	Thoracic	**Normal**
		Dysfunction
	Scapula	**Normal**
		Winging

ASIS, Anterior superior iliac spine; *DSM,* directional susceptibility to movement; *ITB,* iliotibial band; *MMT,* manual muscle test; *PIP,* proximal interphalangeal; *PICR,* path of the instantaneous center of rotation; *PSIS,* posterior superior iliac spine; *SLR,* straight-leg raise; *TFL,* tensor fascia lata; *TFL-ITB,* tensor fascia lata–iliotibial band.

CRITERIA	IMPAIRMENT	DSM
Unable to maintain test position with maximum resistance, but can after 10 to 15 degrees of position change	Middle trapezius muscle—long	
Unable to tolerate maximum resistance at any point in range of motion	Middle trapezius muscle—weak	
Shoulder girdle elevates with application of maximum resistance	Upper trapezius muscle—dominant	
Scapula downwardly rotates or humerus medially rotates	Rhomboid muscles—dominant	
If scapulae are markedly abducted approximately 4", the manual muscle test of rhomboid muscle is indicated		
Head neutral, cervical spine slightly inward curve Levator scapulae—not prominent		
Cervical extension, prominence of levator scapula	Neck extensor muscles—short Levator scapulae muscles—short	
Slight outward curve		
Increased outward curve	Thoracic paraspinal muscles—long Rectus abdominis muscle—short	Rotation
Asymmetric; scoliosis	Abdominal muscle imbalance	Rotation
Flat on thorax Positioned between T2-7, approximately 3 inches from spine		
	Serratus anterior muscle—weak and long	

Movement Impairments: Upper Quarter Examination — cont'd

TEST	SEGMENT	FAULT
Quadruped tests — cont'd		
Alignment—cont'd		
	Glenohumeral	Normal
		Dysfunction
	Lumbar spine	Normal
	Hip joint	Normal
	Ankle	Normal
Rocking backward toward heels		Normal
	Cervical	Dysfunction

ASIS, Anterior superior iliac spine; *DSM*, directional susceptibility to movement; *ITB*, iliotibial band; *MMT*, manual muscle test; *PIP*, proximal interphalangeal; *PICR*, path of the instantaneous center of rotation; *PSIS*, posterior superior iliac spine; *SLR*, straight-leg raise; *TFL*, tensor fascia lata; *TFL-ITB*, tensor fascia lata–iliotibial band.

CRITERIA	IMPAIRMENT	DSM
Abducted more than 3¼" from spine	Serratus anterior muscle—short Rhomboid and trapezius muscles—may be short	
Adducted less than 2½" from spine	Serratus anterior muscle—long Rhomboid muscles—may be short	
Shoulders flexed to 90 degrees with no rotation or abduction Elbows extended		
Glenohumeral joint medially rotated	Medial rotator muscles—short	Medial rotation
Glenohumeral abduction	Deltoid muscle—short and stiff	
Flat or level; no pain		
90 degree-angle between femur and pelvis Neutral rotation, abduction/adduction		
Plantarflexed with dorsum of foot almost on supporting surface		
Head and neck remain level Scapulae maintain a relatively constant position on thorax as they upwardly rotate and slightly abduct and the shoulder flexes Thoracic and lumbar spine maintain a constant alignment as the hips flex		
Levator scapulae muscle definition—notably prominent	Levator scapulae muscles—dominant as neck extensors	Cervical extension
Extension of cervical spine and head	Levator scapulae muscles—short and dominant	Cervical extension

Movement Impairments: Upper Quarter Examination—cont'd

TEST	SEGMENT	FAULT
Quadruped tests — cont'd		
Rocking backward toward heels—cont'd		
	Scapula	Dysfunction
	Glenohumerus	Dysfunction
	Thoracic spine	Dysfunction
Rocking forward		Normal
		Dysfunction
Shoulder flexion (see Figure 6-11)		Normal
	Thoracic spine	Dysfunction

ASIS, Anterior superior iliac spine; *DSM,* directional susceptibility to movement; *ITB,* iliotibial band; *MMT,* manual muscle test; *PIP,* proximal interphalangeal; *PICR,* path of the instantaneous center of rotation; *PSIS,* posterior superior iliac spine; *SLR,* straight-leg raise; *TFL,* tensor fascia lata; *TFL-ITB,* tensor fascia lata–iliotibial band.

CRITERIA	IMPAIRMENT	DSM
Rotation of cervical spine and head	Ipsilateral levator scapulae muscles—short Contralateral upper trapezius muscle—dominant	Cervical rotation
Elevation of shoulder girdle (shrugging motion)	Levator scapulae, rhomboid, upper trapezius muscles—short and stiff Lower trapezius muscle—long and weak	
Excessive scapular abduction	Serratus anterior muscle—short and dominant Trapezius muscle—long and weak	
Insufficient scapular upward rotation	Rhomboid muscles—short and stiff	
Depression of shoulder girdle	Latissimus dorsi muscles—short and stiff	
Humeral medial rotation	Latissimus dorsi, medial rotator muscles—short	Medial rotation
Flexion/depression of thorax	Rectus abdominis muscle—short	Flexion/rotation
Unilateral rotation of thorax, rib cage Prominence increases unilaterally	Oblique abdominal muscle—imbalanced	
Scapula stay flat on thorax as weight on upper extremity increases		
Scapula wing	Serratus anterior muscle—long and weak	
Thoracic and lumbar spines remain motionless		
Rotation of thoracic spine more than ½" with shoulder flexion	Abdominal muscle—poor control	Rotation

Movement Impairments: Upper Quarter Examination—cont'd

TEST	SEGMENT	FAULT

Standing: facing wall tests

Shoulder abduction to 135 degrees

	SEGMENT	FAULT
		Normal
	Starting position with ulnar side of hand against wall	
	Slide arms up wall	
	Lift arms off wall by adducting scapula	
	Slide arms up to 145 degrees of abduction; then lift arms off wall by adducting scapula	
		Dysfunction

ASIS, Anterior superior iliac spine; *DSM,* directional susceptibility to movement; *ITB,* iliotibial band; *MMT,* manual muscle test; *PIP,* proximal interphalangeal; *PICR,* path of the instantaneous center of rotation; *PSIS,* posterior superior iliac spine; *SLR,* straight-leg raise; *TFL,* tensor fascia lata; *TFL-ITB,* tensor fascia lata–iliotibial band.

CRITERIA	IMPAIRMENT	DSM
Starting with shoulders laterally rotated, elbows flexed, ulnar side of hand against wall Slide arms up wall to 135 degrees of abduction Scapula abducts and upwardly rotates Adduct scapula to lift arms off wall		
Unable to abduct to 135 degrees with adequate scapular upward rotation	Trapezius, serratus anterior muscles—long and weak	

Movement Impairments: Upper Quarter Examination — cont'd

TEST	SEGMENT	FAULT
Standing: facing wall tests — cont'd		
Shoulder abduction to 135 degrees—cont'd		
Shoulder flexion to 170 degrees		Normal
		Dysfunction
Shoulder flexion to 170 degrees while shrugging shoulders		Normal

ASIS, Anterior superior iliac spine; *DSM,* directional susceptibility to movement; *ITB,* iliotibial band; *MMT,* manual muscle test; *PIP,* proximal interphalangeal; *PICR,* path of the instantaneous center of rotation; *PSIS,* posterior superior iliac spine; *SLR,* straight-leg raise; *TFL,* tensor fascia lata; *TFL-ITB,* tensor fascia lata–iliotibial band.

CRITERIA	IMPAIRMENT	DSM
Unable to adduct scapula on completion of shoulder abduction	Trapezius muscle—long and weak	
Starting with arms at side, elbows flexed, ulnar side of hand against the wall, flex shoulders while extending elbow Shoulder flexes to 170 degrees with upward rotation and abduction of scapula		
Less than 170 degrees of shoulder flexion	Pectoralis minor, latissimus dorsi muscles—short	
Shoulders remain depressed	Pectoralis minor, latissimus dorsi muscles—short Upper trapezius muscle—long and weak	
Unable to adduct scapula on completion of flexion	Trapezius muscle—long and weak Pectoralis minor muscle—short	
Starting with arms at side, elbows flexed, ulnar side of hand against the wall, flex and shrug shoulders while extending elbow Shoulder flexes to 170 degrees with upward rotation and abduction of scapula with top of shoulder close to ears		

Movement Impairments: Upper Quarter Examination—cont'd

TEST	SEGMENT	FAULT
Standing: facing wall tests—cont'd		
Shoulder flexion to 170 degrees while shrugging shoulders—cont'd		Dysfunction
Standing: back to wall tests		
Flatten back with arms at sides		Normal
		Muscle dysfunction
Flatten back with shoulders flexed to 180 degrees		Normal
		Muscle dysfunction

Inman VT, Ralston HJ, Todd F: *Human walking*, Baltimore, 1981, Waverly Press.
Kendall FP, McCreary EK, Provance PK: *Muscles: testing and function*, ed 4, Baltimore, 1993, Williams and Wilkins.

ASIS, Anterior superior iliac spine; *DSM*, directional susceptibility to movement; *ITB*, iliotibial band; *MMT*, manual muscle test; *PIP*, proximal interphalangeal; *PICR*, path of the instantaneous center of rotation; *PSIS*, posterior superior iliac spine; *SLR*, straight-leg raise; *TFL*, tensor fascia lata; *TFL-ITB*, tensor fascia lata–iliotibial band.

CRITERIA	IMPAIRMENT	DSM
Unable to shrug shoulders during flexion motion	**Upper trapezius muscle—long and weak** **Rhomboid, latissimus dorsi, pectoralis minor muscles—short and stiff**	
Able to flatten lumbar spine without thoracic flexion (depressing chest) **Hips and knees are flexed**		
Chest depresses as attempt to flatten lumbar spine	**Rectus abdominis muscle—short and dominant**	
Able to flatten lumbar spine while maintaining maximum shoulder flexion		
Unable to flatten lumbar spine unless chest elevates and lumbar spine extends	**Latissimus dorsi, pectoralis major, minor muscles—short and stiff**	

Movement Impairments: Upper Quarter Examination — cont'd

POSITION	TEST	DYSFUNCTION STRUCTURAL VARIATION		SCAPULAR SYNDROMES				HUMERAL SYNDROMES			
				DR	DP	AB	WG	AN	SP	HO	MR
Standing	**Alignment** Head and neck	❏ Extended ❏ Forward ❏ Flat ❏ Pain									
	Passive elevation	❏ Pain decreased ❏ Pain same ❏ Pain increased									
	Thoracic spine	❏ Kyphosis ❏ Flat ❏ Scoliosis—rib	R L								
	Infrasternal angle	❏ < 75 degrees ❏ > 100 degrees									
	Lumbar spine	❏ Flat ❏ Lordotic									
	Scapula	❏ Downwardly rotated	R L	☐	☐	☐	☐				
		❏ Depressed	R L								
		❏ Abducted	R L								
		❏ Adducted	R L								
		❏ Winging/tilt	R L								
		❏ Elevated	R L								
	Humerus	❏ Anterior	R L					☐	☐	☐	☐
		❏ Superior	R L								
		❏ Medially rotated	R L								
		❏ Laterally rotated	R L								
		❏ Abducted	R L								
	Shoulder flexion— elevation	❏ < 180 degrees of motion	R L	☐	☐	☐	☐	☐	☐	☐	☐
	Scapula	❏ Inferior angle < midthorax	R L	☐	☐	☐	☐	☐	☐	☐	☐
		❏ < 60 upward rotation	R L								
		❏ Deficient elevation	R L								
		❏ Excessive elevation	R L								
		❏ Excessive abduction	R L								
		❏ Winging	R L								

AB, Abduction; *AN,* anterior glide; *DP,* depression; *HO,* hypomobility; *MR,* medial rotation; *SP,* superior glide: *WG,* winging/tilt.

POSITION	TEST	DYSFUNCTION STRUCTURAL VARIATION		SCAPULAR SYNDROME				HUMERAL SYNDROMES			
				DR	DP	AB	WG	AN	SP	HO	MR
Standing —cont'd	Shoulder flexion— humerus	❏ Anterior glide R L ❏ Superior glide R L ❏ Medial rotation R L ❏ < 170 degrees R L						❏	❏	❏	❏
	Shoulder extension return from flexion	❏ > Depression R L		❏	❏	❏	❏				
	Scapula	❏ > Down rotation R L ❏ > Adduction R L									
	Humerus	❏ Anterior glide R L						❏			
	Shoulder abduction	❏ Inferior angle < midthorax R L		❏	❏	❏	❏				
	Scapula	❏ < 60 upward rotation R L ❏ Deficient elevation R L ❏ Excessive elevation R L ❏ Excessive abduction R L ❏ Winging R L									
	Humerus	❏ Superior glide R L ❏ Anterior glide R L ❏ < Lateral rotation R L ❏ < 120 degrees R L						❏	❏	❏	❏
	Shoulder adduction— return from abduction	❏ Winging R L		❏	❏	❏	❏				
	Scapula	❏ > Depression R L ❏ > Downward rotation R L ❏ > Adduction R L									
	Humerus	❏ Superior glide R L							❏		
Supine	Pectoralis minor length	❏ Short R L ❏ Stiff R L		❏	❏	❏	❏				
	Biceps—short head	❏ Short R L ❏ Stiff R L									
	Shoulder flexion Latissimus dorsi—length	❏ Short R L ❏ Stiff R L									

Movement Impairments: Upper Quarter Examination—cont'd

POSITION	TEST	DYSFUNCTION STRUCTURAL VARIATION		SCAPULAR SYNDROME				HUMERAL SYNDROMES			
				DR	DP	AB	WG	AN	SP	HO	MR
Supine—cont'd	Lumbar spine	☐ Extension	R L								
	Teres major—length	☐ Short	R L								
		☐ Stiff	R L								
	Humeral head	☐ Anterior glide	R L					☐	☐	☐	☐
		☐ Superior glide	R L								
		☐ Medial rotation	R L								
		☐ < 120 degrees	R L								
	Pectoralis major—length Sternal	☐ Short	R L	☐	☐	☐	☐				
		☐ Stiff	R L								
	Clavicular	☐ Short	R L								
		☐ Stiff	R L								
		☐ Long	R L								
	Humeral head	☐ Anterior glide	R L					☐	☐	☐	☐
		☐ Superior glide	R L								
		☐ Medial rotation	R L								
		☐ < 120 degrees	R L								
	Shoulder—lateral rotation	☐ < 90 degrees	R L								
		☐ Stiff									
	Humeral head	☐ Anterior glide	R L								
		☐ Superior glide	R L					☐	☐	☐	☐
	Shoulder medial rotation	☐ < 70 degrees rotation	R L								
	Scapula	☐ Anterior tilt	R L				☐				
	Humeral head	☐ Anterior glide	R L								
		☐ Superior glide	R L					☐	☐	☐	☐
Prone	Shoulder medial rotation	☐ < 70 degrees rotation	R L							☐	
	Scapula	☐ Anterior tilts	R L	☐							
		☐ Elevates	R L								
	Humeral head	☐ Anterior glide	R L					☐			
	Muscle performance	☐ Weak/long R 3 3+ 4- 4 4+/5 L 3 3+ 4- 4 4+/5									

AB, Abduction; *AN*, anterior glide; *DP*; depression; *HO*, hypomobility; *MR*, medial rotation; *SP*, superior glide: *WG*; winging/tilt.

Lower Abdominal Muscle Exercise Progression

This exercise is often indicated for patients with low back pain because it is designed to improve the performance of the external oblique muscles, which are important for control of posterior pelvic tilt and combined with the contralateral internal oblique, control of pelvic rotation. These muscles help to prevent the accessory or compensatory motions of the pelvis and spine that occur during movements of the lower extremity. The way the exercise is performed also helps to improve the performance of the transversus abdominis muscle that stabilizes the lumbar spine. An important consideration is that this exercise also necessitates participation of the hip flexors. Because contraction of the iliopsoas, in particular, creates compressive and anterior shear forces on the lumbar spine, the exercise must be carefully taught and performed and used with caution. Clinical observation has shown that more women than men have weak lower abdominal muscles. The proportionally larger pelvis and lower extremities of women as compared with men contributes to this situation. Pregnancy also contributes to weakness of the abdominal muscles when this is not addressed with postpartum exercises. This exercise should not be used if the patient has acute low back pain; easier forms of lower abdominal muscle exercise, such as heel slides, should be initiated. The patient should not have symptoms while performing the exercise.

Purposes

- To improve the performance of the lower abdominal, external oblique, rectus abdominis, and transversus abdominis muscles
- To learn to contract the abdominal muscles to prevent motions of the spine during movements of the lower extremities

Correct Performance

This is a series of nine exercises of progressively increasing difficulty. The patient starts in a position of hip and knee flexion (hook lying). The patient contracts his or her abdominal muscles by pulling his or her navel toward the spine and then performs the motions described in each level. The patient must maintain the contraction of the abdominal muscles avoiding distention of the abdomen and keeping the back flat.

1. Level 0.3 (E1)—Lift one foot with the other foot on the floor.
2. Level 0.4 (E2)—Hold one knee to the chest, and lift the other foot.
3. Level 0.5—Lightly hold one knee toward the chest, and lift the other foot.
4. Level 1A—Flex the hip to greater than 90 degrees, and lift the other foot.
5. Level 1B—Flex the hip to 90 degrees, and lift the other foot.
6. Level 2—Flex one hip to 90 degrees, and lift and slide the other foot to extend the hip and knee.
7. Level 3—Flex one hip to 90 degrees, lift the foot, and extend the leg without touching the supporting surface.
8. Level 4—Slide both feet along the supporting surface into extension, and return to flexion.
9. Level 5—Lift both feet off the supporting surface, flex the hips to 90 degrees, extend the knees, and lower both lower extremities to the supporting surface.

Once the patient can correctly perform 10 repetitions at the easiest level, he or she progresses to the next level and stops performing the previous exercise. Each exercise starts in the supine position, lying on a table or floor mat with the hips and knees flexed and the feet on the floor. The patient should be able to move the leg without moving (arching) the back. The back should be held flat (no curve) against the floor during extremity motion. If unable to keep the back flat, the patient should hold it in a constant position, without motion, during the exercise. The patient should breathe normally during the exercise. He or she should exhale when moving the second leg. The patient should place the fingertips on each side of the abdomen, just above the pelvis and below the rib cage, to monitor the contraction of the external oblique muscles. The abdomen should stay flat and not distend.

LEVEL 0.3 (E1)

- Lying in the position indicated, the patient contracts the abdominal muscles, flattening the abdomen and reducing the arch in the lumbar spine. To achieve this the patient is instructed to "pull the navel in toward the spine."
- The patient flexes one hip while keeping the knee flexed. By having the hip flexed more than 90 degrees, the weight of the thigh is assisting the posterior pelvic tilt and maintaining a flat lumbar spine.
- The patient returns the lower extremity to the starting position and repeats the exercise with the other lower extremity.
- The patient is cautioned not to push the nonmoving foot into the supporting surface because this will substitute hip extension for abdominal muscle action. The back must remain flat, and there should not be symptoms during performance of the exercise. Some patients may be barely able to lift the foot before having to immediately return it to the starting position.

LEVEL 0.4 (E2)

- Lying in the position indicated, the patient contracts the abdominal muscles, flattening the abdomen and reducing the arch in the lumbar spine. To achieve this, the patient is instructed to "pull the navel in toward the spine."
- The patient flexes one hip and uses the hands to hold the knee to the chest. While maintaining the contraction of the abdominal muscles, he or she flexes the other hip (lifts the foot off the supporting surface). The patient holds for a count of three and then returns the leg to the starting position and rests. He or she performs the exercise with the other lower extremity.
- The patient repeats the exercise five to six times if the back remains flat and he or she remains symptom free.
- If the patient is able to use just one hand to hold the knee to the chest, he or she should use the other hand to palpate the abdominal muscles.
- Some patients may be able to perform this level correctly and not level 0.3. If this is the case, they should start with this series.

LEVEL 0.5

- Lying in the position indicated, the patient contracts the abdominal muscles, flattening the abdomen and reducing the arch in the lumbar spine. To achieve this the patient is instructed to "pull the navel in toward the spine."
- The patient flexes one hip and uses one hand to hold the knee to the chest but holds it less firmly than in the previous level, requiring more abdominal activity. While maintaining the contraction of the abdominal muscles, he or she flexes the other hip (lifts the foot off the supporting surface). The patient holds for a count of three and then returns the leg to the starting position and rests.

He or she performs the exercise with the other lower extremity.

- The patient should repeat the exercise five to six times if the back remains flat and he or she remains symptom free. The patient should perform with the other extremity in the same manner.
- As a progression, the patient holds the hip in less flexion and less firmly as gauged by the effect on the back and on the symptoms.

LEVEL 1A

- Lying in the position indicated, the patient contracts the abdominal muscles, flattening the abdomen and reducing the arch in the lumbar spine. To achieve this the patient is instructed to "pull the navel in toward the spine." Contraction of the abdominals should be maintained while moving the lower

extremity. If the patient is slow in performing the exercise, he or she should relax the abdominal muscles after lifting the first leg and then contract them again before lifting the second leg.

- The patient flexes one hip to greater than 90 degrees by lifting the foot from the table. By having the hip flexed more than 90 degrees, the weight of the thigh is assisting the posterior pelvic tilt and maintaining a flat lumbar spine. Optimally, the flexed extremity will maintain this position with minimal contraction of the hip flexor muscles. At this point the patient contracts the abdominal muscles and flexes the other hip by lifting the foot off the table.
- If the patient's back begins to arch while lifting the second leg, he or she lowers the leg, relaxes, and tries again. The patient maintains the contraction of the abdominal muscles and constant position of the spine while lowering the legs, one at a time, to the starting position.
- The exercise is repeated by starting the sequence with the opposite leg.

LEVEL 1A

- Starting from the position indicated above, the patient contracts the abdominal muscles and holds the spine constant while flexing one hip to 90 degrees (vertical position of the thigh with the foot lifted from the table).
- The patient contracts the abdominal muscles and lifts the other leg to the same position. While maintaining the contraction of the abdominal muscles, the patient lowers the legs one at a time to the starting position.
- If the patient performs the exercise slowly, he or she may need to relax the abdominal muscles before lowering the legs and then contract them again to lower them.
- The exercise is repeated by starting the sequence with the opposite leg. The patient repeats the exercise, alternating legs, until he or she can perform it correctly 10 times. The patient can then progress to Level 1B.

LEVEL 1B

- Starting from the position indicated in Level 1, the patient contracts the abdominal muscles and flexes the hip to 90 degrees, lifting the foot from the table.
- While maintaining the contraction of the abdominal muscles and a constant back position, the patient lifts the other leg up to the same position. Maintaining one leg at 90 degrees, the patient places the other heel on the table and slowly slides the heel along the table until the hip and knee are extended.

- The leg is then returned to the starting position by sliding the heel along the table. The patient continues to hold the abdomen flat and back in a constant position while repeating the extension motion with the other leg and returning it to the starting position.
- The patient repeats the exercise, alternating legs, until he or she can perform it correctly 10 times. The patient can then progress to Level 2.

LEVEL 2

- Starting from the supine position of hip and knee flexion described in Level 1, the patient contracts the abdominal muscles and maintains a constant back position. The patient flexes the hip to 90 degrees, lifting the foot from the table.
- While maintaining the contraction of the abdominal muscles and a constant back position, the patient lifts the other leg up to the same position. Maintaining one hip at 90 degrees, the patient extends the hip and knee while holding the foot off the table until the hip and knee are resting in an extended position on the table.
- The patient returns the leg to the hip and knee flexed position. While maintaining the contraction of the abdominal muscles and a constant back position, the patient extends and lowers the other leg and then returns it to the 90-degree position. The exercise is repeated, alternating legs.

Most patients have adequate strength and control of their abdominal muscles if they can complete this level successfully. Progression to a higher level is not necessary for remediation of a pain problem. Further increases in the level of difficulty of these exercises should be primarily for improved levels of fitness. If indicated, this exercise is repeated until the patient can perform it correctly 10 times, and then he or she progresses to Level 3.

LEVEL 3

- The patient begins the exercise in the supine position with both legs in extension.
- The patient contracts the abdominal muscles to decrease the lumbar curve and to maintain this lumbar position while sliding his or her heels along the table, flexing both hips and knees while bringing them toward the chest.
- Once the hips and knees are flexed, the patient pauses, reinforces the abdominal contraction, and slides both legs back into extension. Maintaining the position of the lumbar spine is extremely important.
- The exercise is repeated until the patient can perform it correctly 10 times before progressing to Level 4.

LEVEL 4

- The patient begins this exercise in the lower extremity extended position described in Level 3.
- The patient begins by contracting the abdominal muscles to flatten the lumbar spine and to maintain the spine motionless while simultaneously flexing the hips and knees, lifting both feet off the table to bring the hips to 90 degrees.
- The patient reinforces the contraction of the abdominal muscles, extends the knees, and lowers the lower extremities to the table. He or she must be able to maintain a flat lumbar spine while performing this exercise.

Special Considerations

- In the presence of an increased lumbar curve or excessive lumbar flexibility into extension (extension DSM), the emphasis of the program is maintaining a flat lumbar spine while performing the exercises. These exercises are not recommended when the patient has symptoms when lying supine with the hips and knees in extension. The exercise sequence for these patients should begin with the heel slide exercise.
- In the presence of a flat back but with poor control by the abdominal muscles, the lumbar spine should remain still, but flattening of the lumbar spine should not be emphasized. This exercise is particularly indicated for patients with a sway-back posture in which the external obliques and the iliopsoas are long.
- Patients can test 100% for upper and lower abdominal muscle strength and still have poor control of pelvic rotation during unilateral lower extremity motion.
- Often patients who have strong rectus abdominis muscles have weak external obliques. This is believed to be because the rectus abdominis has been the primary muscle producing posterior pelvic tilt and its performance becomes more optimal than that of the external obliques. Because the rectus abdominis muscle cannot control rotation as it runs parallel to the axis of rotation, improving the performance of the external obliques is important because they participate with the internal oblique muscles for the control of pelvic rotation.
- Women should be advised not to push their head into the supporting surface. This type of inappropriate stabilization can occur in women who have very weak abdominal muscles or who have a small upper body and a large lower body.

Trunk-Curl Sit-Up (Upper Abdominal Progression)

Purpose

To strengthen the upper abdominal muscles (internal obliques and rectus abdominis)

Commentary

This exercise is seldom prescribed for patients with low back pain. The main indication for this exercise is for physical fitness. The primary muscle groups participating in this exercise are the internal obliques and rectus abdominis for the trunk-curl, with the addition of the hip flexors for the sit-up phase and the external oblique muscles for posterior pelvic tilt. This exercise is more difficult for men than for women because of the higher center of gravity in men than women. This is such a popular exercise many people have been using it as part of their fitness program without the proper individual examination and guidance for correct performance.

Physical therapists should be very familiar with all of the considerations of correct performance of this exercise to address frequently encountered errors. One of the important considerations is the degree of spinal flexibility of the patient. If the patient has excessive spinal flexibility, he or she will be able to flex the spine through a large range of motion before the initiation of the hip flexion phase. If the patient's spinal flexibility is limited, he or she will only be able to flex through a limited range of motion before the initiation of hip flexion. As the patient's program is progressed in difficulty, the therapist must be sure that the patient flexes to the same point in the range before progressing to more advanced exercises.

There are two main factors that can make this exercise unsafe. One factor is the anterior shear stress exerted on the lumbar spine produced by contraction of the hip flexor muscles, particularly the iliopsoas. That is why the abdominal muscles must have enough strength to maintain flexion of the spine at the time of the hip flexor contraction. If the patient's trunk extends as the hip flexion phase is initiated, he or she should perform an easier level of the exercise to protect the spine. The other factor is excessive lumbar flexion at the end of the sit-up phase. When the exercise is performed with the hips and knees flexed, the axis of rotation is shifted from the hip joints to the lumbar spine. The patient also must contract the hip extensors more strongly when the hips and knees are flexed than when they are extended. The hip extensor contraction is to prevent the feet from coming off the supporting surface when the hip flexors are contracting to flex the trunk. This is consistent with the shorter lever arm created by hip and knee flexion and the decrease in passive stabilization of the distal attachments of the hip

flexor muscles. At the end of the sit-up phase, the hips are in approximately 100 to 120 degrees of flexion depending on the degree of hip flexion that the patient assumes for the starting position. If the sit-up is performed with the hips and knees extended, the hips only have to flex to 80 degrees at the end of the sit-up motion.

The safest but not the best way to perform this exercise is to limit the movement to a trunk-curl and have the hips and knees flexed. This does not place maximum demands on the internal obliques because those demands are made when the hip flexors contract, producing anterior pelvic tilt while the trunk is flexing. At this point, the upper abdominal muscles experience the greatest demands to maintain flexion of the spine and posterior pelvic tilt.

Correct Performance

This exercise is a progression of four levels:

1. Level 1A—Trunk-curl only; spinal flexion; easy
2. Level 1B—Trunk-curl with sit-up; spinal and hip flexion; with arms extended; moderate
3. Level 2—Trunk-curl with sit-up; spinal and hip flexion; with arms folded on the chest; difficult
4. Level 3—Trunk-curl with sit-up; spinal and hip flexion; with hands on top of head; most difficult

With a careful analysis by a physical therapist, the following method is preferred:

- The patient assumes a supine position with hips and knees in extension. A small pillow may be placed under the knees. To limit the anterior shear on the lumbar spine, the spine must become flat and remain flat during the trunk curl motion.
- The patient must curl to the limit of his or her spine's flexibility.
- The patient begins with the level established by the physical therapist's testing and proceeds to Level 1A when he or she can perform the exercise correctly 10 times.

LEVEL 1A

- The patient flexes the shoulders to 45 degrees with the elbows extended, as if to reach toward the feet.
- The patient lifts his or her head by bringing the chin toward the neck and slowly curling the trunk (flexing the spine). The correct movement of the head is to reverse the cervical curve by bringing the chin toward the neck.
- The patient must avoid excessive flexion of the lower cervical spine and translation motion of the vertebrae that can occur if the patient is attempting to bring the chin to the chest. He or she must not lead with the face, as if looking upward, because that motion is cervical extension.

- The patient must flex the thoracic and lumbar spines to the limit of their flexibility. He or she stops just before the initiation of the hip flexion phase.
  LEVEL 1B
- The patient flexes the shoulders to 45 degrees with the elbows extended, as if to reach toward the feet.
- The patient lifts his or her head by bringing the chin toward the neck and slowly curling the trunk (flexing the spine). The correct movement of the head is to reverse the cervical curve by bringing the chin toward the neck.
- The patient must avoid excessive flexion of the lower cervical spine and translation motion of the vertebrae that can occur if the patient is attempting to bring the chin to the chest. He or she must not lead with the face, as if looking upward, because that motion is cervical extension.
- The patient must flex the thoracic and lumbar spines to the limit of their flexibility and maintain this position as he or she completes the hip flexion motion (sit-up).
  LEVEL 2
- The patient flexes (folds) the arms across his or her chest, flexes the cervical spine by bringing the chin toward the neck and slowly curls the trunk as he or she comes to a sitting position. The trunk curl is maintained throughout the movement.
- The exercise is repeated correctly 10 times before progressing to Level 3.
  LEVEL 3
- The patient places both hands on top of the head and flexes the cervical spine by bringing his or her chin toward the neck and slowly curling the trunk to the limit of his or her spine's flexibility. The patient maintains this position as he or she comes to the sitting position. The trunk curl is maintained throughout the movement.
- Care should be taken to be sure that the patient is not pushing down on his or her head and compressing the cervical spine as he or she curls the trunk.
- The patient should avoid bringing the elbows forward (horizontal adduction) during the trunk curl because this decreases the effort required.

Special Considerations

- Patients with a thoracic kyphosis should not perform this exercise because it emphasizes maximum thoracic flexion. This exercise is contraindicated for patients with osteoporosis because the trunk flexion increases their risk of compression fractures.
- This exercise is contraindicated for patients with cervical disease because of the stress on the cervical spine.
- This exercise is contraindicated for conditions in which compression of the lumbar vertebrae is undesirable, such as low back pain.
- Patients with spondylolisthesis should not perform the hip flexion phase.
- Patients with excessive lumbar flexion should be carefully monitored and should do the exercise with their hips and knees extended.
- Patients with very limited spinal flexion should not do this exercise because of the exaggerated hip flexion phase. (The duration of the hip flexion phase exceeds that of the trunk flexion phase.)

Hip Abduction/Lateral Rotation From Hip Flexed Flexed Position

Purposes

- To learn to move the femur without moving the spine or pelvis
- To improve the control by the abdominal muscles in order to prevent pelvic and lumbar rotation associated with hip motion
- To stretch the hip adductor muscles
- To improve performance of the abdominal muscles, specifically isometric control of pelvic rotation

Correct Performance

LEVEL 1

- The patient starts with one hip and knee extended and the other hip and knee flexed. He or she places the hands on the pelvis (in the region of the ASIS) to monitor any motion. The patient is instructed to contract the abdominal muscles by "pulling the navel in toward the spine."
- The patient lets the flexed lower extremity move slowly into hip lateral rotation/abduction. The patient stops when he or she experiences symptoms or feels the pelvis begin to rotate. If the pelvis remains stationary, he or she allows the hip to abduct/laterally rotate as far as possible by relaxing the adductor muscles. The patient adducts and medially rotates the hip, returning to the starting position.
- The patient repeats the exercise, trying to increase the hip range while preventing pelvic rotation by contracting the abdominal muscles. The exercise can be repeated with the same extremity before switching to the contralateral lower extremity.

Special Considerations

If the patient has minimal abduction without pelvic motion or has pain, it might be necessary to put pillows along the outside of the leg to allow the leg to relax against a support to prevent pelvic motion or pain.

LEVEL 2. When the patient is able to perform the full range of motion without pain or pelvic rotation, the following progression is suggested:

1. Hip abduction/lateral rotation, then extend knee. The patient contracts the abdominal muscles and lets the flexed lower extremity move into abduction/lateral rotation. At the end of the range, the patient extends the knee joint and tries to prevent the pelvic rotation forces that are increased by the longer lever of the extended knee. The patient flexes the knee and returns to the starting position.

2. Hip abduction/lateral rotation, then extend knee and perform hip flexion/adduction.

The patient contracts the abdominal muscles and lets the flexed lower extremity move into abduction/lateral rotation. At the end of the range, the patient extends the knee followed by hip flexion/adduction, returning the leg to the midline and flexing the knee to return to the starting position. The patient repeats the exercise 5 to 10 times with one extremity, and then the exercise is performed with the other lower extremity.

Straight-Leg Raises (Hip Flexion With Knee Extended)

Purposes
- To strengthen the hip flexor and abdominal muscles
- To stretch the hamstring muscles

Correct Performance
A. Knee extended with hip flexion and return to starting position
   1. The patient lies supine on a table or mat with both legs extended and in neutral rotation.
   2. The patient contracts his or her abdominal muscles to flatten the lumbar spine and flexes one hip with the knee extended, raising the leg from the table.
   3. The patient lowers the leg to the table while maintaining contraction of the abdominal muscles. The patient should not push down (hip extension) against the table with the nonmoving leg because it decreases the demands on the abdominal muscles.
   4. The patient should monitor motion of the pelvic crests to be sure that rotation does not occur.
B. Straight-leg lowering (Knee flexed with hip flexion and knee extended during return to hip extension in neutral rotation.)
   1. The patient contracts the abdominal muscles to flatten the lumbar spine; flexes the hip and knee, bringing his knee to the chest; and extends the knee while maintaining hip flexion. The patient may use his or her hands to hold the thigh so that the hip remains flexed to 90 degrees.
   2. Keeping the knee extended and the lumbar spine flat, the patient lowers the leg to the starting position.

Special Considerations
- The patient should not perform this exercise if it causes pain.
- If the iliopsoas is particularly weak, the patient should laterally rotate the femur before performing hip flexion.
- If the tensor fascia lata is weak, the patient should medially rotate and abduct the femur before performing hip flexion.
- If the patient has weak abdominal muscles ($< 2/5$), then he or she should flex one hip and knee to place the foot on the table. Then, while performing the straight-leg raise with the other leg, the patient should push the foot into the supporting surface to reduce the demands on the abdominal muscles and the anterior shear force on the spine associated with the hip flexor contraction.

Hip Flexor Stretch (Two-Joint)

Purposes
- To stretch the hip flexor, tensor fascia lata, rectus femoris, and iliopsoas muscles
- To correct the compensatory anterior pelvic tilt or rotation motion of the lumbar spine and the pelvis associated with shortness or stiffness of the hip flexor muscles
- To correct the compensatory lateral rotation motion of the tibia associated with shortness of the tensor fascia lata

Correct Performance
- The patient begins by lying close to the end of a firm table with both knees held to the chest and the lumbar spine flat. The position on the table should be such that when the thigh is in contact with the table, one half of its length should extend beyond the table.
- The patient first uses the hands and holds one knee to the chest to maintain a flat, nonflexed lumbar spine and then lowers the other limp into hip extension. Upon completion of the motion, with the lumbar spine flat and the thigh in contact with the table, the hip should be in 10 degrees of extension. The hip flexors should elongate enough to permit 10 degrees of extension.

- While holding one knee to the chest, the patient lowers the other limb into hip extension so that the thigh touches the table. The hip should be in neutral position, and the tibia should be in neutral rotation.
- If the tensor fascia lata is short, the range into hip extension will increase if the hip is abducted. If pelvic tilt is associated with the hip extension, abducting the hip will alleviate the pelvic tilt or delay its onset. If the rectus femoris muscle is short, the hip will not be completely extended when the hip is abducted and passive extension of the knee will increase the range into hip extension. If the hip is still not completely extended, the iliopsoas is short. Sometimes laterally rotating the hip will increase the hip extension, which further supports the belief that the iliopsoas is short.

The following are modifications that must be made in the test when shortness is present in the muscles that are listed or the lumbar spine is more flexible than the tested muscles are extensible:

1. *Tensor fascia lata shortness and stiffness.* The patient should allow the hip to abduct as the thigh is lowered into hip extension. At the end of the range of hip extension or when the thigh is in contact with the table, the patient should adduct the hip, being sure not to substitute with hip medial rotation. The patient should stop if he or she feels pain in the area of the knee. The patient should keep the pelvis from tilting anteriorly or rotating. If the knee is the most flexible segment and there is compensatory tibial lateral rotation during the adduction motion, then the patient should medially rotate the tibia (turn the foot inward) and maintain this position while adducting the hip. The stretch should be maintained for 20 to 30 seconds. The patient then returns the thigh to the abducted position and repeats the motion.
2. *Rectus femoris shortness and stiffness.* With the hip in maximum extension and the knee extended, the patient should flex the knee and allow the hip to extend. The stretch should be maintained for 20 to 30 seconds. The patient then returns to the starting position by extending the knee and repeats the motion.
3. *Iliopsoas shortness and stiffness.* The patient should allow the hip to extend as far as possible. While keeping the pelvis and lumbar spine from tilting anteriorly or rotating, the patient allows the weight of the lower limb to stretch the hip flexor. The patient should prevent hip lateral rotation. After allowing the hip to stretch for 20 to 30 seconds, the patient returns to the starting position and repeats the motion.

Special Considerations

A. This exercise is not often recommended because of the problem with finding a suitable surface for performing the exercise. The other exercises that stretch the hip flexors are usually sufficient and this one is not necessary. If the patient maintains an active exercise program that involves the use of the hip flexors in a shortened position, this exercise may be necessary. In most patients with musculoskeletal pain, the primary problem is the lack of suitable control of segments that become sites of compensatory motion. As explained in other sections of this text, the most important requirement for correction is to increase the stiffness or control by muscles that permit the compensatory motion. Other exercises that are used to stretch the hip flexors and to improve the control of abdominal stabilizing muscles are as follows:
   1. Supine
      a. Knee to chest with leg slides
      b. Bilateral hip and knee extension while maintaining a posterior pelvic tilt
   2. Side lying—Hip adduction/extension with lateral rotation
   3. Prone
      a. Knee flexion
      b. Hip extension with knee extended and flexed
      c. Hip lateral and medial rotation

B. The muscle groups that are most frequently short are the tensor fascia lata–iliotibial band, anterior gluteus medius, and gluteus minimus, which are the hip flexor, abductor, medial rotator muscles. Relatively few patients have shortness of the iliopsoas muscle as compared with those with shortness of the tensor fascia lata and its abductor synergists. Because these hip flexors are abductors, allowing abduction and reassessing the range into hip extension is important to determine which hip flexors are short.

C. In the presence of iliopsoas shortness, some patients will laterally rotate the hip to reduce the stretch on the iliopsoas. The other muscle that laterally rotates the hip is the sartorius, but because this muscle flexes the knee, there will be resistance to passive knee extension when this muscle is short. Shortness of the sartorius is not very common.

Latissimus Dorsi and Scapulohumeral Muscle Stretch (Shoulder Flexion/Elevation With Elbow Extended)

Purposes
- To stretch the latissimus dorsi
- To stretch the teres major and the teres minor
- To increase range of motion of shoulder flexion

Correct Performance

The patient begins in the supine position with the hips and the knees flexed, the lumbar spine flat, and arms at the side.

A. Latissimus dorsi
   1. The patient keeps the elbows extended while flexing both shoulders. He or she should keep the arms close to the ears and maintain shoulder lateral rotation (olecranons pointing toward the ceiling). The back must remain flat against the table.
   2. The patient holds at the end of the range for 5 to 10 seconds and then returns the arms to his or her sides.
B. Teres major and teres minor
   1. The patient performs as in A, except that once the shoulder has flexed to 90 degrees, the patient uses the opposite hand to hold the inferior angle of the scapula against the chest wall. This will prevent excessive anterior or lateral excursion of the scapula as he or she continues to flex the shoulder. The inferior angle of the scapula should not abduct more than the mid-axillary border of the thorax or more than $1/2$ inch laterally.
   2. Once maximum shoulder flexion has been reached, the patient should hold this position for 5 to 10 seconds to let the weight of the arm stretch the teres muscles.
   3. The patient repeats the exercise, alternating extremities after 10 repetitions.
C. Glenohumeral dysfunction. The patient performs as above, except that he or she first flexes the elbow and then initiates shoulder flexion, allowing the elbow to extend after the shoulder flexes to 90 degrees. The patient may need to place a pillow above the shoulder alongside his or her head and slide the hand along a pillow during the phase of shoulder flexion from 90 degrees to 180 degrees.

Special Considerations

- Patients with a kyphosis may need to place a pillow under their thoracic spine and head.
- If the patient has a large thorax and restricted scapular motion, the supine position may interfere with the scapular rotation. The patient may need to actively abduct and upwardly rotate the scapula, particularly if he or she notes pinching in the area of the acromion.

Shoulder Abduction

Purposes

- To stretch the pectoralis major muscle
- To strengthen the abdominal muscles

Correct Performance

The patient assumes a starting position of flexion of the hips and knees with the lumbar spine flat and arms at the sides.

A. Pectoralis major stretch
   1. The patient maintains elbow extension and abducts the shoulders, bringing the arms overhead so that the final position is 120 degrees of abduction, with the arms resting on the table.
   2. The patient should hold this position for 5 to 10 seconds and then lower the arms to the sides, trying to keep the scapulae adducted on the thorax.
B. Abdominal muscle strengthening with upper extremity motion.
   1. The starting position is 120 degrees of shoulder abduction. The patient uses a weight that provides appropriate resistance in his or her hand and horizontally adducts the shoulder, moving in a direction toward the opposite hip. The motion can cease when the arm is vertical. The patient contracts the abdominal muscles and maintains the contraction as he or she lifts and lowers the weights.
   2. The patient repeats the exercise with the opposite extremity.
   3. The patient can also perform the exercise with weights in both hands.

Special Considerations

- If the patient has a kyphosis, he or she may need to place a pillow under the thorax and will not be able to bring the arm back to the table.
- More often, the sternal portion of the pectoralis major is the shorter segment, whereas the clavicular portion is more frequently longer.

Shoulder Abduction in Lateral Rotation With Elbows Flexed

Purposes

- To improve the performance of the lateral rotator and the abductor muscles
- To stretch the medial rotator muscles, primarily the latissimus dorsi and pectoralis major
- To assist in stretch of the pectoralis minor muscle

Correct Performance

- The patient begins the exercise in a position of flexion of the hips and knees with the arms at the sides.
- The patient flexes the elbows, externally rotates the shoulders, and abducts the shoulders by sliding the arms over the head. The patient should keep the arms in contact with the table for an effective stretch of the medial rotator muscles.

Special Considerations
The patient should not experience pain in the area of the acromion.

Shoulder Rotation
MEDIAL ROTATION
Purposes
- To stretch the lateral rotators of the shoulder
- To eliminate compensatory anterior tilt of the scapula with shoulder rotation
- To eliminate compensatory anterior glide of the humeral head during medial rotation of the shoulder
- To improve performance of the lateral rotator muscles of the shoulder

Correct Performance
- The patient begins the exercise with the hips and knees flexed to stabilize the thorax or with the lower extremities in extension. The shoulder is abducted to 90 degrees and is in neutral rotation with the elbow flexed to 90 degrees.
- A folded towel can be placed under the arm, if needed, to lift the arm and align the humerus in the plane of the scapula. The patient uses the opposite hand to hold the shoulder down onto the table, preventing anterior motion of the head of the humerus or anterior tilt of the scapula as the exercise is performed.
- The patient medially rotates the humerus, allowing the forearm to drop toward the table without lifting the shoulder girdle from the table. The patient stops the movement if pain occurs or if the shoulder girdle or the humeral head lifts from the table.
- The arm is returned to the starting position and the movement is repeated slowly 6 to 10 times until maximum range has been achieved without pain or compensatory motions.
- The exercise is repeated with the other arm.

Special Considerations
- If the range of motion is markedly limited and resists stretching, a small weight can be used to assist the stretch. The weight should be heavy enough to exert a rotational effect on the shoulder but light enough so that the patient does not have to actively hold the weight to prevent medial rotation.
- Limited medial rotation range or greater relative flexibility of the scapular or the glenohumeral motion is quite common. Shortness or stiffness of the lateral rotators is believed to be a precursor and a contributor to impingement pain problems.

- After the patient is able to perform the motion correctly, the addition of weights can be used to strengthen the lateral rotator muscles.

LATERAL ROTATION
Purposes
- To stretch the shoulder medial rotator muscles
- To train the humerus to move independently of the scapula
- To improve the performance of the medial rotator muscles

Correct Performance
- The patient is positioned in the same manner as described above for medial rotation.
- The patient laterally rotates the humerus while maintaining a constant position of the scapula and not allowing the head of the humerus to move anteriorly against the hand.
- The arm is returned to the starting position, and the movement is repeated slowly until maximum rotation range has been achieved without pain or compensatory motions. The exercise is repeated 6 to 10 times and then performed with the other arm.
- After correct performance is achieved, the addition of weights can be used to strengthen the medial rotators.

Special Considerations
- Excessive range of lateral rotation is more common than excessive range of medial rotation. When the range is excessive, the anterior glide of the humeral head is also excessive.
- Limited lateral rotation range is not a common finding when the shoulder is only flexed or abducted to 90 degrees.
- If the patient has pain at 90 degrees of abduction, the degree of abduction should be decreased. Supporting the arm on a towel and positioning the shoulder in some degree of horizontal flexion, which is usually in the plane of the scapula (30 degrees in the frontal plane), is another method of reducing pain at the glenohumeral joint.

HORIZONTAL ADDUCTION
Purpose
To stretch the scapulohumeral muscles

Correct Performance
- The patient begins the exercise in a position of hip and knee flexion recommended to stabilize the thorax or with the legs in extension. From the starting position of 90 degrees of abduction, the patient passively horizontally adducts the shoulder.

- When the shoulder is in a position of 90 degrees of flexion, the patient should passively adduct the humerus (pull across the chest) using the other hand by applying pressure at the olecranon.
- The patient holds the humerus in this position for 5 to 10 seconds, releases, and then pulls again. During the stretch, the scapula must remain in contact with the table. The patient should feel a pull in the posterior shoulder girdle muscles but should stop if pain occurs in the shoulder joint.
- The exercise is repeated 6 to 10 times and then performed with the other arm.

Special Considerations

- When the scapulohumeral muscles are short, there is often compensatory scapular motion. Therefore the scapula needs to be stabilized during the motion.
- If anterior joint pain is present, the patient can exert a posterior pressure on the olecranon as he or she passively adducts the humerus. Ensuring that the shoulder flexor muscles are relaxed can also help to alleviate symptoms.

Pectoralis Minor Stretching

Purposes

- To stretch the pectoralis minor muscle on the anterior chest
- To decrease anterior tilt of the scapula
- To improve the mobility of the scapula

Correct Performance

The patient begins the exercise with the hips and knees in flexion so that the back is flat and the arms are at the sides.

A. Assisted stretch (lying on back)
1. The patient begins the exercise in a supine position on a firm surface with the arms at the sides. The assistant stands at the side of the table and places the "heels," or thenar portions of the hands, over the coracoid processes of both scapulae. (Bilateral stretch usually minimizes the rotation of the thorax that can occur with unilateral stretching.) Often it is easier for the assistant if his or her hands are crossed (e.g., so that his or her right hand applies pressure to the patient's right shoulder).
2. Pressure is applied in the direction of the muscle fibers, towards but not directly on the head of the humerus, pushing the shoulder away from the body and down toward the table. The pressure is held for 5 to 10 seconds, released, and repeated. The patient should be experiencing a stretching feeling on the chest but not pain at the area of direct pressure.

B. Self-stretch (lying on back)
1. The patient rolls toward the side to be stretched.
2. The patient applies pressure to the coracoid process to fix the scapula against the floor. While maintaining the pressure on the coracoid process, the patient rotates the trunk away from the shoulder.

C. Assisted stretch (lying face down)
1. The patient is lying face down with arms at the side. The assistant stands at the side and reaches from the top of the shoulder to place his or her fingers in the crease on the front of the shoulder. The other hand reaches through the axilla to place the fingers also on the crease of the shoulder. The assistant then lifts up on the shoulder and leans back at the same time to stretch the muscle.
2. The therapist should not pull on the arm. The stretch should be felt on the chest and not in the shoulder joint.

Special Considerations

- The acromial end of the spine of the scapula should be able to touch the table with the stretch applied by the therapist.
- If the patient has a thoracic kyphosis, the scapula may not reach the table during the stretching.

Side-Lying Exercises (Lower Extremity)

Hip Lateral Rotation

Purposes

- To improve the performance of the hip lateral rotator muscles (gluteus medius and maximus, piriformis, obturator externis and internis, gemellus superior and inferior, and quadratus femoris)
- To learn to differentiate the movement of the hip from that of the pelvis

Correct Performance

- The patient begins the exercise lying with trunk and pelvis perpendicular to the table and the pelvis in neutral tilt. The hip and the knee of the bottom leg should be flexed. The top leg should be in the same alignment, supported on a pillow placed between the knees.
- The patient slowly laterally rotates the hip of the top leg, being sure not to allow the pelvis to rotate. The patient holds this position for 3 to 5 seconds and then returns to the starting position.
- The patient repeats the exercise 5 to 10 times. The motion should only occur in the hip joint. The pelvis and trunk should not move. After 5 to 10 repetitions, the patient rolls onto the other side and repeats the exercise with the opposite leg.

Special Considerations

- The most common error is simultaneous pelvic rotation with hip rotation.
- The patient can start with the pelvis rotated forward to facilitate the use of the posterior hip lateral rotators versus the sartorius, so that the posterior muscles will be working against gravity.
- For the patient who has back pain when lying on the side, a folded towel placed at the waist level just above the iliac crest will often alleviate the pain by eliminating the spinal curvature associated with the side-lying position.

Hip Abduction With and Without Lateral Rotation

LEVEL 1: HIP ABDUCTION WITHOUT LATERAL ROTATION

Purposes

- To improve the performance of the gluteus medius muscles
- To improve the performance of the lateral abdominal muscles. If the primary reason for the exercise is to improve the performance of the lateral abdominal muscles, the hip lateral rotation is not important; if the patient has an anteverted hip, then this exercise is more appropriate than the one with lateral rotation
- To enable the patient to learn to perform hip motion independent of pelvic motion

Correct Performance

- The patient begins with the trunk and pelvis rotated slightly forward, perpendicular to the table, with the pelvis in neutral tilt. The hip and the knee of the bottom leg should be flexed. The hip and the knee of the top leg should be in 45 degrees of flexion, supported on a pillow placed between the knees.
- The patient slowly abducts the entire lower extremity, lifting it off the pillow without rotating the femur or pushing down against the table with the lower leg. The patient holds the hip in abduction for 3 to 5 seconds and then slowly returns it to the pillow.

Special Considerations

- The patient may need a folded towel under the side, placed at waist level above the iliac crest to align the spine, if he or she has back pain in the side-lying position.
- The patient should not perform a lateral pelvic tilt either during the abduction phase or during the return phase to the starting position.
- The degree of hip and knee flexion can be adjusted to increase or decrease the length of the lever

arm to accommodate to the strength of the patient's hip abductors.
- The hip can be placed in more flexion to alleviate pain that the patient may experience when abducting the hip.

LEVEL 2: HIP ABDUCTION WITH LATERAL ROTATION

Purposes

- To improve the performance of the gluteus medius and hip lateral rotator muscles
- To learn to move the hip joint without motion of the pelvis
- To improve the performance of the lateral abdominal muscles

Correct Performance

- The patient begins the exercise in the supine position with the trunk and pelvis rotated slightly forward and perpendicular to the table with the pelvis in neutral tilt. The hip and knee of the bottom lower extremity should be flexed. The hip and knee of the top leg should be in 45 degrees of flexion and supported on a pillow placed between the knees.
- The patient laterally rotates and abducts the upper leg, lifting it from the pillow, holding the abducted position for 3 to 10 seconds and slowly returning the leg to the pillow.

Special Considerations

- The patient can place his or her hand on the pelvis to monitor and ensure that the pelvis does not move during the motion.
- The patient should avoid abducting the lower leg (pushing it into the table), which would indicate that the contralateral hip abductor muscles are providing the stabilization of the pelvis rather than the lateral abdominal muscles.

LEVEL 3: HIP ABDUCTION

Purposes

- To strengthen the posterior gluteus medius and hip lateral rotator muscles (This exercise can be used as a progression of the Level 2 exercise. The knee extension increases the length of the lever arm and the difficulty of the exercise.)
- To stretch the iliotibial band by adducting (lowering) the leg toward the table

Correct Performance

- The patient assumes a position with the trunk and the pelvis rotated slightly forward and the pelvis in neutral tilt. The hip and knee of the bottom extremity should be flexed. The hip and knee of

the top lower extremity should be extended and resting on the lower leg.
- The patient laterally rotates the hip and turns the entire leg outward so that the knee faces slightly upward. He or she then abducts and slightly extends the hip. The pelvis and trunk should not move, and the patient should not abduct (push down) the lower leg.
- The patient holds the leg up for 3 to 5 seconds and then, maintaining the external rotation, slowly lowers the leg to the table. The hip should only adduct 15 degrees, and the leg may not touch the table.

Special Considerations
- The therapist should be sure that the patient does not have hip antetorsion so that excessive lateral rotation is not expected of the patient.
- If the patient has excessive length of the hip abductors, he or she should begin with the upper leg supported on a pillow between the knees and only lower the leg to the pillow so that the hip abductors are not allowed to assume a lengthened position.
- Women are more likely to have excessive length of the hip abductors because of their wide pelvis and habit of sleeping on the side with the upper hip flexed and adducted. This sleeping position should be corrected with a pillow between the legs and a folded towel under the waist.

TENSOR FASCIA LATA—(ILIOTIBIAL BAND STRETCH) REMOVE THE PARENTHESES
Purpose
To stretch lateral structures of the hip

Correct Performance
- The patient assumes a position with the trunk and pelvis perpendicular to the table and the pelvis in neutral tilt. The hip and the knee of the bottom lower extremity should be flexed. The hip of the top lower extremity should be extended, and the knee should be flexed about 20 degrees. In some patients the exercise is more effective if the knee is flexed to 90 degrees than when it is flexed to 20 degrees.
- The patient laterally rotates and slightly abducts and extends the hip of the upper leg. While maintaining the hip in lateral rotation and extension, the patient allows the top lower extremity to adduct toward the table. The patient allows the leg to hang unsupported for at least 10 to 15 seconds. The pelvis must not laterally tilt, and the hip must not flex.
- The leg is returned to the starting position.

Special Considerations
If the patient has knee joint instability, the knee should be completely extended when performing this exercise.

Hip Adduction for Strengthening
Purposes
- To strengthen the hip adductor muscles
- To stretch the iliotibial band

Correct Performance
- The patient assumes a position with the trunk and pelvis perpendicular to the supporting surface. The hip and knee of the bottom lower extremity are extended while the hip of the upper leg is flexed and laterally rotated. The knee is flexed so that the foot can rest on the supporting surface.
- The patient adducts the lower leg as high as possible without allowing the pelvis to move. The position of adduction is held for 3 to 5 seconds, and then the leg is returned to the starting position to repeat the exercise.

Special Considerations
Another position for this exercise is to maintain the top lower extremity in hip and knee extension. In this position, the hip abductors of the top leg will also be contracting while the patient adducts the lower leg.

Side-Lying Exercises (Upper Extremity)
Shoulder Flexion, Lateral Rotation, and Scapular Adduction
SHOULDER FLEXION
Purpose
To strengthen weak shoulder flexors in a gravity-lessened position

Correct Performance
- The patient assumes a side-lying position with the hips and knees flexed and the trunk perpendicular to the supporting surface. Pillows are placed in front of the patient's chest so that the patient's arm and forearm can rest on the pillows with the elbow at shoulder height.
- The patient rests the upper extremity on the pillows with the elbow flexed. The patient flexes the shoulder by sliding his or her arm over his or her head and extending the elbow as the shoulder is flexed.
- The patient holds this position for 5 to 10 seconds before returning to the starting position.

Special Considerations
- The patient should also "think about" upwardly rotating the scapula during the motion.

- The patient should avoid excessive scapular elevation during the flexion motion.

SCAPULAR ADDUCTION (TRAPEZIUS MUSCLE EXERCISE)

Purpose

To improve the performance of the middle and lower trapezius muscles

Correct Performance

- In the side-lying position, the patient's hips and knees are flexed and the trunk is perpendicular to the supporting surface. Pillows are placed in front of the patient's chest so that the patient's arm and forearm can rest on the pillows. The shoulder should be flexed about 120 degrees and the elbow about 20 degrees.
- The patient upwardly rotates and adducts the scapula. He or she initiates the motion with upward rotation. The second phase of the motion is scapular adduction.

Special Considerations

The most common substitution for scapular adduction is depression of the scapula using the latissimus dorsi muscle.

SHOULDER ROTATION

Purpose

To provide resistive exercise to the shoulder lateral rotator muscles when the patient is unable to abduct the shoulder sufficiently (90 degrees) to perform rotation exercises comfortably in the prone position

Correct Performance

- The patient assumes a side-lying position with the hips and knees flexed and the trunk perpendicular to the supporting surface. Pillows are placed in front of the patient's chest so that the patient's forearm can rest on the pillows.
- The patient's arm is resting on the lateral side of the thorax, and the elbow is flexed to 90 degrees with the forearm pronated so that the palm faces the pillow. The patient laterally rotates the shoulder by lifting his or her hand off the pillow.
- At the end of his or her active range, the patient maintains the position for 5 to 10 seconds and returns the arm to the pillow.

Special Considerations

The patient should not move the scapula but should move the arm as though there is an axle running through the longitudinal axis of the humerus. The tendency is to adduct the scapula rather than laterally rotating the humerus.

Scapular Abduction and Upward Rotation

Purpose

To improve the motion of the scapulae when performing shoulder joint motions

Correct Performance

- The patient assumes a side-lying position with the hips and knees flexed and the trunk perpendicular to the supporting surface. Pillows are placed in front of the patient's chest so that the patient's arm and forearm can rest on the pillows with the elbow at shoulder height.
- The shoulder is positioned in approximately 100 degrees of flexion with the elbow flexed about 45 degrees. The patient emphasizes abducting and upwardly rotating the scapula while performing shoulder flexion by sliding the arm along the pillows. The emphasis should be placed on the scapular motion, and minimal emphasis should be placed on the completion of glenohumeral flexion.

Special Considerations

The therapist ensures that the patient does not abduct without upwardly rotating the scapula. The emphasis of this exercise is to improve the performance of the serratus anterior muscle.

Prone Exercises (Lower Extremity)

Knee Flexion

Purposes

- To stretch the rectus femoris and the tensor fascia lata muscles
- To prevent compensatory motion of the pelvis and spine during stretching of the rectus femoris and tensor fascia lata muscles
- To improve the performance of the abdominal muscles in providing isometric control of the pelvis

Correct Performance

- The patient assumes a prone position with the hips extended and in neutral abduction/adduction and rotation. The knees are extended. The upper extremities can be positioned in any comfortable position.
- The patient contracts the abdominal muscles and flexes one knee as far as possible while keeping the pelvis and thigh stationary. The patient can monitor the degree of pelvic motion by either placing the hands on the buttocks or the finger tips under the ASIS.
- If the patient is unable to prevent the pelvic motion while contracting the abdominal muscles,

he or she should stop the knee flexion at that point. Another alternative is to place a pillow under the patient's abdomen but not under the hip joints.

- The patient returns the leg to the starting position of knee extension and performs the same exercise with the other leg. The exercise is repeated, alternating legs.

Special Considerations

- In patients with shortness or stiffness of the tensor fascia lata muscle and iliotibial band, pelvic motion can be prevented by placing the limb in 15 to 20 degrees of hip abduction before starting the knee flexion motion.
- If the tibia laterally rotates during knee flexion, the patient can medially rotate the tibia during flexion or flex both knees at the same time while keeping both knees and ankles together to decrease the tibial rotation.

Hip Rotation

Purposes

- To stretch the hip rotator muscles
- To train the patient to rotate the thigh at the hip joint without allowing the pelvis to move

Correct Performance

- The patient lies prone with hips and knees extended and hips in neutral rotation, neutral abduction, and adduction. A small pillow may be used under the patient's waistline (but not hips) if the prone position causes an increase in the patient's symptoms or if excessive lumbar extension is noted.
- The patient contacts the abdominal muscles and flexes one knee. While keeping the pelvis still, the patient rotates the hip laterally and then medially. If the range is limited, the patient holds the position for 5 to 10 seconds and then returns the leg to the midline. The exercise is performed in the same manner with the opposite leg.
- While performing the rotation motion with the hip, the patient monitors the pelvis to prevent motion. The patient can do this by either placing both hands on the buttocks or with the finger tips of both hands placed beneath the ASIS. If the patient feels motion of the pelvis while rotating the thigh, he or she can attempt to control the pelvis by contracting the abdominal muscles.

Special Considerations

- If lateral rotation of the tibia occurs during hip lateral rotation, the patient should rotate the foot medially (tibial medial rotation) while performing the hip motion. The tibial rotation is caused by

tightness of the tensor fascia lata-iliotibial band (TFL-ITB) and excessive flexibility of the knee joint.

- If the knee is unstable and marked movement of the tibia is noted, this exercise may be contraindicated because the movement may be a lateral glide of the tibia on the femur.
- If the greater trochanter makes a large excursion during hip lateral rotation, the therapist can control it by placing a hand on the thigh below the buttock and restricting the motion of the greater trochanter. This faulty pattern of femoral motion is believed to be the hip flexing secondary to the shortness of the TFL-ITB.
- If the patient has hip antetorsion or retrotorsion, the therapist may only recommend one direction of rotation.

Hip Extension With Knee Extended

Purposes

- To strengthen the gluteus maximus and hamstring muscles
- To train the patient to initiate the motion with the gluteus maximus muscle and increase its participation while decreasing the use of the hamstrings during hip extension
- To improve the control of the proximal femur so that the greater trochanter maintains a constant position and does not move excessively in an anterior glide during extension
- To stretch the iliopsoas muscle

Correct Performance

- The patient assumes a prone position with hips and knees extended. The hips are in neutral rotation and neutral abduction/adduction. A small pillow may be used under the waistline (but not hips) if the prone position increases the patient's symptoms or if there is excessive lumbar extension.
- The patient extends and slightly lateral rotates the hip while maintaining knee extension. The patient should "think about" contracting the gluteus maximus muscle to initiate the motion. The pelvis should remain in contact with the table. The hip extension range is only 10 degrees.
- The patient monitors the position of the pelvis by placing both hands on the buttocks or with the fingertips of both hands under the ASIS. If pelvic tilt or rotation is felt, the patient contracts the abdominal muscles before extending the hip to prevent pelvic motion.
- The patient holds the leg in extension for 3 to 5 seconds and slowly returns the leg to the table and performs the exercise with the opposite leg. The exercise is repeated, alternating legs.

Special Considerations

- If the patient is in hip extension while standing, the therapist should use a pillow under the abdomen to allow the hip to be more flexed. The patient should not extend the hip more than 10 degrees.
- The patient must not substitute lumbar extension for hip extension.
- Contraction of the gluteus maximus muscle should occur before or simultaneously with the hamstring contraction.
- If the greater trochanter moves anteriorly during hip extension, the patient should laterally rotate the hip by contracting the gluteal muscles before initiating the extension movement.

Hip Extension With Knee Flexed

Purposes

- To improve the performance of the gluteus maximus muscle
- To stretch the hip flexor muscles

Correct Performance

- The patient assumes the same starting position described for the previous exercise.
- The patient flexes one knee to approximately 125 degrees. Ideally the patient should be able to relax the hamstrings, and the weight of the leg should keep the knee flexed. The patient then slightly laterally rotates and extends the hip 10 degrees. The patient holds the leg in extension for 5 to 10 seconds and then slowly lowers it to the table. He or she repeats the exercise with the same leg before performing with the other side.
- The patient should be instructed to prevent pelvic motion or hip flexion (pushing into table) with the contralateral limb. The patient should monitor pelvic motion by placing the finger tips of both hands on the ASIS. If pelvic tilt or rotation occurs, the patient contracts the abdominal muscles by "pulling the navel in toward the spine" before initiating hip extension.

Special Considerations

- Because the rectus femoris muscle is maximally stretched in this position, the tendency to extend the lumbar spine during hip extension is increased and thus the patient must be carefully monitored.
- Patients who have anterior pelvic tilt in standing often have difficulty using their gluteus maximus muscles at the end of the range and will readily substitute with lumbar extension at the last phase of the movement. These patients need this exercise because they also do not extend the hip sufficiently on return from forward bending.

- A pillow may be placed under the abdomen, but if that is necessary, this level may be too difficult for the patient.
- If the patient has to contract the hamstrings to keep the knee flexed, he should use a strap around his leg that he can hold with his hand to keep the knee passively flexed.

Hip Abduction

Purposes

- To improve the performance of the gluteus medius and other hip abductor muscles
- To train the patient to move the femur at the hip joint without moving the pelvis or spine

Correct Performance

- The patient assumes a prone position with hips and knees extended and hips in neutral abduction/adduction and rotation.
- The patient abducts the hip by sliding the leg out to the side as far as possible without tilting the pelvis or moving the spine. The patient holds the position for 5 to 10 seconds and then slowly returns the leg to the midline position.
- The patient can monitor the pelvis for movement by placing the hands on the buttocks or the finger tips on the anterior superior spine. The patient repeats the exercise with the other leg and alternates legs when continuing the exercise.

Special Considerations

- Because this is a gravity-lessened exercise, it can be used when the posterior gluteus medius muscle is very weak. Because the patient is prone, he or she uses the extensor hip abductor more than the flexor abductors.
- This exercise is also good for initiating improved use of the hip extensors without the tendency for the patient to extend the lumbar spine, which occurs with hip extension.

Isometric Hip Lateral Rotation With Hips Abducted and Knees Flexed

Purposes

- To improve the performance of the hip lateral rotator muscles
- To assist in shortening elongated hip lateral rotator muscles

Correct Performance

- The patient lies prone with knees flexed and hips abducted and laterally rotated so that the medial borders of both feet touch.
- The patient performs isometric hip lateral rotation by pushing the feet together for 5 to 10 seconds

and then relaxing them. The patient continues to push and relax the legs for the desired number of repetitions and then returns the legs to the extended position on the table.

Special Considerations
It is possible to substitute hip flexion/medial rotation for lateral rotation; therefore the therapist should be sure to observe a change in contour of the gluteal muscles when the patient is performing the isometric contraction. The patient should also be taught to contract the gluteal muscles when performing the exercise.

Isometric Gluteus Maximus Contraction

Purpose
To improve the performance of the gluteus maximus muscles

Correct Performance
Patient lies prone and tightens the buttock muscles. Patient should think about the legs turning outward while contracting the buttock muscles, holding for 5 to 10 seconds.

Special Considerations
If the patient has a flat lumbar spine, this exercise should be used cautiously to avoid contributing to the lumbar flexion.

Prone Exercises (Upper Extremity)

Back Extensor Activation (Shoulder Flexion to Elicit Back Extensor Muscle Activity)

Purpose
To improve the performance of the back extensor muscles

Correct Performance
The patient lies face down on a table so that his or her arm hangs over the edge of the table. The patient flexes his shoulder from 90 to 170 degrees.

Special Considerations
- The patient should avoid back extension motion.
- The patient should avoid any rotation of the spine.
- The shoulder flexion range should not elicit pain on the top of the shoulder.

Shoulder Flexion

Purposes
- To improve the movement of the scapula
- To improve the performance of the serratus anterior muscle

Correct Performance
- Two pillows are placed lengthwise on the table. The patient lies in the prone position on top of the pillows with the lower extremities in extension. The arms are positioned on the table at the sides with the shoulders in extension and the elbows flexed so the forearms rest on the table. Towel rolls may need to be placed under the shoulders to correct positioning of the scapula.
- The patient flexes one shoulder while extending the elbow by sliding the arm up over the head. As the patient advances the arm, he or she is trying to emphasize the abduction and upward rotation of the scapula rather than thinking about lifting the weight of the arm. The patient visualizes a string running from the elbow to the inferior angle of the scapula, pulling the scapula out into abduction as the arm advances. The patient should not focus on achieving maximum shoulder flexion but should concentrate on the movement of the scapula.
- The patient returns the arm to the starting position before repeating the exercise with the opposite arm.

Special Considerations
- This is a gravity-lessened exercise and should be the easiest position for performing scapular motion. Because the weight of the thorax is not resting on the scapula, the scapula should move more easily than if performed in the supine position.
- In this position, the therapist can observe the motion of the scapula to ensure that the desired movement pattern is occurring. The therapist can also assist the scapula if there is resistance to the movement from the rhomboid muscles.

Trapezius Muscle Exercise Progression
LEVEL 1: HANDS ON HEAD
Purpose
To improve the performance of the middle and lower trapezius muscles

Correct Performance
- The patient begins in the prone position with shoulders and elbows flexed and hands on the head. Towel rolls are placed under each shoulder to correct any anterior tilt of the scapulae.
- The patient lifts the arms by adducting the scapulae. The patient should visualize a diagonal movement of the scapulae. The patient should not let the shoulders shrug, and he or she should hold the position for 5 to 10 seconds and then relax.

Special Considerations

The common movement impairments are flexing the humerus without adducting the scapulae and depressing the shoulder girdle with the latissimus dorsi instead of depressing the scapulae with the lower trapezius.

LEVEL 2: SCAPULAR ADDUCTION FROM SHOULDER ABDUCTION WITH ELBOW FLEXED

Purpose

To improve the performance of the middle and the lower trapezius muscles

Correct Performance

- The patient assumes a prone position with the arms overhead and the elbows flexed.
- The patient adducts the scapulae by bringing the shoulder blades toward the spine. If the lower trapezius muscle action is being emphasized, the patient should also be instructed to pull the scapula down and towards the spine. The patient should lift the arm and hand while contracting the trapezius muscle. The hand should remain slightly higher than the elbow to emphasize lateral rotation.

Special Considerations

- The patient should not shrug the shoulder as he or she lifts the arm.
- The scapula should not downwardly rotate, which would suggest rhomboid action.

LEVEL 3: SCAPULAR ADDUCTION FROM SHOULDER ABDUCTION WITH ELBOW EXTENDED

Purpose

To improve the performance of the middle and lower trapezius muscles

Correct Performance

- The patient lies prone with the shoulders abducted to 120 degrees and the elbows extended with the forearms in a neutral position and the thumbs pointing upward.
- The patient adducts the scapulae by bringing the shoulder blades back and down toward the spine while lifting the arms from the table (1 to 2 inches). The patient holds the arms for 5 to 10 seconds and then relaxes and lowers them to the table.
- This exercise can also be performed with one arm at a time as well as with both arms simultaneously.

Special Considerations

- The patient should not elevate (shrug) the shoulder when lifting the arm (upper trapezius substitution).

- The hand should stay higher than the arm.
- There should not be pain in the area of the acromion.
- The patient should not depress the shoulder girdle by substituting the latissimus dorsi for the lower trapezius.

Shoulder Rotation

Purposes

- To improve the performance of the shoulder rotators
- To train the patient to move the humerus without moving the scapula during the appropriate part of the range

LATERAL ROTATION

Correct Performance

- The patient begins in the prone position on a bed or table with the shoulder abducted to 90 degrees, the elbow flexed to 90 degrees, and the forearm hanging over the edge of the table. Folded towels should be placed under the proximal humerus to position the scapula and humerus in correct alignment. The scapula should not be abducted or tilted anteriorly, and the humerus should be in the plane of the scapula.
- The patient slowly laterally rotates the humerus at the glenohumeral joint so that the forearm moves toward his or her head. There should not be any movement of the scapula when the patient rotates the humerus. To assist the patient in isolating humeral movement, he or she is instructed to concentrate on letting the upper arm "turn about a fixed axis" rather than letting the scapula and humerus move together as a unit. The patient holds the motion for 5 to 10 seconds and slowly returns the arm to the starting position.

MEDIAL ROTATION

Correct Performance

- The patient assumes the same position as listed in the previous exercise.
- The patient medially rotates the humerus so that the forearm moves toward the hip. The patient is instructed to do this by letting the humerus "turn about a fixed axis" without any movement of the scapula. The patient holds the maximum range achieved for 5 to 10 seconds and then slowly returns the arm to the neutral position.

Special Considerations

Often the scapulae will abduct and move toward the humerus during lateral rotation because the lateral rotator action is not adequately counterbalanced by the scapular adductor muscles. If the patient reduces the "effort" during lateral rotation, the scapular movement will be diminished.

END-RANGE MEDIAL ROTATION

If improving the performance of the subscapularis muscle is the focus of the exercise, then the most important part of this exercise is the movement at the end of the medial rotation range.

Correct Performance

- Pillows can be placed lengthwise under the patient so that the forearm and hand can be placed on the table when the shoulder is maximally medially rotated with the elbow flexed. Then the patient extends the elbow slightly while maintaining maximum medial rotation. The isometric control of the medial rotators is easier to achieve than the concentric activity.
- The patient can allow the shoulder to laterally rotate a few degrees and then medially rotate and return to the starting position. The patient repeats the exercise as necessary, gradually increasing the lateral and medial rotation ranges.

Quadruped Exercises

Quadruped Rocking

Purposes

- To decrease the compressive forces on the spine in patients with low back pain
- To assist in correcting rotational malalignments of the spine (The lack of compressive forces with symmetric four-point support provided by the quadruped position enables the spine to self-adjust to a more structurally normal alignment. When rocking backward, the slight distraction on the spine and the associated stretch on the erector spinae muscles assist in correction of the alignment.)
- To alleviate low back pain
- To stretch the one-joint hip extensor muscles (gluteus maximus, piriformis, etc.) and to address any differences in the relative stiffness of these muscles compared with the back extensor muscles and their effect on compensatory pelvic and spinal rotation
- To assist in decreasing compensatory flexibility of the lumbar spine associated with hip extensor stiffness or shortness
- To assist in correction of thoracic kyphosis; the lack of compressive forces allows the thoracic spine to reverse its exaggerated flexion curvature

- To shorten and improve the performance of the thoracic back extensors
- To stretch the short extensors of the lumbar spine
- To improve the patient's "sense" of the correct alignment of the trunk
- To improve the performance of the serratus anterior muscle
- To train the patient to perform flexion and extension of the hips without moving the spine
- To improve the posterior glide of the femur in the acetabulum
- To improve the posterior glide of the humeral head
- To increase shoulder flexion range of motion
- To stretch the levator scapulae muscle

Correct Performance

- The patient assumes a comfortable position on the hands and knees. The head should be level with the shoulders, the shoulders should be centered over the hands, the spine should be flat, the hip joints should be centered over the knees, the hip joints should be at 90 degrees, and the ankles should be plantar flexed. The knees should be comfortably apart and in the same plane.
- The therapist corrects the patient's alignment faults. The patient practices assuming the correct pain-free position.
- If the patient has an extension syndrome or pain with contraction of the hip flexors, the patient should push back toward his or her heels with the hands rather than flex the hips to rock backward in order to avoid psoas contraction.
- The patient assumes the correct position and then rocks backward as far as directed. The motion should occur in the hip and shoulder joints only, not the back. The back should remain straight and still. The shoulders should flex as the patient flexes the hips beyond 100 degrees. The patient should stop if he or she experiences pain and return to the starting position.
- The head and neck should not extend when the patient rocks backward. If the head and cervical spine extend during the rocking backward motion, then the patient should pull the chin toward the neck and maintain the contraction of the neck flexors while rocking backward. The extension is the result of levator scapulae shortness. As the scapulae are upwardly rotating, the levator is being stretched bilaterally, which causes cervical and head extension.

Special Considerations

- In the presence of asymmetric stiffness of the hip extensors, the patient may have to laterally rotate and abduct the hip with the stiff muscles so that the pelvis will remain level during the rocking backward movement. With repetitions of the movement, the stiffness should decrease and the hip joint alignment can be repositioned appropriately.

- If the patient has unilateral or bilateral hip ante-torsion and the hips are in the anatomically neutral alignment, the hips may not flex sufficiently to keep the pelvis level. The patient should medially rotate the hip or hips with antetorsion to correct the motion.
- If spinal rotation occurs as the patient begins to flex the hips, this can also be the result of asymmetric stiffness of the hips, which is evident in either pelvic rotation or lateral tilt. The therapist should adjust the patient's hip joint position accordingly. Spinal rotation is the result of asymmetric length of the paraspinal muscles. Often when the patient rocks backward, the rotation increases. The therapist should apply counter pressure to the spine as the patient rocks backward. Repetition of the rocking backward with the counter pressure can correct the asymmetry. The therapist should be sure that the counter pressure is not causing symptoms.
- If the patient has a large abdomen or heavy thighs, he or she will not be able to rock backward as far without compensatory hip and lumbar flexion.
- If the patient with back pain is markedly obese with a very large abdomen, the pendulous abdomen will likely contribute to anterior shear forces in this position and make this exercise contraindicated.
- If the patient has cardiac disease, this position may be too stressful for cardiac output and must be used with caution.
- If the patient has knee dysfunction, the range into hip and knee flexion can be limited.
- Hip joint disease with limited hip flexion will contribute to compensatory pelvic and lumbar rotation. The therapist should limit the excursion to avoid excessive flexibility of the lumbar spine.

ROCKING FORWARD

This exercise is rarely used because of the undesirable stresses associated with end range extension of the lumbar spine.

Purposes

- To improve lumbar flexibility into extension
- To improve the performance of the abdominal muscles
- To improve the performance of the hip flexor muscles

- To improve the performance of the serratus anterior muscles

Correct Performance

- This movement is rarely used.
- The patient begins in the quadruped position as described previously. The patient rocks backward as far as possible and then flexes the shoulders as far as possible so that the arms are maximally stretched in front of the body.
- To rock forward, the patient should keep the elbows straight and rock forward as far as instructed by the therapist. He or she should contract the abdominal muscles while rocking forward.

Special Considerations

- The patient must have good strength and control of the abdominal muscles if he or she is going to rock all the way forward. Look for even distribution of spinal extension. Avoid extension at one or two segments. If the patient's abdominal muscles are weak, he or she may have excessive lumbar extension, particularly at the lumbosacral junction.
- The patient should not rock beyond the point at which the scapulae begin to wing. Winging of the scapulae indicate that the load imposed by the weight of the trunk exceeds the capacity of the serratus to maintain the scapulae against the thorax. Shortness of the scapulohumeral muscles and insufficient counterstabilization by the trapezius and rhomboids also contribute to the winging of the scapula.
- When rocking forward, the patient is probably using the hip flexor muscles to control the rate and degree of hip extension, which may contribute to the pain problem.

Limb Movement in the Quadruped Position

SHOULDER FLEXION

Purposes

- To increase the demands on the abdominal muscles to prevent trunk rotation while the arm is in motion
- To improve the performance of the back extensor muscles
- To improve balance control

Correct Performance

- The patient assumes the quadruped position as described previously. The patient contracts the abdominal muscles by pulling his or her navel toward the spine to prevent rotation of the trunk while flexing his or her humerus with the elbow extended. If the spine starts to rotate immediately upon initiating shoulder flexion, then the patient may have to limit the arm movement to barely lifting his or her hand off the supporting surface by flexing the elbow while contracting the abdominal muscles. This modification should enable the patient to control the associated movement impairment.

- The patient lifts the arm as far towards 170 degrees of shoulder flexion as possible without the occurrence of pain or trunk rotation. This position is held for 5 to 10 seconds, and then the arm is returned to the starting position.
- The patient repeats the exercise, alternating arms.

Special Considerations

- The primary objective is to prevent asymmetric or exaggerated trunk rotation. As mentioned previously, the lever that the patient is lifting can be adjusted by having the patient flex the elbow rather than flex the shoulder to decrease the demands on the abdominal muscles and back extensors. The instructions are based on the patient's ability to control the rotation.
- The back extensor activity should be bilateral or may be slightly greater contralaterally as indicated by change in the muscle contour.
- If the patient flexes the hips more than 90 degrees, he or she will decrease the demands on the abdominal muscles and back extensors. This is another method of adjusting the demands of the exercise or can be a way in which the patient is unaware that he or she is modifying the exercise and decreasing its demands.

HIP EXTENSION
Purposes

- To improve the performance of the abdominal muscles and back extensors in controlling trunk and pelvic rotation
- To improve the performance of the hip extensor muscles of both the weight-bearing limb and the non–weight-bearing limb
- To improve balance control

Correct Performance

HIP EXTENSION WITH KNEE FLEXED. The patient assumes the quadruped position as described previously with the hips slightly adducted so that during single lower limb support there will be less tendency for the pelvis to rotate. The patient contracts his abdominal muscles by pulling his or her navel toward the spine. The patient keeps the knee flexed and extends the hip while maintaining a constant position of the pelvis and spine.

The patient must not extend the spine. The motion must be limited to the hip joint.

HIP AND KNEE EXTENSION. To increase the level of difficulty of the exercise, the patient can extend the knee while extending the hip. The patient holds the final position for 5 to 10 seconds before returning to the starting position and progressing to the other leg.

Special Considerations

As with the other exercises, the purpose of this exercise is for the patient to be able to maintain a constant position of the pelvis and spine during extremity movements. The therapist must determine the appropriate level of difficulty for the patient to achieve this objective. The patient must not extend the lumbar spine so that he or she will avoid end-range extension.

HIP AND KNEE EXTENSION WITH SHOULDER FLEXION
Purposes

- To improve the performance of the abdominal and back extensor muscles
- To improve balance control

Correct Performance

- The patient is instructed to initially contract the abdominal muscles by "pulling the navel in toward the spine" and then flexing one shoulder while keeping the elbow extended. The patient then extends the contralateral hip and knee while maintaining a constant position of the pelvis and spine.
- For a more advanced level of performance, the patient contracts the abdominal muscles and then simultaneously flexes the shoulder and extends the hip and knee.
- The exercise is then performed with the other arm and leg.

Special Considerations

- The patient should be able to perform single limb movements without spinal motion before attempting this exercise.
- The patient must be carefully instructed not to allow pelvic or spinal rotation during the limb movement. Most often patients cannot completely extend the hip without rotating the pelvis.
- Many patients perform this exercise incorrectly because it is commonly used in exercise classes. They must be carefully instructed regarding the correct technique.

Cervical Flexion and Extension
Purposes

- To stretch the neck extensor muscles, including the levator scapulae

- To improve the performance of the neck extensor muscles
- To assist the patient in learning to extend the cervical spine correctly and avoid posterior shear forces
- To assist the patient in learning to reverse the cervical curve for flexion rather than moving excessively at the lower cervical segments
- To learn to move in the correct segments of the cervical spine

Correct Performance

The patient assumes the quadruped position as described previously. With the cervical spine in the normal cervical alignment, the patient is instructed to bring the chin toward the neck to reverse the cervical curvature. The patient holds this position for 5 to 10 seconds and then extends the cervical spine by "thinking about rotating his head about a rod running through the center of his or her head. The therapist is attempting to teach the patient to perform a rotational movement in the sagittal plane." The axis should be in the middle of the cervical vertebrae.

Special Considerations

- In some patients, marked asymmetry may be noted between the muscle bulk on the left and right sides of the cervical spine. Such asymmetry can be associated with swimming strokes performed with consistent head turning to one side only.
- In some patients the levator scapulae muscles may appear prominent in this position. This is interpreted as dominance of the levator scapula as a neck extensor and insufficient participation by the intrinsic neck extensor muscles.
- Some patients will perform extension with excessive movement of the lower cervical segments and insufficient participation of the upper segments.

Cervical Rotation

Purposes

- To improve the performance of the cervical rotator muscles
- To train the patient to rotate the head and neck correctly, about a fixed axis, rather than the combination motions of extension/rotation or lateral flexion/rotation

Correct Performance

The patient assumes the quadruped position as described previously. Starting from the neutral position of the cervical spine, the patient rotates his or her head to one side as far as possible without pain. The patient is instructed to "think about rotating about a rod running longitudinally through the head and neck." The patient

is to avoid any type of twisting motion. He or she should hold the position for 5 to 10 seconds and then rotate to the opposite side.

Special Considerations

The patient should not have any pain in the neck in this position and should stop the motion at the point that he or she experiences pain. The levator scapulae muscles should not appear prominent.

Sitting Exercises

Knee Extension and Ankle Dorsiflexion

Purposes

- To stretch the hamstrings and the calf muscles
- To correct muscle length discrepancies between the medial and lateral hamstring muscles
- To train the patient to control compensatory lumbar flexion and rotation associated with stretch of the hamstrings
- To train the patient to use the anterior tibialis muscle and to avoid use of the extensor digitorum longus, which can become a dominant dorsiflexor of the ankle
- To stretch the peroneal muscles
- To train the patient to avoid inappropriate recruitment of the tensor fascia lata muscles
- To train the patient to avoid excessive recruitment of the hip flexors to maintain the sitting position or during knee extension
- To train the patient to avoid hip medial rotation during knee extension
- To train the patient to avoid inappropriate cocontraction of the quadriceps and hamstring muscles
- To correct faulty lateral glide of the patella
- To improve the performance of the quadriceps and ankle dorsiflexor muscles
- To shorten and improve the performance of the lumbar back extensor muscles
- To train the patient to avoid lateral rotation of the tibia during knee extension

Correct Performance

- The patient assumes a sitting position, preferably in a chair with a straight back. The hip joint is flexed to 90 degrees, the pelvis is vertical, and the lumbar spine is flat.
- The patient slowly extends one knee as far as possible without pain and without posterior tilting or rotation of the pelvis or flexion or rotation of the spine. If sitting with the back supported, he or she can be instructed to extend the upper back against the chair (isometric extension) while extending the knee. The

patient's hip should be maintained in neutral rotation. He or she should not have any contraction of the tensor fascia lata or hamstring muscles. When the knee is at maximum extension, the patient dorsiflexes the ankle, pointing the foot toward the knee. While dorsiflexing the ankle, the patient should avoid leading with the toes or everting the foot. The patient holds the position for 5 to 10 seconds and returns the leg to the starting position.

- The exercise is repeated, alternating the legs.

Special Considerations

- If the medial hamstrings are stiffer than the lateral hamstrings, the patient will medially rotate the hip during knee extension. However, when instructed to maintain neutral rotation, the patient will be able to extend the knee through the full range. If the medial hamstrings are short, the knee extension will be limited when the patient maintains neutral rotation.
- If the patient extends the hip during knee extension, which will be evident by the depression of the thigh into the seat of the chair, he or she is probably co-contracting with the hamstrings. Passive extension of the knee will confirm or refute this hypothesis. If the patient is co-contracting the hamstrings, he or she should make an "easy" effort to extend the knee. A useful verbal cue is to ask the patient to think about "using only two fibers of the quadriceps" to extend the knee. This contraction pattern is often seen in patients who have frequently performed resisted knee extension exercises.
- If the patient displays pelvic or lumbar rotation during knee extension, abducting the hip before beginning the exercise often decreases the compensatory rotation. The stiffness or shortness of the gluteus maximus/iliotibial band is believed to be a contributing factor to this pattern.
- If the patient has patella alta or excessive lateral glide, he or she can stretch the shortened structures by assisting the gliding of the patella as the knee returns from extension to flexion.
- The best way of assessing the rotation of the thigh is by having the therapist place his or her hands on the top of the patient's thigh during knee extension. If the patient medially rotates the hip during knee extension, there are two possible contributing factors: (1) shortness or stiffness of the medial hamstrings and (2) inappropriate recruitment of the tensor fascia lata. The patient will need to decrease the active effort of knee extension to eliminate the tensor fascia lata contraction.
- The patient with hammer toes will most likely initiate ankle dorsiflexion with the toe extensor muscles, and he or she should be trained to move at the ankle and not at the toes. The patient with a pronated foot often everts the foot while dorsiflexing the ankle. If the patient inverts instead of everts, he or she will feel a stretch along the lateral side of the leg because of stretch of the peroneal muscles.
- If the patient has limited ankle dorsiflexion, he or she can use a towel under the ball of the foot and pull on the towel with the hands to passively dorsiflex the ankle.

Hip Flexion

Purposes

- To improve the performance of the iliopsoas muscle
- To increase the range into hip flexion
- To improve the isometric control of trunk rotation by the abdominal muscles, particularly if there is asymmetric strength as seen with scoliosis

Correct Performance

- The patient is seated with the hips at 90 degrees, the spine and pelvis erect, and the arms resting at the sides of the thighs. The patient is instructed to passively flex the hip by lifting the thigh toward the chest with his or her hands while keeping the spine and pelvis motionless. The exercise is performed passively to minimize the recruitment of the tensor fascia lata, sartorius, and rectus femoris muscles. At the end of the range of hip flexion, the patient contracts the hip flexors to maintain the flexion position and releases the hand support of the thigh. He or she tries to maintain the hip in a constant position for 5 to 10 seconds.
- If the patient is able to do this easily, then he or she is instructed to push with his or her hand against the knee, resisting the contraction of the hip flexor muscles for 3 to 5 seconds. The patient should be careful to keep the knee close to the midline and the thigh in neutral hip rotation. In some cases the patient may slightly laterally rotate the hip to further isolate the iliopsoas muscle.
- The patient slowly lowers the leg to the starting position and repeats the exercise, alternating the legs.

Special Considerations

- This exercise is used primarily for patients who have hip pain associated with a weak or long iliopsoas muscle.
- This exercise is much easier to perform if one foot is touching the ground rather than when the patient is sitting on a table with both feet unsupported.

- This exercise requires support from the trunk muscles and can be used as a corrective exercise when there is asymmetric strength, as in patients with scoliosis.
- This exercise should be used with caution in patients with low back pain because of the compressive forces associated with iliopsoas contraction. In the sitting position, the anterior shear forces associated with contraction of the iliopsoas should be less than in the supine position.

Standing Exercises

Shoulder Flexion (Back Against Wall)
Purposes
- To provide an orientation for normal alignment of the head, shoulders, and spine
- To decrease thoracic kyphosis or depressed chest
- To improve the performance of the shoulder flexor, pectoralis major, anterior deltoid, scapulohumeral, serratus anterior, and trapezius muscles
- To improve the control of glenohumeral lateral rotation by the teres minor, infraspinatus, and posterior deltoid muscles
- To stretch the latissimus dorsi muscle
- To improve the performance of the abdominal muscles
- To improve the technique of the return from glenohumeral joint flexion avoiding anterior tilt or abduction of scapula or thoracic flexion

LEVEL 1: ELBOWS FLEXED
Correct Performance
- The patient assumes a position with the back, shoulders, and buttocks against the wall. The head should be in line with the shoulders. To bring the back of the head against the wall, the patient should avoid cervical extension, bring the chin toward the neck, and think about lifting the chest to bring the head and shoulders back to the wall. The feet should be apart with the heels about 3 inches away from the wall. The arms are at the sides with the cubital fossae facing anteriorly and the palms of the hands facing the sides of the body.
- The patient flexes the elbows, maintaining neutral rotation of the shoulder joint, and flexes the shoulders. After reaching 90 degrees of shoulder flexion, the patient extends the elbows while completing the motion of shoulder flexion as far as possible without pain. The patient should not shrug the shoulders (unless specifically instructed to do so) while flexing them, and he or she should try to keep the olecranon pointing anteriorly,

which emphasizes lateral rotation. The patient should not allow the low back to extend. The patient can contract the abdominal muscles before he or she begins the motion to prevent the extension, or he or she can contract them upon completion of maximum shoulder flexion.
- The patient should hold the final position for 5 to 10 seconds and then reverse the movement pattern to return to the starting position. The patient should be careful to not allow the scapulae to tilt anteriorly or to flex the thorax, but he or she should try to move primarily in the glenohumeral joint.

Special Considerations
- Because the elbow flexed position decreases the length of the lever that is being moved, this exercise is preferred if the patient has excessive superior glide of the humerus or inadequate upward rotation of the scapula.
- The patient should stop the motion if he or she feels pain in the area of the acromion. Women 50 years of age and older are especially susceptible to developing impingement pain with this exercise, particularly if they have large breasts, dropped shoulders, and deep indentations on their shoulders from bra straps. The patient can continue to perform the exercise but will need to stop the motion at the onset of pain. The patient should do repetitions of the exercises facing the wall which is more effective in depressing the humeral head during flexion.
- If the patient has a marked thoracic kyphosis, he or she will not be able to place the back of the head against the wall or be able to touch the wall with his or her arms at the completion of shoulder flexion. This patient should be advised that this is not the goal of the exercise in his or her case.
- If the patient has shoulder pain and a depressed chest or a thoracic kyphosis, the patient should attempt to reach the maximum pain-free range of shoulder flexion even though there is associated trunk motion. At the completion of the motion, the patient should contract the abdominal muscles to decrease the compensatory lumbar extension. The action of the external oblique abdominal muscles should be emphasized so that the patient is attempting to flatten the abdomen by narrowing his infrasternal angle and not allowing flexion of the thoracic spine and associated depression of the chest.
- This exercise is also helpful in training the patient to avoid excessive superior glide of the humerus during flexion because a limited portion of the deltoid is participating. In contrast, when the patient

performs abduction the entire deltoid muscle is participating, therefore markedly increasing the superior glide forces acting on the humerus.

LEVEL 2: ELBOWS EXTENDED
Correct Performance
Starting from the position described in Level 1, the patient flexes the shoulders while maintaining elbow extension. While attempting to achieve the maximum pain-free range of flexion, the patient keeps the eyes level, avoiding cervical extension or tilting the head backward. The patient maintains this position for 5 to 10 seconds while contracting the abdominal muscles and tries to flatten the back against the wall. The patient extends the shoulders slowly, lowering the arms to the sides, being careful to keep the shoulders against the wall.

Special Considerations
This exercise is a progression of the Level 1 exercise because the extended elbow position increases the length of the lever that is being moved and increases the demands on the shoulder girdle muscles. The patient should be able to perform the previous level in an optimal manner before progressing to this exercise.

Shoulder Abduction (Back Against Wall)
Purposes
- To provide an orientation for normal alignment of the head, shoulders, and spine
- To decrease a thoracic kyphosis or depressed chest
- To lengthen the pectoralis major muscle
- To improve the performance of the trapezius muscle
- To train the patient to move the humerus without associated movement of the scapula and thorax during the return to neutral from shoulder flexion/ abduction

Correct Performance
- The patient assumes a position with the back, head, shoulders, and buttocks against the wall. The feet should be apart with the heels about 3 inches from the wall. The arms are at the side with the cubital fossae facing anteriorly and the palms of the hands facing the sides of the body.
- The patient flexes the elbows and then flexes and abducts the shoulders (diagonal movement) to 90 degrees of abduction with the elbows flexed. The scapulae and arms should be in contact with the wall. The patient slowly extends the elbows and elevates the shoulder by sliding the arms over his or her head. The patient keeps the arms in contact

with the wall while achieving the maximum range of elevation. The patient holds this position for 5 to 10 seconds while contracting the abdominal muscles, pulling the abdomen up and in so that the back flattens against the wall. The patient reverses the movement to return to the starting position of the arms at the sides.

Special Considerations
- If the patient has a thoracic kyphosis, he or she will not be able to get the arms back to the wall and should be advised not to extend the back to attempt to do so.
- If the patient has shortness of the pectoralis major or minor muscles, he or she may need to practice the movement of assuming the correct starting position of 90 degrees of abduction with the elbows flexed. The patient should try to have his or her shoulders stretch as broad as possible. Until this position can be assumed easily, the patient should not attempt to increase the degrees of abduction.
- If the patient experiences pain in the shoulder joint while attempting to achieve the position of 90 degrees of abduction, he or she can actively adduct the scapulae while moving the arms, which often alleviates this problem because it alleviates the impingement of the humerus on the posterior aspect of the glenoid.
- The therapist should monitor the patient's glenohumeral joint to ensure that the humerus does not glide superiorly during the motion. If the humerus fails to maintain a constant axis of rotation, the therapist should suspect over-pull by the deltoid or shortness of the scapulohumeral capsular muscles.

Shoulder Flexion (Other Than Back Against Wall)
Three methods are described that address different performance problems and in some situations are part of a progression to improve range of motion or control of scapular and glenohumeral motions.
Purposes
- To increase the range of shoulder flexion
- To improve the performance of the serratus anterior muscle
- To improve the performance of the shoulder flexor muscles
- To reduce compensatory elevation of the shoulder girdle during shoulder flexion
- To encourage depression of the head of the humerus during shoulder flexion

FACING WALL

This method is best suited for improving the mobility of the glenohumeral joint when the patient has restricted range of motion or excessive humeral superior glide. Another indication is marked weakness of the shoulder flexor muscles, such as with rotator cuff tears.

Correct Performance

- The patient stands close to the wall with the feet comfortably apart. The shoulders are in a neutral position and the elbows are flexed with the ulnar side of the forearms and hands against the wall.
- With the ulnar border of his hands against the wall, the patient flexes the shoulders by sliding the hands along the wall. The patient should exert some pressure against the wall with the hands to create a force of depression and posterior glide at the humeral heads. The humerus should not medially rotate during the flexion motion. The patient should stop the motion when he or she experiences pain in the region of the acromion. The exercise is performed with one arm in the presence of a primary glenohumeral dysfunction and bilaterally if scapular dysfunction is the primary problem. The final position should be held for 5 to 10 seconds before reversing the movement to return to the starting position.

Special Considerations

- If the patient has pain during active shoulder flexion, then he or she can use the contralateral hand to passively flex the shoulder while leaning into the wall, putting pressure against the hand of the painful shoulder to depress and posteriorly glide the humeral head.
- If the humerus medially rotates during flexion, the patient can use the contralateral hand at the lateral aspect of the olecranon to direct the elbow medially to maintain humeral lateral rotation and to prevent abduction.
- If the patient has marked weakness of the rotator cuff muscles, then he or she can use the contralateral hand to assist the shoulder flexion motion. If the complete range can be achieved, the patient can then lift the hand away from the wall, hold the arm in the vertical position, and lower the arm by sliding it back down the wall. This procedure uses the mechanical advantage of not having to lift the weight of the arm, because the vertical position reduces the weight of the extremity, and using eccentric contraction, which requires less development of active muscle tension to control the extremity.

- To emphasize the performance of the serratus anterior muscle, the patient should be instructed in how to "think about" abducting and upwardly rotating the scapula as the shoulder is flexed. The patient should not be concerned as much with the range of shoulder flexion as with the motion of the scapula. The therapist can assist the scapular motion passively, which also provides an indication of the resistance to scapular upward rotation from muscles such as the rhomboids.

STANDING IN DOORWAY

This method is used to increase the range of shoulder flexion motion.

Correct Performance

The patient stands in a doorway so that his or her body is slightly forward of the doorway and the elbow is in full flexion with the forearm and hand resting against the door frame. The patient flexes the shoulder by sliding the ulnar side of the forearm up the door frame. The patient should push his or her hand into the door frame while sliding the hand up the door frame into full shoulder flexion and elbow extension. The position of the body forward of the shoulder and the resistance of the surface assists the patient in depressing and posteriorly gliding the humeral head and thus achieving the full range of shoulder flexion.

Special Considerations

- If necessary, the patient can assist with the contralateral hand.
- The patient should not shrug the shoulder unless he or she has a depressed shoulder and the therapist is attempting to improve the performance of the upper trapezius muscle.

SIDE OF BODY AGAINST WALL

This method is used to assist the patient in maintaining or regaining range of motion through lateral rotation range of motion that has been compromised by rotator cuff dysfunction or capsular restriction.

Correct Performance

The patient stands with one side of the body close to the wall and has the shoulder in lateral rotation with the elbow fully flexed and the dorsal aspect of the forearm and hand against the wall. The patient slides the arm up the wall into flexion with elbow extension. This positioning assists the patient in maintaining shoulder lateral rotation throughout the movement.

Special Considerations

The degree of lateral rotation range that is imposed on the shoulder can be gauged by the distance that the patient stands away from the wall.

Shoulder Abduction (Facing Wall and Trapezius Exercises)

Purposes

- To improve the performance of the upper trapezius muscle
- To improve the performance of the lower trapezius muscle
- To increase the range of scapular upward rotation
- To improve the control of humeral lateral rotation

Correct Performance

- *Trapezius.* The patient stands close to and facing the wall. The elbows should be flexed with the arms at the side of the body rather than in front of the body. The position requires lateral rotation of the humerus and adduction of the scapulae. The ulnar side of the forearm and hand should be against the wall.
- *Upper trapezius.* The patient is instructed to abduct the shoulders by sliding the forearms and hands up the wall. The motion follows the path of a diagonal. When the shoulders are abducted to 90 degrees, the patient should shrug his or her shoulders (bring the acromions toward the ears) while continuing the abduction/elevation motion. The shrugging motion is used to elicit activity of the upper trapezius. At the completion of the abduction motion, the patient should lift the hands off the wall by adducting the scapulae. The patient should hold this position for 5 to 10 seconds.
- *Lower trapezius.* The patient is instructed to abduct the shoulders by sliding the forearms and hands up the wall until he or she reaches a diagonally overhead position. The patient then lifts the hands off the wall by adducting and depressing the scapulae. He or she should hold this position for 5 to 10 seconds and then reverse the motion to return to the starting position. The patient can also return the hands to the wall while maintaining the abducted/elevated shoulder position and then repeat the scapular motion of adduction and depression.

Special Considerations

- The therapist should ensure that the patient is adducting the scapula and not just moving at the glenohumeral joint or depressing the shoulder girdle with the latissimus dorsi muscle.

- The patient can also be instructed to adduct the scapulae without the depression component if the shoulders are not posturally elevated.

Walking Exercises

Control of Hip and Knee Medial Rotation

LIMITING PELVIC ROTATION

Purposes

- To prevent excessive rotation of the pelvis and lumbar spine
- To improve control by the abdominal muscles of the rotation of the pelvis and spine

Correct Performance

- The patient begins with an erect standing posture, looking straight ahead with the feet pointing slightly outward.
- The patient is instructed to contract the abdominal muscles by "pulling the navel in toward the spine." The patient may also place the hands on the iliac crests to monitor the movements of the pelvis. The patient then practices walking while trying to prevent pelvic rotation. Often it is necessary for the patient to take smaller steps, particularly if the hip flexors are short and the abdominal muscles are weak.

Special Considerations

The patient should not perform bilateral contraction of the gluteal muscles to posteriorly tilt the pelvis because this limits the ability to flex the hip.

LIMITING HIP MEDIAL ROTATION

Purposes

- To prevent excessive hip medial rotation during the stance phase of gait
- To prevent excessive medial rotation at the knee during stance phase of gait
- To prevent excessive ankle pronation associated with excessive hip medial rotation

Correct Performance

- The patient begins with an erect standing posture, looking straight ahead with the feet pointing slightly outward.
- At heel strike of the affected extremity, the patient is instructed to contract the gluteal muscle to prevent excessive hip medial rotation.

Special Considerations

The patient should not hyperextend the knee at heel strike, but he or she should allow the normal knee flexion to occur. As the body moves over the foot, the knee should extend.

Limiting Hip Adduction

Purposes
- To prevent excessive hip adduction during the stance phase of gait
- To prevent lateral trunk flexion associated with a weak gluteus medius muscle
- To improve the performance of the gluteus medius muscle

Correct Performance
- The patient begins with an erect standing posture, looking straight ahead with the feet pointing slightly outward.
- At heel strike the patient contracts the gluteal muscles, avoiding lateral trunk flexion to the same side, and maintains the contraction throughout the entire stance phase.

Special Considerations
- Lateral trunk flexion to the stance side is considered a sign of greater weakness of the gluteus medius muscle than hip adduction (drop). In this case, the patient may need a cane.
- The broader shoulders of men make it possible to have only a slight amount of lateral trunk flexion that alleviates the load on the hip abductors. This must be carefully observed by the physical therapist.

Preventing Knee Hyperextension

Purposes
- To prevent hyperextension of the knee in order to reduce the strain on the posterior knee joint
- To reduce the stress at the hip joint associated with the knee hyperextension
- To improve the performance of the quadriceps muscles

Correct Performance
- The patient begins with an erect standing posture, looking straight ahead with the feet pointing slightly outward.
- At heel strike the patient is instructed not to let the knee hyperextend. As the patient brings the body forward into midstance, he or she pushes the ball of the foot into the floor to increase the use of the plantar flexor muscles.

Special Considerations
The plantar flexor muscles assist in controlling the advance of the tibia during heel strike to midstance. Often the use of the plantar flexor muscles aids the control at the knee and helps to prevent the hyperextension at the knee. The timing is important because if the patient contracts his plantar flexor muscles too early, it will contribute to the hyperextension.

Limiting Knee Rotation

Purpose
To teach the patient to be aware of and to control the position of the knee when his or her weight is shifted onto the stance leg

Correct Performance
- The patient begins with an erect standing posture, looking straight ahead with the feet pointing slightly outward.
- The patient steps forward with the foot slightly turned outward. As the patient sets the heel down, he or she contracts the gluteal muscles to prevent medial rotation or hyperextension of the knee. As the patient shifts his or her weight forward and rolls over the foot, he or she needs to press the ball of the foot into the floor. The knee should be in slight flexion at heel contact and pointing straight ahead as the shift occurs. The knee then extends as the body moves forward over the foot and the gait progresses from heel contact to foot flat.

Special Considerations
- Some medial rotation of the hip and knee is normal. Excessive rotation is important to identify.
- The therapist should differentiate between medial rotation of the entire lower extremity when the femur and tibia maintain a relatively constant relationship and when the femur is rotating excessively with respect to the tibia.
- Hip antetorsion contributes to the appearance of excessive hip medial rotation. This is a structural factor and should not be considered a dysfunctional position.

Ankle Plantar Flexion

Purposes
- To correct the lack of participation of the plantar flexor muscles during the heel strike to the foot flat phase of gait
- To correct the lack of participation of the plantar flexor muscles during the foot flat to toe off phase of gait

Correct Performance
- The patient begins with an erect standing posture, looking straight ahead with the feet pointing slightly outward.

- At heel strike the patient thinks about pushing back on the floor to control the advance of the knee. From foot flat to toe off the patient contracts the plantar flexors to push the ball of the foot into the floor and lifts the heel.

Special Considerations

- Patients with knee pain often can be helped by increasing plantar flexor activity from heel strike to foot flat.

- Patients who look like they have a shuffling gait often will benefit from instruction in increasing their push-off.
- Patients with Achilles tendonitis also often need instruction in correct push-off. If the forefoot flexors are particularly strong and calf muscles test weak, the patient should be instructed to "lift the heels" and not to "go up on the toes."

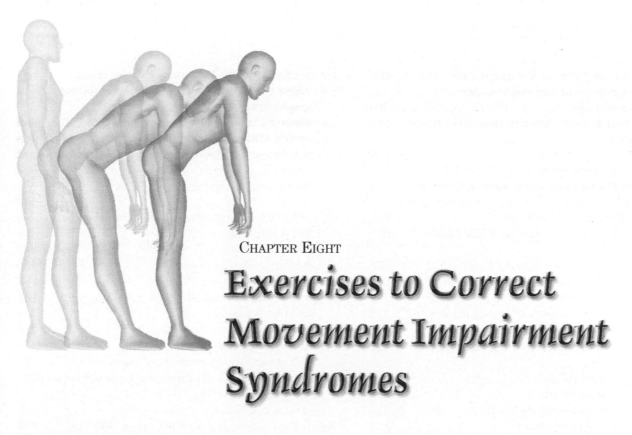

CHAPTER EIGHT

Exercises to Correct Movement Impairment Syndromes

Forward Bending: Hip Flexion With Flat Lumbar Spine   **403**
    Level 1: With hand support   403
    Level 2: Without hand support   403
Forward Bending With Spinal and Hip Flexion   **404**
Lateral Spinal Flexion—Side-Bending Position   **404**
Single-Leg Stance: Unilateral Hip and Knee Flexion   **405**
Hip and Knee Extension With Contralateral Hip and Knee Maximally Flexed   **406**
Hip and Knee Extension From Hip and Knee Flexion   **407**
Hip and Knee Flexion From Passive and Active Hip and Knee Extension   **408**
Hip and Knee Flexion With Sliding Heel From Hip and Knee Extension   **409**
Lower Abdominal Progression—Unilateral Hip Flexion   **409**
    Level 0.3: Lift one foot with alternate foot on floor   409
Lower Abdominal Progression—Hip and Knee Held to Chest During Hip Flexion   **410**
    Level 0.4: Hold knee to chest and lift the alternate foot   410
    Level 0.5: Lightly hold one knee toward chest and lift the alternate foot   410
Lower Abdominal Progression—Hip and Knee Flexion With Alternate Foot Unsupported   **411**
    Level 1A: Hip flexed to greater than 90 degrees and the alternate foot lifted   411

    Level 1B: Hip flexed to 90 degrees and lift the alternate foot   411
Lower Abdominal Progression—Hip and Knee Extension   **411**
Lower Abdominal Progression—Hip and Knee Extension   **412**
    Level 2: One hip flexed to 90 degrees, the alternate foot lifted and slid to extend the hip and knee   413
    Level 3: One hip flexed to 90 degrees, foot lifted and then extend without the leg touching the supporting surface   413
Lower Abdominal Progression: Bilateral Hip and Knee Flexion   **413**
    Level 4: Slide both feet along the supporting surface into extension and return to flexion   413
    Level 5: Lift both feet off the supporting surface; with hips flexed to 90 degrees, extend the knees and lower both lower extremities to the supporting surface   413
Upper Abdominal Progression: Trunk Curl–Sit Up   **414**
    Level 1A: Trunk curl: spinal flexion (easiest)   414
    Level 1B: Trunk curl–sit up: spinal and hip flexion (least difficult)   414
    Level 2: Trunk curl–sit up: spinal and hip flexion (difficult)   414
    Level 3: Trunk curl–sit up: spinal and hip flexion (most difficult)   414
Hip Abduction–Lateral Rotation From Flexion Position: Bent Knee Fallouts   **415**
    Level 1   415

Hip Abduction–Lateral Rotation From Flexion Position: Knee Extended   416
   Level 2 (difficult)   416
Straight-Leg Raises: Hip Flexion With Knee Extended   417
Two-Joint Hip Flexor Stretch   418
Shoulder Flexion—Elevation With Elbow Extended and Latissimus Dorsi Muscle Stretch   419
Shoulder Flexion/Abduction   420
Shoulder Flexion—Elevation With Elbow Flexed   420
Shoulder Abduction—Gravity Lessened   421
Shoulder Rotation—Supine Horizontal Adduction (Flexion)   422
   Medial rotation—stretch of lateral rotator muscles   422
   Lateral rotation—stretch of medial rotator muscles   422
   Horizontal adduction   422
Pectoralis Minor Stretch   423
   Assisted stretch—lying on back   423
   Self stretch—lying on back   423
   Assisted stretch—lying face down   423
Hip Lateral Rotation—Side-Lying Position   424
Hip Abduction With and Without Lateral Rotation—Side-Lying Position   425
   Level 1: Hip abduction with lateral rotation   425
   Level 2: Hip abduction with lateral rotation   425
   Level 3: Hip abduction   426
   Tensor fascia lata–iliotibial band stretch   426
Hip Adduction for Strengthening—Side-Lying Position   426
Shoulder Flexion, Lateral Rotation, and Scapular Adduction—Side-Lying Position   427
   Shoulder flexion   427
   Scapular adduction (trapezius muscle exercise)   427
   Shoulder rotation   427
Knee Flexion—Face-Lying Position   428
Hip Rotation—Face-Lying Position   429
Hip Extension With Knee Extended—Face-Lying Position   430
Hip Extension With Knee Flexed—Face-Lying Position   431
Hip Abduction—Face-Lying Position   432
Isometric Hip Lateral Rotation With Hips Abducted and Knees Flexed   433

Isometric Gluteus Maximus Contraction   433
Shoulder Flexion to Elicit Back Extensor Muscle Activity—Face-Lying Position   434
Shoulder Flexion—Face-Lying Position   434
Trapezius Muscle Exercise Progression—Face-Lying Position   435
   Level 1   435
   Level 2   435
   Level 3   435
Shoulder Rotation—Face-Lying Position   436
   Lateral Rotation   436
   Medial Rotation   436
   End-Range Medial Rotation   436
Rocking—Quadruped Position   437
Limb Movement—Quadruped Position   438
   Shoulder flexion   438
   Hip extension with knee flexion   438
   Hip and knee extension   438
   Hip/knee extension with shoulder flexion   438
Head and Cervical Flexion and Extension—Quadruped Position   439
   Cervical rotation   439
Knee Extension and Dorsiflexion—Sitting Position   440
Hip Flexion—Sitting Position   441
Shoulder Flexion—Standing With Back Against the Wall   442
   Shoulder flexion with elbow flexion   442
   Shoulder flexion with elbow extension   442
Shoulder Abduction—Standing With Back Against the Wall   443
Shoulder Flexion—Standing Facing Wall   444
   Facing wall   444
   Standing in doorway   444
   Standing with side of body against wall   444
Shoulder Abduction—Standing Facing Wall—Trapezius Exercises   445
   Upper trapezius   445
   Trapezius   445
   Lower trapezius   445
Control of Hip and Knee Medial Rotation During Walking   446
Preventing Knee Hyperextension During Walking   447
Ankle Plantar Flexion   447

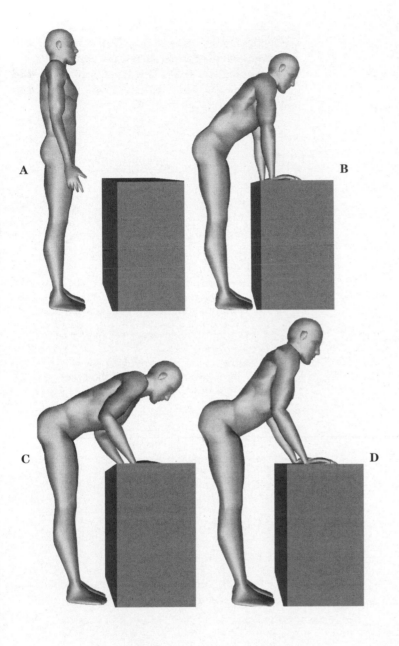

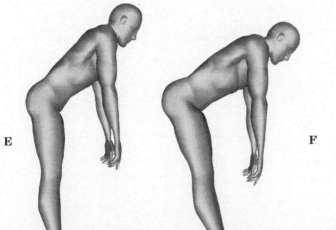

Forward Bending: Hip Flexion With Flat Lumbar Spine (Figures A-F)

Purposes:
- To decrease low back flexibility
- To increase hip joint flexibility
- To improve ability to move in hips without excessive bending of the lumbar spine
- To improve the performance of the gluteal muscles

Starting position: Stand with feet spaced comfortably apart.

Level 1: **With hand support** *(see Figures A-D)*

Method: ❑ Perform variation if box is checked

Down
Place your hands on a table
Try to put the weight of your upper body on your hands
Bend in the hip joints; "think about sticking your seat out"
Do not bend your back
Do not arch your back (see *incorrect* posture in Figure D)
❑ Bend in the knee joints
Let your elbows bend
Bend as far as possible or STOP if pain is experienced

Return
Tighten your buttocks muscles
Move in your hips throughout the return to an erect position
Avoid swaying pelvis forward

Repetitions: _____

Level 2: **Without hand support** *(see Figures E-F)*

Reach toward the floor with your hands as you bend forward in the hip joints
Continue as instructed in "Level 1: With hand support"

Repetitions: _____

Copyright © 2002 by Mosby, Inc. May be copied for patient use only.

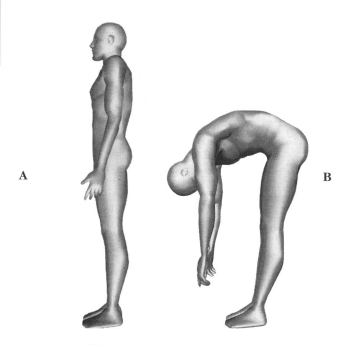

A　　B

Forward Bending With Spinal and Hip Flexion (Figures A-B)

Purposes: • To increase thoracic or lumbar flexibility
• To improve the performance of the gluteal muscles

Starting position: Stand with feet spaced comfortably apart.

Method: ❏ Perform variation if box is checked

❏ Let your upper and lower back bend as you bend forward
❏ Try to bend in just your low back as you bend forward
❏ Contract your abdominal muscles as you bend forward
　 Return by contracting the gluteal muscles
　 Move in the hip joints and move throughout the return to the erect position

Repetitions: _____

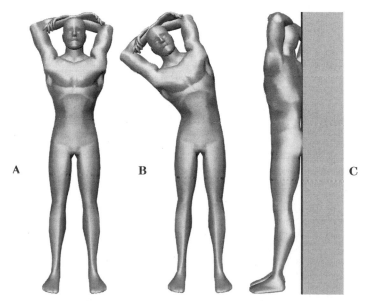

A　　　B　　　C

Lateral Spinal Flexion — Side-Bending Position (Figures A-C)

Purposes: • To increase the flexibility of the paraspinal muscles
• To increase the flexibility of the abdominal muscles
• To decrease the excessive flexibility of some spinal segments

Starting position: Stand with both feet spaced comfortably apart. Raise arms overhead and clasp hands together.

Method: ❏ Perform variation if box is checked

　 Stand with your back against a wall to avoid rotating
　 Place your hands on the top of your head (see Figure A)
　 Lean to the side (see Figure B)
　 Think about TILTING your shoulders rather than moving from your waist; STOP if pain is experienced
　 Return to an erect standing position
❏ Take a deep breath and lift your chest
❏ Place your hand on your side at waist level and continue as before

Repetitions: _____

Copyright © 2002 by Mosby, Inc. May be copied for patient use only.

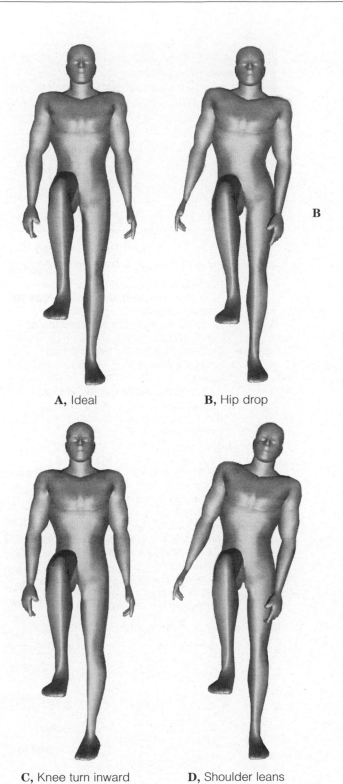

A, Ideal   **B,** Hip drop

B

C, Knee turn inward   **D,** Shoulder leans

Single-Leg Stance: Unilateral Hip and Knee Flexion (Figures A-D)

Purposes: • To improve the performance of the gluteal hip muscles
• To improve the isometric control by the abdominal muscles
• To prevent compensatory movements of the hip, pelvis, and spine
• To prevent the thigh from turning inward

Starting position: Stand with both feet relatively close together to keep from shifting to the side of the stance leg.

Method: ❏ Perform variation if box is checked

Shift your weight to stance leg
Tighten your buttock muscle on the side of your stance leg
Lift your alternate thigh in front of your body while bending your knee
❏ Contract your abdominal muscles
❏ Keep your pelvis level
❏ Place your hands on your pelvis to monitor your movement
❏ Do not let your opposite hip drop (see Figure B)
❏ Do not let your knee turn inward (see Figure C)
❏ Do not let your shoulders lean to the side (see Figure D); keep your trunk still
❏ Do not let your ankle pronate (i.e., arch collapsed or turned in)

Repetitions: _____

Copyright © 2002 by Mosby, Inc. May be copied for patient use only.

Hip and Knee Extension With Contralateral Hip and Knee Maximally Flexed (Figures A-C)

Purposes:
- To stretch the hip flexor muscles
- To improve the control of the pelvis by the abdominal muscles

Starting position: Bend hips and knees; feet are on the floor.

A

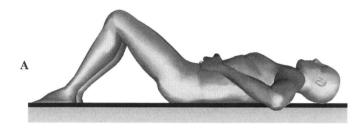

B

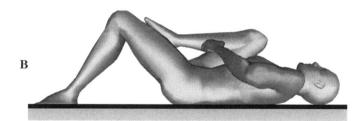

C

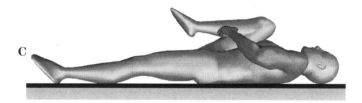

Method: ❑ Perform variation if box is checked

   Place fingers on abdominal muscles (i.e., on outside of abdomen between pelvis and ribs)
   Contract your abdominal muscles by pulling your "navel toward your spine"
   Lift one knee toward your chest
   Use your hand to hold your knee to your chest
   If necessary, reinforce abdominal contraction
   Slide your other leg down, STOP if pain is experienced in your back

❑ Slide your leg down, while contracting your abdominal muscles
   STOP if pelvis tilts; return to the starting position

❑ Place your hand on your pelvis; and prevent forward tilting movement of your pelvis

❑ Slide your leg out to side; with repetitions, bring your leg in toward your other leg
   Return by sliding your leg back to the starting position while contracting your abdominal muscles

Repetitions: _____ Repeat with your alternate leg

Copyright © 2002 by Mosby, Inc. May be copied for patient use only.

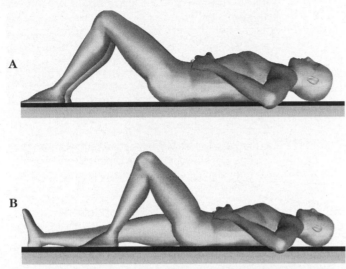

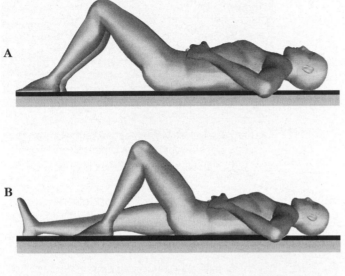

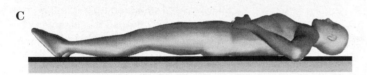

Hip and Knee Extension From Hip and Knee Flexion (Figures A-C)

Purposes: • To improve the control of pelvic tilt by the abdominal muscles
• To stretch the hip flexors

Starting position: Bend hips and knees; feet are on the floor.

Method: ❏ Perform variation if box is checked

Place your fingers on your abdominal muscles (i.e., outside of abdomen between your pelvis and ribs)
Contract your abdominal muscles by "pulling your navel toward your spine"
Slide one leg down while keeping your pelvis from moving
If you experience no pain, slide your alternate leg down
Return by sliding one leg back at a time; make certain to contract your abdominal muscles
❏ Place a pillow under your upper back and head

Repetitions: _____

Copyright © 2002 by Mosby, Inc. May be copied for patient use only.

Hip and Knee Flexion From Passive and Active Hip and Knee Extension (Figures A-C)

Purposes:
- To increase hip flexion flexibility
- To stretch the hip extensors (gluteus maximus and piriformis)
- To improve the isometric control of the pelvis by the abdominal muscles
- To move the lower extremities without pain

Starting position: *Passive:* Lie on your back with one leg straight and the other hip and knee bent. *Active:* Lie on your back with both legs straight.

A

B

C

D

E

Method: ❏ Perform variation if box is checked

Passive (see Figures A-B)
❏ Use _____ hand(s) or _____ towel(s) under thigh to pull knee to chest
❏ Be sure to relax the hip muscles as you pull your knee to your chest
  STOP if you experience pain in your groin or back
❏ Place a towel with a few folds under your low back
❏ Lower your leg so that your foot is on the table and your hip and knee are still bent
❏ Repeat with the same leg _____ times
❏ Perform with your alternate leg as above _____ times
❏ Place a pillow under your upper back and head

Active (see Figures C-E)
❏ Contract your abdominal muscles by pulling "your navel toward your spine"
❏ Slide your foot along a table to bend your hip and knee and place your foot on table
❏ Use your hip muscles to bring your knee to your chest
❏ Use your hands to pull your knee to your chest when your thigh is vertical or your hip is at 90 degrees
❏ Do not push down with your alternate leg
❏ Lower leg and return to starting position
❏ Return your leg to the starting position
❏ Place pillow under upper back and head

Repetitions: _____

Alternate legs: _____

Copyright © 2002 by Mosby, Inc. May be copied for patient use only.

Hip and Knee Flexion With Sliding Heel From Hip and Knee Extension (Figures A-B)

Purposes:
- To improve the performance of the abdominal muscles in controlling pelvic motion
- To stretch the hip flexor muscles

Starting position: Lie on the back with legs straight.

Method: ❏ Perform variation if box is checked

Place your hands on your abdominal muscles (i.e., outside of your abdomen between pelvis and ribs)
Contract your abdominal muscles by "pulling your navel to your spine"
Slide one foot along the table until your hip and knee are bent and your foot is resting on the table
Relax
Contract your abdominal muscles
Slide your foot down, returning it to the rest position
Repeat the movement with your alternate leg
❏ Place a pillow under your upper back and head

Repetitions: _____

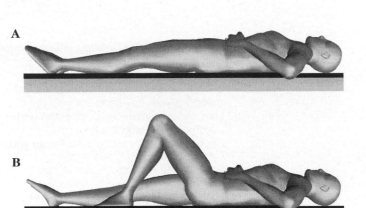

A

B

Lower Abdominal Progression — Unilateral Hip Flexion (Figures A-B)

Purposes:
- To improve the performance of abdominal muscles (external obliques, rectus abdominis, transversus)
- To learn to prevent lumbar spine motions associated with leg motion

Starting position: Bend your hips and knees with your feet on floor. Place your fingers on your abdominal muscles (i.e., outside of abdomen between pelvis and ribs).

Level 0.3: Lift one foot with alternate foot on floor

Method: ❏ Perform variation if box is checked

Contract your abdominal muscles by "pulling your navel toward your spine"
Lift one foot off the table
Maintain your abdominal contraction and lower your foot back to the table
❏ If pain is experienced, push down into table with one foot, while lifting the alternate foot off the table
❏ Use a pillow under upper back and head
Repeat the movement with your alternate foot

Repetitions: _____

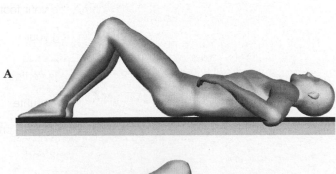

A

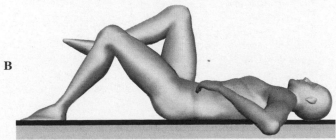

B

Copyright © 2002 by Mosby, Inc. May be copied for patient use only.

Lower Abdominal Progression — Hip and Knee Held to Chest During Hip Flexion (Figures A-B)

Purposes:
- To improve the isometric performance of the abdominal muscles (e.g., external obliques, rectus abdominis, transversus)
- To move the lower extremity without movement of the spine or pelvis

Starting position: Bend hips and knees with feet on floor.

A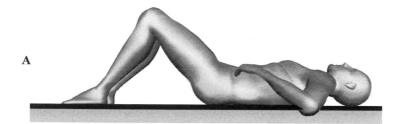

B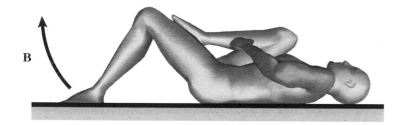

❑ Perform variation if box is checked

Level 0.4: Hold knee to chest and lift the alternate foot

Method:
Contract your abdominal muscles by "pulling your navel toward your spine"
Lift one knee toward your chest
Hold your knee toward your chest with your hand
If able to hold your knee with one hand, place your alternate hand on the abdominal muscle (i.e., outside of abdomen between your pelvis and ribs)
Make certain your abdominal muscles are contracted
Lift your alternate foot off the table
Lower your foot to the table while maintaining a contraction of your abdominal muscles
Repeat _____ times
Repeat this movement with your alternate leg

Repetitions: _____

❑ Perform variation if box is checked

Level 0.5: Lightly hold one knee toward chest and lift the alternate foot

❑ Start if no pain is experienced when performing previous level 10 times
❑ Do not hold your knee toward your chest as lightly as previously while lifting your leg off table
❑ Let your knee move away from your chest and hold it lightly with your hand while lifting your leg off the table

Repetitions: _____

Copyright © 2002 by Mosby, Inc. May be copied for patient use only.

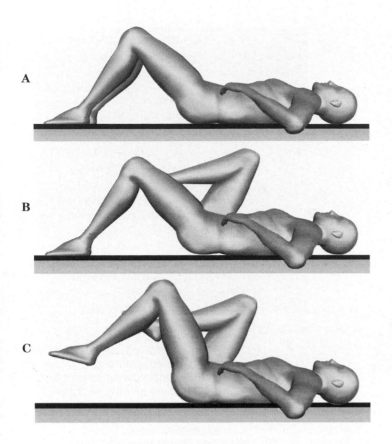

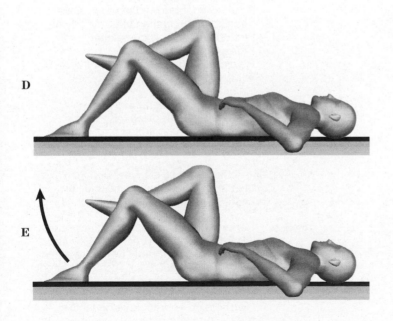

Lower Abdominal Progression—Hip and Knee Flexion With Alternate Foot Unsupported (Figures A-E)

Purposes:
- To improve the performance of the abdominal muscles (e.g., external obliques, rectus abdominis, and transversus)
- To move the lower limb without moving the pelvis or spine

Starting position: Bend hips and knees with feet on floor. Place fingers on abdominal muscles (i.e., outside of abdomen between pelvis and ribs).

Level 1A: Hip flexed to greater than 90 degrees and the alternate foot lifted *(Figures A-C)*

Method: Contract abdominal muscles by "pulling navel toward spine"
Lift one foot off the floor and bring your knee toward your chest to more than 90 degrees
If necessary, contract your abdominal muscles again
Lift the alternate foot off the floor
Do not let your back move
Lower your last leg lifted while maintaining the abdominal contraction
Lower your alternate leg back to the starting position
Repeat starting with your alternate leg

Level 1B: Hip flexed to 90 degrees and lift the alternate foot *(Figures D-E)*

Method: Contract abdominal muscles by "pulling navel toward spine"
Lift one foot off the floor and stop when your hip is bent 90 degrees and your thigh is pointing toward ceiling
If necessary, again contract your abdominal muscles
Lift the alternate foot off the table
Do not let your back move
Lower your last leg lifted so it returns to starting position
Lower your alternate leg to the starting position

Repetitions: _____

Copyright © 2002 by Mosby, Inc. May be copied for patient use only.

Lower Abdominal Progression—Hip and Knee Extension (Figures A-D)

Purposes:
- To improve the isometric performance of the abdominal muscles (e.g., external obliques, rectus abdominis, transversus)
- To move your leg without movement of your spine or pelvis

Starting position: Bend hips and knees with feet on floor. Place fingers on your abdominal muscles (i.e., outside abdomen between pelvis and ribs).

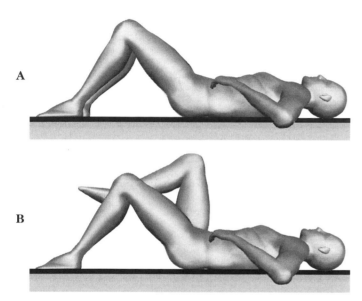

A

B

Level 2: One hip flexed to 90 degrees, the alternate foot lifted and slid to extend the hip and knee (see Figures A-B)

Method: ❏ Perform variation if box is checked

Contract abdominal muscles by "pulling your navel toward your spine"
Lift one leg up until your hip is bent to 90 degrees and your thigh is pointing toward ceiling
If necessary, reinforce the contraction of your abdominal muscles
Do not let your abdomen distend
Do not push your head back into supporting surface
Breathe
Lift your alternate foot off the table
Slide your foot down the table, while lightly touching the table
Straighten your leg completely
❏ Relax
Reinforce your abdominal contraction
Slide your foot back to the starting position
❏ Repeat with the same leg
❏ Lower your nonmoving leg to table, so both feet are on table
❏ Repeat starting with your opposite leg

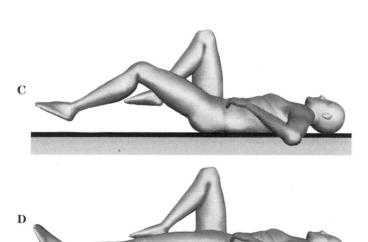

C

D

Level 3: One hip flexed to 90 degrees, foot lifted and then extend without the leg touching the supporting surface (see Figures C-D)

Method: Perform the same movements as outlined in Level 2 except the following:
Hold your foot off table while straightening your leg out
Set your leg down on table
Bring your leg back to starting position by holding your foot off the table
Make certain to contract your abdominal muscles
Do not let your back move
Repeat with the opposite leg

Repetitions: _____

Copyright © 2002 by Mosby, Inc. May be copied for patient use only.

Lower Abdominal Progression: Bilateral Hip and Knee Flexion (Figures A-B)

Purpose:
- To improve the performance of the abdominal muscles (e.g., external obliques, rectus abdominis, transversus)

Starting position: Lie down with both hips and knees straight.

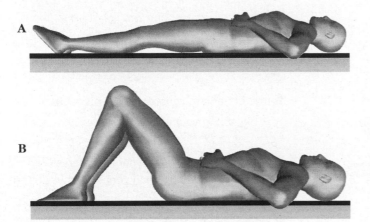

Level 4: Slide both feet along the supporting surface into extension and return to flexion

Method: Contract your abdominal muscles by "pulling your abdomen toward your spine"
Bend your hips and knees and slide your heels along the table
Lift both feet off table when your hips are bent to 90 degrees
Reverse the movement to return to the starting position

Repetitions: _____

Level 5: Lift both feet off the supporting surface; with hips flexed to 90 degrees, extend the knees and lower both lower extremities to the supporting surface

Method: Contract your abdominal muscles by "pulling your abdomen toward your spine"
Bend your hips and knees by lifting both your feet off the table and bringing your knees to your chest
Hold your hips at 90 degrees and straighten your knees
Lower your legs to the table, returning to starting position

Repetitions: _____

Copyright © 2002 by Mosby, Inc. May be copied for patient use only.

Upper Abdominal Progression: Trunk Curl–Sit Up (Figures A-D)

Purpose:
- To improve the performance of the upper abdominal muscles (e.g., internal obliques, rectus abdominis)

Starting position: Bend hips and knees with a pillow under your knees and with your arms in front of body (see Figure A). Straighten hips and knees, and position arms in front of body (see Figure B).

A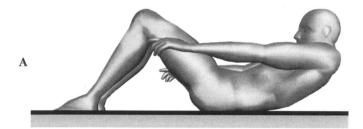

Level 1A: Trunk curl: spinal flexion (easiest)

Method: ❏ Perform variation if box is checked

Bring your chin toward your the base of your neck
Curl your trunk as far as possible
Stop just before your hips start to bend or your feet lift off table

B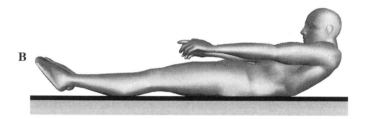

Level 1B: Trunk curl–sit up: spinal and hip flexion (least difficult)

Method: ❏ Perform variation if box is checked

Bring chin toward your the base of your neck
Curl your trunk as far as possible
Maintain the curl
Continue until sitting up

C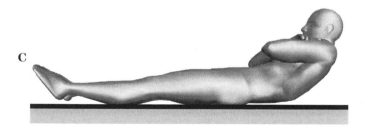

Level 2: Trunk curl–sit up: spinal and hip flexion (difficult)

Method: ❏ Perform variation if box is checked

Fold your arms on your chest (see Figure C)
Bring your chin toward your your the base of your neck
Curl your trunk as far as possible
Maintain the curl
Continue until sitting up

D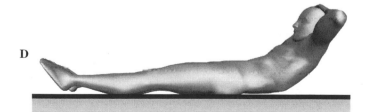

Level 3: Trunk curl-sit up: spinal and hip flexion (most difficult)

Method: ❏ Perform variation if box is checked

Place hands on top of head (not behind head) (see Figure D)
Bring chin toward your the base of your neck
Curl trunk as far as possible
Maintain the curl
Continue until sitting up

Repetitions: _____

Copyright © 2002 by Mosby, Inc. May be copied for patient use only.

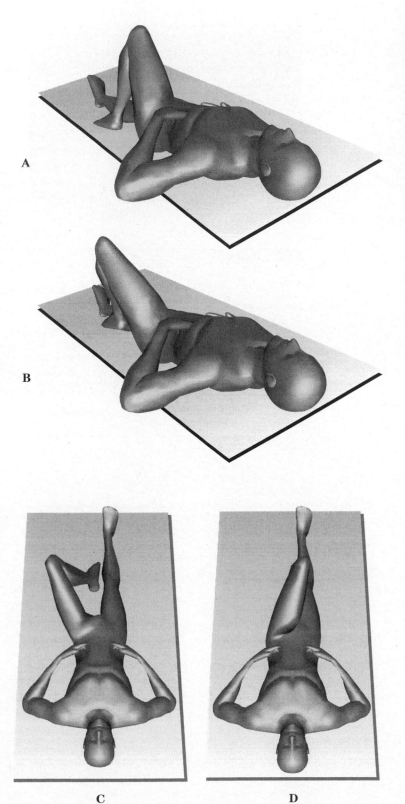

A

B

C   D

Hip Abduction—Lateral Rotation From Flexion Position: Bent Knee Fallouts (Figures A-D)

Purposes:
- To improve the isometric performance of the abdominal muscles in preventing pelvic rotation
- To move the leg without moving the pelvis
- To stretch the hip adductor muscles (e.g., inner thigh muscles)

Starting position: Place hands on pelvis. Bend one knee with foot on the floor. Straighten alternate leg. Place a pillow along side the leg that is bent.

Level 1

Method: ❑ Perform variation if box is checked

Contract your abdominal muscles by pulling "your navel toward your spine"
Let your knee move toward, outside, and away from your body (see Figures B-C)
Keep your pelvis still
Bring your knee back to the starting position

❑ Bring your knee toward the inside of your body toward your opposite leg (see Figure D)
Return to the starting position
Repeat the movement _____ times
Perform with alternate leg

❑ Place pillow under the knee of the leg that is straight

❑ Place a pillow along side the leg that is bent at the level of the knee

Repetitions: _____

Copyright © 2002 by Mosby, Inc. May be copied for patient use only.

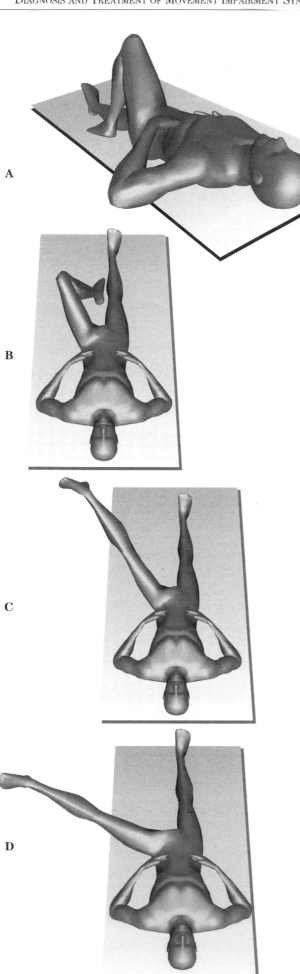

A

B

C

D

Hip Abduction — Lateral Rotation From Flexion Position: Knee Extended (Figures A-D)

Purposes:
- To improve the isometric performance of the abdominal muscles, controlling rotation of the pelvis
- To move leg without movement of pelvis or spine

Starting position: Place your hands on your pelvis. Straighten one leg. Bend one hip and knee with your foot on floor.

Level 2 (Difficult)

Method: ❑ Perform variation if box is checked

Contract your abdominal muscles by "pulling your navel toward your spine"

Let your knee move away from your body (see Figure B)

From that position, straighten your knee (see Figure C)

Try not to push down with your non-moving leg

❑ Bend your knee

❑ Return to the starting position

❑ Repeat straightening and bending your knee while maintaining this position of your leg _____ times

❑ Return to the starting position

❑ Repeat as above

❑ Straighten your knee, keep your knee straight, and bring your leg toward opposite shoulder by moving at hip (see Figure D)

Repeat the movement with your alternate leg

Copyright © 2002 by Mosby, Inc. May be copied for patient use only.

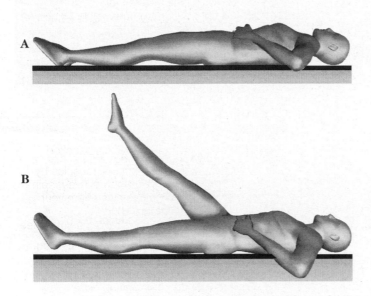

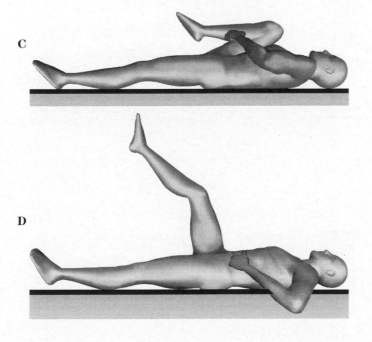

Straight-Leg Raises: Hip Flexion With Knee Extended (Figures A-D)

Purposes: • To improve the performance of the abdominal muscles
- To improve the performance of the hip flexor muscles
- To stretch the hamstring muscles

Starting position: Straighten hips and knees. Place fingers on abdominal muscles (i.e., outside of abdomen between pelvis and ribs).

Method: ❑ Perform variation if box is checked

Contract your abdominal muscles by "pulling your navel toward your spine"
Keep your knee straight
Raise your leg straight up while keeping your knee straight
Do not push down with your nonmoving extremity
Lower your leg back to the starting position while keeping your abdominal muscles contracted

OR

❑ Bend your hip and knee, bringing your knee toward your chest (see Figure C)
❑ Straighten your knee while keeping your hip at 90 degrees (i.e., thigh pointing toward ceiling) (see Figure D)
❑ Hold your thigh with your hand, while straightening your knee
❑ Keep your knee straight and lower your leg back to the starting position
Repeat the movement with your alternate leg

Repetitions: _____

Copyright © 2002 by Mosby, Inc. May be copied for patient use only.

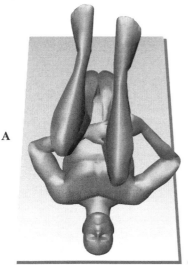

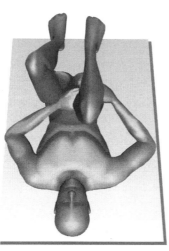

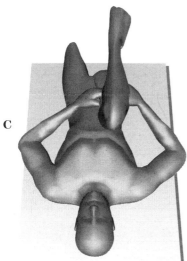

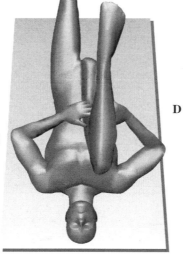

A

B

C

D

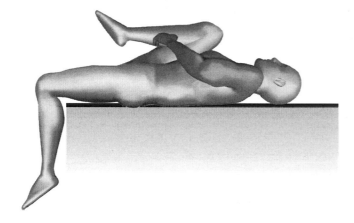

E

Two-Joint Hip Flexor Stretch (Figures A-E)

Purposes:
- To stretch the hip flexors (e.g., tensor fascia lata, rectus femoris, iliopsoas)
- To prevent compensatory anterior pelvic tilt or rotation
- To prevent compensatory tibial rotation

Starting position: Lie on a hard table with your back flat. Bring both knees to your chest, but hold only one knee to your chest with your hands.

Method:
- ❏ Perform variation if box is checked

    Hold one knee to your chest to keep your back flat and your pelvis from moving

    Contract your abdominal muscles by "pulling your navel toward your spine"

    Lower your alternate leg, allowing it to go out to the side

- ❏ Turn your foot in toward your alternate foot to prevent rotation of your leg

    Lower your leg all the way to the table; if possible, make certain your back does not move

    Pull your thigh in toward your alternate leg

    Hold position for 20 to 30 seconds, and then allow your leg to go out to the side again

    Do not let your thigh turn inward

    STOP pulling your thigh toward the alternate leg at the point pain is experienced in your knee

- ❏ Repeat; pull in _____ times
- ❏ If your thigh does not reach the table, let your leg hang for 20 to 30 seconds; make certain to keep your back flat

    Repeat this movement with your alternate leg

Repetitions: _____

Copyright © 2002 by Mosby, Inc. May be copied for patient use only.

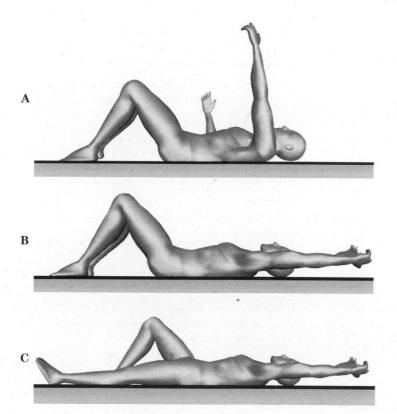

A

B

C

Shoulder Flexion—Elevation With Elbow Extended and Latissimus Dorsi Muscle Stretch (Figures A-C)

Purposes:
- To stretch the latissimus dorsi muscles
- To increase the flexibility of the pectoralis major muscle
- To increase shoulder joint motion
- To decrease the upper back curve
- To improve the performance of the abdominal muscles

Starting position: Bend hips and knees with feet on floor, arms at side.

Method: ❑ Perform variation if box is checked

❑ Contract abdominal muscles by "pulling your navel toward your spine"

❑ Raise one arm overhead as far as possible, STOP if any pain or discomfort is experienced on the top of your shoulder

❑ Raise both arms overhead as far as possible, STOP if any pain or discomfort is experienced on the top of your shoulder

❑ Use _____ pounds in _____ one hand

❑ Use _____ pounds in _____ both hands

❑ Let your weight pull your arm toward the table for _____ seconds

❑ Slide one leg down while keeping your arms overhead and your back flat (see Figure B)

❑ Slide your alternate leg down so both legs will be straight; maintain your arms overhead and your back flat (see Figure C)

Repetitions: _____

Copyright © 2002 by Mosby, Inc. May be copied for patient use only.

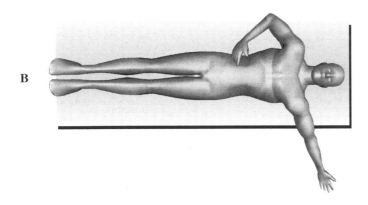

A

B

Shoulder Flexion/Abduction (Figures A-B)

Purpose: • To improve the performance of the abdominal muscles

Starting position: Bend hips and knees with feet on floor, arms at side.

Method: ❑ Perform variation if box is checked

Bend your hips and knees with feet on floor
❑ Hold _____ pound in _____ one hand
❑ Hold _____ pounds in _____ both hands
Raise your arm(s) overhead and out to the side
Contract your abdominal muscles by "pulling your navel toward your spine"
❑ Lift your arm(s) so that it(they) are moving toward the ceiling in a direction toward the opposite hip
Keep your elbows straight
❑ Stop when your arm is vertical and return it to an overhead position

Repetitions: _____

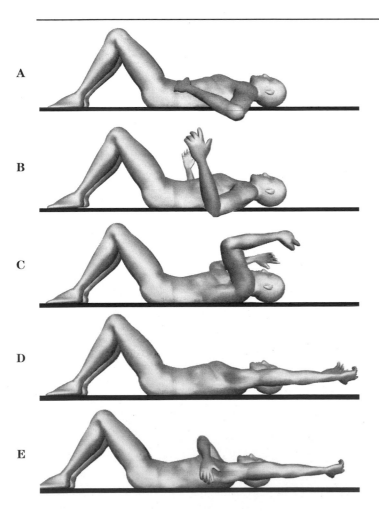

A

B

C

D

E

Shoulder Flexion—Elevation With Elbow Flexed (Figures A-E)

Purpose: • To increase shoulder joint motion

Starting position: Bend hips and knees with feet on floor and arms at side.

Method: ❑ Perform variation if box is checked

Bend elbow and lift at shoulder joint to bring your arm overhead
Straighten your elbow as the arm moves toward an overhead position
❑ Place a pillow along side of the head and slide your arm along pillow
❑ STOP if pain is experienced on top of your shoulder
❑ Use your alternate hand placed on elbow to push down on the arm as it is moving overhead
❑ Stretch your shoulder blade muscles
Lift the arm to be stretched to 90 degrees
Hold outside of your shoulder blade with your alternate hand to prevent it from moving
Continue to lift your arm overhead while restraining your shoulder blade

Repetitions: _____

Copyright © 2002 by Mosby, Inc. May be copied for patient use only.

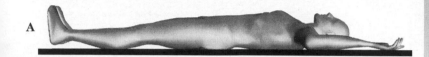

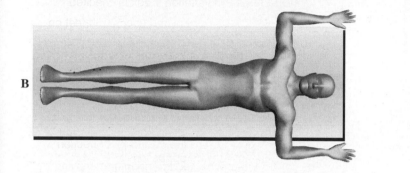

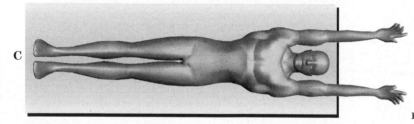

Shoulder Abduction — Gravity Lessened (Figures A-C)

Purposes:
- To increase shoulder joint motion
- To improve the performance of the muscles from the shoulder blade to the arm
- To stretch the pectoralis major muscle
- To stretch the shoulder medial rotator muscles

Starting position: Hips and knees can be straight or bent with feet on floor. Move arms away from body at shoulder level with your elbow bent to 90 degrees.

Method: ❏ Perform variation if box is checked

Slide your arms overhead toward your ears
❏ Place a pillow next to your head and under your arm, slide your arm along the pillow
❏ Contract your abdominal muscles STOP if pain is experienced at the top of your shoulder
❏ Do not shrug your shoulders while moving your arms
❏ Shrug your shoulders while moving your arms

Repetitions: _____

Copyright © 2002 by Mosby, Inc. May be copied for patient use only.

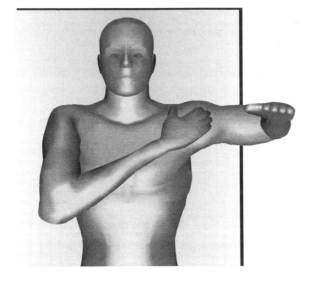

A

Shoulder Rotation — Supine Horizontal Adduction (Flexion) (Figures A-D)

Purposes:
- To increase the range of motion of shoulder rotation
- To prevent compensatory movement of shoulder blade during arm motion
- To prevent compensatory movement of the top of the arm during arm motion
- To improve the performance of the shoulder rotator muscles

Starting position: Hips and knees can be straight or bent with arm at shoulder level with elbow bent to 90 degrees. Place opposite hand on shoulder to prevent it from moving as the arm moves. Place a folded towel under the upper arm and elbow if recommended by therapist.

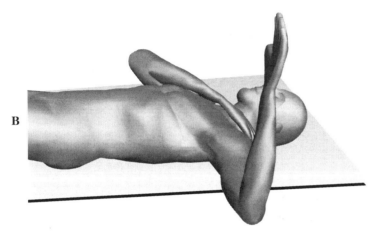

B

Medial rotation—stretch of lateral rotator muscles
(see Figure C)

Method: Move hand toward hip, keeping shoulder or top of arm bone from moving by Pressure from opposite hand
- Position arm at _____ degrees, not at 90 degrees
- Hold _____ pounds of weight in your hand; let your weight pull your hand down toward the table
  STOP if pain is experienced in your shoulder joint
  Do not let your elbow straighten
  Return to the starting position
  Repeat _____ times

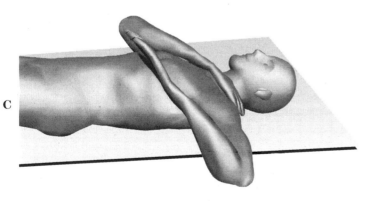

C

Lateral rotation—stretch of medial rotator muscles
(see Figure D)

Method: Let your hand move toward your head, keeping the top of your arm bone from pushing into your restraining hand
- Position your arm at _____ degrees, not at 90 degrees
- Hold _____ pounds weight in hand; let weight pull hand toward table
  STOP if pain is experienced in your shoulder joint
  Return to starting position
  Repeat _____ times

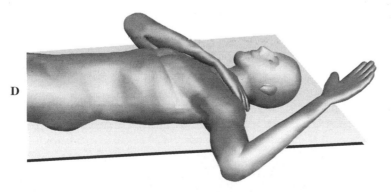

D

Horizontal adduction

Method: Lift your arm, keep your shoulder blade on the table, and bring your arm in front of your body
  When your arm is in front of your body, with your elbow pointing toward ceiling, use your alternate hand to pull your arm farther across your body toward the opposite shoulder
- Use your hand to push your arm down toward the table as you move
- Keep your shoulder blade flat against the table
  Repeat _____ times

Copyright © 2002 by Mosby, Inc. May be copied for patient use only

Pectoralis Minor Stretch

Purpose: • To stretch the pectoralis minor muscle

Starting position: Hips and knees can be bent with feet on floor, or legs can be straight. Arms are at the side.

❑ Perform variation if box is checked

Assisted stretch—lying on back

Method: Assistant places the palm of his or her hand in the crease of your shoulder, not on your arm bone (see figure)

Assistant applies pressure in a direction that is away from your chest and toward the table (i.e., a diagonal away from your body in a downward direction)

Apply pressure for _____ seconds

Try to keep your chest from moving

Stretch should be felt on your chest and not at your shoulder joint

❑ Assistant uses one hand on both of your shoulders, crossing your hands so that if standing on the patient's right side, the assistant's left hand will be on the patient's left shoulder and the assistant's right hand will be on the patient's right shoulder

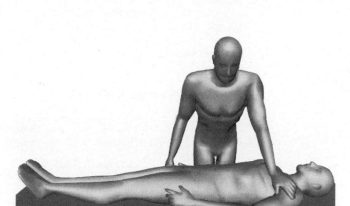

Self stretch—lying on back

Method: Roll your trunk toward your shoulder to be stretched so that your shoulder blade is held firmly against floor

Use the palm of your opposite hand to apply pressure at the crease of your shoulder

Rotate your trunk away from your shoulder

Assisted stretch—lying face down

Method: While lying face down with arms at side, assistant stands at your side and reaches from the top of your shoulder to place his or her fingers in the crease on front of your shoulder

Your alternate hand reaches through the arm pit to place your fingers also on the crease of your shoulder

Assistant then lifts up on your shoulder and leans back at the same time to stretch the muscle

DO NOT PULL on your arm, the stretch should be felt on your chest and not in your shoulder joint

Repetitions: _____

Copyright © 2002 by Mosby, Inc. May be copied for patient use only.

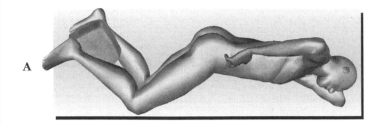

A

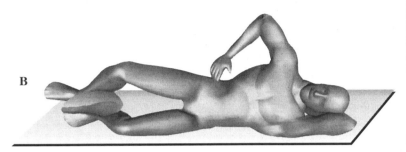

B

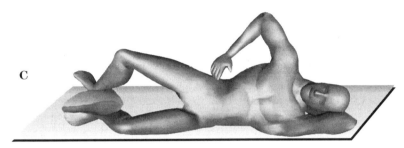

C

Hip Lateral Rotation—Side-Lying Position (Figures A-C)

Purposes:
- To improve the performance of the hip lateral rotator muscles
- To move the hip without moving the pelvis
- To improve the isometric performance of the lateral abdominal muscles

Starting position: Lay on the side with bottom hip and knee bent. Rotate your pelvis slightly forward. Bend your top hip and knee and rest on the bottom leg or on a pillow. Place hand on your pelvis.

❑ Perform variation if box is checked

Method: ❑ Place a pillow between your knees or ankles
Rotate your top leg so that your knee turns upward
Move in hip joint only
Do not let your pelvis rotate

Repetitions: _____

Copyright © 2002 by Mosby, Inc. May be copied for patient use only

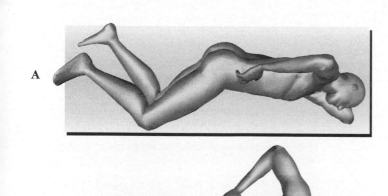

A

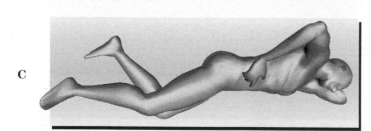

B

C

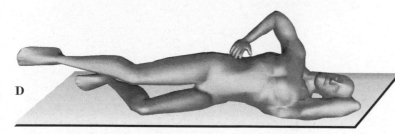

D

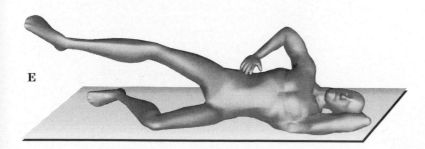

E

Hip Abduction With and Without Lateral Rotation — Side-Lying Position (Figures A-H)

Purposes:
- To improve the performance of the hip abductor muscles
- To stretch the hip abductor muscles (tensor fascia lata–iliotibial band)
- To improve the isometric performance of the lateral abdominal muscles
- To move in the hip joint without movement of the pelvis

Starting position: Bottom hip and knee is bent while lying on the side. The pelvis is rotated slightly forward. The hand can be on pelvis or on the area of the gluteus medius muscle.

❑ Perform variation if box is checked

Level 1: **Hip abduction with lateral rotation**
(see Figures A-B)

Method: Bend your top hip and knee about 45 degrees
Slightly rotate knee so knee cap is pointing slightly upward; lift your thigh at hip joint
❑ Place pillow between your knees
❑ Place a folded towel under your waist
❑ Place your hands on pelvis to keep your pelvis from moving
❑ Place your fingers on gluteus medius muscle
Do not lift high
Do not push down with your bottom leg
Lower your leg to the starting position

Level 2: **Hip abduction with lateral rotation**
(see Figures C-E)

Method: Slightly bend hip and knee of top leg
Slightly rotate your top leg so knee is pointing slightly upward while lifting your thigh at hip joint up and back
❑ Place a pillow between your knees
❑ Place a folded towel under your waist
❑ Place your hand on your pelvis to monitor for movement
❑ Place your fingers on your gluteus medius muscle
Do not let your pelvis tilt
Do not push down with your bottom leg
Lower your leg to the starting position

Copyright © 2002 by Mosby, Inc. May be copied for patient use only.

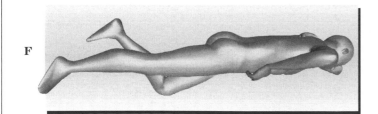

F

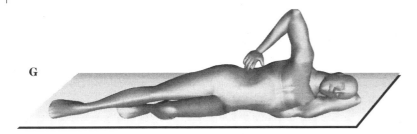

G

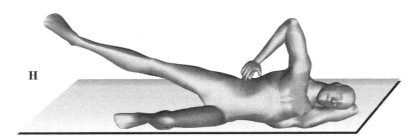

H

Level 3: Hip abduction (see Figures F-H)

Method: Straighten hip and knee
- ❏ Place your hand on your pelvis to monitor for movement
- ❏ Place your fingers on the gluteus medius muscle, keeping your hip back; lift your leg upward toward the ceiling

Do not lift your leg high
Do not let your knee turn inward
Do not let your pelvis tilt
Do not push down with your bottom leg
Lower your leg to the starting position

Tensor fascia lata–iliotibial band stretch (see Figures F-G)

Method: Place your hand on your pelvis to monitor for movement
Position your leg slightly forward
Straighten your knee; turn it up slightly
Lift your leg upward toward the ceiling
Bring your leg backward, moving at hip so that the leg is slightly behind the body
Do not allow your pelvis to move or your back to arch when bringing the hip back
Lower your leg toward the table
Do not let your pelvis move
If your leg does not lower 15 degrees below level of hip joint, relax the hip muscles except for those used to keep your leg turned up; allow your leg to hang for 15 to 20 seconds
Relax your leg and repeat the movements

Repetitions: _____

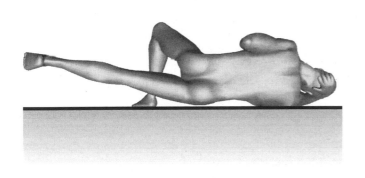

Hip Adduction for Strengthening— Side-Lying Position

Purposes:
- To improve the performance of the hip adductor (inner thigh) muscles
- To stretch the hip abductor muscles

Starting position: Lay on the side of the leg that is to be exercised. Straighten hip and knee. Hold your pelvis and trunk perpendicular to the supporting surface. Rotate the top leg at the hip; your knee is bent so your foot is on the floor in front of your bottom leg. Place the hand of your arm on top of your body on the floor to stabilize your trunk.

Method: ❏ Perform variation if box is checked

Keep your knee straight and knee cap pointing straight ahead
Lift your bottom leg up toward the top leg
- ❏ Straighten your hip and knee of the top leg; hold it up parallel to the bottom leg; bring your bottom leg up to meet your top leg
Return your bottom leg to the starting position

Repetitions: _____

Copyright © 2002 by Mosby, Inc. May be copied for patient use only.

Shoulder Flexion, Lateral Rotation, and Scapular Adduction — Side-Lying Position (Figures A-C)

Purposes:
- To improve the performance of the shoulder muscles that raise the arm overhead
- To improve the performance of the shoulder muscle that rotates the arm
- To increase the motion of the shoulder blade
- To improve the performance of the trapezius muscle

Starting position: While lying on side, hips and knees are bent. Arm is at shoulder level with elbow flexed and resting on pillow.

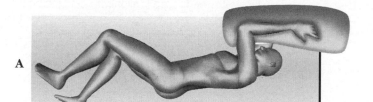

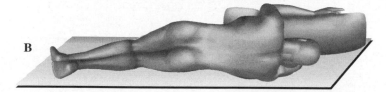

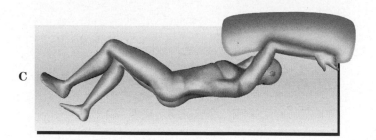

❑ Perform variation if box is checked

Shoulder flexion *(see Figures A-C)*

Method: Slide your arm overhead as far as possible
Straighten your elbow as your arm moves overhead
❑ Try to move your shoulder blade upward and toward the front of your body
Slide your arm back to the starting position
Do not shrug your shoulder

❑ Perform variation if box is checked

Scapular adduction (trapezius muscle exercise) *(see Figure C)*

Method: Rest your arm on a pillow in a slightly overhead position
❑ Pull your shoulder blade toward your spine (see Figure B)
❑ Lift your arm off the pillow by pulling your shoulder blade toward your spine

❑ Perform variation if box is checked

Shoulder rotation

Method: Rest your upper arm on the side of your body
Bend your elbow to 90 degrees
Rest your forearm against your abdomen
Keep your upper arm still and raise your forearm and hand toward the ceiling by rotating in your shoulder joint
Return your forearm and hand to the starting position

Repetitions: _____

Copyright © 2002 by Mosby, Inc. May be copied for patient use only.

A

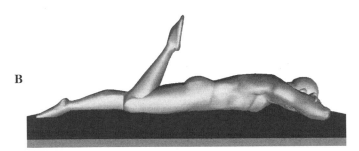

B

C

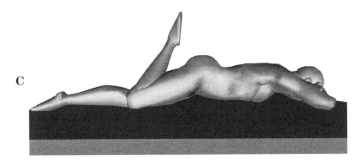

Knee Flexion—Face-Lying Position (Figures A-C)

Purposes:
- To decrease the compensatory motion of the pelvis and spine
- To increase the flexibility and stretch the quadriceps and tensor fascia lata muscles
- To improve the performance of the abdominal muscles

Starting position: Lay face down with your legs straight and relatively close together.

Method: ❑ Perform variation if box is checked

Tighten your abdominal muscles by "pulling your navel toward your spine"
Bend your knee
Do not let your pelvis move (see *incorrect* posture in Figure C)
Do not pull hard, which can cause a cramp in the back of your thigh
Return your leg to the starting position
❑ Place a pillow under your abdomen
❑ Place your hands on your buttocks or on the bones in front of your pelvis to monitor movement of your pelvis
Repeat with your alternate leg

Repetitions: _____

Copyright © 2002 by Mosby, Inc. May be copied for patient use only.

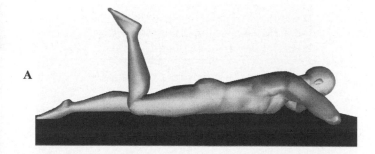

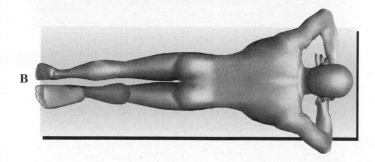

Hip Rotation — Face-Lying Position (Figures A-D)

Purposes:
- To decrease the compensatory motion of the pelvis during hip motion
- To improve the flexibility and stretch the hip rotator muscles
- To improve the performance of the abdominal muscles

Starting position: Lay face down with legs straight and relatively close together.

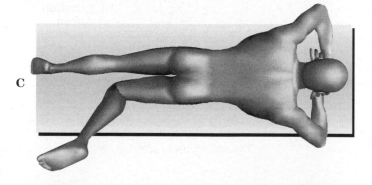

Method: ❑ Perform variation if box is checked

    ❑ Place a pillow under your abdomen
    ❑ Place your hands on your buttocks or on the bones on the front of your pelvis to monitor the movement of your pelvis

    Contract your abdominal muscles by "pulling your navel toward the spine"

    Bend your knee to 90 degrees (leg is vertical) (see Figure A)

    Rotate your hip by allowing your foot to move in toward your alternate leg (see Figure C) and then away from the opposite leg (see Figure D)

    Keep your pelvis still

    Repeat the motion _____ times with one leg

    Return to the starting position

    Repeat the motion with your alternate leg

Repetitions: _____

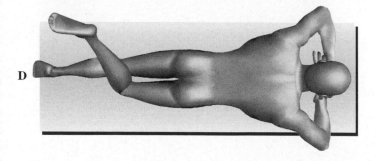

Copyright © 2002 by Mosby, Inc. May be copied for patient use only.

Hip Extension With Knee Extended — Face-Lying Position (Figures A-B)

Purposes:
- To improve the performance of the gluteus maximus and hamstring muscles
- To stretch the hip flexor muscles
- To improve the performance of the back extensor muscles
- To improve the performance of the abdominal muscles

Starting position: Lying face down with legs straight and relatively close together.

Method: ❏ Perform variation if box is checked

Contract your abdominal muscles by "pulling your abdomen toward your navel"

To lift your entire leg off the supporting surface, think about turning your leg slightly outward as you contract your buttock (gluteal) muscle

Do not let your pelvis move

Do not lift your leg high (only 10 degrees of hip motion in this direction)

Hold position for a count of 3 to 10 seconds

Return your leg to the starting position

❏ Place pillow under abdomen

❏ Place your fingers on the bones on the front of pelvis to monitor pelvic motion

Repeat with your alternate leg

Repetitions: _____

A

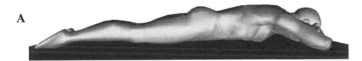

B

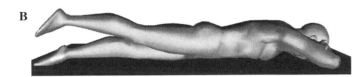

Copyright © 2002 by Mosby, Inc. May be copied for patient use only

Hip Extension With Knee Flexed— Face-Lying Position (Figures A-B)

Purposes:
- To improve the performance of the gluteus maximus muscle
- To stretch the hip flexor muscles
- To improve the performance of the back extensor muscles
- To improve the performance of the abdominal muscles

Starting position: Lie face down with legs extended and relatively close together.

Method: ❑ Perform variation if box is checked

Bend your knee; if possible, let your leg rest on thigh to relax hamstring muscles
❑ Place your leg against the seat of chair or your foot against the wall
Contract your abdominal muscles by "pulling your navel toward your spine"
Contract buttock (gluteal) muscles to lift your thigh off the supporting surface
Do not lift your thigh high (only 10 degrees of motion in this direction)
Do not let your pelvis move
Hold this position for 3 to 10 seconds
Return to the rest position
❑ Place a pillow under your abdomen
❑ Place your fingers on the bones on front of your pelvis to monitor pelvic motion
Repeat with your alternate leg

Repetitions: _____

A

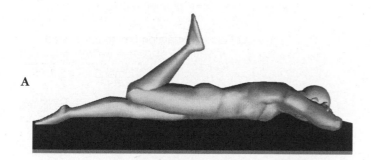

B

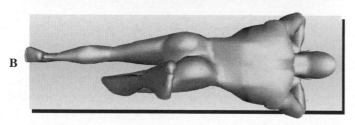

Copyright © 2002 by Mosby, Inc. May be copied for patient use only.

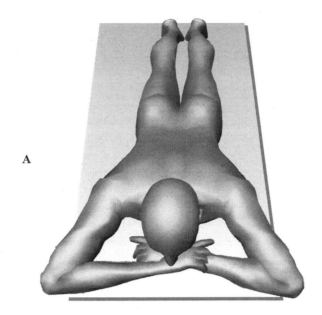

A

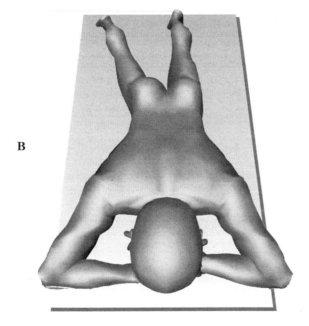

B

Hip Abduction—Face-Lying Position (Figures A-B)

Purposes: • To improve performance of hip abductor and gluteus medius muscles
• To improve the performance of the hip extensor muscles
• To improve the performance of the hip adductor muscles

Starting position: Lay face down with your legs straight and relatively close together.

Method: ❑ Perform variation if box is checked

❑ Place a pillow under your abdomen
❑ Place your fingers on the bones on front of your pelvis to monitor the movement
Contract your buttock muscle to slide your leg out to the side
Do not let your pelvis move
Return your leg to the starting position
Repeat with your alternate leg

Repetitions: _____

Copyright © 2002 by Mosby, Inc. May be copied for patient use only.

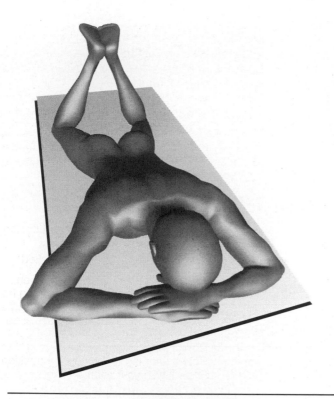

Isometric Hip Lateral Rotation With Hips Abducted and Knees Flexed

Purpose: • To improve the performance of the hip lateral rotator muscles

Starting position: Lay face down with knees apart and bent. Allow the hips to rotate so that your feet touch.

Method: ❑ Perform variation if box is checked

❑ Place a pillow under your abdomen
From the starting position, push your feet together by tightening your buttocks
Hold position for 5 to 10 seconds
Relax and repeat movement

Repetitions: _____

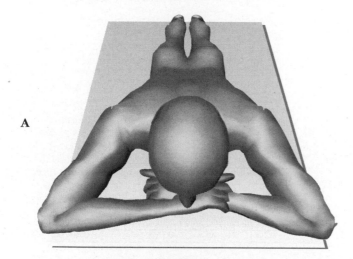

A

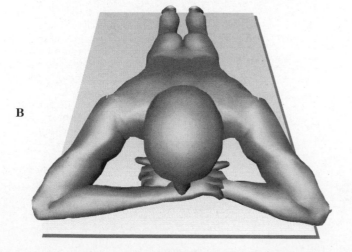

B

Isometric Gluteus Maximus Contraction (Figures A-B)

Purpose: • To improve the performance of the gluteus maximus muscles

Starting position: Lay face down with legs straight and relatively close together.

Method: ❑ Perform variation if box is checked

Tighten your buttocks muscles
"Think about" your legs turning outward while contracting your buttocks muscles
Hold position for 5 to 10 seconds
Relax

Repetitions: _____

Copyright © 2002 by Mosby, Inc. May be copied for patient use only.

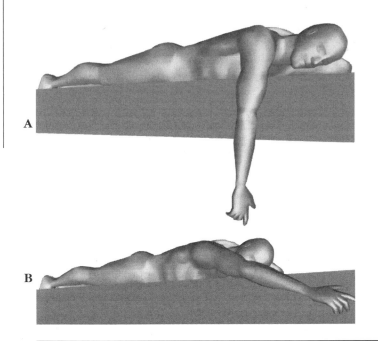

Shoulder Flexion to Elicit Back Extensor Muscle Activity—Face-Lying Position (Figures A-B)

Purpose: • To improve the performance of the back extensor muscles

Starting position: Lay face down on a table near the edge so that the arm hangs over the edge of table.

Method: Lift the arm up to the overhead position

Hold position for 5 to 10 seconds
Return to the rest position
Repeat with the same arm
Repeat with the opposite arm

Repetitions: _____

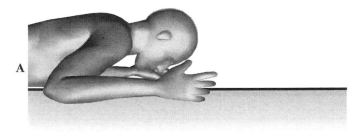

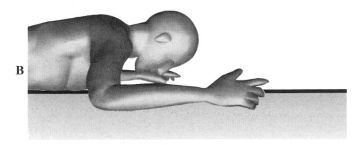

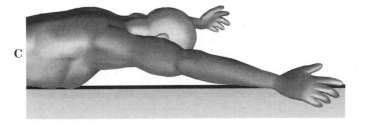

Shoulder Flexion—Face-Lying Position (Figures A-C)

Purposes: • To increase the range of shoulder flexion
• To improve the performance of the shoulder flexor muscles
• To improve the movement of the shoulder blade by serratus anterior muscle

Starting position: Face-lying position with enough pillows under the upper body and pelvis to ensure that the arms with the elbows bent can be comfortably placed alongside the body. The little finger side of the forearm and hand should be in contact with the supporting surface. The forehead can be supported with a folded towel.

Method: ❑ Perform variation if box is checked

Slide your arms overhead, STOP if pain is experienced on top of your shoulder
❑ Think about moving your shoulder blade so that the bottom of it moves forward and up; motion will be as though a string is tied from your elbow to the bottom of the shoulder blade
❑ When your elbow is directly under your shoulder, place some weight on your elbow as you continue the sliding movement; STOP if pain is experienced in your shoulder joint
Do not let your elbows move away from your sides as you slide your arms overhead

Repetitions: _____

Copyright © 2002 by Mosby, Inc. May be copied for patient use only.

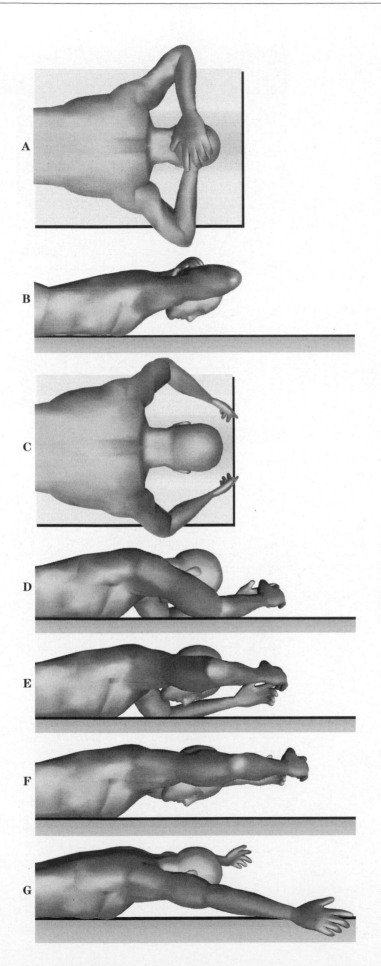

Copyright © 2002 by Mosby, Inc. May be copied for patient use only.

Trapezius Muscle Exercise Progression— Face-Lying Position (Figures A-G)

Purpose: • To improve the performance of the trapezius muscle

❑ Perform variation if box is checked

Level 1 *(see Figures A-B)*

Starting position: Face down with arms overhead, elbows bent, and hands on back of head.

Method: ❑ Place a pillow under your chest
Lift your elbows by pulling your shoulder blades together
Hold position for 5 to 10 seconds
Let your elbows return to starting position

Level 2 *(see Figures C-F)*

Starting position: Face down with arms overhead, elbows bent, hands resting by head with the thumb pointing upward.

Method: ❑ Place a pillow under your chest
Lift your arms by pulling your shoulder blades together
Keep your hand higher than your elbow
Hold position for 5 to 10 seconds
Let your arms return to the rest position

Level 3 *(see Figure G)*

Starting position: Face down with arms overhead and slightly out to side, elbows straight, and thumbs pointing toward ceiling.

Method: ❑ Place a pillow under your chest
Lift your arms by pulling your shoulder blades together and slightly downward
Keep your hand higher than your elbow
Hold position for 5 to 10 seconds
Let your arms return to rest position

Repetitions: _____

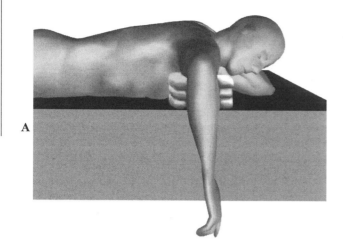

A

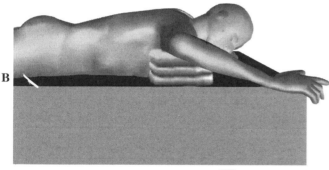

B

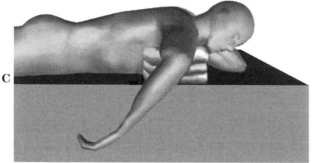

C

Shoulder Rotation—Face-Lying Position (Figures A-C)

Purpose: • To improve the performance of the shoulder rotator muscles

Starting position: Face down on a table or bed with the upper arm at shoulder level and resting on towels. Elbow is bent and forearm is hanging over the edge of the table (see Figure A).

❏ Perform variation if box is checked

Lateral Rotation *(see Figure B)*

Method: Turn hand up toward your head
Imagine that you are rotating your forearm about an axle running through your upper arm
Do not let your shoulder blade move
Do not lift your arm off the towels
Hold the position at the end of the range for 5 to 10 seconds
❏ Hold a _____ pound weight in your hand

Medial Rotation *(see Figure C)*

Method: Turn your hand down toward your hip
Imagine that you are rotating your forearm about an axle that runs through your upper arm
Do not lift your upper arm off the towels
Hold position at the end of the range for 5 to 10 seconds
❏ Hold a _____ pound weight in your hand

End-Range Medial Rotation

Starting position: Face down on table lying on two pillows with upper arm at shoulder level supported by towels. Elbow is bent with forearm rotated toward hip and hand resting on the table.

Method: Keep your upper arm still while straightening your elbow just enough so that your hand is no longer resting on the table
Hold position for 5 to 10 seconds
If you have difficulty holding your hand in this position, return it to the table
If you can control your forearm and hand, let your forearm rotate toward the floor and then rotate it back toward your hip
Do not lift your upper arm off the towels

Repetitions: _____

Copyright © 2002 by Mosby, Inc. May be copied for patient use only.

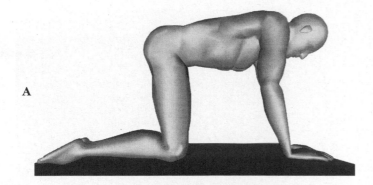

A

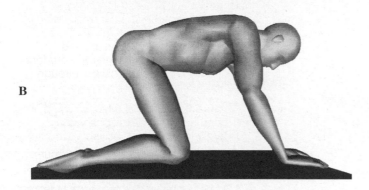

B

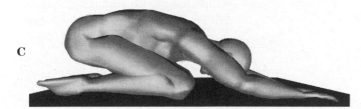

C

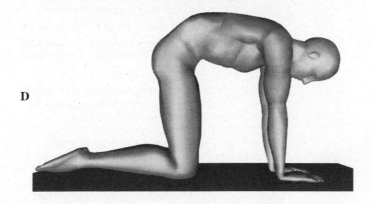

D

Rocking—Quadruped Position (Figures A-D)

Purposes:
- To decrease the compression forces acting on the spine
- To improve the flexibility and stretch of the buttock hip muscles
- To improve the hip bending motion
- To decrease the outward bending of the lower back
- To decrease the outward curve of the upper back
- To reverse the inward curve of the lower back
- To decrease the rotation of the spine
- To improve the performance of the serratus anterior muscle

Starting position: While on hands and knees with feet pointing away from body, center hips over the knees, which are a few inches apart. Position the hips at a 90-degree angle, spine straight, shoulders centered over hands, and head in line with the body.

Method: ❑ Perform variation if box is checked

   Keep spine straight
   Rock backward toward your heels by moving in hip joint; "think about aiming your buttocks toward the ceiling"
   STOP if any pain is experienced
❑ Rock backward part of the way toward your heels (see Figure B)
❑ Rock backward as far as possible toward your heels (see Figure C)
❑ Do not let your back arch upward (see *incorrect* posture in Figure D)
❑ Push back with hands, and do not tighten hip muscles
❑ Stretch your arms out once you have rocked back as far as possible; keep your spine straight
❑ Arch your spine upward (see Figure D)
❑ Let your spine arch inward
❑ Put your knees farther apart
❑ Let your knees turn outward and your feet turn inward
   Return to the rest position
❑ Rock forward while contracting your abdominal muscles

Repetitions: _____

Copyright © 2002 by Mosby, Inc. May be copied for patient use only.

Limb Movement — Quadruped Position (Figures A-C)

Purposes:
- To improve the performance of abdominal muscles
- To improve the control of the spine in preventing rotation
- To improve balance control
- To improve the control of the pelvis

Starting position: While on hands and knees with feet pointing away from body, center hips over the knees, which are a few inches apart. Position the hips at a 90-degree angle, spine straight, shoulders centered over hands, and head in line with the body.

❑ Perform variation if box is checked

Shoulder flexion (see Figure A)

Method: Contract abdominal muscles by "pulling your navel toward your spine"
❑ Barely lift your hand off the supporting surface by bending your elbow
❑ Lift one arm overhead and hold position for 5 to 10 seconds
Do not let your trunk move when lifting your arm
Return hand to the supporting surface
Repeat movement with your other hand

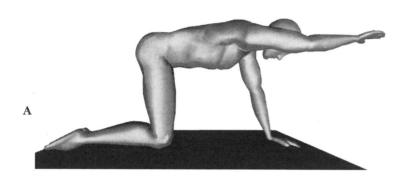

A

Hip extension with knee flexion

Method: Contract your abdominal muscles by "pulling your navel toward your spine"
Keep your knee bent and lift your leg at the hip backward
Do not let your pelvis or spine move
Hold position for 3 to 10 seconds
Return to the starting position
Repeat with your alternate leg

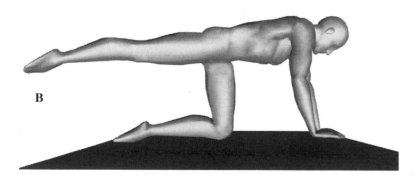

B

Hip and knee extension (see Figure B)

Method: Contract your abdominal muscles by "pulling your navel toward your spine"
Lift your leg backward so that your hip and knee straighten
Do not let your pelvis or spine move
Hold position for 3 to 10 seconds
Return to the starting position
Repeat with the alternate leg

Hip/knee extension with shoulder flexion (see Figure C)

Method: Contract your abdominal muscles by "pulling your navel toward your spine"
Lift your opposite leg and arm at the same time
Lift leg backward and over head
Do not let your pelvis or spine move
Hold position for 3 to 10 seconds
Return to the starting position
Repeat with your opposite arm and leg

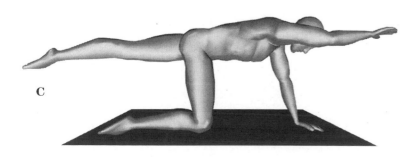

C

Repetitions: _____

Copyright © 2002 by Mosby, Inc. May be copied for patient use only.

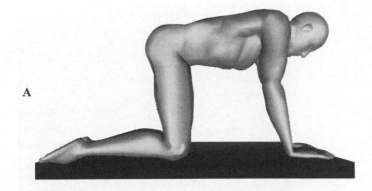

A

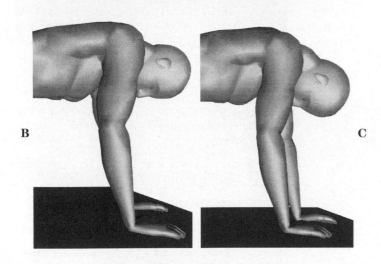

B

C

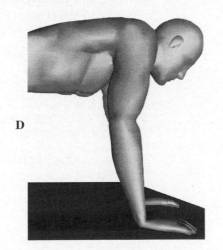

D

Head and Cervical Flexion and Extension— Quadruped Position (Figures A-D)

Purposes:
- To improve the performance of the neck extensors and flexors
- To stretch the levator scapulae muscles
- To improve the control of neck motion

Starting position: While on hands and knees with feet pointing away from body, center hips over knees, which are a few inches apart. Position the hips at a 90-degree angle, spine straight, shoulders centered over hands, and head in line with the body.

❏ Perform variation if box is checked

Method: Bring your chin down toward the base of your neck (see Figure B)

Do not let your neck drop forward in the area where it attaches to the body (see Figure C)

Lift your head up to slightly above the starting position (see *incorrect* posture in Figure D)

Do not lift your head all the way up

❏ Perform variation if box is checked

Cervical rotation

Method: From the starting position with the head and neck straight and level with the body, turn head to one side

Do not twist your head but imagine turning your head around a rod that is running directly through the center of your head

Return to the starting position

Repeat turning in the opposite direction

Repetitions: _____

Copyright © 2002 by Mosby, Inc. May be copied for patient use only.

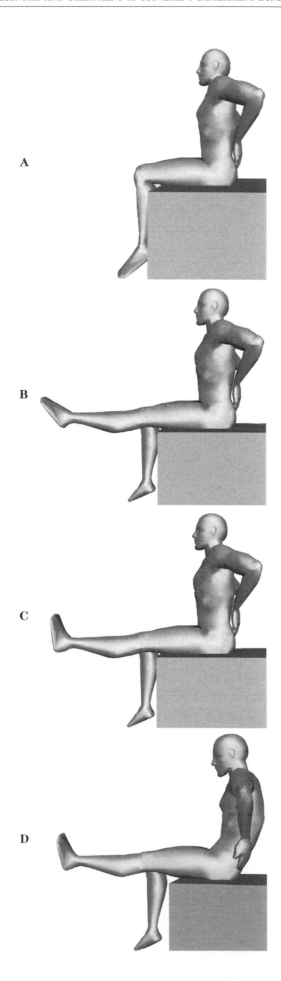

A

B

C

D

Knee Extension and Dorsiflexion—Sitting Position (Figures A-D)

Purposes:
- To improve the length of the hamstring muscles
- To improve the control of the back extensor muscles
- To decrease the tendency for the back to bend outward
- To control undesirable hip rotation during knee movement
- To stretch the muscles attaching to the knee cap
- To stretch the calf muscles
- To improve the control by the muscles that lift the ankle

Starting position: Sit on a chair with a preferably straight back. Hips should be at a right-angle with the trunk and shoulders in line with the hips. Both feet can be on the floor. If the chair does not have a back, back should be monitored for motion (see Figure A).

Method: ❏ Perform variation if box is checked

❏ Push the upper back into the chair without letting it move
Straighten your knee as far as possible (see Figure B)
Move at your ankle to point your toes toward your knee (see Figure C)
Do not let your back bend outward (see *incorrect* Figure D)
Do not lead with your toes when pointing your foot

❏ Do lead with your big toe side when pointing your foot

❏ Hold a towel in your hands, place the towel around the ball of your foot, pull your foot toward your knee with your hands
Do not let your thigh lift off the supporting surface
Do not let your thigh turn inward

❏ Think about using as little of the muscle on the front of the thigh as possible
Hold position for 5 to 10 seconds
Return to the starting position

❏ As your leg goes down, place your fingers and thumb on the outside of your knee cap, and guide your knee cap down and slightly inward as your knee returns to the starting position

Repetitions: _____

Copyright © 2002 by Mosby, Inc. May be copied for patient use only.

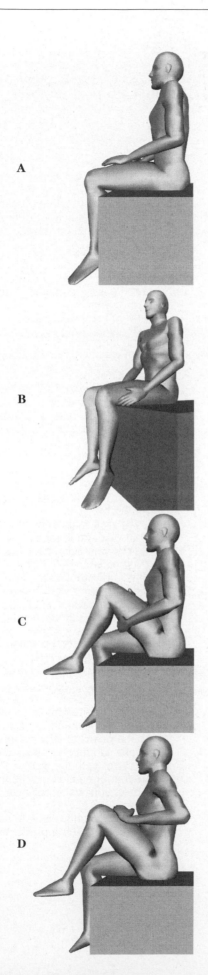

A

B

C

D

Hip Flexion — Sitting Position (Figures A-D)

Purposes:
- To improve the performance of the muscles that lift the leg toward the chest
- To improve the control by the trunk muscles
- To stretch the muscles on the back of the hip

Starting position: Sit on a chair, preferably with a straight back. The hips should be at a right angle with the trunk and shoulders in line with the hips. Both feet can be on the floor.

Method: ❏ Perform variation if box is checked

   Use both hands to lift your thigh as high as possible without causing pain (see Figure B)

   Do not use your hip muscles while lifting your thigh

   After lifting your thigh as far as possible, release the hold by hands and use your hip muscles

   Hold your thigh in this position for 5 to 10 seconds (see Figure D)

   Let your thigh return to the starting position

❏ Hold your thigh up, and push your thigh with your hand (isometric) for 5 to 10 seconds

❏ Repeat movement with your alternate leg

Repetitions: _____

Copyright © 2002 by Mosby, Inc. May be copied for patient use only.

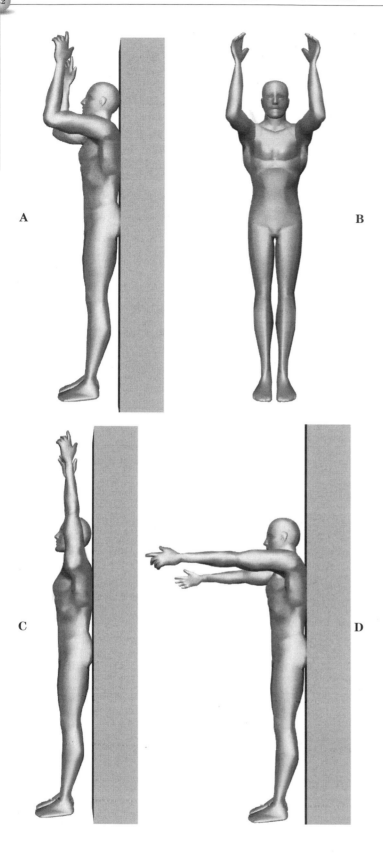

A

B

C

D

Shoulder Flexion — Standing With Back Against the Wall (Figures A-D)

Purposes:
- To improve the performance of the trapezius muscle
- To stretch the latissimus dorsi muscle
- To increase the range-of-shoulder motion
- To improve the control of the shoulder lateral rotator muscles
- To improve the alignment of the upper back

Starting position: Stand with back against the wall. Heels are approximately 3 inches away from the wall. Arms are at side of body.

Shoulder flexion with elbow flexion

Method: ❑ Perform variation if box is checked

   Bend your elbows
   Bring your arms forward so that your elbows face forward
   Bring your arms overhead, allowing your elbows to straighten as your arm goes overhead
   Try to bring your hands and arms back against the wall
   Keep your arms close to your head
   Do not let your back arch or pull away from the wall
❑ Contract your abdominal muscles to flatten your low back against the wall
   Hold the position for 5 to 10 seconds
   You should NOT experience any pain at the top of the shoulder; STOP the motion before the point of experiencing pain
❑ Take a deep breath, and repeat _____ times
   Return to the starting position

Shoulder flexion with elbow extension

Method: ❑ Perform variation if box is checked

   Keep elbows straight
   Raise arms overhead
   Keep the palms of your hands facing upward and then backward, as your arms approach the wall
   Keep your arms close to the head
   Do not let your back pull away from the wall
   Hold the position for 5 to 10 seconds
   Return to the starting position

Repetitions: _____

Copyright © 2002 by Mosby, Inc. May be copied for patient use only.

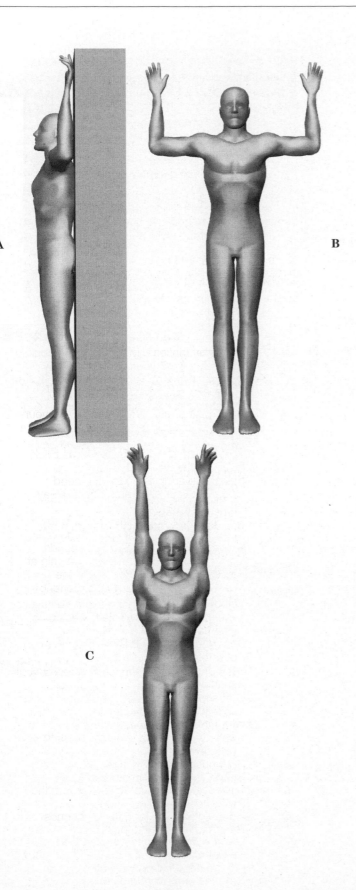

A

B

C

Shoulder Abduction — Standing With Back Against the Wall (Figures A-C)

Purposes: • To improve the performance of the trapezius muscle
• To increase the range-of-shoulder motion
• To stretch the pectoralis major muscle

Starting position: Stand with back against the wall. Heels are approximately 3 inches away from the wall. Arms are at side of body.

Method: ❏ Perform variation if box is checked

Raise your arms to shoulder level
Bend elbows 90 degrees
Touch the wall with your arms, forearms, and hands
❏ Bring your arms back to the wall, but do not force them to touch the wall
Slide your arms up the wall toward your head
Straighten your elbows as your arms move overhead
Bring your arms close to your head
STOP if pain is experienced on top of your shoulder
❏ Contract your abdominal muscles to flatten your back against the wall
Hold position for 5 to 10 seconds
Return your arms to shoulder-level position

Repetitions: _____

Copyright © 2002 by Mosby, Inc. May be copied for patient use only.

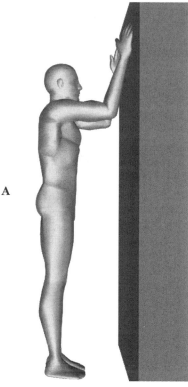

A

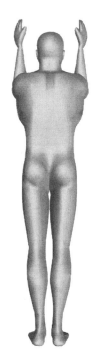

B

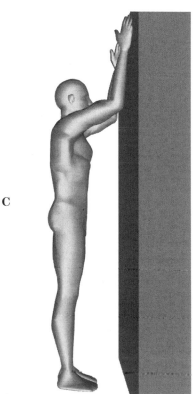

C

Shoulder Flexion — Standing Facing Wall (Figures A-C)

Purposes:
- To increase range-of-shoulder flexion
- To improve the performance of the trapezius muscle
- To improve the performance of the shoulder lateral rotator muscles

Starting position: Stand facing the wall as close as possible with elbows bent and the side of the forearm and little finger side of the hand against the wall.

❏ Perform variation if box is checked

Facing wall

Method: Slide hand(s) up wall until overhead
STOP if pain is experienced on top of shoulder
❏ With your arm(s) over your head, lift your arms off the wall by pulling your shoulder blades toward your spine
❏ Do not let your shoulder shrug as you slide your arm overhead
❏ Pull shoulder blades toward your spine and down
❏ Keep your elbow facing the wall as you move your arm overhead; do not let it turn outward
❏ Use your alternate hand either under the elbow of the arm to be exercised or by grasping the wrist to help lift the affected arm overhead
❏ Use your alternate hand to keep the elbow from turning outward
Return to the starting position

Standing in doorway

Method: Place your body in the doorway, bend your elbow, the palm of hand should be facing your body, place the little finger side of your hand against the wall
Slide your hand up the wall as high as possible
STOP if pain is experienced on top of your shoulder
❏ With arm overhead, lean body into doorway, so that the arm is farther overhead
❏ With the arm overhead, lift the arm off the wall by pulling the shoulder blade toward your spine
Hold position for 5 to 10 seconds
Return your hands to the wall and slide them down
Return to the starting position

Standing with side of body against wall

Method: Stand with the arm to be exercised, next to a wall with the elbow bent and the back of the hand facing the wall
Slide the arm overhead
Hold position for 5 to 10 seconds
If painful, move a small distance away from the wall
Return to the starting position

Repetitions: _____

Copyright © 2002 by Mosby, Inc. May be copied for patient use only.

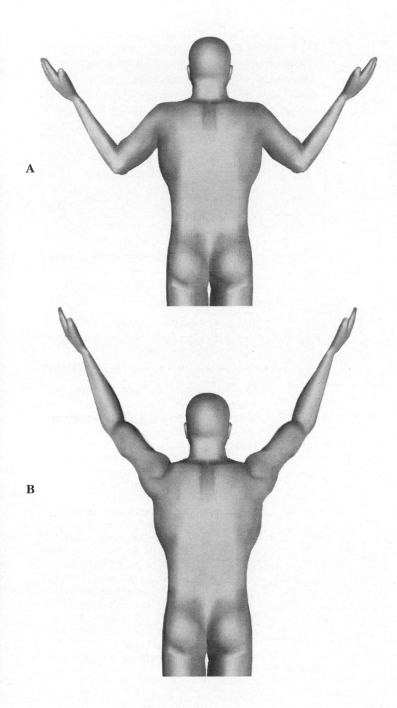

A

B

Shoulder Abduction—Standing Facing Wall—Trapezius Exercises (Figures A-B)

Purposes:
- To improve the performance of the trapezius muscle
- To increase range-of-shoulder motion

Starting position: Stand close to and face the wall with the elbows bent and the little finger side of the hand against the wall. Arms should be out to the side with the elbows closer to the body than the hands.

Upper trapezius

Method: Slide your hands up the wall to the overhead position but slightly out to the side, rather than straight up close to your head

When your upper arm is at shoulder level, shrug your shoulders as you continue to slide your hands up the wall

When your arms are as straight as they can go:
- Lift your arms off the wall by pulling your shoulder blades toward spine
- Hold the position for 5 to 10 seconds
- Return your hands back against the wall and slide them back to the starting position

Trapezius

Method: Slide your hands up the wall to the overhead position but slightly out to the side, rather than straight up and close to your head

Do not shrug your shoulders as you slide your arms overhead

When your arms are as straight as possible

Lift your hands off the wall by pulling your shoulder blades toward your spine

Hold the position for 5 to 10 seconds

Return your hands to the wall and slide them back to the starting position

Lower trapezius

Method: Slide your hands up the wall to the overhead position but slightly out to side rather than straight up close to your head

Do not shrug your shoulders as you slide your hands up the wall

When your hands are overhead, lift them off the wall by pulling your shoulder blades toward your spine and down

Hold the position for 5 to 10 seconds

Return your hands to the wall and slide them back down to the starting position

Repetitions: _____

Copyright © 2002 by Mosby, Inc. May be copied for patient use only.

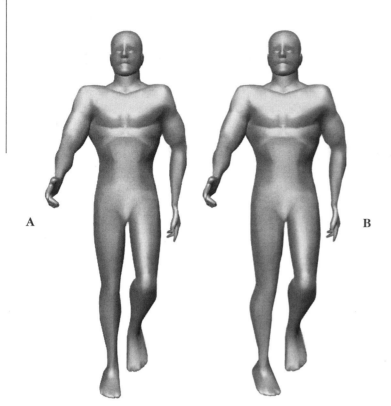

A   B

Control of Hip and Knee Medial Rotation During Walking (Figures A-B)

Purposes:
- To improve the performance of the hip lateral rotators
- To reduce the excessive hip medial rotation
- To reduce the stress on the knee joint associated with excessive medial rotation
- To reduce the stress on the arch of the foot associated with medial rotation
- To reduce the stress on the big toe associated with excessive medial rotation

Starting position: Stand and prepare to take a step with the affected leg.

Method: ❑ Perform variation if box is checked

When walking, as the heel hits the ground, tighten the gluteal muscle to ensure that the knee does not turn but points straight ahead as you place weight on your leg

As you bring your body over your leg, strongly contract your gluteal muscle

Do not let your knee turn in (see *incorrect* posture in Figure B)

As you continue to bring your body forward over your foot, be sure your knee goes in a line over your second toe and not over the inside of your big toe

❑ Do not let the arch of your foot collapse as your body comes over your foot

❑ Try to tighten the muscles of your foot so that your arch does not collapse

Relax your gluteal muscle after your body comes forward over your foot and foot leave the ground

Repeat movement with each step

Repetitions: _____

Copyright © 2002 by Mosby, Inc. May be copied for patient use only.

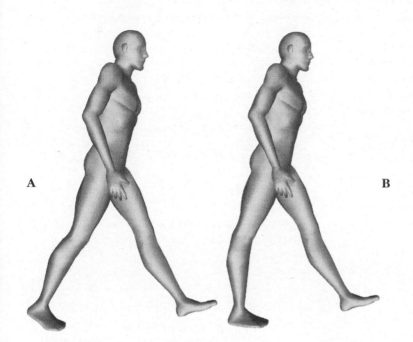

A B

Preventing Knee Hyperextension During Walking (Figures A-B)

Purposes: • To prevent the knee from bending backward when walking

Starting position: Stand and prepare to take a step with the affected leg.

Method: When walking as your body comes over your knee:

Move toward the toe of your foot, lift your heel by contracting the muscles in the calf of your leg (see Figure A)

Do not let your knee bend backward (it will probably feel as though your knee is bent) (see *incorrect* posture in Figure B)

Relax your calf and knee muscles as your toes come off the ground

Repeat with each step

Repetitions: _____

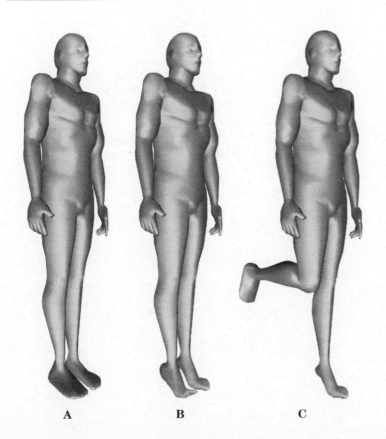

A B C

Ankle Plantar Flexion (Figures A-C)

Purpose: • To improve the performance of the muscles of the calf of the leg

Starting position: Stand with feet comfortably apart. Stand with front of foot on edge of step. Stand with front of foot on edge of step but with support under the heels, which allows the heels to be lower than the front of the foot.

Method: ❏ Perform variation if box is checked

Lift heels to go up on the ball of your foot

Go as high as possible

Hold position for 5 to 10 seconds

Return to the starting position

❏ Lift one foot off the ground by bending your knee

❏ While standing on one leg, lift your heel by contracting the muscles of the calf of your leg so that you are standing on the ball of your foot

❏ Hold the position for 5 to 10 seconds

Return to the starting position

Repetitions: _____ with each leg

Copyright © 2002 by Mosby, Inc. May be copied for patient use only.

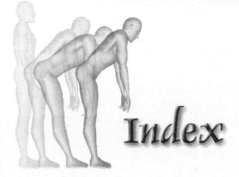

Index

A

Abdominal muscles
  actions of, 69-73l
  lower, exercise progression for, 373-375
  shortness of, 61*f*
  upper, exercise progression for. *See* Trunk-curl sit-up
Acetabulum, 15
Acromioclavicular joint pain, 218
Acromion, humerus anterior of, 200*f*
Actin, 17
Adduction, shoulder, 25*f*
Adductor brevis, 138
Adductor longus, 138
Adductor magnus, 138
Adhesions, 6
Alignment, 3, 146*t*
  assessment of structural variations and acquired
      impairments, 82-84
  in femoral accessory motion hypermobility, 166*t*
  in femoral hypomobility with superior glide, 169
  in femoral lateral glide syndrome with short-axis
      distraction, 171*t*
  in hip extension syndromes, 161*t*
  in humeral hypomobility syndrome, 241
  in humeral superior glide syndrome, 234-235
  in scapular abduction syndrome, 226
  in scapular winging syndrome, 228
  lumbopelvic, 52, 54*f*
  of humerus, normal, 198-199
  of scapula, 219*t*
    normal, 195-198
  of shoulders, normal, 194-195
  quadruped tests for, 304-308, 304*f*
  sitting tests for, 310
  spinal, variations in, 80*f*
  standing movement tests for, 320-321
  upper quarter examinations for, 328-332
  upper quarter tests for, 350-352
Alignment test, 264-268
American Physical Therapy Association, 3
Angle of inclination, 127, 129*f*
Angle of torsion, 125
Ankle dorsiflexion, knee extension and, in corrective
      exercises, 393-394
Ankle plantar flexion, in corrective exercise, 399-400
Ankle, anterior leg muscles affecting, 140-142
Ankle, in leg length discrepancies, 125

Annulus of disk, 62
Anterior superior iliac spine (ASIS), 52, 122
Antetorsion, 125, 127*f*
Anteversion. *See* Antetorsion
Arms, and scapular alignment
Arthrokinematics, 6, 44, 45
ASIS. *See* Anterior superior iliac spine
Asymmetry
  in lumbar spine, 62
  of iliac crest, 124*f*
  of medial rotational range, 127
  spinal, assessment of, 82
Atrophy, 16, 17*f*, 18-19
Axiohumeral, 211
Axioscapular, 209

B

Back. *See* Spine, lumbar
Back muscles, superficial, 65*f*, 66*f*. *See also* Specific muscles
Bending. *See* Flexion
Biceps femoris, 139*f*
Bilateral hip/knee flexion (partial squat), 268-270
Biomechanical element impairments, 41-46
  dynamics: relationship between motion and forces
      producing motion, 44-45
  kinematics and impairments of joint function, 45-46
  kinesiopathologic model applied to patellofemoral joint
      dysfunction, 46
  statics: effects of gravitational forces, 42-44
Biomechanics, 42
Bowing, tibial, 129*f*
Bowlegs. *See* Genu varum
Breasts, large
  and scapular alignment, 219
  in scapular abduction syndrome, 226
Bucket-handle derangement, 45*f*
Bursitis, in scapula, 225

C

Capsulitis, adhesive, 234
Central nervous system dysfunction, 2
Cerebral vascular accident, 11
Cervical flexion and extension, in corrective exercise,
      392-393
Charlie Chaplin gait, 125

Page numbers followed by *f* indicate figures; *t*, tables.

Classification, need for, 7-8
Clavicle, 210
Compensatory relative flexibility, 30-31
Compression, 108
    of lumbar spine, 63-64
    of supraspinatus tendon, 215*f*
Contraction
    eccentric, patterns of, 40-41
    isometric, 70
Coxa varum, 127
Craig's test,
Craig test, 126, 128*f*
Curls, 71, 72, 73*f*
Curvature, lumbar, 52, 54*f. See also* Spine, lumbar,
        movement impairment syndromes of
Cycling, effects of, 13
Cyclists, and femoral accessory motion hypermobility, 167

D

Deep calf muscles, 141
Deltoid, 212
Deltoid contractile inefficiency, 214*f*
Depression, scapular, 213*f*
Diagnosis and intervention, key to, 15
Differential Diagnosis in Physical Therapy, 76
Diplegia, spastic, 144
Directional susceptibility to movement (DSM), 4, 44, 78, 121
Disk
    annulus of, 62
    degeneration of, 61
    degenerative disease of, 74, 75-76
    intervertebral, herniation of, 74, 76, 77*f*
Disk disease, degenerative, 74, 75-76
Distraction, long axis, 135
Double knee to chest test, 274, 274*f*, 321
DSM. *See* Directional susceptibility to movement
Dynamics, 42
Dynamics: relationship between motion and forces
        producing motion, 44-45
Dysfunction, spinal, causes of, 51

E

Electromyography, and hamstring and abdominal muscles,
        36, 38*f*
Elongation, prolonged, effects of, 23
EMG. *See* Electromyography
Entrapment, 6
Erector spinae, 65-67, 136
Examination format, 4
Examinations, for lower and upper quarter movement
        impairment, 263-366. *See also* Movement
        impairments, lower and upper quarter
        examinations for

Exercise, role of, in muscle atrophy, 18
Exercises, corrective, 4-5, 367-400
    for improvement of abdominal muscles, 69-71, 72-73
    for movement impairment syndromes, 401-447
        ankle plantar flexion, 447
        face-lying position
            hip abduction, 432
            hip extension with knee extended, 430
            hip extension with knee flexed, 431
            hip rotation, 429
            knee flexion, 428
            shoulder flexion, flexion to elicit back extensor
                muscle activity, 434
            shoulder rotation, 436
            trapezius muscle exercise progression, 435
        forward bending
            with hip flexion and flat lumbar spine, 403
            with spinal and hip flexion, 404
        hip abduction, with lateral rotation from flexion
                position
            bent knee fallouts, 415
            knee extended, 416
        hip and knee extension
            from hip and knee flexion, 407
            with contralateral hip and knee maximally flexed,
                406
        hip and knee flexion
            from passive and active hip and knee extension,
                408
            with sliding heel from hip and knee extension,
                409
        isometric
            gluteus maximus contraction, 433
            hip lateral rotation with hips abducted and knees
                flexed, 433
        lower abdominal progression
            with bilateral hip and knee flexion, 413
            with hip and knee extension, 412
            with hip and knee flexion with alternate foot
                unsupported, 411
            with hip and knee held to chest during hip flexion,
                410
            with unilateral hip flexion, 409
        pectoralis minor stretch, 423
        quadruped position
            head and cervical flexion and extension, 439
            limb movement, 438
            rocking, 437
        side bending with lateral spinal flexion, 404
        shoulder abduction with gravity lessened, 421
        shoulder flexion
            elevation with elbow extended and latissimus dorsi
                muscle stretch, 419
            elevation with elbow flexed, 420
        two-joint hip flexor stretch, 418

Exercises, corrective—cont'd
    for movement impairment syndromes—cont'd
        shoulder flexion/abduction, 420
        shoulder rotation, supine horizontal adduction, 422
        side-lying position
            hip abduction with and without lateral rotation, 425
            hip adduction for strengthening, 426
            hip lateral rotation, 424
            shoulder flexion, lateral rotation, and scapular
                adduction, 427
        single-leg stance with unilateral hip and knee flexion,
            405
        sitting position
            hip flexion, 441
            knee extension and dorsiflexion, 440
        standing facing wall
            shoulder abduction—trapezius exercises, 445
            shoulder flexion, 444
        standing with back against the wall
            shoulder abduction, 443
            shoulder flexion, 442
        straight-leg raises
            hip flexion with knee extended, 417
        upper abdominal progression with trunk curl–sit up,
            414
        walking
            control of hip and knee medial rotation, 446
            preventing knee hyperextension, 447
    in prone position, 385-390
        back extensor activation, 388-389
        gluteus maximus contraction, isometric, 388
        hip abduction, 387
        hip extension, 387
        isometric hip lateral rotation with hips abducted and
            knees flexed, 387-388
        knee flexion, 385-387
        shoulder rotation, 389-390
        trapezius muscle exercise progression, 388-389
    in quadruped position, 390-393
    in side-lying position, 382-385
    in sitting position, 393-395
    in standing position, 368-370, 395-398
    in supine position, 371-382
        control of pelvic rotation with lower extremity
            abduction/lateral rotation, 377-378
        control of pelvis with lower-extremity motion, 371-372
        gluteus maximus stretch, 372
        hip and knee flexion, sliding heel from hip and knee
            extension, 372
        hip flexor stretch, 371, 378-379
        latissimus dorsi and scapulohumeral muscle stretch,
            379-380
        lower abdominal exercise progression, 373-375
        pectoralis minor stretching, 382
        shoulder abduction with lateral rotation, 380-381

Exercises, corrective—cont'd
    in supine position—cont'd
        shoulder rotation, 381-382
        straight leg raises, 378
        trunk-curl sit-up (upper abdominal progression),
            376-377
    prone, 385-393
    side-lying, 382-385
    walking, 398-399
Extension
    of hip, 124
    of lumbar spine, normal and impairments of, 60-61
    lumbar, test for, 321
Extensor digitorum longus, 141, 142f
External oblique, 69-71, 70f, 135

F

Facet joint synovitis, 74
Facet syndrome, 74
Fascitis, iliotibial band, 154
Femoral accessory hypermobility syndrome, 188-189
Femoral accessory motion hypermobility, 166-168
    case presentation, 167-168
Femoral anterior glide syndrome, 144-151, 176-177
    case presentations, 148-151
    confirming tests, 147
    intervention, 147-148
    movement impairments, 145-146, 145f
    muscle and recruitment pattern impairments, 147
    relative flexibility and stiffness impairments, 146
    symptoms and pain, 144-145
    with lateral rotation, 151-154
        case presentation in, 153-154
        intervention, 152-153
    with lateral rotation syndrome, 180
    with medial rotation syndrome, 178-179
    with superior glide, 168-171, 186-187
        case presentation in, 170-171
        confirming tests, 169
        flexibility and stiffness impairments, 169
        intervention, 169-170
        movement impairments, 170
        muscle and recruitment pattern impairments, 169
        symptoms and pain, 170
    with short-axis distraction, 171-174
        case presentation, 172-174
        confirming tests, 172
        flexibility and stiffness impairments, 172
        intervention, 172
        movement impairments, 171
        muscle and recruitment pattern impairments, 172
        symptoms and pain, 171
Femur, 15
Flat thoracic spine, 199

Flexibility
    and stiffness, impairments, 90
    compensatory relative, 30-31
Flexion
    glenohumeral, 220f
    of lumbar spine, normal and impairments of, 58-60
    lateral, assessment of, 76
        in hip joint, 125
        normal and impairments of, 63, 64f
    of hip, 124
    of shoulder, 202f, 209f-210f
        increased, 212f
Flexor digitorum brevis, 143f
Flexor digitorum longus, 142
Foot
    lateral leg muscles affecting, 142
    muscles attached to, 143-144
    pronated, and hallux valgum, 370
    rigid, 43f
Force, muscular, 16
Force couple, scapular, 207f
Forces, static, on posture, 42-44, 42f. See also Gravity,
        effects of, on muscle use
Forward bending
    alignments in, 61f. See also Spine, lumbar, motions of,
        flexion
    assessment of, 76
    curled, in corrective exercise, 369
    in corrective exercise, 368
Forward bending test, 270-272, 320
Frozen shoulder, 241

G

Gait
    alterations in muscular strategies during, 35
    antalgic, 130
    assessment of, 82
    normal, 26
    tests of, 318-319
Gastrocnemius, 140
Gemelli, superior and inferior, 138
Genu recurvatum, 42, 134
Genu valgum, 125, 132f, 370
Genu varum, 44, 129, 130f, 131f, 370
Glenohumeral capsule, posterior, stiffness of, 216f
Glenohumeral hypomobility, 260-261
Glenohumeral joint, 13f
Glenoid, motion of, 206
Glide, in hip joint, 135
Gluteus maximus, 15, 16, 137
Gluteus maximus contraction, isometric, in corrective
        exercise, 388

Gluteus maximus stretch in corrective exercise, 371-372
Gluteus minimus, 138
Gracilis, 138
Gravity, effects of, on muscle use, 42-44

H

Hallux valgum, pronated foot and, 370
Hammer toes, 141
Hamstring and abdominal muscles, interaction of, 36
Hamstring muscles, 26, 139f
    dominance of, over abdominal muscles, 36-37, 37f
    evaluation of, 28
    stretching of, 124
Hamstring strain, 164
Hemiparesis, 11
Hemiplegia, 144
Herniation, of intervertebral disk, 74, 76, 77f
Hip
    antetorsion in, 34, 34f
    control of, and knee medial rotation, in corrective
        exercise, 398-399
    extension of, in prone position, 16f
    medial muscles affecting, 138
    motions of, 134-135
    movement impairment syndromes of, 121-191
        femoral anterior glide syndrome, 144-151
        femoral anterior glide syndrome with lateral rotation,
            151-154
        frequency of, 122t
        hip adduction syndrome, 154-161
        motions of hip, 134-135
        muscular actions of, 135-144
        normal alignment of hip, 121-134
        specific impairments, 144-175
    muscular actions of, 135-144
        anterior leg muscles affecting ankle, 140-142
        anterior muscles affecting hip and knee, 138
        anterior muscles affecting the hip joint, 136-137
        anterior trunk muscles affecting the pelvis, 135-136
        lateral leg muscles affecting foot, 142
        median muscles affecting the hip, 138
        muscle and movement impairments, 143-144
        muscles attached to foot, 143-144
        posterior leg muscles affecting foot, 142
        posterior leg muscles affecting knee and ankle, 140
        posterior muscles affecting the hip joint, 137-138
        posterior muscles affecting the pelvis, 136
    normal alignment of, 122-134
        hip joint, 123-129
        knee joint in, 129-134
Hip, retrotorsion in, 34-35, 34f, 129f
Hip, rotation of, 135

Hip abduction
    in corrective exercise, 387
    with and without lateral rotation, 383-384
    with associated lateral pelvic tilt, assessment of, 78
Hip abduction/lateral rotation from flexion, assessment of,
        78
Hip abduction/lateral rotation test, 292-296, 292f
Hip abduction/lateral rotation with hip flexed, 288-290, 288f
Hip adduction, 370
    assessment of, 78-79
Hip adduction syndrome, 154-161, 180-181, 182-183
    case presentations, 156-161
    confirming tests, 155
    femoral accessory motion hypermobility, 166-168
    femoral hypomobility with superior glide, 168-171
    femoral lateral glide syndrome with short-axis
            distraction, 171-174
    flexibility and stiffness impairments, 155
    hip extension with knee extension syndrome, 161-164
    hip lateral rotation syndrome, 164-166
    intervention, 155-156
    movement impairments, 155
    muscle and recruitment pattern impairments, 155
    symptoms and pain, 154-155
    with medial rotation, 182-183
Hip adduction tests, 296
Hip and knee, muscles affecting, 138
Hip and knee flexion
    active, assessment of, 78
    in supine position, 372
    limited range of, in standing position, 370
Hip antetorsion, unilateral, 124
Hip extension, 134
    assessment of, 80-81
    evaluation of, 28, 29f
Hip extension with knee extended test, 302, 302f
Hip extension with knee extension, 184-185
Hip extension with knee extension syndrome, 161-164
    case presentation, 162-164
    confirming tests, 162
    flexibility and stiffness impairments, 162
    intervention, 162
    movement impairments, 161
    muscle and recruitment pattern impairments, 162
    muscle length and strength impairments, 162
    symptoms and pain, 161
Hip extension with knee flexed
    in corrective exercise, 387
    test, 302-304, 302f
Hip extension with medial rotation, 186
Hip flexion, 134
    assessment of, 79f, 82f
    with knee extended, assessment of, 78

Hip flexor length, assessment of, 77-78
Hip flexor length test, 276-278, 276f
Hip flexor length test, supine, 321
Hip flexor strategy pattern, 144
Hip flexor stretch, in corrective exercise, 371, 378-379
Hip flexors, evaluation of, 28
Hip joint
    accessory motions of, 135
    anterior muscles affecting, 136-137
    assessment of, 124-128
Hip joint angle, 122
Hip joint motions, 134-135
Hip joint test, 321
Hip lateral rotation
    assessment of, 78
    in corrective exercise, 382-383
Hip lateral rotation syndrome, 164-166,190
    case presentation, 165-166
Hip lateral rotation test, 300, 300f
Hip medial rotation, excessive, 370
Hip medial rotation test, 298-300, 298f
Hip rotation
    assessment of, 80
    isometric lateral, in corrective exercise, 387-388
Hip rotation test, sitting, 314
Hip test, 302
Hip/knee flex partial squat test, 321
Hips/knees extension test, 322
Hips/knees flexion test, 321
Humeral anterior glide, 254-255
Humeral anterior glide syndrome, 232-234
Humeral hypomobility syndrome, 241-244
    case presentation, 243-244
    confirming tests, 241
    treatment, 241-243
Humeral superior glide, 256-257
Humeral superior glide syndrome, 234-237
    case presentation, 236-237
    confirming tests, 235-236
    muscle impairments, 235
    treatment, 236
Humerus
    abducted and medially rotated, 201f
    Humerus, alignment of, normal and impaired, 198-199
    Humerus, laterally rotated, 201f
    movement impairment syndromes of, 231-244
        humeral anterior glide syndrome, 232-234
        humeral hypomobility syndrome, 241-244
        humeral superior glide syndrome, 234-237
        shoulder medial rotation syndrome, 237-240
    neutral rotation of, 199f
Humerus anterior of acromion, 200f
Hyperextension

Hyperextension—cont'd
    in gymnasts, 61
    in knee joint, 129
Hypermobility, in low back, 74
Hypertrophy, 16, 17*f*, 19, 29

I

IAR. *See* Instantaneous axes of rotation
ICR. *See* Instantaneous center of rotation
Iliopsoas, 26, 68-69, 68*f*, 135, 136
Iliopsoas test, 286-288
Iliotibial band (ITB), 131
Illness, acute phase of, 1
Imbalances in control of one joint, 143*t*
Impairments in biomechanical elements. *See* Biomechanical
        element impairments
Impairments, 10
    of muscle and movement, 143-144
    of shoulder alignment, 195, 195*f*
Impingement, 6
Impingement syndrome, 234, 235*f*
    of shoulders, 213, 216
Inclination, angle of, 127, 129*f*
Infraspinatus, 215
Instability, spinal, 74, 75
Instantaneous axes of rotation (IAR), 58*f*, 59*f*
Instantaneous center of rotation (ICR), 12
Internal oblique, 71-72, 135
Interspinales, 67
Intertransversarii, 67
ITB. *See* Iliotibial band

J

Joint, lumbosacral, 61
Joint dysfunction, 2
Joint function, impairments of, and kinematics, 45-46
Joint mobility, evaluation of, 2
Joints, accessory movements of, 44-45

K

Kinematics, 42, 44-45, 46
Kinesiologic model of movement, 9-10, 10*f*
Kinesiopathologic model applied to patellofemoral joint
        dysfunction, 46
Kinesiopathologic model of movement, 4, 14*f*, 12-16, 12*f*
Kinetics, 44
Knee and ankle, posterior leg muscles affecting, 140
Knee extension
    and ankle dorsiflexion, in corrective exercises, 393-394
    assessment of, 82

Knee flexion, assessment of, 80
Knee flexion test, 298, 298*f*
Knee hyperextension, prevention of, in corrective exercise,
        399
Knee. *See also* Knee joint
    anterior muscles affecting hip and, 138
    hyperextension of, 43, 122, 43*f*, 123*f*
    medial rotation of, and control of hip in corrective
        exercise, 398-399
    normal flexion of, 46*f*
    posterior muscles affecting hip and, 139-141
Knee joint
    hyperextension of, 129
    in normal alignment of hip, 129-134
        frontal plane, 129-134
        sagittal plane, 129
    valgus and varus deformities in 130*f*
    varus of, 44*f*
Knee joint test, 321
Knee rotation, limiting, in corrective exercise, 399
Knock-knees. *See* Genu valgus
Kyphosis, thoracic, 82, 199, 205, 219, 226, 196*f*

L

Lateral rotators, test of length of, 216*f*
Latissimus dorsi, 31, 65, 211
    and scapulohumeral muscle stretch, 379-380
    length assessment of, 212*f*
Leg muscles anterior, affecting the ankle, 140-142
Leg muscles, posterior, affecting knee and ankle, 140
Length-tension relationship in muscle, 24*f*
Levator scapula, 207
Limb movement in quadruped position, 391-392
Load, excessive, 5
Lordosis, lumbar, 82, 90
Low back, movement impairment syndromes of, 74-107
    compression, 108
    lumbar extension syndrome, 88-93
    lumbar flexion syndrome, 103-107
    lumbar rotation syndrome, 93-98
    lumbar rotation-extension syndrome with or without
        radiating symptoms, 74-88
    lumbar rotation-flexion syndrome, 98-103
    sacroiliac dysfunction, 107-108
Lower abdominal muscle exercise progression, 373-375
Lower abdominal, external oblique, and rectus abdominis
        performance, 280-282, 282*f*
Lower quarter examination, checklist for, 320-328
Lumbar extension syndrome, 88-93
    alignment in, 89
    case presentations in, 91-93
    diagnosis and treatment of, 112-113

Lumbar extension syndrome—cont'd
    movement impairments in, 89-90
    symptoms and pain in, 89
    treatment of, 90-91
Lumbar flexion syndrome, 105-111
    alignment in, 105
    case presentations in, 105-107
    confirming tests for, 105
    diagnosis and treatment of, 110-111
    excessive flexibility in, 104*f*
    flexibility and stiffness impairments in, 105
    movement impairments in, 103
    muscle and recruitment pattern impairments in, 105
    symptoms and pain, 103
    treatment of, 105
Lumbar rotation syndrome, 93-98
    alignment in, 93
    case presentations in, 95-98
    confirming tests, 95
    diagnosis and treatment of, 114-115
    flexibility and stiffness impairments in, 94-95
    movement impairments in, 93-94
    muscle and recruitment impairments in, 95
    symptoms and pain, 93
    treatment of, 95
Lumbar rotation with extension, diagnosis and treatment of,
        118-119
Lumbar rotation with flexion, diagnosis and treatment of,
        116-117
Lumbar rotation-extension syndrome with or without
        radiating symptoms
    alignment: structural variations and acquired
        impairments, 82-84
    case presentations, 84-88
    movement impairments, 76-82
    symptoms and pain, 74-76
Lumbar rotation-flexion syndrome, 98-103
    alignment: structural variations and acquired
        impairments, 99
    case presentations in, 100-103
    confirming tests, 100
    flexibility and stiffness impairments, 99
    movement impairments in, 98-99
    muscle recruitment pattern impairments, 99-100
    symptoms and pain, 98
    treatment of, 100
Lumbar spine. *See* Spine, lumbar, movement impairment
        syndromes of

M

Magnetic resonance imaging (MRI), 107
    of shoulder, 214-215

Manual muscle testing (MMT), 155
Metatarsophalangeal (MTP) joints, 142
Microtrauma, 3, 5
MMT. *See* Manual muscle testing
Motion
    and forces producing motion, relationship between, 44-45
    synergists for, 143
Motions of lumbar spine, 57-74
Motor unit loss, 1
Movement impairment syndrome, 5. *See also* MPS;
        Movement impairments
Movement impairment syndromes, 3, 5-7
    of hip, 121-191. *See also* Hip, movement impairment
        syndromes of
    of shoulder girdle, 193-244. *See also* Shoulder girdle,
        movement impairment syndromes of
Movement impairments, 15
    in lumbar extension syndrome, 89-90
    lower and upper quarter examination for, 263-366
        lower quarter examinations, 264-327
            gait, tests for, 318-319
            prone tests, 296-304
            quadruped tests, 304-310
            side-lying tests, 292-296
            sitting tests, 310-315
            standing tests, 264-268, 316-317
            standing movement tests, 268-274
            supine tests, 274-292
        upper quarter examinations, 328-366
            checklist for, 362-366
            prone tests, 344-350
            quadruped tests, 350-354
            standing tests, 328-338
            standing: back to wall tests, 360
            standing: facing wall tests, 356-360
            supine tests, 338-344
Movement, 3
    as underlying cause of pain syndromes, 3-4
    components of, multiple impairments of, 47, 48*f*
    concepts and principles of, 9-50
        base element impairments of the muscular system,
            16-33
        base element impairments of skeletal system:
            structural variations in joint alignment during,
            34-46
        kinesiologic model of, 9-10
        kinesiopathologic model of, 12-16
        multiple impairments of components of movement, 47
        pathokinesiologic model of, 10-12
        support element impairments of, 47
    impairments of, in low back, 76-82
    kinesiopathologic model of, 4
    models of. *See* Specific Models
    repeated, 13

Movement—cont'd
    repetitive, cumulative effects of, 12
Movement patterns, of shoulder girdle, 201-206
Movement system balance (MSB) concept, 3
Movement system, focus on, 2-3
MPS. *See* Musculoskeletal pain syndromes
MRI. *See* Magnetic resonance imaging
MSB. *See* Movement system balance
MTP. *See* Metatarsophalangeal (MTP) joints
Multifidus, 35, 67
Muscle
    atrophy of, clinical relevance of, 18-19
    contractile capacity of, factors affecting, 16
    lengthened, secondary to anatomic adaptation—addition
        of sarcomeres, 23-26
    shortened, caused by anatomic adaptation, loss of
        sarcomeres, 26-28
    skeletal, structure of, 17
    stretching of, 26
    synergistic
        altered dominance in recruitment patterns in, 35-39
            upper trapezius, dominance of, 35-36
            hamstring, dominance of, over abdominal muscles,
                36-37, 37*f*
            examples of, 37-39
        dissociated length changes in, 28
        length imbalances in, 28t
Muscle and movement impairments, 143-144
Muscle fibers, factors affecting, 16
Muscle length, 19-34
    impairments of
        compensatory relative flexibility, 30-31
        dissociated length changes in synergistic muscles, 28
        increased muscle length related to strain, 20-23
        lengthened muscle secondary to anatomic adaptation,
            23-26
        muscle and soft-tissue stiffness, 28-33, 33*f*
        over-stretch weakness, 19
        shortened muscle cause by anatomic adaptation—loss
            of sarcomeres, 26-28
    mechanisms for lengthening, 19
Muscle length adaptation, anatomic, 23*f*
Muscle performance, weakness in, 15
Muscle strength
    decreased, 17-19
    impairments of, 16-19
    increased, from hypertrophy, 19
Muscle testing, manual, 1, 2
Muscle weakness, causes of, 17
Muscles. *See* Specific muscles
Muscular system, base element impairment of, 16-33
    muscle length, 19-33
    muscle strength, impairments of, 16-19

Muscular system, base element impairments of, 16-33
Musculoskeletal pain syndrome (MPS), 26
    cause identification versus symptom reduction, 7
    diagnosis and management of, 5-6
    prevalence of, 5
    structures affected by, 6
    treatment approaches based on intervention, 6-7
Myelocele, meningeal, 144
Myosin, 17

N

Neck pain, 218
Nervous system, modular element impairments of, 35-41
    eccentric contraction, patterns of, 40-41
    recruitment and relative flexibility, 39-40
    recruitment patterns, altered, 35
    recruitment patterns of synergistic muscles, altered
        dominance in, 35-39
    role of, in the activation of muscle, 2
Neuromuscular and skeletal systems, peripheral,
        dysfunction of, 1-2
NUSTEP conference, 2

O

Obesity, with large thorax, 219
Obturator internus and externus, 138
Optotrak, 18*f*
Osteoarthritis of lumbar spine, 74,76
Osteokinematics, 45
Osteoporosis, 368

P

Pain, localized, terms commonly used to describe, 5
Pain, musculoskeletal. *See also* Musculoskeletal pain
        syndrome
Pain syndromes, movement as cause of, 3-4
Path of instantaneous center of rotation (PICR), 12, 12*f*
Pathokinesiologic model of movement, 10-12, 11*f*
Pathokinesiology, 10
Pathology, Implications for the Physical Therapist, 76
Pectineus, 138
Pectoralis major, 211, 212*f*
Pectoralis minor, 210
    attachments of, 210*f*
    length of, upper quarter test for, 338-340
    shortness of, 210, 211*f*
    stretching of, 382
Pelvic girdle motions, 134
Pelvis
    abduction of, 135

Pelvis—cont'd
    adduction of, 135
    anterior trunk muscles affecting, 135-136
    control of, with lower extremity motion in corrective
        exercise, 371
    faulty alignment of, 55*f*
    female, variation in, 123
    hip, and thigh, muscles of, 137*f*
    in normal alignment of hip, 122-124
    posterior muscles affecting, 136
    tests for, 321
    tilt of, exaggerated, 39-40, 40*t*
Peroneus brevis, 142
Peroneus longus, 142
Peroneus longus and brevis, 142*f*
Peroneus tertius, 142
PGM. *See* Posterior gluteus medius
Physical therapy (PT), evolution of, 1
Physical therapy profession, future growth of, 3
PICR. *See* Path of instantaneous center of rotation
Piriformis, 15, 16, 138
Piriformis syndrome, 138, 154
Poliomyelitis, 1
Position effects, assessment of, 81, 82
Position test, 264
    prone, 296
    side-lying, 292
Posterior gluteus medius, 125, 134
Posterior superior iliac spine (PSIS), 52, 122
Posture
    alterations in 42*f*, 43*f*
    habits of, correction of, 91
Postures, sustained, 13
Prone position, tests for assessment during, 80-81
Prone tests, 296-304, 323-324, 364-365
    hip extension with knee extended, 302, 302*f*
    hip extension with knee flexed, 302-304, 302*f*
    hip lateral rotation, 300, 300*f*
    hip medial rotation, 298-300, 298*f*
    position, 296
PT. *See* Physical therapy

Q

Quadratus lumborum, 67-68, 136
Quadriceps femoris, 138
Quadruped position, 365-366
    corrective exercises in, 390-393
    tests for assessment during, 81
Quadruped tests, 304-310, 324-325
    alignment, 304-308, 304*f*
    rocking backward toward heels, 308
    rocking forward test, 308
    shoulder flexion, 310, 310*f*

R

Range of motion, 58
Recovery phase, 1
Recruitment and relative flexibility, 39-40
Recruitment patterns, altered, 35
Rectus abdominis, 69, 73, 135, 136*f*
Rectus femoris, 31, 137, 138, 139*f*
Repetitive use injuries, 5
Retrotorsion, 125
Retroversion. *See* Retrotorsion
Return from forward bending test, 272
Rhomboid, 208
Rhomboid dominance, test for, 205, 206*f*, 350
Rocking, assessment of motion, 81
Rocking, quadruped, 390-391
Rocking backward toward heels, upper quarter test,
        352-354
Rocking backward toward heels test, 308
Rocking forward test, 308
Rocking forward, upper quarter test, 354
Rolling, tests for assessment during, 84
Rotation
    assessment of, 77, 83-84
    impaired, 79*f*
    lumbar, 61-63
    of hip, 135
    of pelvis, 134
    pelvic, assessment of, 123*f*-124
    standing movement tests for, 321
    tibiofemoral, excessive, 126*f*
Rotation of lumbar spine, normal and impairments of,
        61-63
Rotator cuff, 205*f*, 212
Rotator cuff tear, 218, 234
Rotator cuff tendinopathy or impingement, 218

S

Sacroiliac dysfunction (SI), 107-108
Sarcomeres, 16
    addition of, 23-26
    loss of, 26-28
Sartorius, 137
Scapula
    abducted, and humeral rotation, 215*f*
    adducted, 196*f*, 209-210
    alignment of, normal and impaired, 195-198
    bursitis in 225
    downwardly rotated, 219*t*
    elevation of, 208*f*
    excessive abduction of, 202*f*, 225*f*
    glossary of motions of, 199, 201
    insufficient rotation of, 220*f*

Scapula—cont'd
   movement impairment syndromes of, 216-244
      alignment and movement, relationship between, 216-217
      scapular abduction syndrome, 225-228
      scapular depression syndrome, 223-225
      scapular downward rotation syndrome, 217-222
      scapular syndrome, criteria for diagnosis of, 217
      scapular winging syndrome, 228-230, 229*f*
   tendinopathy in, 225
   tilted, 197*f*
   winged, 198*f*
   winging of, 41*f*, 203, 204*f*
Scapulae, adducted, 23
Scapular abduction, 250-251
Scapular abduction syndrome, 225-228
   case presentation, 227-228
   confirming tests, 226
   movement pattern impairments, 225-226
   muscle impairments, 226
   symptoms, pain problems, and associated diagnoses, 225
   treatment of, 226-227
Scapular depression, 248-249
Scapular depression syndrome, 223-225
   case presentation, 224-225
   treatment of, 224
Scapular downward rotation syndrome, 217-222, 234
   case presentation, 222-223
   confirming tests, 221
   muscle impairments, 219-221
   relative flexibility and stiffness impairments, 219
   symptoms, problems, and associated diagnoses, 217-218
   treatment of, 221-222
Scapular downward rotation, 246-247
Scapular winging and tilting, 252-253
Scapular winging syndrome, 228-230, 229*f*
Scapulohumeral, 212-216
Scapulothoracic joint, 13*f*
Sciatica, 42, 158, 199, 219, 226, 228
Semimembranosus, 139
Semitendinosus, 139
Serratus anterior, 23, 208
Shoulder
   abducted forward, 197*f*
   alignment of, normal and impaired, 194-195
   depressed, 223*f*
   frozen, 241
   magnetic resonance imaging of, 214-215
Shoulder abduction
   in corrective exercises, 396, 398
      with lateral rotation, 380-381
   upper quarter tests for, 336-338
Shoulder extension, upper quarter examinations for, 334-335

Shoulder flexion, 209*f*-210*f*
   assessment of, 81
   in corrective exercise, 395-398
   upper quarter examinations for, 332-334
   upper quarter tests for, 340-342, 354
Shoulder flexion, lateral rotation, and scapular adduction in corrective exercise, 384-385
Shoulder flexion test, 310, 310*f*
Shoulder flexion to 180 degrees, assessment of, 78
Shoulder girdle
   motions of, 199-206
   movement patterns, 201-206
   movement impairment syndromes
      and motions of shoulder girdle, 199-206
      of humerus, 231-244
      of scapula, 216-230
      muscular actions of shoulder girdle, 206-216
      normal alignment of shoulder girdle, 194-199
   muscles of, 208*f*
   muscular actions of, 206-216
      scapulohumeral muscles, 212-216
      thoracohumeral muscles, 211-212
      thoracoscapular muscles, 206-211
   normal and impaired alignment of
      humerus, 198-199
      scapula, 195-198
      shoulders, 194-195
      thoracic spine, 199
Shoulder lateral rotation, upper quarter tests for, 346-348, 346*f*
Shoulder medial rotation, 258-259
Shoulder medial rotation syndrome
   case presentation, 240
   confirming tests, 238, 239*f*
   movement pattern impairments, 238
   muscle impairments, 238
   muscle length and strength impairments, 238
   relative flexibility and stiffness impairments, 238
   symptoms, pain problems, and associated diagnoses, 237-238
   treatment of, 238-239
Shoulder medial rotation, upper quarter tests for, 344, 344*f*
Shoulder rotation in corrective exercise, 381-382, 389-390
SI. *See* Sacroiliac dysfunction
Side bending. *See also* Flexion, lateral
   impaired, 78*f*
   in corrective exercise, 369
Side bending test, 272, 320-321
Side-lying tests, 292-296, 323
   hip abduction/lateral rotation, 292-296, 292*f*
   hip adduction, 296
   position, 292
Single leg stance test, 77, 270, 321

Single-leg standing, in corrective exercise, 369-370

Sitting

normal alignment and impairments of lumbar spine
during, 54-57

tests for assessment during, 82, 84

Sitting hip flexion test, 314, 314*f*

Sitting knee extension and ankle dorsiflexion, 310-313, 310*f*

Sitting position, corrective exercises in, 393-395

Sitting tests, 310-315, 325-326

alignment, 310

hip rotation, 314

sitting hip flexion, 314, 314*f*

sitting knee extension and ankle dorsiflexion, 310-313,
310*f*

Sitting to standing, tests for assessment during, 84

Skeletal system, base element impairments of, structural
variations in joint alignment, 34-35, 34*f*

Skeletal systems, neuromuscular and, peripheral,
dysfunction of, 1-2

SLR. *See* Straight leg raise test

Soleus, 140, 142

Spinal rotation test, 274

Spine, degenerative conditions of, 74. *See also* Lumbar
rotation-extension syndrome with or without
radiating symptoms

Spine, lumbar

assessment of, 53*f*

motions of, 57-74

compression, 63-64

extension of lumbar spine, 60-61

flexion, 58-60, 63, 64*f*

path of instantaneous center of rotation (PICR), 57-58

return from flexion, 60

rotation, 61-63

translation, 63

movement impairment syndromes of, 51-119. *See also*
Specific impairment syndrome

muscular actions of, 65-74

abdominal muscles, 69-73

back muscles, 65-69

sitting, 54-57

standing, 52-54, 52*f*, 53*f*, 54*f*, 55*f*

normal alignment of the lumbar spine, 52-57

osteoarthritis of, 74, 76

test for, 322

Spine

movement impairment syndromes of, 45

shape of, 52*f*

thoracic, 199

PSIS. *See* Superior posterior iliac spine

Spondylolisthesis, 63, 74, 75

Stair climbing, tests for assessment during, 84

Standing, normal alignment and impairments of lumbar
spine during, 52-54, 52*f*, 53*f*, 54*f*, 55*f*

Standing, tests for assessment during, 76-77, 82-83, 84

back to wall tests, 360

facing wall tests, upper quarter examination, 356-360,
356*f*, 358*f*

Standing movement tests, 268-274, 320-321

bilateral hip/knee flexion (partial squat), 268-270

forward bending, 270-272

return from forward bending, 272

side bending, 272

single-leg stance, 270

spinal rotation, 274

Standing position, corrective exercises in, 368-370

Standing tests, 263-268, 316-317, 320, 362-363

alignment, 264-268

back to wall, 316, 316*f*

position, 264

Statics, effects of gravitational forces, 42-44

Stenosis, spinal, 74-75

Sternoclavicular joint pain, 218

Sternocleidomastoid, 58

Stiffness, 28-33, 30*f*, 33*f*

anatomic variations due to, 33*f*

clinical relevance of, 32

lumbar spinal, 61, 63

variations in, 30-31, 33*f*

Straight-leg raise, assessment of, 78

Straight leg raise test, 284-286, 284*f*

Straight-leg raises, in corrective exercises, 378

Straight-leg raising, 37

Strain

and decreased muscle strength, 19

increased muscle length secondary to, 20-23, 21*f*

of right thoracoscapular muscles, 22*f*

Stress, tissue response to, 46*f*

Stress requirement, 3

Stretching, passive, effects of, 26. *See also* Specific exercises

Subluxation, humeral, 218, 225

Subscapularis, 215

hypertrophy of, 198

Supine position

corrective exercises in, 371-382

tests for assessment during, 77-78

Supine test, lower abdominal, external oblique, and rectus
abdominis performance, 280-282, 280*f*

Supine tests, 274-292, 321-322, 363-364

double knee to chest, 274, 274*f*

hip abduction/lateral rotation with hip flexed, 288-290,
288*f*

hip flexor length test, 276-278, 276*f*

iliopsoas test, 286-288

straight leg raise test, 284-286, 284*f*

trunk curl-sit up, 282-284, 282*f*

unilateral hip and knee flexion (single knee to chest),
290-292, 290*f*

Support elements, impairment of, 47-48
Supraspinatus, 214
Supraspinatus tendon, compression of, 215f
Swayback posture, 37, 137, 139f
Symptom source and restricted use approach, 6
System-focused approach, 6

T

Taping, in treatment of muscle strain, 22, 22f
Tendinitis, calcific, 234
Tendinopathy, 194
   in scapula, 225
     supraspinatus, 234
Tensor fascia lata (TFL), 15, 28, 63
Tensor fascia lata–iliotibial band (TFL-ITB), 128, 128f, 136f
Tensor fascia lata–iliotibial band stretch, 384
Teres major, 216
Teres minor, 215
Tests. *See* Examinations for lower and upper quarter
        movement impairment; Specific tests
TFL-ITB. *See* Tensor fascia lata–iliotibial band
TFL. *See* Tensor fascia lata
Thixotropy, 29
Thoracic outlet or neural entrapment, 218. *See also* Thoracic
        outlet syndrome
Thoracic outlet syndrome, 210
Thoracic spine, alignment of, 199
Thoracohumeral muscles, 211-212
   strain of, 22f
Thorax, large, in scapular abduction syndrome, 226
Tibial varum. *See* Genu varum
Tibialis anterior, 140, 141, 142f
Tibialis posterior, 142
Tilt
   of scapula, 252-253
   pelvic, 134
     assessment of, 122, 123f
Titin, 29
Torsion
   angle of, 125
   tests of, 127

Torsion, tibial, 131, 132f, 133f, 134f
Translation motion, 63
Transversus abdominis, 35, 73, 135
Trapezius, 207
   upper quarter tests for, 348-350
Trapezius muscle exercise progression, 388-389
Trandelenburg test, 155
Tribology, 12
Trochanter, greater, 16
Trunk-curl sit-up in corrective exercise, 376-377
Trunk curl-sit up test, 282-284, 282f

U

Unilateral hip and knee flexion (single knee to chest) test,
     290-292, 290f
Unilateral hip/knee flexion test, 322-323
Upper trapezius, dominance of, 35-36

V

Vastus intermedius, 138
Vastus lateralis, 138
Vastus medialis oblique (VMO), 46, 138
Vertebrae. *See* Spine, lumbar
VMO. *See* Vastus medialis oblique

W

Walking
   corrective exercises in, 398-399
   tests for assessment during, 82, 84
Weakness
   consequences of, 1
   muscle, causes of, 17
   over-stretch, 19
     case presentation, 20
Winging of scapula, 252-253, 41f
Wolff's law, 43
Wrist flexion during finger extension, 40, 41f